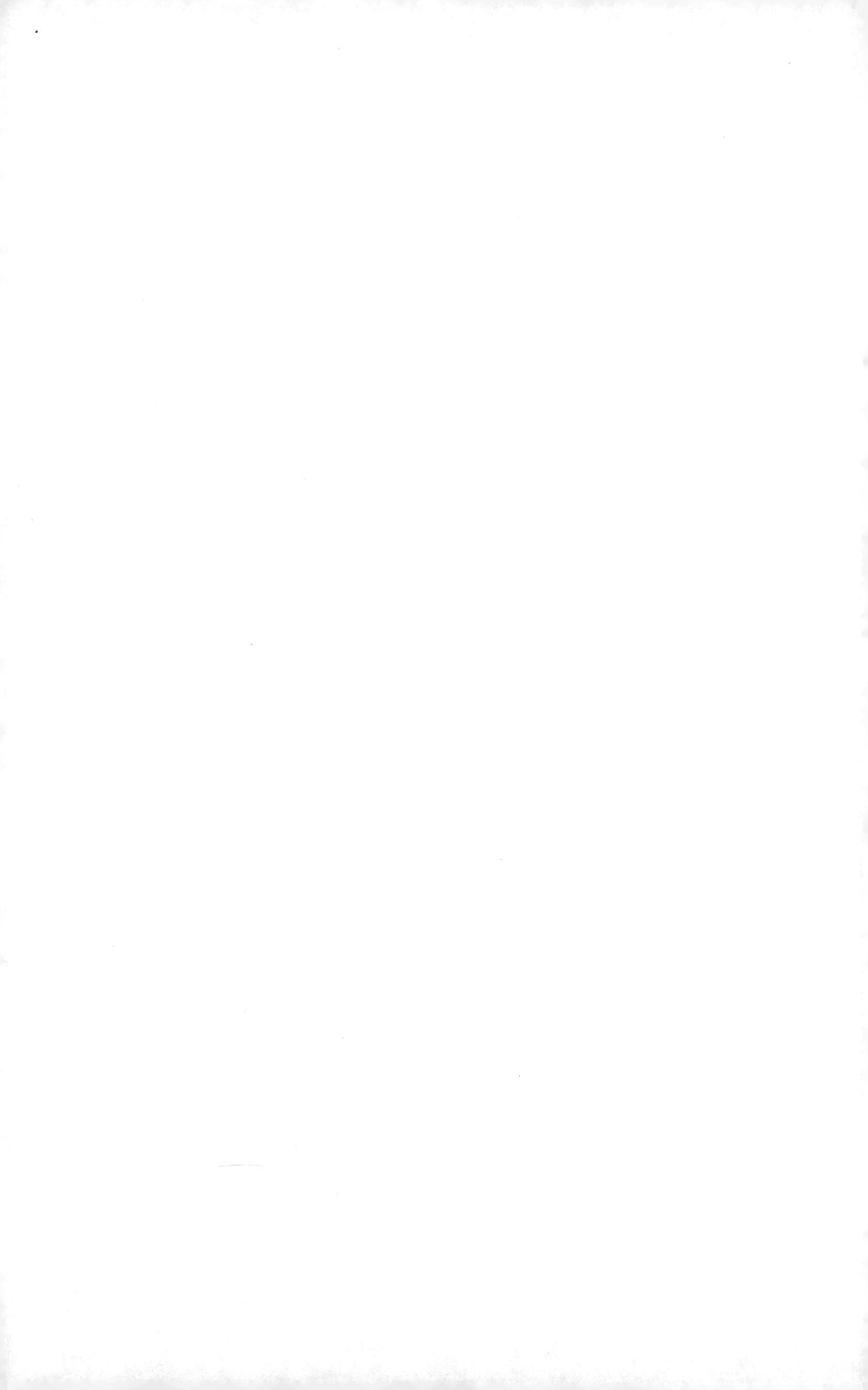

# Vitamin E

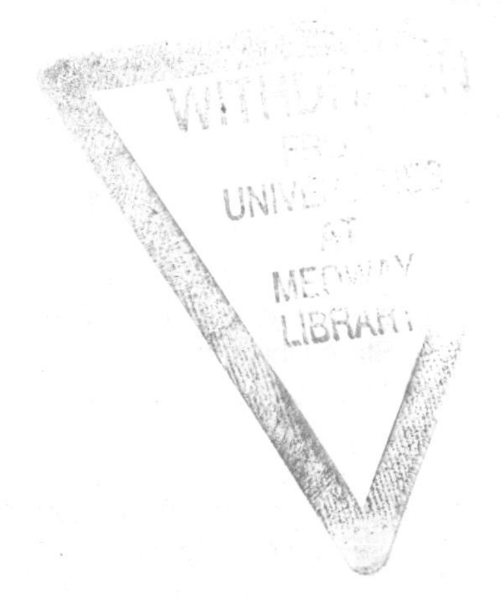

# FOOD SCIENCE AND TECHNOLOGY

*A Series of Monographs, Textbooks, and Reference Books*



1. Flavor Research: Principles and Techniques, *R. Teranishi, I. Hornstein, P. Issenberg, and E. L. Wick*
2. Principles of Enzymology for the Food Sciences, *John R. Whitaker*
3. Low-Temperature Preservation of Foods and Living Matter, *Owen R. Fennema, William D. Powrie, and Elmer H. Marth*
4. Principles of Food Science
   Part I: Food Chemistry, *edited by Owen R. Fennema*
   Part II: Physical Principles of Food Preservation, *Marcus Karel, Owen R. Fennema, and Daryl B. Lund*
5. Food Emulsions, *edited by Stig E. Friberg*
6. Nutritional and Safety Aspects of Food Processing, *edited by Steven R. Tannenbaum*
7. Flavor Research: Recent Advances, *edited by R. Teranishi, Robert A. Flath, and Hiroshi Sugisawa*
8. Computer-Aided Techniques in Food Technology, *edited by Israel Saguy*

9. Handbook of Tropical Foods, *edited by Harvey T. Chan*
10. Antimicrobials in Foods, *edited by Alfred Larry Branen and P. Michael Davidson*
11. Food Constituents and Food Residues: Their Chromatographic Determination, *edited by James F. Lawrence*
12. Aspartame: Physiology and Biochemistry, *edited by Lewis D. Stegink and L. J. Filer, Jr.*
13. Handbook of Vitamins: Nutritional, Biochemical, and Clinical Aspects, *edited by Lawrence J. Machlin*
14. Starch Conversion Technology, *edited by G. M. A. van Beynum and J. A. Roels*
15. Food Chemistry: Second Edition, Revised and Expanded, *edited by Owen R. Fennema*
16. Sensory Evaluation of Food: Statistical Methods and Procedures, *Michael O'Mahony*
17. Alternative Sweeteners, *edited by Lyn O'Brien Nabors and Robert C. Gelardi*
18. Citrus Fruits and Their Products: Analysis and Technology, *S. V. Ting and Russell L. Rouseff*
19. Engineering Properties of Foods, *edited by M. A. Rao and S. S. H. Rizvi*
20. Umami: A Basic Taste, *edited by Yojiro Kawamura and Morley R. Kare*
21. Food Biotechnology, *edited by Dietrich Knorr*
22. Food Texture: Instrumental and Sensory Measurement, *edited by Howard R. Moskowitz*
23. Seafoods and Fish Oils in Human Health and Disease, *John E. Kinsella*
24. Postharvest Physiology of Vegetables, *edited by J. Weichmann*
25. Handbook of Dietary Fiber: An Applied Approach, *Mark L. Dreher*
26. Food Toxicology, Parts A and B, *Jose M. Concon*
27. Modern Carbohydrate Chemistry, *Roger W. Binkley*
28. Trace Minerals in Foods, *edited by Kenneth T. Smith*
29. Protein Quality and the Effects of Processing, *edited by R. Dixon Phillips and John W. Finley*
30. Adulteration of Fruit Juice Beverages, *edited by Steven Nagy, John A. Attaway, and Martha E. Rhodes*
31. Foodborne Bacterial Pathogens, *edited by Michael P. Doyle*
32. Legumes: Chemistry, Technology, and Human Nutrition, *edited by Ruth H. Matthews*
33. Industrialization of Indigenous Fermented Foods, *edited by Keith H. Steinkraus*
34. International Food Regulation Handbook: Policy • Science • Law, *edited by Roger D. Middlekauff and Philippe Shubik*
35. Food Additives, *edited by A. Larry Branen, P. Michael Davidson, and Seppo Salminen*
36. Safety of Irradiated Foods, *J. F. Diehl*

37. Omega-3 Fatty Acids in Health and Disease, *edited by Robert S. Lees and Marcus Karel*
38. Food Emulsions: Second Edition, Revised and Expanded, *edited by Kåre Larsson and Stig E. Friberg*
39. Seafood: Effects of Technology on Nutrition, *George M. Pigott and Barbee W. Tucker*
40. Handbook of Vitamins: Second Edition, Revised and Expanded, *edited by Lawrence J. Machlin*
41. Handbook of Cereal Science and Technology, *Klaus J. Lorenz and Karel Kulp*
42. Food Processing Operations and Scale-Up, *Kenneth J. Valentas, Leon Levine, and J. Peter Clark*
43. Fish Quality Control by Computer Vision, *edited by L. F. Pau and R. Olafsson*
44. Volatile Compounds in Foods and Beverages, *edited by Henk Maarse*
45. Instrumental Methods for Quality Assurance in Foods, *edited by Daniel Y. C. Fung and Richard F. Matthews*
46. *Listeria*, Listeriosis, and Food Safety, *Elliot T. Ryser and Elmer H. Marth*
47. Acesulfame-K, *edited by D. G. Mayer and F. H. Kemper*
48. Alternative Sweeteners: Second Edition, Revised and Expanded, *edited by Lyn O'Brien Nabors and Robert C. Gelardi*
49. Food Extrusion Science and Technology, *edited by Jozef L. Kokini, Chi-Tang Ho, and Mukund V. Karwe*
50. Surimi Technology, *edited by Tyre C. Lanier and Chong M. Lee*
51. Handbook of Food Engineering, *edited by Dennis R. Heldman and Daryl B. Lund*
52. Food Analysis by HPLC, *edited by Leo M. L. Nollet*
53. Fatty Acids in Foods and Their Health Implications, *edited by Ching Kuang Chow*
54. *Clostridium botulinum*: Ecology and Control in Foods, *edited by Andreas H. W. Hauschild and Karen L. Dodds*
55. Cereals in Breadmaking: A Molecular Colloidal Approach, *Ann-Charlotte Eliasson and Kåre Larsson*
56. Low-Calorie Foods Handbook, *edited by Aaron M. Altschul*
57. Antimicrobials in Foods: Second Edition, Revised and Expanded, *edited by P. Michael Davidson and Alfred Larry Branen*
58. Lactic Acid Bacteria, *edited by Seppo Salminen and Atte von Wright*
59. Rice Science and Technology, *edited by Wayne E. Marshall and James I. Wadsworth*
60. Food Biosensor Analysis, *edited by Gabriele Wagner and George G. Guilbault*
61. Principles of Enzymology for the Food Sciences: Second Edition, *John R. Whitaker*
62. Carbohydrate Polyesters as Fat Substitutes, *edited by Casimir C. Akoh and Barry G. Swanson*
63. Engineering Properties of Foods: Second Edition, Revised and Expanded, *edited by M. A. Rao and S. S. H. Rizvi*

64. Handbook of Brewing, *edited by William A. Hardwick*
65. Analyzing Food for Nutrition Labeling and Hazardous Contaminants, *edited by Ike J. Jeon and William G. Ikins*
66. Ingredient Interactions: Effects on Food Quality, *edited by Anilkumar G. Gaonkar*
67. Food Polysaccharides and Their Applications, *edited by Alistair M. Stephen*
68. Safety of Irradiated Foods: Second Edition, Revised and Expanded, *J. F. Diehl*
69. Nutrition Labeling Handbook, *edited by Ralph Shapiro*
70. Handbook of Fruit Science and Technology: Production, Composition, Storage, and Processing, *edited by D. K. Salunkhe and S. S. Kadam*
71. Food Antioxidants: Technological, Toxicological, and Health Perspectives, *edited by D. L. Madhavi, S. S. Deshpande, and D. K. Salunkhe*
72. Freezing Effects on Food Quality, *edited by Lester E. Jeremiah*
73. Handbook of Indigenous Fermented Foods: Second Edition, Revised and Expanded, *edited by Keith H. Steinkraus*
74. Carbohydrates in Food, *edited by Ann-Charlotte Eliasson*
75. Baked Goods Freshness: Technology, Evaluation, and Inhibition of Staling, *edited by Ronald E. Hebeda and Henry F. Zobel*
76. Food Chemistry: Third Edition, *edited by Owen R. Fennema*
77. Handbook of Food Analysis: Volumes 1 and 2, *edited by Leo M. L. Nollet*
78. Computerized Control Systems in the Food Industry, *edited by Gauri S. Mittal*
79. Techniques for Analyzing Food Aroma, *edited by Ray Marsili*
80. Food Proteins and Their Applications, *edited by Srinivasan Damodaran and Alain Paraf*
81. Food Emulsions: Third Edition, Revised and Expanded, *edited by Stig E. Friberg and Kåre Larsson*
82. Nonthermal Preservation of Foods, *Gustavo V. Barbosa-Cánovas, Usha R. Pothakamury, Enrique Palou, and Barry G. Swanson*
83. Milk and Dairy Product Technology, *Edgar Spreer*
84. Applied Dairy Microbiology, *edited by Elmer H. Marth and James L. Steele*
85. Lactic Acid Bacteria: Microbiology and Functional Aspects: Second Edition, Revised and Expanded, *edited by Seppo Salminen and Atte von Wright*
86. Handbook of Vegetable Science and Technology: Production, Composition, Storage, and Processing, *edited by D. K. Salunkhe and S. S. Kadam*
87. Polysaccharide Association Structures in Food, *edited by Reginald H. Walter*
88. Food Lipids: Chemistry, Nutrition, and Biotechnology, *edited by Casimir C. Akoh and David B. Min*
89. Spice Science and Technology, *Kenji Hirasa and Mitsuo Takemasa*

90. Dairy Technology: Principles of Milk Properties and Processes, *P. Walstra, T. J. Geurts, A. Noomen, A. Jellema, and M. A. J. S. van Boekel*
91. Coloring of Food, Drugs, and Cosmetics, *Gisbert Otterstätter*
92. *Listeria*, Listeriosis, and Food Safety: Second Edition, Revised and Expanded, *edited by Elliot T. Ryser and Elmer H. Marth*
93. Complex Carbohydrates in Foods, *edited by Susan Sungsoo Cho, Leon Prosky, and Mark Dreher*
94. Handbook of Food Preservation, *edited by M. Shafiur Rahman*
95. International Food Safety Handbook: Science, International Regulation, and Control, *edited by Kees van der Heijden, Maged Younes, Lawrence Fishbein, and Sanford Miller*
96. Fatty Acids in Foods and Their Health Implications: Second Edition, Revised and Expanded, *edited by Ching Kuang Chow*
97. Seafood Enzymes: Utilization and Influence on Postharvest Seafood Quality, *edited by Norman F. Haard and Benjamin K. Simpson*
98. Safe Handling of Foods, *edited by Jeffrey M. Farber and Ewen C. D. Todd*
99. Handbook of Cereal Science and Technology: Second Edition, Revised and Expanded, *edited by Karel Kulp and Joseph G. Ponte, Jr.*
100. Food Analysis by HPLC: Second Edition, Revised and Expanded, *edited by Leo M. L. Nollet*
101. Surimi and Surimi Seafood, *edited by Jae W. Park*
102. Drug Residues in Foods: Pharmacology, Food Safety, and Analysis, *Nickos A. Botsoglou and Dimitrios J. Fletouris*
103. Seafood and Freshwater Toxins: Pharmacology, Physiology, and Detection, *edited by Luis M. Botana*
104. Handbook of Nutrition and Diet, *Babasaheb B. Desai*
105. Nondestructive Food Evaluation: Techniques to Analyze Properties and Quality, *edited by Sundaram Gunasekaran*
106. Green Tea: Health Benefits and Applications, *Yukihiko Hara*
107. Food Processing Operations Modeling: Design and Analysis, *edited by Joseph Irudayaraj*
108. Wine Microbiology: Science and Technology, *Claudio Delfini and Joseph V. Formica*
109. Handbook of Microwave Technology for Food Applications, *edited by Ashim K. Datta and Ramaswamy C. Anantheswaran*
110. Applied Dairy Microbiology: Second Edition, Revised and Expanded, *edited by Elmer H. Marth and James L. Steele*
111. Transport Properties of Foods, *George D. Saravacos and Zacharias B. Maroulis*
112. Alternative Sweeteners: Third Edition, Revised and Expanded, *edited by Lyn O'Brien Nabors*
113. Handbook of Dietary Fiber, *edited by Susan Sungsoo Cho and Mark L. Dreher*
114. Control of Foodborne Microorganisms, *edited by Vijay K. Juneja and John N. Sofos*
115. Flavor, Fragrance, and Odor Analysis, *edited by Ray Marsili*

116. Food Additives: Second Edition, Revised and Expanded, *edited by A. Larry Branen, P. Michael Davidson, Seppo Salminen, and John H. Thorngate, III*
117. Food Lipids: Chemistry, Nutrition, and Biotechnology: Second Edition, Revised and Expanded, *edited by Casimir C. Akoh and David B. Min*
118. Food Protein Analysis: Quantitative Effects on Processing, *R. K. Owusu-Apenten*
119. Handbook of Food Toxicology, *S. S. Deshpande*
120. Food Plant Sanitation, *edited by Y. H. Hui, Bernard L. Bruinsma, J. Richard Gorham, Wai-Kit Nip, Phillip S. Tong, and Phil Ventresca*
121. Physical Chemistry of Foods, *Pieter Walstra*
122. Handbook of Food Enzymology, *edited by John R. Whitaker, Alphons G. J. Voragen, and Dominic W. S. Wong*
123. Postharvest Physiology and Pathology of Vegetables: Second Edition, Revised and Expanded, *edited by Jerry A. Bartz and Jeffrey K. Brecht*
124. Characterization of Cereals and Flours: Properties, Analysis, and Applications, *edited by Gönül Kaletunç and Kenneth J. Breslauer*
125. International Handbook of Foodborne Pathogens, *edited by Marianne D. Miliotis and Jeffrey W. Bier*
126. Food Process Design, *Zacharias B. Maroulis and George D. Saravacos*
127. Handbook of Dough Fermentations, *edited by Karel Kulp and Klaus Lorenz*
128. Extraction Optimization in Food Engineering, *edited by Constantina Tzia and George Liadakis*
129. Physical Principles of Food Preservation: Second Edition, Revised and Expanded, *Marcus Karel and Daryl B. Lund*
130. Handbook of Vegetable Preservation and Processing, *edited by Y. H. Hui, Sue Ghazala, Dee M. Graham, K. D. Murrell, and Wai-Kit Nip*
131. Handbook of Flavor Characterization: Sensory Analysis, Chemistry, and Physiology, *edited by Kathryn D. Deibler and Jeannine Delwiche*
132. Food Emulsions: Fourth Edition, Revised and Expanded, *edited by Stig E. Friberg, Kåre Larsson, and Johan Sjöblom*
133. Handbook of Frozen Foods, *edited by Y. H. Hui, Paul Cornillon, Isabel Guerrero Legarreta, Miang H. Lim, K. D. Murrell, and Wai-Kit Nip*
134. Handbook of Food and Beverage Fermentation Technology, *edited by Y. H. Hui, Lisbeth Meunier-Goddik, Åse Solvejg Hansen, Jytte Josephsen, Wai-Kit Nip, Peggy S. Stanfield, and Fidel Toldrá*
135. Genetic Variation in Taste Sensitivity, *edited by John Prescott and Beverly J. Tepper*
136. Industrialization of Indigenous Fermented Foods: Second Edition, Revised and Expanded, *edited by Keith H. Steinkraus*
137. Vitamin E: Food Chemistry, Composition, and Analysis, *Ronald Eitenmiller and Junsoo Lee*
138. Handbook of Food Analysis: Second Edition, Revised and Expanded: Volumes 1, 2, and 3, *edited by Leo M. L. Nollet*

139. Lactic Acid Bacteria: Microbiological and Functional Aspects, Third Edition, Revised and Expanded, *edited by Seppo Salminen, Atte von Wright, and Arthur Ouwehand*
140. Fat Crystal Networks, *Alejandro G. Marangoni*
141. Novel Food Processing Technologies, *edited by Gustavo V. Barbosa-Cánovas, M. Soledad Tapia, and M. Pilar Cano*

*Additional Volumes in Preparation*

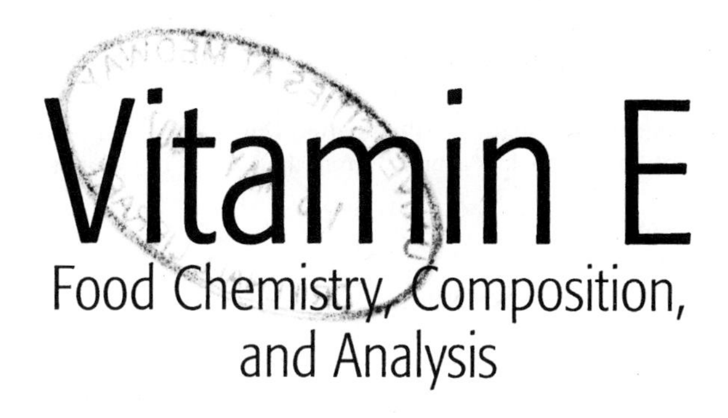

# Vitamin E

## Food Chemistry, Composition, and Analysis

Ronald Eitenmiller
*University of Georgia*
*Athens, Georgia, U.S.A.*

Junsoo Lee
*Chungbuk National University*
*Chungbuk, Korea*

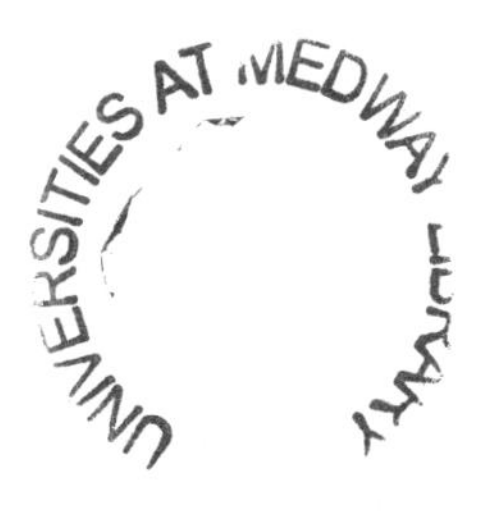


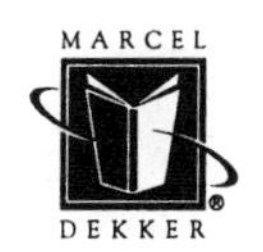


MARCEL DEKKER, INC. NEW YORK • BASEL

**Library of Congress Cataloging-in-Publication Data**
A catalog record for this book is available from the Library of Congress.

**ISBN: 0-8247-0688-9**

This book is printed on acid-free paper.



**Headquarters**
Marcel Dekker, Inc., 270 Madison Avenue, New York, NY 10016, U.S.A.
tel: 212-696-9000; fax: 212-685-4540

**Distribution and Customer Service**
Marcel Dekker, Inc., Cimarron Road, Monticello, New York 12701, U.S.A.
tel: 800-228-1160; fax: 845-796-1772

**Eastern Hemisphere Distribution**
Marcel Dekker AG, Hutgasse 4, Postfach 812, CH-4001 Basel, Switzerland
tel: 41-61-260-6300; fax: 41-61-260-6333

**World Wide Web**
http://www.dekker.com

The publisher offers discounts on this book when ordered in bulk quantities. For more information, write to Special Sales/Professional Marketing at the headquarters address above.



Current printing (last digit):

10 9 8 7 6 5 4 3 2 1

**PRINTED IN THE UNITED STATES OF AMERICA**

# Preface

Knowledge about vitamin E has expanded so rapidly over the past few decades that it is difficult for anyone to keep up with even a few of the general areas pertinent to the vitamin—chemistry, nutrition, metabolism, genetics, functional impact on disease onset and severity, pharmacology, regulations, food technology, and food composition and analytical challenges, to name a few. Our careers in food science and technology are focused on food composition and analysis. We have been privileged to play a role in improving the availability of food composition information on vitamin E and, in some ways, the analytical capability for its assay. Interaction with the food industry, the U.S. Department of Agriculture Nutrient Data Laboratory, the U.S. Food and Drug Administration, and various international organizations concerned with food composition has opened many avenues for research, none of which has been more satisfying or challenging than work on vitamin E.

The overall objective of this book is to provide insight into the vast body of scientific information available on vitamin E related to food science and technology; thus, the emphasis is on food chemistry, food composition, and food analysis. At the same time, these topics are intertwined with the food delivery system, basic nutrition, food regulations, the functional food and pharmaceutical industries, and the excellent efforts of scientists worldwide who are unraveling the subtleties of vitamin E biochemistry. While our primary goal is to provide a resource useful to food scientists, we hope scientists and students in others fields will find the book helpful.

## ACKNOWLEDGMENT

This book would not have been possible without the help of Ms. Huan Huan Huang, Dr. Lin Ye, and Dr. Ji-Yeon Chun. We sincerely thank them for their diligent efforts.

*Ronald Eitenmiller*
*Junsoo Lee*

# Contents

# List of Abbreviations

| | |
|---|---|
| $\lambda$ | Wavelength |
| $\mu g$ | Microgram |
| $\mu L$ | Microliter |
| $\mu m$ | Micrometer |
| $\varepsilon$ | Molar absorptivity |
| $\alpha$-T | $\alpha$-tocopherol |
| $\beta$-T | $\beta$-tocopherol |
| $\gamma$-T | $\gamma$-tocopherol |
| $\delta$-T | $\delta$-tocopherol |
| $\alpha$-T3 | $\alpha$-tocotrienol |
| $\beta$-T3 | $\beta$-tocotrienol |
| $\gamma$-T3 | $\gamma$-tocotrienol |
| $\delta$-T3 | $\delta$-tocotrienol |
| $\alpha$-TAC | *all-rac*-$\alpha$-tocopheryl acetate |
| $\alpha$-TTP | $\alpha$-tocopherol transfer protein |
| A | Acetone |
| ACNA | Atlanta Center for Nutrient Analysis, U.S. Food and Drug Administration |

| | |
|---|---|
| AI | Adequate Intake |
| AIM-NDBS | Architecture and Integration Management, Nutrient Data Bank System |
| $AlCl_3$ | Aluminum trichloride |
| *all-rac*-$\alpha$-T | *all-rac*-$\alpha$-tocopherol |
| AMD | Age-related macular degeneration |
| An V | p-Anisidine value |
| AOCS | American Oil Chemists' Society |
| AOM | Active oxygen method |
| AREDS | Age-Related Cataract and Vision Loss Study |
| ASAP | Antioxidant Supplementation in Atherosclerosis Prevention Study |
| ATBC | Alpha-Tocopherol, Beta Carotene Cancer Prevention Study |
| AVED | Ataxia with vitamin E deficiency |
| $BF_3$ | Boron trifluoride |
| BHA | Butylated hydroxyanisole |
| CC | Confidence code |
| CE | Capillary electrophoresis |
| CEC | Capillary electrochromatography |
| CFR | Code of Federal Regulations |
| CHAOS | Cambridge Heart Antioxidant Study |
| $CHCl_3$ | Chloroform |
| $CH_2Cl_2$ | Methylene chloride |
| CLAS | Cholesterol Lowering Atherosclerosis Study |
| CPSII | Cancer Prevention Study II |
| CRM | Certified reference material |
| CSFII | Continuing Survey of Food Intakes by Individuals |
| CVD | Cardiovascular disease |
| CZE | Capillary zone electrophoresis |
| DIPE | Diisopropyl ether |
| DL | Detection limit |
| $E^{o'}$ | Reduction potential |
| EAR | Estimated average requirement |
| EC | Electrochemical detector |

| | |
|---|---|
| $E_{1cm}^{1\%}$ | Specific extinction coefficient |
| EDCCS | Eye Disease Care Control Study |
| EKC | Electrokinetic chromatography |
| ELSD | Evaporative light scattering detector |
| EQ | Ethoxyquin |
| $Et_2O$ | Diethyl ether |
| EtOAC | Ethyl acetate |
| EtOH | Ethanol |
| $E_M$ | Emission |
| $E_X$ | Excitation |
| FDA | United States Food and Drug Administration |
| FFA | Free fatty acids |
| FID | Flame ionization detector |
| FLD | Fluorescence detector |
| FLO | Fresh linseed oil |
| FSIS | Food Safety and Inspection Service |
| FSO | Fresh sunflower oil |
| GC | Gas chromatography |
| GC-MS | Gas chromatography–mass spectrometry |
| GISSI | Gruppo Italiano per lo Studio della Sopravviverza nell'Infarcto Micardio Prevention Study |
| GM | *M. gluteus medius* |
| GMP | Good manufacturing practice |
| GPC | Gel permeation chromatography |
| GRAS | Generally recognized as safe |
| GSH | Glutathione |
| GSSH | Reduced glutathione |
| HAC | Acetic acid |
| HDL cholesterol | High density lipoprotein cholesterol |
| Hex | Hexane |
| HLE | a-TAC supplemented heated linseed oil |
| HLO | Heated linseed oil |
| HMG-CoA reductase | 3-hydroxy-3-methyl glutaryl coenzyme A reductase |
| HMSO | Her Majesty's Stationery Office |
| $HNO_2$ | Nitrous acid |
| $HO_2^{\cdot}$ | Hydroperoxyl radical |

| | |
|---|---|
| $H_2O_2$ | Hydrogen peroxide |
| HOCl | Hypochlorous acid |
| HOPE | Heart Outcomes Prevention Evaluation |
| HP-GPC | High-performance gel permeation chromatography |
| HPLC | High-performance liquid chromatography |
| HPPDase | p-hydroxyphenylpyruvic acid dioxygenase |
| HPS | MRC/BHF Heart Protection Study |
| HPSEC | High-performance size-exclusion chromatography |
| HSBO | Hydrogenated soybean oil |
| HSE | $\alpha$-TAC supplemented heated sunflower oil |
| HSO | Heated sunflower oil |
| INFOODS | The International Network of Food Data Systems |
| IPA | Isopropyl alcohol |
| IS | Internal standards |
| IT | Induction time |
| IU | International unit |
| LC | Liquid chromatography |
| LCE | Low-cost extruder cooker |
| LC/MS | Liquid chromatography/mass spectrometry |
| LC-MS/MS | Liquid chromatography–tandem mass spectrometry |
| LD | *M. longissimus dorsi* |
| LL | *M. longissimus lumborum* |
| $LO^{\cdot}$ | Alkoxy radical |
| $LO_2^{\cdot}$ | Peroxy radical |
| LOAEL | Lowest observed adverse effect level |
| LOD | Limit of detection |
| LDL cholesterol | Low-density lipoprotein cholesterol |
| LOQ | Limit of quantitation |
| LT | *M. longissimus thoracis* |
| M | Molar |
| MAP | Modified atmosphere packaging |
| MDA | Malondialdehyde |
| MeCN | Acetonitrile |
| MEEKC | Microemulsion electrokinetic capillary chromatography |
| MEKC | Micellar electrokinetic chromatography |
| MeOH | Methanol |

| | |
|---|---|
| MetMb | Metmyoglobin |
| mg $\alpha$-TE | Milligram a-tocopherol equivalent |
| mL | Milliliter |
| mm | Millimeter |
| mM | Millimolar |
| mmol | Millimole |
| MP | Mobile phase |
| MRP | Maillard reaction products |
| MS | Mass spectrometry |
| MSPD | Matrix solid phase extraction |
| MTBE | Methyl-*tert*-butyl ether |
| MUFA | Monounsaturated fatty acid |
| mV | Millivolt |
| $NaClO_4$ | Sodium perchlorate |
| $NADP^+$ | Oxidized nicotinamide adenine dinucleotide phosphate |
| NADPH | Reduced nicotinamide adenine dinucleotide phosphate |
| NaOAC | Sodium acetate |
| NCI | National Cancer Institute |
| NHANES I | First National Health and Nutrition Examination Survey |
| NHANES II | Second National Health and Nutrition Examination Survey |
| NIST | National Institute of Standards and Technology |
| NLEA | Nutrition Labeling and Education Act of 1990 |
| NLT | Not less than |
| NMT | Not more than |
| nm | Nanometer |
| nmol | Nanomole |
| $NO^{\cdot}$ | Nitric oxide |
| $NO_2^{\cdot}$ | Nitrogen dioxide |
| $NO_2^+$ | Nitronium cation |
| $N_2O_3$ | Dinitrogen trioxide |
| $N_2O_4$ | Dinitrogen tetroxide |
| NOAEL | No observed adverse effect level |
| NOS | Nitric oxide synthetase |
| NP-HPLC | Normal-phase high-performance liquid chromatography |

| | |
|---|---|
| NRC | National Research Council |
| $O^{\cdot}$ | Superoxide |
| $^{1}O_2$ | Singlet oxygen |
| $O_3$ | Ozone |
| ODPVA | Octadecanoyl polyvinyl alcohol |
| ODS | Octadecylsilica |
| $OH^{\cdot}$ | Hydroxy radical |
| $ONOO^-$ | Peroxynitrate |
| ONOOH | Peroxynitrous acid |
| PE | Petroleum ether |
| PF | Protection factor |
| pg | Picogram |
| PKC | Protein kinase C |
| PL | Phospholipid |
| PM | *M. psoas* major |
| PMC | 2,2,5,7,8-pentamethyl-6-chromanol |
| POLA | Pathologies Oculaires Lies à l' Age |
| ppb | Parts per billion |
| ppm | Parts per million |
| PPP | Primary Prevention Project |
| PSE | Pale, soft, exudative |
| PUFA | Polyunsaturated fatty acid |
| PV | Peroxide value |
| QI | Quality index |
| QL | Quantitation limit |
| $R^{\cdot}$ | Alkyl radical |
| RB | Refined bleached oil |
| RBC | Red blood cell |
| RDA | Recommended dietary allowance |
| RH | Relative humidity |
| RNS | Reactive nitrogen species |
| $ROO^{\cdot}$ | Peroxy radical |
| ROOH | Hydroperoxide |
| ROONO | Alkyl peroxynitrates |
| ROS | Reactive oxygen species |

| | |
|---|---|
| RP-HPLC | Reversed-phase high-performance liquid chromatography |
| $RSD_R$ | Relative standard deviation (reproducibility) |
| RSM | Response surface methodology |
| SFA | Saturated fatty acid |
| SFC | Supercritical fluid chromatography |
| SFC/MS | Supercritical fluid chromatography/mass spectrometry |
| SFE | Supercritical fluid extraction |
| SM | *M. semimembranosus* |
| SPACE | Secondary Prevention with Antioxidants of Cardiovascular Disease in Endstage Renal Disease |
| SPE | Solid-phase extraction |
| SRM | Standard reference material |
| SSA | Significant scientific agreement |
| TAG | Triacylglyceride |
| TBA | Thiobarbituric acid values |
| TBARS | Thiobarbituric acid reactive substance |
| TBHQ | Tertiary butylhydroquinone |
| tBME | *tert*-butylmethyl ether |
| $TDA^+$ | Tetradecyl ammonium ion |
| TDT | Thermal Death Time |
| TG | Triglyceride |
| THBP | Trihydroxybutyrophenone |
| THF | Tetrahydrofuran |
| TLC | Thin-layer chromatography |
| TMHQ | Trimethylhydroquinone |
| TPGSNF | *RRR*-$\alpha$-tocopheryl polyethylene glycol 1000 succinate |
| TRF | Tocotrienol-rich fraction |
| $TRF_{25}$ | Tocotrienol rich fraction of rice bran |
| UF | Uncertainty factor |
| UHT | Ultrahigh-temperature |
| UL | Tolerable upper intake level |
| USDA | United States Department of Agriculture |
| USP | United States Pharmacopeia |

| | |
|---|---|
| UV | Ultraviolet |
| UV-B | Ultraviolet B |
| UV/VIS | Ultraviolet/visible |
| V | Volt |
| VECAT | Vitamin E, Cataract, and Age-Related Maculopathy Trial |
| VLDL | Very-low-density lipoproteins |
| WOF | Warmed-over flavor |
| $ZnCl_2$ | Zinc chloride |

# 1

# Vitamin E: Chemistry and Biochemistry

## 1.1. INTRODUCTION

Vitamin E and other antioxidant components of the diet (vitamin C, carotenoids, selenium, flavonoids, and several others) have been put to the forefront of the medical and nutrition sciences because of significant advances in understanding of the relationship of oxidative stress in its various forms to the onset and/or control of many chronic diseases. Since these disease states including coronary heart disease and cancer are focus points for consumer health interests and the medical community, dietary antioxidant components are highly recognized and sought after by the consumer. Of the many such dietary components, vitamin E has commanded most interest because of its availability, strong marketing potential, overall health impact, and central role in preventing oxidation at the cellular level.

Vitamin E was discovered and characterized as a fat-soluble nutritional factor during reproductive studies with rats. Evans and Bishop published these observations in 1922 (1). First named *factor X* and the *antisterility factor*, the vitamin was later designated vitamin E by Bishop, since its discovery closely followed the discovery of vitamin D. A vitamin E active compound was isolated from wheat germ oil in 1936 (2). At this point, the Evans research group named the compound *α-tocopherol* (α-T) from the Greek words *tocos* (birth) and *ferein* (bringing), relating to its essentiality for rats to bear young. The *ol* suffix denotes that the compound is an alcohol (3). Other notable events in the early history of vitamin E include the isolation of $\beta$- and $\gamma$-tocopherol ($\beta$-, $\gamma$-T) from vegetable oil in 1937 (4), determination of the structure of $\alpha$-T in 1938 (5,6), synthesis of $\alpha$-T in 1938 (7), recognition of the antioxidant activity of the tocopherols (8), recognition that $\alpha$-T was the most effective tocopherol in prevention of vitamin E deficiency (4), isolation of $\delta$-tocopherol ($\delta$-T) from soybean oil in 1947 (9), identification of the four naturally occurring tocotrienols ($\alpha$-T3, $\beta$-T3, $\gamma$-T3, $\delta$-T3) (10,11), and documentation of naturally occurring tocopherols and tocotrienols in foods (12–20). Many excellent reviews cover all aspects of vitamin E knowledge. Each review has many outstanding qualities, anyone interested in the early history of vitamin E should read the publication of the Symposium on Vitamin E and Metabolism in honor of Professor H. M. Evans (21).

## 1.2. CHEMISTRY OF VITAMIN E

### 1.2.1. Structure

*Vitamin E* is the collective term for fat-soluble 6-hydroxychroman compounds that exhibit the biological activity of $\alpha$-T measured by the rat resorption–gestation assay. Tocol (Figure 1.1) (2-methyl-2-(4′,8′,12′-trimethyltridecyl)-chroman-6-ol) is generally considered the parent compound of the tocopherols. Accepted nomenclature has been set by the IUPAC-IUB Joint Commission on Nomenclature (22–24).

Naturally occurring vitamin E consists of $\alpha$-, $\beta$-, $\gamma$-, and $\delta$-T and the corresponding $\alpha$-, $\beta$-, $\gamma$-, and $\delta$-T3 (Figure 1.1). The tocopherols are characterized by the 6-chromanol ring structure methylated to varying degrees at the 5, 7, and 8 positions. At position 2, there is a $C_{16}$ saturated side chain. The tocotrienols are unsaturated at the 3′, 7′, and 11′ positions of the side chain. The specific tocopherols and tocotrienols, therefore, differ by the number and positions of the methyl groups on the 6-chromanol ring. $\alpha$-Tocopherol and $\alpha$-T3 are trimethylated; $\beta$-T, $\beta$-T3, $\gamma$-T, and $\gamma$-T3 are dimethylated; and $\delta$-T and $\delta$-T3 are monomethylated (Figure 1.1). Trivial and chemical names are given in Table 1.1.

### 1.2.2. Stereochemistry

The tocopherols possess three asymmetric carbons (chiral centers) at position 2 of the chromanol ring and at positions 4′ and 8′ of the phytyl side chain. Synthetic $\alpha$-T (*all-rac-$\alpha$*-T) is a racemic mixture of equal parts of each stereoisomer. Therefore, each tocopherol has eight ($2^3$) possible optical isomers. Only *RRR*-tocopherols are found in nature. The eight isomers of *all-rac-$\alpha$*-T

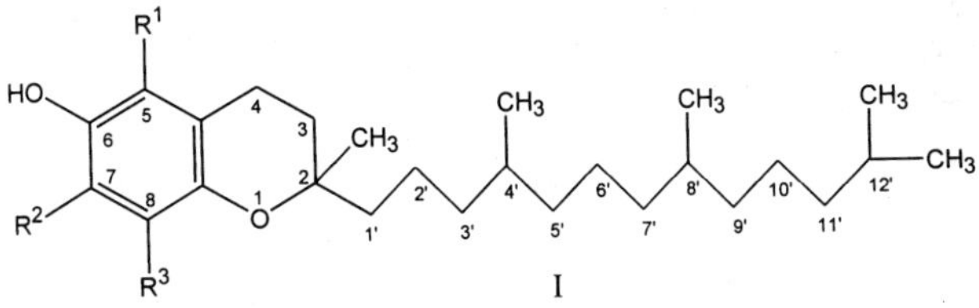

I

| | |
|---|---|
| $R^1 = R^2 = R^3 = H$ | Tocol |
| $R^1 = R^2 = R^3 = CH_3$ | α–Tocopherol |
| $R^1 = R^3 = CH_3$; $R^2 = H$ | β-Tocopherol |
| $R^1 = H$; $R^2 = R^3 = CH_3$ | γ–Tocopherol |
| $R^1 = R^2 = H$; $R^3 = CH_3$ | δ-Tocopherol |

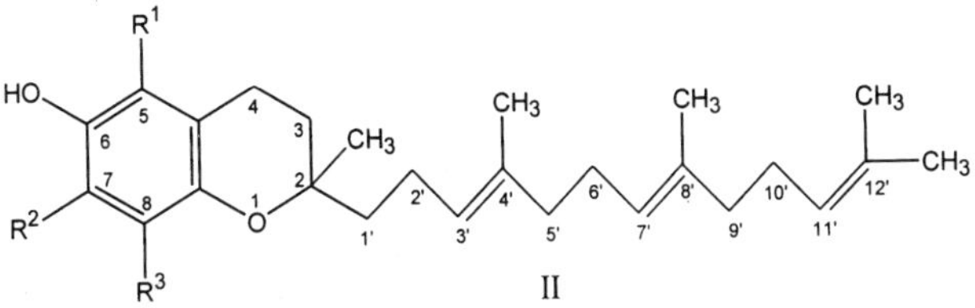

II

| | |
|---|---|
| $R^1 = R^2 = R^3 = H$ | Tocotrienol |
| $R^1 = R^2 = R^3 = CH_3$ | α–Tocotrienol |
| $R^1 = R^3 = CH_3$; $R^2 = H$ | β-Tocotrienol |
| $R^1 = H$; $R^2 = R^3 = CH_3$ | γ–Tocotrienol |
| $R^1 = R^2 = H$; $R^3 = CH_3$ | δ-Tocotrienol |

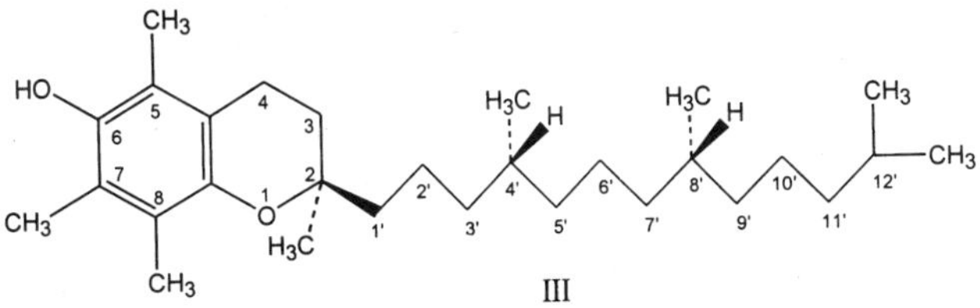

III

(2 R 4' R 8' R) α–Tocopherol
RRR - α - Tocopherol

**FIGURE 1.1** Structures of tocopherols and tocotrienols.

**TABLE 1.1** Trivial and Chemical Names of the Tocopherols and Tocotrienols

| Tocopherols | | | | | |
|---|---|---|---|---|---|
| | | | Ring position | | |
| Trivial name | Chemical name | Abbreviation | $R^1$ | $R^2$ | $R^3$ |
| Tocol | 2-Methyl-2-(4′,8′,12′-trimethyltridecyl) chroman-6-ol | — | H | H | H |
| α-Tocopherol | 5,7,8-Trimethyltocol | α-T | $CH_3$ | $CH_3$ | $CH_3$ |
| β-Tocopherol | 5,8-Dimethyltocol | β-T | $CH_3$ | H | $CH_3$ |
| γ-Tocopherol | 7,8-Dimethyltocol | γ-T | H | $CH_3$ | $CH_3$ |
| δ-Tocopherol | 8-Methyltocol | δ-T | H | H | $CH_3$ |

| Tocotrienols | | | | | |
|---|---|---|---|---|---|
| | | | Ring position | | |
| Trivial name | Chemical name | Abbreviation | $R^1$ | $R^2$ | $R^3$ |
| Tocol | 2-Methyl-2-(4′,8′,12′-trimethyltrideca-3′,7′,11′-trienyl) chroman-6-ol | — | H | H | H |
| α-Tocotrienol | 5,7,8-Trimethyltocotrienol | α-T3 | $CH_3$ | $CH_3$ | $CH_3$ |
| β-Tocotrienol | 5,8-Dimethyltocotrienol | β-T3 | $CH_3$ | H | $CH_3$ |
| γ-Tocotrienol | 7,8-Dimethyltocotrienol | γ-T3 | H | $CH_3$ | $CH_3$ |
| δ-Tocotrienol | 8-Methyltocotrienol | δ-T3 | H | H | $CH_3$ |

(*RRR*-, RSR-, RRS-, RSS-, SRR-, SSR-, SRS-, and SSS-) are depicted in Figure 1.2. As discussed more completely in Chapter 2, only the *2R*-stereoisomeric forms (*RRR*-, RSR-, RRS-, and RSS) of $\alpha$-T are considered active forms of vitamin E for the human (25). Chemical synthesis of the tocopherols is discussed in Section 1.2.5.

The tocotrienols arising from 2-methyl-2-(4′,8′,12′-trimethyltrideca-3′,7′,11′-trienyl) chroman-6-ol (nonmethylated ring structure) have only one chiral center at position 2. Consequently, only *2R* and *2S* stereoisomers are possible. Unsaturation at positions 3′ and 7′ of the phytyl side chain permits four cis/trans geometric isomers. The eight potential tocotrienol isomers are given in Table 1.2. Only the *2R*, 3′-trans, 7′-trans isomer exists in nature. Isolation and elucidation of the structural properties of the tocotrienols were accomplished in the 1960s by the Pennock and associates and Isler and associates research groups (11,26). Drotleff and Ternes (27). examined hydrogenation of oils and biohydrogenation in the rumen as possible sources for cis/trans isomerization of the tocotrienols but found little evidence of changes in the *2R*, *trans-trans* configuration.

### 1.2.3. Nomenclature Rules

Because of the complexity of tocopherol and tocotrienol nomenclature, the IUPAC-IUB 1981 recommendations are given as presented by the Joint Commission on Biochemical Nomenclature (23).

1. Terms
    a. Vitamin E: The term *vitamin E* should be used as the generic descriptor for all tocol and tocotrienol derivatives exhibiting qualitatively the biological activity of $\alpha$-tocopherol. This term should be used in derived terms such as *vitamin E deficiency*, *vitamin E activity*, and *vitamin E antagonist*.
    b. Tocol: The term *tocol* is the trivial designation for 2-methyl-2-(4′,8′,12′-trimethyltridecyl) chroman-6-ol [Compound I (Figure 1.1)], where $R^1 = R^2 = R^3 = H$).
    c. Tocopherol(s): The term *tocopherol(s)* should be used as a generic descriptor for all mono, di, and trimethyl tocols. Thus, the term is not synonymous with the term *vitamin E*.
2. Compound I (Figure 1.1) ($R^1 = R^2 = R^3 = CH_3$), known as $\alpha$-tocopherol, is designated $\alpha$-tocopherol or 5,7,8-trimethyl tocol.
3. Compound I (Figure 1.1) ($R^1 = R^3 = CH_3$; $R^2 = H$), known as $\beta$-tocopherol, is designated $\beta$-tocopherol or 5,8-dimethyl tocol.
4. Compound I (Figure 1.1) ($R^1 = H$; $R^2 = R^3 = CH_3$), known as $\gamma$-tocopherol, is designated $\gamma$-tocopherol or 7,8-dimethyl tocol.

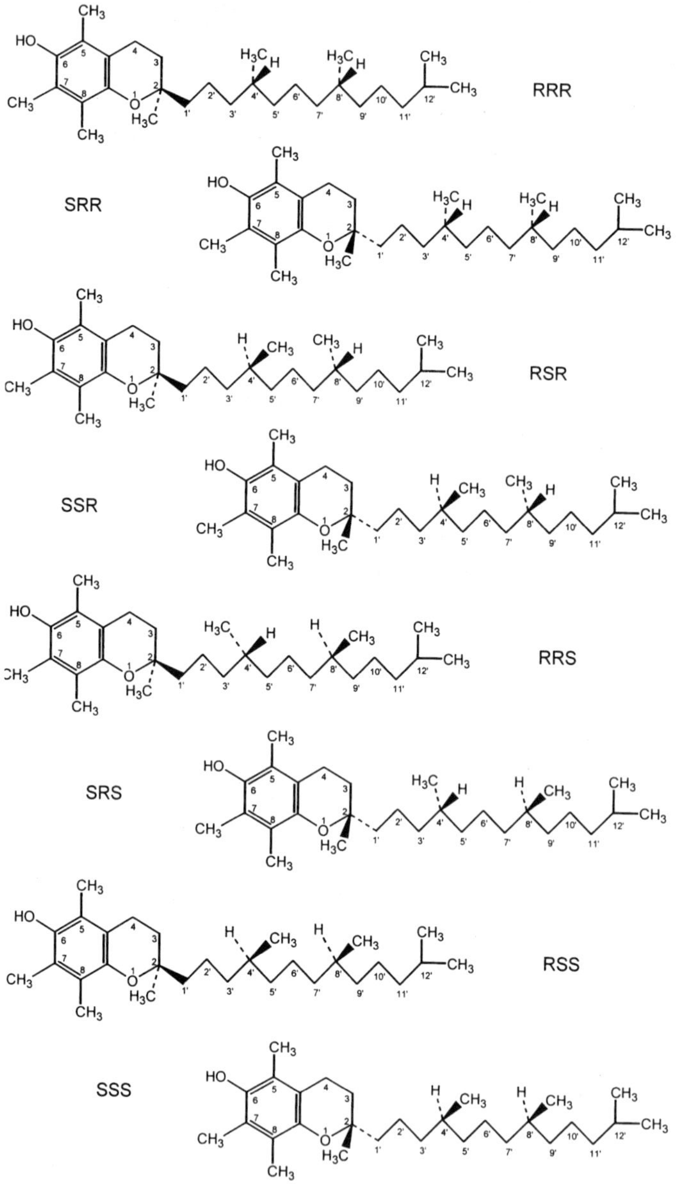

RRR

SRR

RSR

SSR

RRS

SRS

RSS

SSS

**FIGURE 1.2** Stereoisomers of $\alpha$-tocopherol.

**TABLE 1.2** The Eight Possible RS, Cis/Trans Isomers of the Tocotrienols

| R configuration position 2 | S configuration position 2 |
|---|---|
| 2R, 3′cis, 7′cis | 2S, 3′cis, 7′cis |
| 2R, 3′cis, 7′trans | 2S, 3′cis, 7′trans |
| 2R, 3′trans, 7′cis | 2S, 3′trans, 7′cis |
| 2R, 3′trans, 7′trans | 2S, 3′trans, 7′trans |

5. Compound I (Figure 1.1) ($R^1 = R^2 = H$; $R^3 = CH_3$) is known as $\delta$-tocopherol or 8-methyl tocol.
6. Compound II (Figure 1.1) ($R^1 = R^2 = R^3 = H$) 2-methyl-2-(4′,8′,12′-trimethyltrideca-3′,7′,11′-trienyl) chroman-6-ol is designated tocotrienol [only *all-trans* (E,E)-tocotrienols have been found in nature].
7. Compound II (Figure 1.1) ($R^1 = R^2 = R^3 = CH_3$), formerly known as $\zeta$, or $\zeta_2$-tocopherol, is designated 5,7,8-trimethyltocotrienol or $\alpha$-tocotrienol. The name *tocochromanol-3* has also been used.
8. Compound II (Figure 1.1) ($R^1 = R^3 = CH_3$; $R^2 = H$), formerly known as $\varepsilon$-tocopherol, is designated 5,8-dimethyltocotrienol or $\beta$-tocotrienol.
9. Compound II (Figure 1.1) ($R^1 = H$; $R^2 = R^3 = CH_3$), formerly known as $\eta$-tocopherol, is designated 7,8-dimethyltocotrienol or $\gamma$-tocotrienol. The name *plastochromanol-3* has also been used.
10. Compound II (Figure 1.1) ($R^1 = R^2 = H$; $R^3 = CH_3$) is designated 8-methyltocotrienol or $\delta$-tocotrienol.
11. The only naturally occurring stereoisomer of $\alpha$-tocopherol hirtherto discovered [compound III, (Figure 1.1)] has the configuration 2*R*,4′R,8′R according to the sequence rule. Its semisystematic name is, therefore, (2*R*,4′R,8′R)-$\alpha$-tocopherol. The same system can be applied to all other individual stereoisomers of tocopherols.
12. Trivial designations are sometimes desirable to indicate briefly the configuration of important stereoisomers of $\alpha$-tocopherol and especially mixtures of such stereoisomers. Some of these materials are of considerable commercial and therapeutic importance. The use of the following trivial designations for the most important material of this class is recommended.
    a. The $\alpha$-tocopherol mentioned earlier, which has the configuration 2*R*,4′R,8′R, formerly known as *d*-$\alpha$-tocopherol, should be called *RRR*-$\alpha$-tocopherol.
    b. The diastereoisomer of *RRR*-$\alpha$-tocopherol, formerly known as *l*-$\alpha$-tocopherol, being the epimer of *RRR*-$\alpha$-tocopherol at C-2 with the configuration 2*S*,4′R,8′R, should be called 2-*epi*-$\alpha$-tocopherol.

c. A mixture of *RRR*-$\alpha$-tocopherol and 2-*epi*-$\alpha$-tocopherol (obtained by synthesis using phytol and the appropriate achiral hydroquinone derivative) should be called 2-*ambo*-$\alpha$-tocopherol. This mixture was formerly known as *dl*-$\alpha$-tocopherol until the optical activity of phytol was recognized when *dl*-$\alpha$-tocopherol was restricted to *all-rac*-$\alpha$-tocopherol. It is probable that the asymmetric reaction involved in this partial synthesis would only by chance lead to the formation of equimolar proportions. The acetate of 2-*ambo*-$\alpha$-tocopherol (2-*ambo*-$\alpha$-tocopheryl acetate) was the former international standard for vitamin E activity.

d. The reduction product of natural 5,7,8-tocotrienol, in which the double bonds at 3′, 7′, and 11′ are hydrogenated and two new asymmetric centers are created at C-4′ and C-8′, is a mixture in unspecified proportions of four diastereoisometric $\alpha$-tocopherols, having the configurations 2*R*,4′R,8′R; 2*R*,4′S,8′R; 2*R*,4′S,8′S; and 2*R*,4′R,8′S. The material should be called 4′-*ambo*, 8′-*ambo*-$\alpha$-tocopherol.

e. The totally synthetic vitamin E, obtained without any control of stereochemistry, is a mixture in unspecified proportions (in preparations examined, the proportions closely approached equimolar of four racemates or pairs of enantiomers (i.e., eight diastereoisomers). It should be called *all-rac*-$\alpha$-tocopherol (it was formerly known as dl--tocopherol, although this designation was previously used for 2-ambo--tocopherol).

13. Esters of tocopherols and tocotrienols should be called *tocopheryl esters* and *tocotrienyl esters*, respectively (e.g., $\alpha$-tocopheryl acetate, $\alpha$-tocotrienyl acetate).

## 1.2.4. Spectral Properties

Ultraviolet (UV) and fluorescence properties of several vitamin E compounds are given in Table 1.3 (28–32). The UV spectra for tocopherols and tocotrienols in ethanol show maximal absorption between 292 and 298 nm. Minimal absorption occurs between 250 and 260 nm (29,33–36). Esterification at the 6-hydroxyl shifts the absorption to shorter wavelengths; *all-rac*-$\alpha$-tocopheryl acetate shows maximal absorption at 286 nm (28,35,36). Intensity of absorption decreases with esterification. $E_{1cm}^{1\%}$ in ethanol for *all-rac*-$\alpha$-tocopheryl acetate ranges from 40 to 44, compared to 75.8 to 91.4 for the tocopherols and tocotrienols (28).

Excitation of the chroman ring at wavelengths near or at maximal absorption (e.g., 292 nm) produces maximal emission at 320 nm or slightly

**TABLE 1.3** Ultraviolet and Fluorescence Properties of Vitamin E

| | | | Spectral characteristics | | | | |
|---|---|---|---|---|---|---|---|
| | | | Absorbance[b] | | | Fluorescence[c] | |
| Substance[a] | Molar mass | Formula | $\lambda_{max}$ nm | $E^{1\%}_{1cm}$ | $\varepsilon$ | Ex nm | Em nm |
| α-T<br>CAS No. 59-02-9<br>**10159** | 430.71 | $C_{29}H_{50}O_2$ | 292 | 75.8 | [3265] | 295 | 320 |
| β-T<br>CAS No. 148-03-8<br>**9632** | 416.69 | $C_{28}H_{48}O_2$ | 296 | 89.4 | [3725] | 297 | 322 |
| γ-T<br>CAS No. 7616-22-0<br>**9633** | 416.69 | $C_{28}H_{48}O_2$ | 298 | 91.4 | [3809] | 297 | 322 |
| δ-T<br>CAS No. 119-13-1<br>**9634** | 402.66 | $C_{27}H_{46}O_2$ | 298 | 91.2 | [3515] | 297 | 322 |
| α-T3<br>CAS No. 2265-13-4<br>**9636** | 424.67 | $C_{29}H_{44}O_2$ | 292 | 86.0 | [3652] | 290 | 323 |
| β-T3<br>CAS No. 49-23-3<br>**9635** | 410.64 | $C_{28}H_{42}O_2$ | 296 | 86.2 | [3540] | 290 | 323 |
| γ-T3<br>CAS No. 14101-61-2 | 410.64 | $C_{28}H_{42}O_2$ | 297 | 91.0 | [3737] | 290 | 324 |
| δ-T3<br>CAS No. 25612-59-3 | 369.61 | $C_{27}H_{40}O_3$ | 297 | 85.8 | [3403] | 292 | 324 |
| α-Tocopheryl acetate<br>CAS No. 52225-20-4 (dl)<br>CAS No. 58-95-7 (l)<br>**10160** | 472.75 | $C_{31}H_{52}O_3$ | 286 | 40–44 | [1891–2080] | 285 | 310 |
| α-Tocopheryl succinate<br>CAS No. 4345-03-3<br>**1059** | 530.79 | $C_{33}H_{54}O_5$ | 286 | 38.5 | [2044] | — | — |

[a]Common or generic name; CAS No., Chemical Abstract Service number; bold print designates the *Merck Index* (30) monograph number.
[b]Values in brackets are calculated from corresponding $E^{1\%}_{1cm}$ values, in ethanol.
[c]In hexane $\varepsilon$, molar absorptity.
*Source:* Ref. 28.

higher wavelengths (28,29,37). The tocopherols and tocotrienols, therefore, possess strong native fluorescence that provides an ideal specific mode of detection for fluorescence-based liquid chromatographic (LC) methods (Chapter 7). Vitamin E esters show only weak fluorescence compared to the alcohols; however, the fluorescence is strong enough to allow quantitation by LC methods (28).

Characterization of other physicochemical properties of vitamin E including infrared, nuclear magnetic resonance, and mass spectra can be obtained from a variety of literature sources. Characterization studies were reviewed in several of the previously cited publications (33–36).

### 1.2.5. Chemical Synthesis

**1.2.5.1. *all-rac-α*-Tocopherol, 2-*ambo-α*-Tocopherol, and *all-rac-α*-Tocopheryl Esters.** Currently used synthesis routes for the commercial production of vitamin E are based on successful synthesis reactions published in the 1930s. Synthesis follows formation of the chroman ring by a Friedl–Crafts alkylation reaction that attaches the alkyl side chain of phytol, isophytol, or phytyl halides onto the benzene ring of trimethylhydroquinone (TMHQ) and causes subsequent ring closure (38–40). Condensation of TMHQ with phytol yields 2*R*S, 4′R, 8′R-*α*-T (2-*ambo*-*α*-T), and TMHQ reaction with isophytol yields *all-rac*-*α*-T (Figure 1.3) (31,38,39). Current industrial syntheses primarily use the isophytol-TMHQ condensation (38,39). Approximately, 80% of the world production (>25,000 tons) of vitamin E is produced by this synthesis route (39,40). Acid catalysis of the alkylation reaction is required and accomplished by $ZnCl_2$, $BF_3$, $AlCl_3$ or other Lewis acids (39,40). The reaction proceeds through an intermediate carbonium ion formed by the interaction of the catalyst with the reactant donating the side chain. Bonrath et al (40). presented a synthesis of *all-rac*-*α*-T from isophytol and TMHQ using fluorinated NH-acidic catalysts. Compared to traditional $ZnCl_2$/HCl or $BF_3$ catalysts, the imide catalyst provided higher selectivity with small amounts of phytadiene and furan dehydration products, higher yield (up to 94%), milder reaction conditions, lower catalyst requirement (0.1 mol %), decreased waste problems, and higher recovery of the catalyst.

Synthesis of *β*-, *γ*-, and *δ*-T can be accomplished by using the same reaction scheme by altering the placement and number of methyl groups on the hydroquinone ring. Synthesis of *γ*-T would, therefore, require 2,3-dimethyl hydroquinone. However, potential for production of multiple end products due to lack of selectivity makes isolation of the desired product difficult (41).

A large percentage of synthetic *all-rac*-*α*-T is esterified into *all-rac*-*α*-tocopheryl acetate with conversion of smaller quantities into succinate and

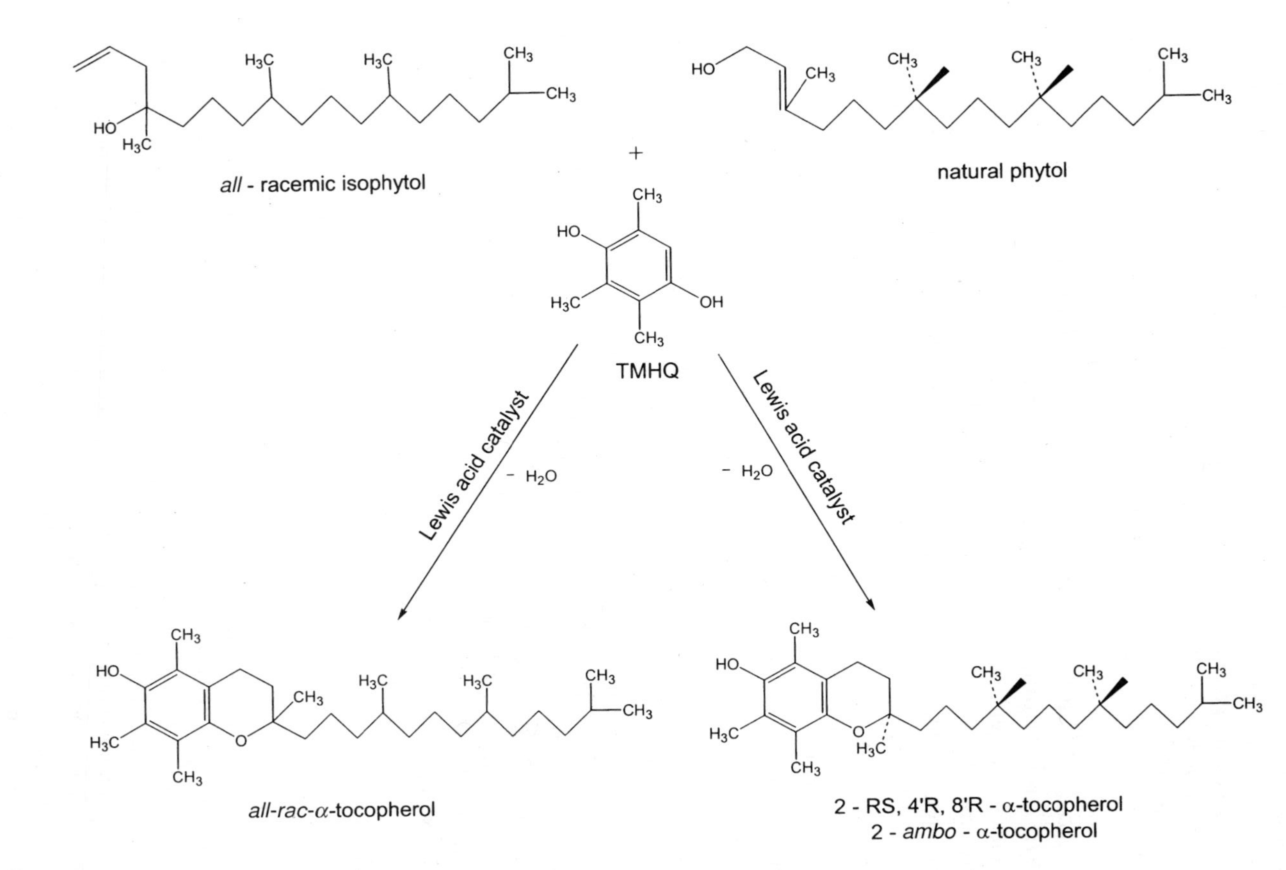


**FIGURE 1.3** Chemical synthesis of *all-rac-* and 2-*ambo*-tocopherol. (Modified from Refs. 31, 38, 39.)

nicotinate esters (39). Fortification of food and supplementation of animal and poultry rations requires stabilization against oxidation by esterification of the 6-hydroxy on the chroman ring. Netscher (39). reported that 71% of the world's production of *all-rac*-$\alpha$-T is utilized by the feed industry, 24% by the pharmaceutical industry, 3% in cosmetics manufacture, and 2% in human food production.

**1.2.5.2. Vitamin E Concentrates, *RRR*-$\alpha$-Tocopherol, and *RRR*-$\alpha$-Tocopheryl Acetate.** Raw material for production of vitamin E concentrates and "natural source" *RRR*-$\alpha$-T is deodorizer distillate obtained as a by-product of the edible oil refining process. The vacuum, high-temperature, and steam-stripping conditions employed during deodorization lead to volatilization of small-molecular-weight substances in the oil. Tocopherols and tocotrienols together with other small-molecular-weight substances such as plant sterols are distilled and concentrated in the distillate (Chapter 5, Section 5.2.1). With the increasing market for functional food ingredients such as vitamin E and sterols, the distillate is now a valuable by-product and source for value-added products. The distillate is amenable to further processing to produce vitamin E concentrates that have a large market and provide the concentrated material containing mixtures of tocopherols for conversion into *RRR*-$\alpha$-T, the preferred form for vitamin supplements for human consumption.

Tocopherol and/or tocotrienol concentrations in distillates are quite variable. The type of oil, the total vitamin E content, and the tocopherol/tocotrienol profile of the oil determine the content and tocopherol/tocotrienol profile of the distillate. Processing of soybean oil yields a distillate similar to the soybean oil in the relative amounts of the tocopherols that are present. Soybean oil distillate is high in $\gamma$-T, and sunflower oil yields a distillate high in $\alpha$-T. Likewise, deodorization of palm oil or rice bran oil produces a distillate high in the tocotrienols. Analyses of distillates from various oils in our laboratory (University of Georgia) have shown vitamin E concentrations as high as 1% by weight (unpublished). Deodorization processes have been optimized to increase levels of vitamin E in the distillate and to maintain levels in oil sufficient to ensure oxidative stability of the oil (42).

Deodorizer distillates, because of the high concentration of tocopherols and/or tocotrienols, provide ideal raw materials for further concentration to produce commercial vitamin E concentrates. Distillates originating from the refining of soybean oil are the most common source of vitamin E concentrates. Vitamin E concentrates are produced by molecular distillation of the distillate or by various other fractionation processes including saponification to remove saponifiable material in combination with molecular distillation (43). Commercial vitamin E concentrates usually range from 30% tocopherol by weight to 90% or above. A 70% concentrate that was analyzed in our laboratory contained 10.6% $\alpha$-T, 0.8% $\beta$-T, 64% $\gamma$-T, and 24.3% $\delta$-T, closely matching the tocopherol profile of refined, bleached, deodorized (RBD) soybean oil (Chapter 8, Table 8.3). Such vitamin E concentrates are widely used by the food industry as natural source antioxidants and by the pharmaceutical and food supplement industries as vitamin E sources. Because of the instability of tocopherols and tocotrienols to oxidation, the usual delivery form to the human is a capsule. Direct addition to food for fortification requires the use of $\alpha$-tocopheryl acetate, which is quite stable to oxidation.

Mixed *RRR*-tocopherols, concentrated and partially purified from the distillate, are methylated to *RRR*-$\alpha$-T. Chemical methylation by halo-, amino-, or hydroxyalkylation converts $\beta$-, $\gamma$- and $\delta$-T into alkylated intermediates that are reduced to *RRR*-$\alpha$-T (Figure 1.4). The industrial process was reviewed by Netscher (39). The *RRR*-$\alpha$-T produced from the mixed tocopherols originating from the edible oil distillates, usually soybean oil distillate, can be used directly in the alcohol form or stabilized toward oxidation by esterification. *RRR*-$\alpha$-tocopheryl acetate is the most common form provided to the pharmaceutical and food industries for products containing natural source *RRR*-$\alpha$-T. Papas (3). provides an excellent description of the use of the term *natural* in relation to $\alpha$-T. *Natural source* indicates that the $\alpha$-T was extracted from natural raw materials (edible oil distillates almost always) and has maintained the molecular structure of *RRR*-$\alpha$-T. Practically all natural source $\alpha$-T is used for human applications. Global usage of natural source *RRR*-$\alpha$-T includes 77% in pharmaceutical products, 14% in food applications, 8% in cosmetics, and only 1% in feeds (39).

**1.2.5.3. Synthesis of *RRR*-$\alpha$-Tocopherol.** The global supply of *RRR*-$\alpha$-T from natural sources (edible oil distillates) does not meet demand. Papas(3). reported that the present annual production capacity is less than 4000 tons per year. With increased manufacturing capacity, availability of deodorizer distillate could become a limiting factor in production of *RRR*-$\alpha$-T. Therefore, stereoselective synthesis of *RRR*-$\alpha$-T has been intensively investigated for several decades, since the biological activity of *RRR*-$\alpha$-T was shown to be higher than that of other stereoisomers of $\alpha$-T and other tocopherols and tocotrienols (44,45). Stereoselective synthesis routes for *RRR*-$\alpha$-T were described in detail by Netscher (38). However, even with a significant research effort, commercially feasible synthesis of *RRR*-$\alpha$-T and other *RRR*-tocopherols has not been achieved (39).

**1.2.5.4. Tocotrienols.** Original syntheses of the tocotrienols were developed by the Isler and colleagues in the 1960s (26,46,47). The procedures were reviewed in detail by Schudel et al (36) and Kasparek (34). Synthesis of

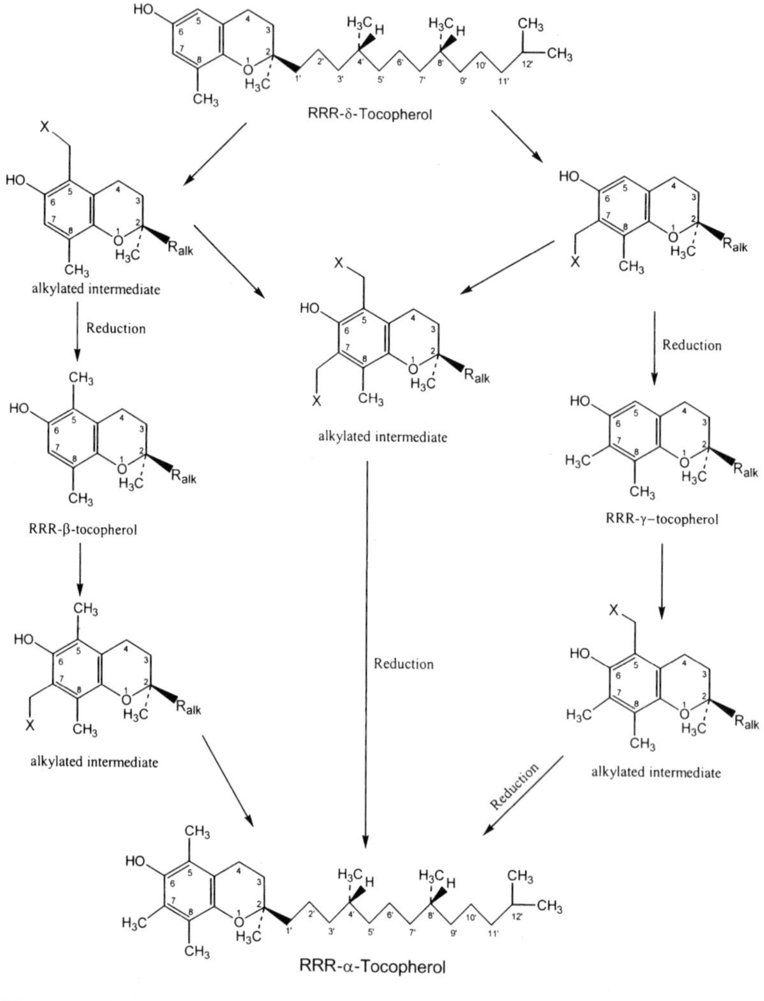

FIGURE 1.4 Conversion of $\beta$-, $\gamma$-, and $\delta$-tocopherol into $\alpha$-tocopherol by methylation. (Modified from Ref. 39.)

$\alpha$-T3 is shown in Figure 1.5. all-*trans*-Geranyllinallol is condensed with TMHQ with boron trifluoride etherate catalyst followed by oxidation with silver oxide to form geranylgeranyl-trimethyl benzoquinone. Ring closure is completed by boiling pyridine to form the chromanel ring. Reduction with sodium in boiling ethanol yields 2*RS*, 3′E, 7′E-$\alpha$-T3, $\beta$-, $\gamma$-, and $\delta$-T3 were synthesized by the same procedure (26,34,46).

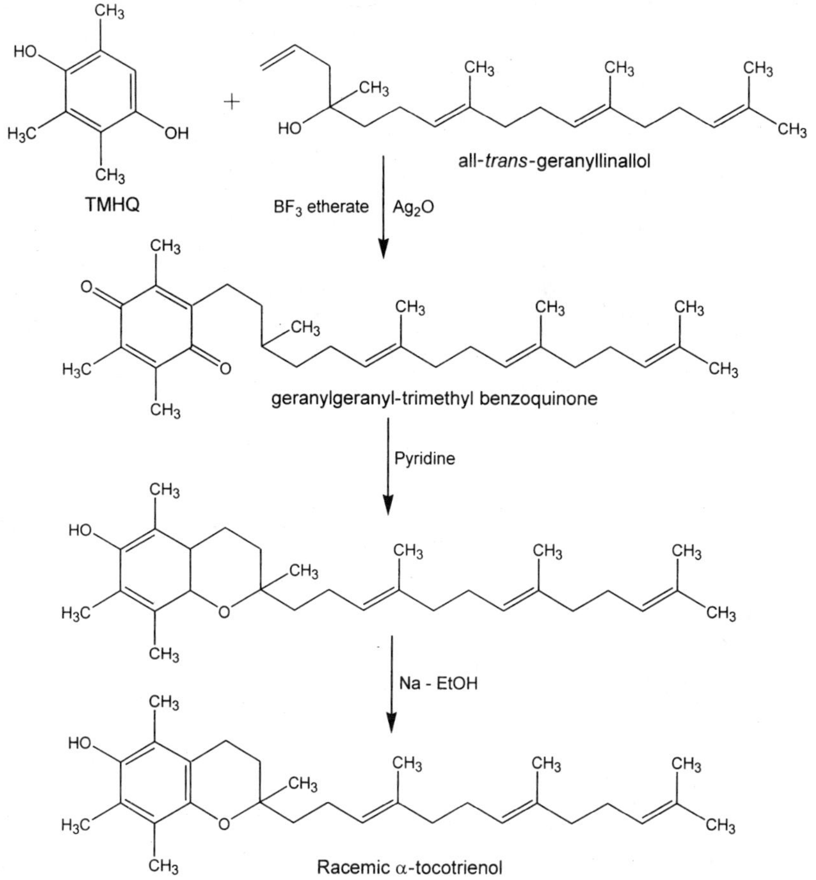

TMHQ + all-*trans*-geranyllinallol

$BF_3$ etherate | $Ag_2O$

geranylgeranyl-trimethyl benzoquinone

Pyridine

Na - EtOH

Racemic α-tocotrienol

**FIGURE 1.5** Chemical synthesis of $\alpha$-tocotrienol. (Modified from Refs. 34, 36.)

## 1.2.6. Commercial Forms

Demand for vitamin E products has rapidly increased over the past two decades. Along with market demand, the number of product types available to the pharmaceutical, food, feed, and cosmetic industries has increased. Technology to manufacture products for specific applications is sophisticated, including microencapsulation and enrobing technologies. For all applications, oxidative stability of the vitamin E product is required. Use of microencapsulation or coatings to protect tocopherols and tocotrienols by forming oxygen barriers allows wider use of nonesterified delivery forms. Microencapsulation through spray drying of the vitamin E in the presence of various carriers imparts specific characteristics to the application form, including water dispersibility of powdered products with good flow characteristics. Commercial forms include the following categories:

1. Pure Standards: Pure standards are readily available for the tocopherols from major chemical suppliers. Tocotrienol standards are less commonly available. The United States Pharmacopeia (USP) standard is *all-rac-α*-tocopheryl acetate. One USP unit of vitamin E activity is defined as the activity of 1 mg of *all-rac-α*-tocopheryl acetate, 0.67 mg of *RRR-α*-T, or 0.74 mg of *RRR-α*-tocopheryl acetate (48). *all-rac-α*-Tocopheryl acetate (USP) is the most commonly used form for fortification of foods and feed and for pharmaceutical use in vitamin supplements. As synthesized, *all-rac-α*-tocopheryl acetate is a viscous, light yellow oil.
2. Oils and Concentrates: Natural source tocopherols, tocotrienols, *RRR-α*-T, and *all-rac-α*-tocopheryl esters are available as pure oils and concentrates diluted with edible oil. Mixed, natural source concentrates range from 20% by weight to 90% by weight mixed tocopherols. Such concentrates are marketed as antioxidants for foods and supplements. Tocopheryl esters in the oil form are primarily used for fortification of food and feed because of their oxidative stability.
3. Dry, Granular Powders: Esters of *RRR-α*-T or *all-rac-α*-T can be absorbed onto silicon dioxide, microcrystalline cellulose, or modified cellulose or spray-dried with suitable carriers such as gelatin, dextrin, and sugars to produce dry, granular powders. These powders have good flow characteristics for use in compressed tablets, chewable tablets, and gelatin capsules. They are not water-dispersible.
4. Water-Dispersible Free-Flowing Powders: Mixed, natural source tocopherols, *RRR-α*-T, and tocopheryl esters are microencapsulated by spray drying the oils with various carriers including gelatin, gum acacia, and carbohydrates such as dextrin, sucrose, or glucose. Vitamin E oil droplets are embedded in a protective matrix that is water-dispersible. Some products are coated with starch or modified starch to enhance water dispersiblity. Flow characteristics are enhanced through addition of silicon dioxide. Water-dispersible dry products are used in vitamin premixes, for fortification of liquids and dry products that will be reconstituted. These formulations are suitable for use in compressed tablets or gelatin matrix multivitamins and mineral supplements.
5. Gelatin Microcapsules: *all-rac-α*-Tocopheryl acetate is available in gelatin microcapsules for cosmetic use.
6. Water-Soluble Vitamin E: Eastman Chemical Company manufactures a water-soluble vitamin E. Chemically, the product is synthesized by

esterification of polyethylene glycol 1000 onto *RRR*-$\alpha$-tocopheryl succinate (49). The compound is marketed as TPGSNF, *RRR*-$\alpha$-tocopheryl polyethylene glycol 1000 succinate. The material is a waxy, yellow solid with the ability, because of its amphiphilic properties, to form miscible micelles in water. Applications include modification of thermal properties of miscible oils, enhancement of vitamin E bioavailability in humans and animals, drug absorption enhancement and provision of a vehicle for drug delivery. The role as an absorption enhancer is beneficial in the treatment of chronic choleostasis (50).

## 1.3. BIOCHEMISTRY OF VITAMIN E

All 6-hydroxychromanols that constitute the vitamin E family are plant products of well-defined biosynthetic routes. All photosynthetic organisms synthesize the vitamin. Synthesis has not been documented in any other organisms, and plant products provide the only natural dietary sources. Early studies concluded that $\alpha$-T is formed in both photosynthetic and nonphotosynthetic tissue of higher plants, concentrated in the chloroplasts (51–52). Other tocopherols and tocotrienols are in higher concentration in nonphotosynthetic tissues (53). In *Calendula officinalis* leaves, $\alpha$-T was only present in chloroplasts, whereas $\gamma$- and $\delta$-T were found in the chloroplasts, mitochondria, and microsomes (54). No tocopherols were present in Golgi membranes and cytosol. Biosynthesis of the tocopherols occurred primarily in the chloroplasts (55–58). Most vitamin E partitions into the lipid phase of the choloroplast membrane with the phytyl side chain embedded within the membrane bilayer (56). Orientation of the vitamin E occurs through interaction of the benzoquinone ring with the carbonyls of triacylglycerol esters (56). Such localization and orientation have been established in mammalian cells as well.

### 1.3.1. Biosynthesis

#### 1.3.1.1. Formation of Homogentisic Acid.

Synthesis of vitamin E by higher plants is quite well understood. Early studies that defined the synthesis were reviewed by Threlfall (52) and Draper (59). Later reviews include those by Hess (56) and Bramley et al. (60), which provide insight into studies that characterize the enzymological features of the biosynthesis. Studies mostly completed in the 1960s identified the shikimic acid pathway present in plants, algae, and bacteria but not in animals (59) as a key pathway yielding homogentisic acid. The pathway (Figure 1.6) proceeds through the *p*-hydroxyphenylpyruvic acid intermediate, forming homogentisic acid, which constitutes the *p*-benzoquinone ring of the chromanol structure. Homogentisic acid provides the

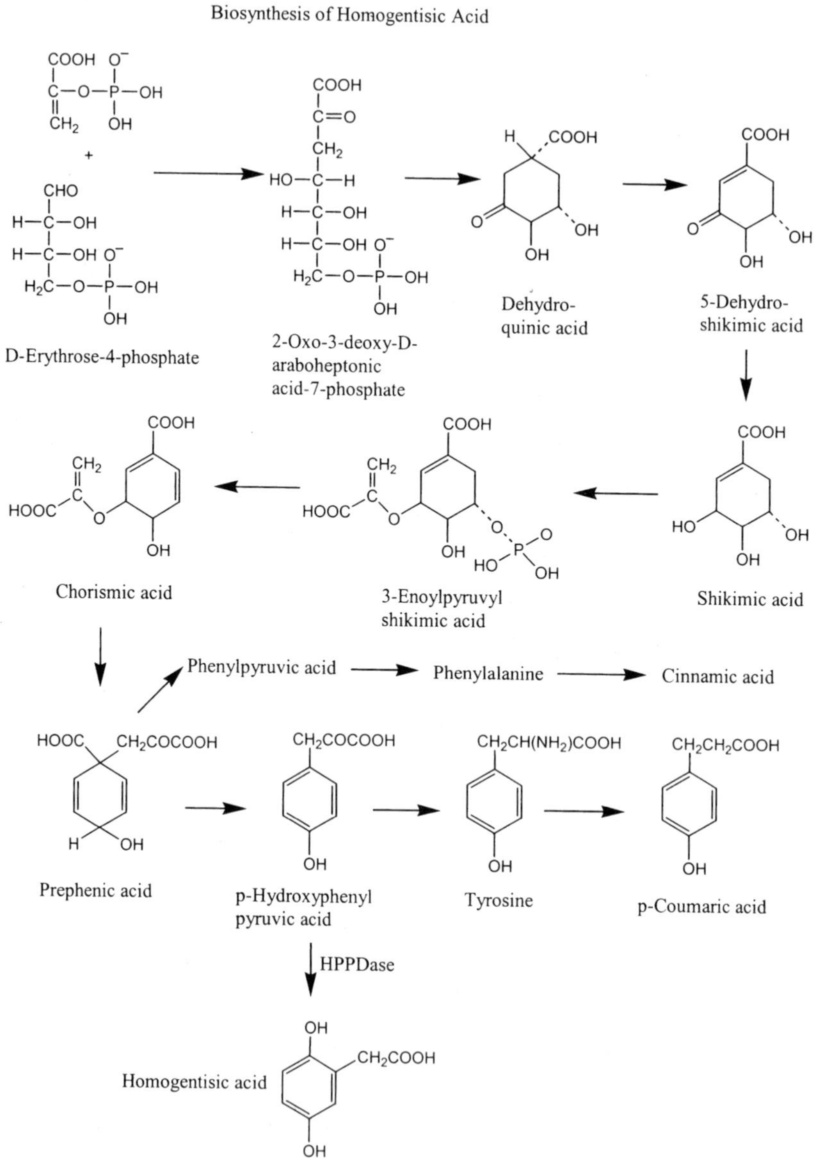

Biosynthesis of Homogentisic Acid

D-Erythrose-4-phosphate

2-Oxo-3-deoxy-D-araboheptonic acid-7-phosphate

Dehydro-quinic acid

5-Dehydro-shikimic acid

Shikimic acid

3-Enoylpyruvyl shikimic acid

Chorismic acid

Phenylpyruvic acid → Phenylalanine → Cinnamic acid

Prephenic acid

p-Hydroxyphenyl pyruvic acid

Tyrosine

p-Coumaric acid

HPPDase

Homogentisic acid

**FIGURE 1.6** Biosynthesis of homogentisic acid. (Modified from Refs. 52,59.)

backbone structure for further formation of the tocopherols and plastoquinones (59). Also, *p*-hydroxyphenylpyruvic acid is converted through tyrosine to ubiquinone. Conversion to homogentisic acid is catalyzed by *p*-hyroxyphenylpyruvic acid dioxygenase (HPPDase, *p*-hydroxyphenylpyruvate: oxygen oxidoreductase, hydroxylating, decarboxylating, EC 1.13.11.27, EC 1.14.2.2). The HPPDase inserts two oxygen molecules, oxidatively decarboxylates, and rearranges the side chain of *p*-hydroxyphenylpyruvic acid to form homogentisic acid (60–63). In mammals, HPPDase functions in the degradation of aromatic amino acids. The subcellular location, purification, and cloning of genes of HPPDase from carrot cells (63) preceded accomplishment of further research with *Arabidopsis* sp. mutants (62).

**1.3.1.2. Conversion of Homogentisic Acid to Tocopherols.** Conversion of homogentisic acid to the tocopherols includes the following steps:

1. Polyprenyltransferase Reaction: Addition of the phytyl side chain results from the reaction of homogentisic acid with phytyl-diphosphate (pyrophosphate) (Figure 1.7). Polyprenyltransferase catalyzes with the simultaneous prenylation reaction, decarboxylation, and release of pyrophosphate to form 2-methyl-6-phytylbenzoquinol, which constitutes the intermediate for synthesis of the tocopherols (60,64). The polyprenyltransferases catalyze condensation reactions of homogentisic acid with phytyl-diphosphate, geranylgeranyl-diphosphate, or solanesyl-diphosphate to form tocopherols, tocotrienols, and plastoquinones, respectively (64). Phytyl-diphosphate also provides the isoprenoid tail for the synthesis of phylloquinones (vitamin $K_1$) and the chlorophylls (52,64–66). Collakova and DellaPenna (64) successfully cloned gene products from *Synechocystis* sp. PCC6803 and *Arabidopsis* sp. that encode polyprenyltransferases specific for tocopherol synthesis. Loci PDS1 and PDS2 that had previously been characterized when mutated, decreased the levels of tocopherols and plastoquinones in *Arabidopsis* sp. The PDS1 locus encodes for p-hydroxyphenylpyruvate dioxygenase. Locus PDS2 was proposed to be responsible for synthesis of a polyprenyltransferase that catalyzes the conversion of homogentisic acid to either 2-methyl-6-phytylbenzoquinol or 2-demethylplastoquinol-9 (62). The PDS1 and PDS2 mutants in *Arabidopsis* sp. were proved to be deficient in plastoquinone and tocopherols (62). The PDS2 mutation was thought to affect a step of the plastoquinone–tocopherol pathway after the HPPDase reaction, most likely the polyprenyltransferase reaction.
2. 2-Methyl-6-Phytylbenzoquinol Methyl Transferase Reaction: 2-Methyl-6-phytylbenzoquinol is methylated by a methyltransferase to form

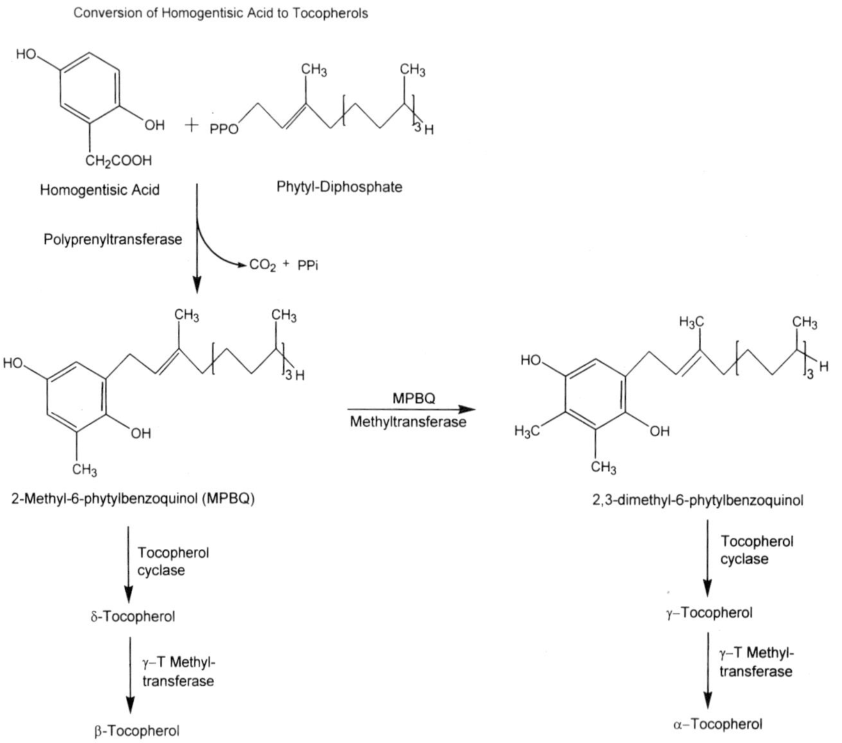

**FIGURE 1.7** Conversion of homogentisic acid to tocopherols by the action of polyprenyltransferase and tocopherol cyclase. (Modified from Refs. 60, 64.)

2,3-dimethyl-6-phytylbenzoquinol. This compound is the immediate precursor of $\gamma$-T (67). In 2002, Shintani et al. (67) identified a putative 2-methyl-6-phytylbenzoquinol methyltransferase gene (SLL0418) from the *Synechocystic* sp. PCC6803 genome that encodes the methyltransferase. The enzyme catalyzes methylation of C-3 of 2-methyl-6-solanyl-benzoquinol in the terminal step of plastoquinone synthesis. The enzyme was described as playing a more important role in determining the tocopherol profile than in determining total tocopherol content (67).

3. Tocopherol Cyclase Reactions: Tocopherol cyclase catalyzes the formation of the $\delta$-T from 2-methyl-6-phytylbenzoquinone and $\gamma$-T from 2,3-dimethyl-6-phytylbenzoquinone (67,68) (Figure 1.7). Tocopherol cyclase from *Anabaena variabilis* (*Cyanobacteria*) blue-green algae was studied in depth by Stocker et al. (68–70). Substrate specificity

is imparted through recognition of the -OH group at C-1 of the hydroquinone, the (E) configuration of the double bond on the side chain, and the length of the side chain on 2-methyl-6-phytylbenzoquinol or 2,3-dimethyl-6-phytylbenzoquinol. Substrates enter the active site of tocopherol cyclase with the recognition of the hydrophobic tail. The enzyme is equally effective in converting 2,3-dimethyl-6-geranylbenzoquinol to $\gamma$-T3 and 2-methyl-6-geranylgeranyl benzoquinol to $\delta$-T3(68). (Figure 1.8).

4. $\gamma$-Tocopherol Methyltransferase Reaction: $\gamma$-Tocopherol and $\delta$-T are methylated by a specific $\gamma$-T methyltransferase at the 5 position of the chromanol ring to yield $\alpha$- and $\beta$-T, respectively. $\alpha$- And $\beta$-methyltransferases have not been identified in nature, and $\alpha$- and $\beta$-T are considered terminal products of the biosynthesis (67). The enzyme was purified and characterized from spinach chloroplasts and *Euglena gracilis* (71–73). Shintani and DellaPenna(74). showed that $\gamma$-T methyltransferase is a primary determinant of the tocopherol composition of seed oils. The $V_{max}$ values of $\gamma$-T methyltransferase from peppers were similar for $\gamma$-, $\delta$-T, and $\gamma$-, $\delta$-T3, but $\beta$-T is not a substrate (75). Overexpression of the $\gamma$-T methyltransferase gene in *Arabidopsis* sp. increased $\alpha$-T content of the oil without decreasing total tocopherol content. A seed of lines overexpressing the largest amount of $\gamma$-T methyltransferase had more than 95% of total tocopherol as $\alpha$-T. To accomplish the preceding research, *Arabidopsis* sp. was transformed with the pDC3-A.t. $\gamma$-T methyltransferase expression construct containing the *Arabidopsis* sp. $\gamma$-T methyltransferase complementary deoxyribonucleic acid (cDNA) driven by the carrot DC3 promoter (71). Understanding of the role and activity of the $\gamma$-T methyltransferase explains why many seed oils contain low $\alpha$-T levels.

**1.3.1.3. Biosynthesis of Tocotrienols.** Condensation of homogentisic acid with geranylgeranyl diphosphate, catalyzed by geranylgeranyltransferase, yields 2-methyl-6-geranylgeranyl benzoquinol, providing the substrate for formation of the tocotrienols (Figure 1.8). The 2-methyl-6-geranylgeranyl benzoquinol intermediate is converted to the respective tocotrienols by action of 2-methyl-6-phytylbenzoquinol methyltransferase. In 2002, investigation of the $\gamma$-T methyltransferase from pepper fruits indicated that methylation capacity of $\delta$- and $\gamma$-T3 is almost equivalent to the capacity to methylate the corresponding tocopherols (75). It has been postulated that enzymes participating in tocopherol and tocotrienol biosynthesis after the phytyltransferase and geranylgeranyltransferase reactions utilize both the phytylated and geranylgeranylated substrates (64,75).

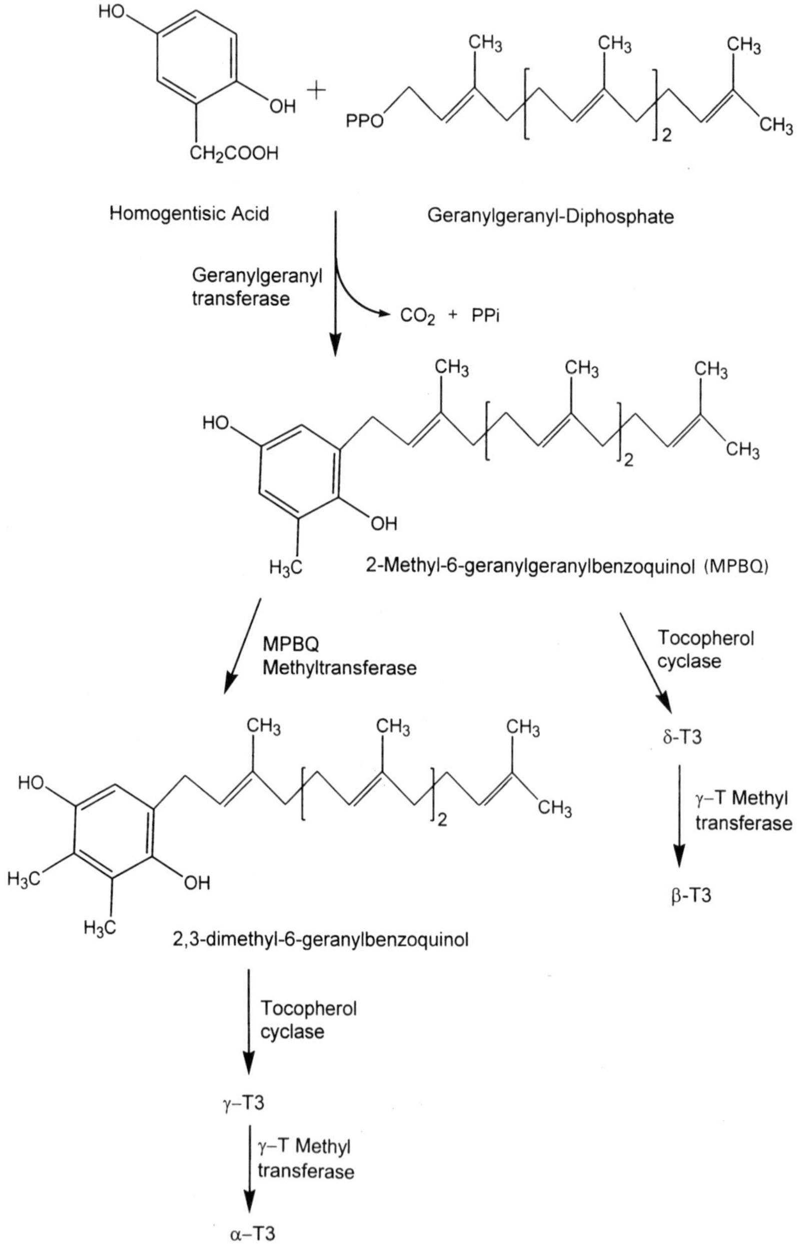

Homogentisic Acid + Geranylgeranyl-Diphosphate

Geranylgeranyl transferase → $CO_2$ + PPi

2-Methyl-6-geranylgeranylbenzoquinol (MPBQ)

MPBQ Methyltransferase

2,3-dimethyl-6-geranylbenzoquinol

Tocopherol cyclase

γ–T3

γ–T Methyl transferase

α–T3

Tocopherol cyclase

δ-T3

γ–T Methyl transferase

β-T3

**FIGURE 1.8** Conversion of homogentisic acid to tocotrienols by the action of geranylgeranyl-transferase, methyltransferase, and tocopherol cyclase. γ-T, γ-tocopherol; γ-T3, γ-tocotrienol; α-T3, α-Tocotrienol. (Modified from Refs. 67, 68.)

#### 1.3.1.4. Increasing α-Tocopherol Levels in Plant Foods.

The more complete understanding of the biosynthetic steps leading to the synthesis of α-T levels in plant foods and the availability of cloned genes of the responsible enzymes have set the stage to increase α-T levels in plant foods. Thus, the nutritional impact of such foods as sources of vitamin E for the human can be increased. Approaches to engineering plants to increase concentration of α-T have been reviewed by Hess (56), Grusak and DellaPenna (76), Hirschberg (77), and DellaPenna (78). Tocopherol biosynthetic enzymes were classified into two groups by Grusak and DellaPenna:

1. Enzymes that predominantly affect quantitative aspects of the pathway (formation and phytylation of homogentisic acid)
2. Enzymes that predominantly affect qualitative aspects of the biosynthesis (cyclization and methylation enzymes)

DellaPenna (78) emphasized that research to improve the nutritional quality of plants is limited by a lack of knowledge of plant metabolism. Because of the breadth of the area, meaningful research requires an interdisciplinary effort involving nutritional biochemistry, food science, plant science, and genetics with expertise in human, animal, and plant molecular biological characteristics. Classical biochemical and genetic approaches to plant improvement are being combined with genomic approaches and rapidly developing molecular biology techniques to help identify genes of plant secondary metabolism pathways significant to improvement of nutritional quality (78). DellaPenna (78) has defined nutritional genomics as the interface between plant biochemistry, genomics, and human nutrition.

γ-Tocopherol methyltransferase that converts γ-T to α-T was considered to be a good molecular target to have a positive impact on α-T levels in plants. Successful manipulation of the γ-T methyltransferase was achieved in *Arabidopsis* sp (71). Overexpression of the γ-T methyltransferase gene shifted oil composition strongly toward α-T. Seeds of the lines overexpressing the gene contained as much as 80 times greater α-T concentrations when compared to normal seeds. Up-regulation of the γ-T methyltransferase was, therefore, proved to be a viable approach to increasing α-T levels in plant foods. The work should be transferable to other oilseed crops that have γ-T as the primary tocopherol. Likewise, success will most likely be forthcoming on engineering plants to produce higher amounts of total tocopherol levels at the quantitative stages of the biosynthesis.

### 1.3.2. Biological Role of Vitamin E

#### 1.3.2.1. Vitamin E and Oxidative Stress.

Vitamin E functions with other lipid- and water-soluble antioxidants to provide living systems an efficient defense against free radicals and the damage that they impart at the cellular level. *Free radicals* are defined as chemical species capable of independent existence that contain one or more unpaired electrons. Free radical generation occurs when organic molecules undergo homolytic cleavage of covalent bonds and each fragment retains one electron of the original bonding electron pair (79). This process produces two free radicals from the parent molecule with net negative charges with the ability to react with an electron of opposite spin from another molecule. Free radical generation also occurs when a nonradical molecule captures an electron from an electron donating molecule. During normal metabolism, a wide array of reactive oxygen species (ROS) and reactive nitrogen species (RNS) are produced (80). The ROS and RNS include both radicals and oxidants capable of generation of free radicals (81,82) (Table 1.4). Oxidants and oxygen radicals formed from triplet oxygen by reaction with other radicals or by photoexcitation, metabolic reactions, irradiation, metal catalysis, or heat are the primary prooxidants that induce oxidative stress in living systems or initiate autoxidative events in raw and processed foods. Reactive nitrogen species, particularly nitric oxide ($NO^{\cdot}$), can contribute to oxidative stress along with ROS. Nitric oxide acts as a biological messenger with regulatory functions in the central nervous, cardiovascular, and immune systems (83). Nitric oxide is synthesized by the oxidation of arginine to $NO^{\cdot}$ by nitric oxide synthetase (NOS; EC 1.14.13.39). The enzyme is highly active in macrophages and neutrophils, in

**TABLE 1.4** Reactive Oxygen and Nitrogen Species

| | |
|---|---|
| Reactive oxgyen species | |
| Radicals | Nonradicals |
| Superoxide, $O_2^{\cdot -}$ | Iron-oxygen complex |
| Hydroxy, $OH^{\bullet}$ | Hydrogen peroxide, $H_2O_2$ |
| Alkoxy, $LO^{\bullet}$ | Singlet oxygen, $^1O_2$ |
| Hydropheroxyl, $HO_2^{\cdot}$ | Ozone, $O_3$ |
| Peroxy, $LO_2^{\cdot}$ | Hypochlorous acid, HOCl |
| Reactive nitrogen species | |
| Radicals | Nonradicals |
| Nitric oxide, $NO^{\cdot}$ | Nitrous acid, $HNO_2$ |
| Nitrogen dioxide, $NO_2^{\cdot}$ | Dinitrogen tetroxide, $N_2O_4$ |
| | Dinitrogen trioxide, $N_2O_3$ |
| | Peroxynitrate, $ONOO^-$ |
| | Peroxynitrous acid, ONOOH |
| | Nitronium cation, $NO_2^+$ |
| | Alkyl peroxynitrates, ROONO |

*Source*: Modified from Refs. 81, 82.

which $NO^{\cdot}$ and superoxide anion ($O_2^{\cdot-}$) are produced during the oxidative burst triggered by inflammation (84).

In cells, ROS are primarily produced in the mitochondria, phagocytes, and peroxisomes and by the cytochrome P-450 enzymes (59,80). Bramley et al. (60) categorized ROS production as follows:

1. Mitochondria: Production of superoxide ($O_2^{\cdot-}$) and hydrogen peroxide ($H_2O_2$) by normal respiration
2. Phagocytes: Production of $O_2^{\cdot-}$, $H_2O_2$, nitric oxide ($NO^{\cdot}$), and hypochlorite ($ClO^-$) in association with the respiratory burst
3. Peroxisomes: Degradation of various substances including fatty acids to yield $H_2O_2$
4. Cytochrome P-450 enzymes: Catalysis of various oxidation reactions
5. Low-wavelength irradiation: Generation of hydroxy radicals ($OH^{\cdot}$) from water
6. Ultraviolet irradiation: Cleavage of the O-O covalent bond in $H_2O_2$ to produce two $OH^{\cdot}$ radicals

**1.3.2.2. Availability of Antioxidants.** Since generation of free radicals occurs in hydrophilic and hydrophobic locations, both water- and lipid-soluble antioxidants are required to limit free radical damage. Important water-soluble antioxidants include ascorbic acid, glutathione (GSH), dihydrolipoate, selenium, iron, and copper sequestering proteins and various enzymes that destroy ROS and oxidants. Specific enzymes that participate in the antioxidant system include catalase, glutathione peroxidase, and superoxide dismutase. Catalase is located in the peroxisomes and catalyzes the conversion of $H_2O_2$ to water and oxygen.

$$2H_2O_2 \longrightarrow 2H_2O + O_2$$

Catalase also interacts with lipid hydroperoxides, yielding alcohols and water.

$$LOOH + 2H^+ \longrightarrow LOH + H_2O$$

Glutathione peroxidase is a selenoenzyme located in the mitochondria and cytoplasm (33). It catalyzes the reduction of $H_2O_2$ to water. The GSH provides the protons with formation of reduced glutathione (GSSH).

$$H_2O_2 + 2GSH \longrightarrow 2H_2O + GSSH$$

Glutathione peroxidase also degrades lipid hydroperoxides to alcohols and water.

$$LOOH + 2GSH \longrightarrow ROH + H_2O + GSSG$$

Superoxide dismutase is present in the mitochondria and cytoplasm. It catalyzes the conversion of superoxide anion to hydrogen peroxide and triplet oxygen.

$$2\dot{O}_2^- + 2H^+ \longrightarrow H_2O_2 + O_2$$

$\alpha$-Tocopherol is the primary lipid-soluble antioxidant in mammalian and plant cells located in the cell membranes and available to protect lipoproteins. It functions as a primary, chain-breaking antioxidant, scavenging peroxy free radicals. Protection of polyunsaturated fatty acids (PUFAs) is facilitated by the greater affinity of lipid-generated free radicals for reaction with $\alpha$-T than with PUFA located in membrane phospholipids. $\alpha$-Tocopherol is an efficient chain-breaking antioxidant since it can rapidly transfer the phenolic $H^+$ to lipid peroxyradicals, while itself becoming a relatively inactive radical—the $\alpha$-tocopheroxyl radical, which is resonance stabilized. The antioxidant mechanisms of vitamin E are discussed in Chapter 3.

An important aspect of the potency of $\alpha$-T as an antioxidant centers on its molecular properties and orientation within the cell membrane. $\alpha$-Tocopherol is recognized as a significant membrane stabilizing component as well as an antioxidant. In the membrane, the phytyl side chain is embedded within the bilayer (see Figure 3.16, Chapter 3) with the chromanol ring and the 6-OH positioned toward the surface of the membrane. Hydrogen bonding and hydrophobic interactions are thought to occur among the chromanol ring, the phytyl tail, and fatty acids. These interactions stabilize the membrane and position the chromanol ring to facilitate hydrogen atom donation to lipid peroxy radicals. Migration of the $\alpha$-tocopheroxyl radical from the lipid bilayer to the surface of the membrane allows regeneration of the $\alpha$-T through interaction with water-soluble reducing agents that act as hydrogen donors to the $\alpha$-tocopheroxyl radical.

Tappel (85) originally suggested that ascorbic acid might reduce $\alpha$-tocopheroxyl radicals back to $\alpha$-T in vivo. This approach led to the recycling theory for vitamin E regeneration, which is still the subject of investigation. Vitamin E recycling by water-soluble reductants explains why a tocopherol molecule can scavenge many radicals (86); however, direct in vivo evidence has been difficult to obtain. The extent of recycling of vitamin E at the cellular level remains unknown (25,87). The most likely hydrogen donors that act in vitro to regenerate vitamin E are ascorbic acid and glutathione (88). Such interactions participate together with $\alpha$-T to provide antioxidant defense as the antioxidant "network" (88–90). Radicals of the water-soluble hydrogen donors would be regenerated through oxidation–reduction cycles back to their nonradical states. A depiction of vitamin E recycling in given in Figure 1.9 (56,90–92).

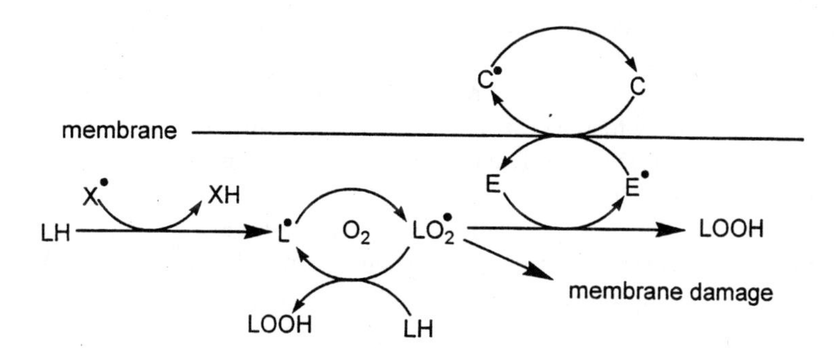


Possible regeneration modes

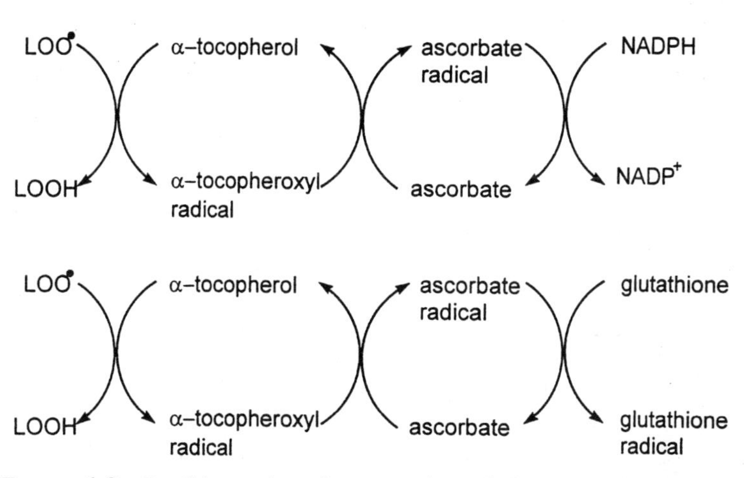


**FIGURE 1.9** Possible modes of regeneration of the $\alpha$-tocopheroxyl radical to $\alpha$-tocopherol; NADPH, reduced nicotinamide adenine dinucleotide phosphate; $NADP^+$, oxidized NADP. (Modified from Refs. 56, 89, 90.)

**1.3.2.3. Antioxidant Activity of the Tocotrienols.** $\alpha$-Tocotrienol is generally considered to be a better radical scavenger than $\alpha$-T. This conclusion, as summarized by several researchers working in the area, is based on the following observations (90,93–97):

1. $\alpha$-Tocotrienol scavenged peroxyl radicals more efficiently than $\alpha$-T in liposomes, protecting against Fe(II) + reduced nicotinamide adenine dinucleotide phosphate (NADPH)-induced peroxidation in rat liver microsomes (93,97).

2. $\alpha$-Tocotrienol protects cytochrome P-450 from oxidation more effectively than $\alpha$-T (93).
3. The $\alpha$-tocotrienoxyl radical is recycled in membranes and lipoproteins faster than the $\alpha$-tocopheroxyl radical. $\alpha$-T3 is located closer to the membrane surface than $\alpha$-T, an arrangement that most likely improves efficiency of recycling (93).
4. $\alpha$-Tocotrienol disorders membrane lipids to a greater extent than $\alpha$-T. A more uniform distribution of $\alpha$-T3 within the membrane increases the chance for collision with free radicals (90).

Preferential selection of *2R*"tags-stereoisomers of -T in the liver by the action of the -T transfer protein (Chapter 2) explains why tocopherols and tocotrienols have lower biological activity (90). Researchers have suggested that increased tissue concentrations of -T3 could provide greater antioxidant protection with increased clinical impact (90,95).

Antioxidant activities of tocotrienols compared to antioxidant activities of $\alpha$-T in a dipalmitoleyl-phosphatidyl choline liposome system as measured by production of luminol are shown in Figure 1.10 (98). The half quenching concentrations ($K_{50}$) were $\alpha$-T, 200 nM; d-$P_{21}$-T3, 14 nM; and d-$P_{25}$-T3, 6 nM.

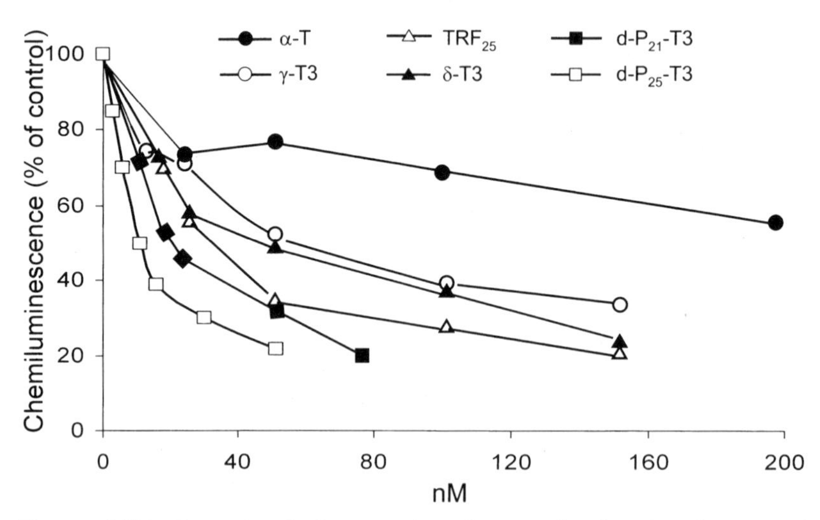


**FIGURE 1.10** Peroxyl radical scavenging of $\alpha$-tocopherol and various tocotrienols found in heat stabilized rice bran. $\alpha$-T, $\alpha$-tocopherol; $\gamma$-T3, tocopherol; $TRF_{25}$, tocotrienol rich fraction. (Modified from Ref. 98.)

Compared to α-T, the tocotrienols were 4–33 times more efficient scavengers of peroxyl radicals in the model system.

### 1.3.2.4. Nonantioxidant Functions of α-Tocopherol and α-Tocotrienol.

*Tocopherols.* Very specific nonantioxidative roles for α-T that cannot be fulfilled by other tocopherols or tocotrienols have been quite recently identified. These functions at the molecular level are under intense study and suggest that the ability of humans to select α-T from the dietary mixture of tocopherols and tocotrienols indicates an evolutionary selection of α-T for nonantioxidant roles (99–101). This evolving aspect of α-T is highly significant to the understanding of the onset of chronic disease at the molecular level. Several critical reviews were published in 2001–2002,(90,99–103). indicating that the knowledge base on molecular control mechanisms attributable to vitamin E is in its infancy.

The varied, nonantioxidant roles for α-T operate through cell signaling at the posttranscriptional level or at the gene expression level. As a modulator of cell signaling, α-T inhibits events leading to inflammation and atherosclerosis. Many cell signaling functions modulated by α-T are through inhibition of protein kinase C (PKC), a family of phospholipid-dependent serine and threonine kinases that participate in regulation of cell growth, death, and stress responsiveness (104). α-Tocopherol does not bind with PKC as do most enzyme inhibitors or inhibit its expression. It acts at the posttranscriptional level by activating protein phosphatase $PP_2A$, which dephosphorylates PKC (105). Specific physiological responses regulated, at least in part, by α-T action on PKC include cell proliferation, platelet adhesion and aggregation, enhancement of immune response, free radical production, and gene expression.

Regulation of gene expression at the transcriptional stage is now accepted as a primary regulatory function of α-T. It is recognized to participate in the up-regulation of the expression of α-topomyosin and the down-regulation of the expression of several genes including those responsible for α-1 collagen and collgenase synthesis, formation of foam cells, α-TTP, and of scavenger receptors of oxidized low-density lipoproteins.

*Tocotrienols.* Specific nonantioxidant actions of α-T3 that are not accomplished by α-T have been identified. As early as 1994, Hendrich et al. (106) suggested that tocotrienols should be considered as a specific group of food components independent of the tocopherols because of their proven biological activities that differ from those of α-T. An inhibitor of cholesterol synthesis in mammalian systems was isolated from barley and proved to be α-T3 (107). Studies with humans given Palmvittee, a tocotrienol-rich fraction from palm oil, indicated that supplementation decreased total cholesterol level in hypercholesterolemic subjects (108,109). Further studies with pigs (110), rats on atherogenic diets (111), and chickens (112) substantiated that tocotrienol supplementation could improve blood lipid profiles.

The cholesterol-lowering ability of α-T3 is attributed to the posttranscriptional suppression of 3-hydroxy-3-methylglutaryl coenzyme A reductase (HMG-CoA reductase). Through a cell signaling mechanism, α-T3 increases cellular levels of farnesol from the precursor, mevalonate, which signals the degradation of HMG-CoA reductase by proteolytic processes (113–115,119).

Qureshi et al. (98,116–118), in addition to studies on tocotrienols from palm oil, defined the ability of a tocotrienol rich fraction ($TRF_{25}$) from rice bran to modify human blood lipid profiles; $TRF_{25}$ is a tocotrienol concentrate prepared from heat stabilized rice bran (180°C under vacuum for 60 min). It consists of 8.7% α-T, 15.5% α-T3, 1.6% β-T3, 39.4% γ-T3, 4.4% δ-T, 5.2% δ-T3, 20.9% desmethyl and didesmethyl tocotrienols, and 4.3% unidentified materials (98). Supplementation of $TRF_{25}$ into the diets of hypercholesterolemic subjects on the American Heart Association Step 1 Diet decreased several blood lipid parameters. At 100 mg $TRF_{25}$ per day, maximal decreases of 20%, 25%, 14%, and 12%, respectively, were noted for total cholesterol, low-density lipoprotein (LDL) cholesterol, apolipoprotein B, and triacylglycerides over 10 weeks. High-density lipoprotein (HDL) and apolipoprotein A1 significantly increased during the supplementation period.

The cholesterol lowering ability of the tocotrienols varies to a large extent by compound. Reported activities are β-T3 < α-T3 < γ-T3 < δ-T3 < desmethyl-T3 < didesmethyl-T3 (116). Desmethyl-T3 and didesmethyl-T3 have been isolated and characterized from the $TRF_{25}$ concentrate from heat stabilized rice bran (98). These tocotrienols differ from other tocotrientols in that no methyl groups are present on the benzene ring of the chroman (Figure 1.11). The two compounds are present in much higher concentrations in heated than in nonheated rice bran and constitute 20.9% by weight of the $TRF_{25}$ concentrate (117). The patented heat treatment (120) of 180°C under vacuum for 60 min produces six novel analogs of the tocotrienols, including the desmethyl- and didesmethyl-T3 forms, which are present in quite large quantities. Chemistry of the heat conversion effects has not been explained.

The subject of tocotrienol inhibition of cholesterol synthesis and ability to modify other significant blood lipid markers of cardiovascular disease has become controversial in recent years with completion of research that did not substantiate the various effects noted by the Qureshi research group (121,122). Mensink et al. (122) reported that tocotrienols did not modify serum lipids, lipoproteins, or platelet function in men with mildly elevated serum lipids. Men with total serum cholesterol between 6.5 and 8.0 mmol/L or lipoprotein (a) levels > 150 mg/L were treated with 140 mg tocotrienols plus 80 mg α-T or with only 80 mg α-T for 6 weeks. Serum LDL cholesterol in the tocotrienol

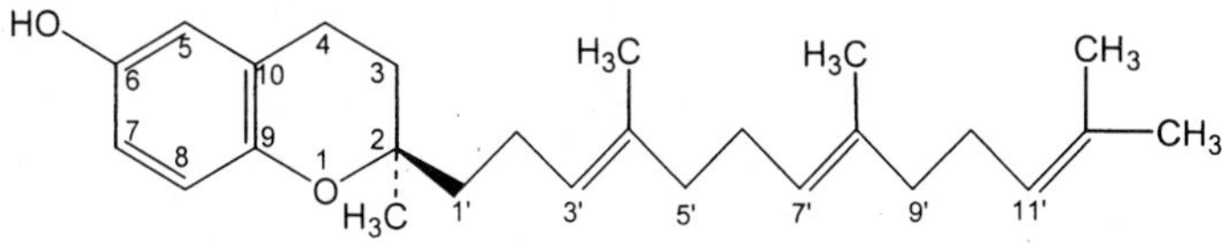

Desmethyl Tocotrienol
d - $P_{21}$ - T3

3, 4-dihydro-2-methyl-2-(4,8,12-trimethyltrideca-3'(E), 7'(E), 11'-trienyl)-2H-1-benzopyran-6-ol

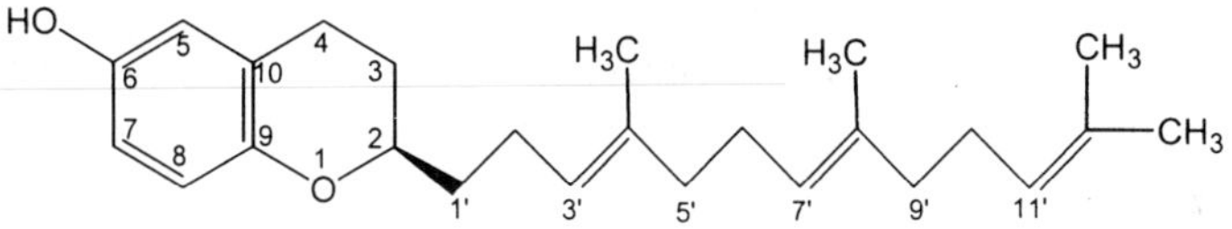

Didesmethyl Tocotrienol
d - $P_{25}$ - T3

3, 4-dihydro-2-(4,8,12-trimethyltrideca-3'(E), 7'(E), 11'-trienyl)-2H-1-benzopyran-6-ol

**FIGURE 1.11** Structures of desmethyl tocotrienol and didesmethyl tocotrienol from heat stabilized rice bran.

group did not change. Changes in HDL cholesterol, triacylglycerols, lipoprotein (a), and lipid peroxide concentrations were similar for the tocotrienol-$\alpha$-T group and the $\alpha$-T group. No effects were noted with platelet function. Additional work using supplementation of diets of hypercholesterolemic individuals with purified tocotrienyl acetates did not decrease serum or LDL cholesterol and lipoprotein B after 8 weeks (123). Subjects in this study were stabilized on an American Heart Association (AHA) Step 1 Diet for 4 weeks before initiation of the supplementation. The Step 1 Diet was maintained throughout the study.

Past research by Qureshi et al (112). showed that tocotrienol preparations that effectively impact HMG-CoA reductase activity contain 15–20% by weight $\alpha$-T and at least 60% $\gamma$- + $\delta$-T3. The Mensink et al. study(122). used a tocotrienol preparation with 37% $\alpha$-T and 42% $\gamma$- + $\delta$-T3. This fact could very well explain the discrepancies in the literature concerning tocotrienol effects on blood lipid profiles. However, Mensink and colleagues' research group stated in 2002 in a critical review that it is "very unlikely that tocotrienols have a cholesterol-lowering effect for the general population" (124).

## REFERENCES

1. Evans, H.M.; Bishop, K.S. On the existence of a hitherto unrecognized dietary factor essential for reproduction. Science **1922**, *56*, 650–651.
2. Evans, H.M.; Emerson, O.H.; Emerson, G.A. The isolation from wheat germ oil of an alcohol alpha-tocopherol, having the properties of vitamin E. J. Biol. Chem. **1936**, *113*, 319–332.
3. Papas, A. *The Vitamin E Factor*; New York: HarperCollins, 1999.
4. Emerson, O.H.; Emerson, G.A.; Mahammad, A.; Evans, H.M. The chemistry of vitamin E: tocopherols from various sources. J. Biol. Chem. **1937**, *122*, 99–107.
5. Fernholz, E. The thermal decompostion of $\alpha$-tocopherol. J. Am. Chem. Soc. **1937**, *59*, 1154–1155.
6. Fernholz, E. On the constitution of alpha-tocopherol. J. Am. Chem. Soc. **1938**, *60*, 700–705.
7. Karrer, P.; Frizsche, H.; Ringier, B.H.; Solomon, A. Synthese des alpha-tocopherol. Helv. Chim. Acta **1938**, *21*, 820–825.
8. Olcott, H.S.; Emerson, O.H. Antioxidants and the autoxidation of fats. IX. The antioxidant properties of tocopherols. J. Am. Chem. Soc. **1937**, *59*, 1008–1009.
9. Stern, M.G.; Robeson, C.D.; Weisler, L.; Baxter, J.G. $\delta$-Tocopherol I: isolation from soybean oil and properties. J. Am. Chem. Soc. **1947**, *69*, 869–874.
10. Pennock, J.F.; Hemming, F.W.; Kerr, J.D. Reassessment of tocopherol chemistry. Biochim. Biophys. Res. Commun. **1964**, *17*, 542–548.
11. Whittle, K.J.; Dunphy, P.J.; Pennock, J.F. The isolation and properties of $\delta$-tocotrienol from *Hevea* latex. Biochem. J. **1966** *100*, 138–145.
12. Harris, P.L.; Quaife, M.L.; Swanson, W.J. Vitamin E content of foods. J. Nutr. **1950** *40*, 367–381.
13. Herting, D.C.; Drury, E.E. Vitamin E content of vegetable oils and fats. J. Nutr. **1963**, *81*, 335–342.
14. Dicks, M.W. Vitamin E content of foods and feeds for human and animal consumption. Bulletin 435, University Wyoming Agric. Exp. Sta, 1965.
15. Booth, V.H.; Bradford, M.P. Tocopherol contents in vegetables and fruits. Br. J. Nutr. **1963**, *17*, 575–581.
16. Slover, H.T. Tocopherols in foods and fats. Lipids **1970**, *6*, 291–296.
17. Draper, H.H. The tocopherols. In *Fat-Soluble Vitamins*; Morton, R.A., Ed.; Pergamon Press: New York, 1970.
18. Ames, S.R. Tocopherols. V. Occurrence in foods. In *The Vitamins*; Sebrell, W.H., Jr, Harris, R.S., Eds.; Academic Press: New York, 1972; Vol. V.
19. Bauernfeind, J.C. Tocopherols in foods. In *Vitamin E: A Comprehensive Treatise*; Machlin, L.J., Ed.; Marcel Dekker: New York, 1980.
20. Sheppard, A.J.; Weihrauch, J.L.; Pennington, J.A.T. The analysis and distribution of vitamin E in vegetable oils and foods. In *Vitamin E in Health and Disease*; Packer, L., Fuchs, J., Eds.; Marcel Dekker: New York, 1992.
21. Symposium on Vitamin E and metabolism in honor of professor H. M. Evans. In *Vitamins and Hormones*; Academic Press: New York, 1962; 375–660.
22. IUPAC-IUB Commission on Biochemical Nomenclature. Nomenclature of tocopherols and related compounds. Recommendations 1973. Eur. J. Biochem. **1974**, *46*, 217–219.

23. IUPAC-IUB Joint Commission on Biochemical Nomenclature (JCBN). Nomenclature of tocopherols and related compounds: recommendations 1981. Eur. J. Biochem. **1982**, *123*, 473–475.
24. AIN Committee on Nomenclature. Nomenclature policy: generic descriptors and trivial names for vitamins and related compounds. J. Nutr. **1990**, *120*, 12–19.
25. Food and Nutrition Board, Institute of Medicine. *Dietary Reference Intakes for Vitamin C, Vitamin E, Selenium, and Carotenoids*; National Academy Press: Washington, DC, 2000.
26. Mayer, H.; Metzger, J.; Isler, O. Die stereochemic von natürlichem γ-tocotrienol (plastochromanol-3), plastochromanol-8 und plastochromemol-8′. Helv. Chim. Acta **1967**, *50*, 1376–1393.
27. Drotleff, A.M.; Ternes, W. Cis/trans isomers of tocotrienols—occurrence and bioavailability. Eur. Food. Res. Technol. **1999**, *210*, 1–8.
28. Eitenmiller, R.R.; Landen, W.O., Jr. *Vitamin Analysis for the Health and Food Sciences*; CRC Press: Boca Raton, FL, 1999; 109–148.
29. Ball, G.F.M. *Fat-Soluble Vitamin Assays in Food Analysis*; Elsevier: New York, 1988; 7–56.
30. Budavari, S. *The Merck Index*, 13th Ed.; Merck and Company: Whitehouse Station, NJ, 2001; 9573–9574.
31. Mino, M.; Nakamura, H.; Diplock, A.T.; Kayden, H.J. Eds. *Vitamin E*; Japan Scientific Souetier Press: Tokyo, 1991; 3–12.
32. Machlin, L.J. Ed. *Handbook of Vitamins*, 2nd Ed.; Marcel Dekker: New York, 1991; 105 pp.
33. Friedrich, W. *Vitamins*; Walter de Gruyter: Berlin, 1988; 215–283.
34. Kasparek, S. Chemistry of tocopherols and tocotrienols. In *Vitamin E: A Comprehensive Treatise*; Machlin, L.J., Ed.; Marcel Dekker: New York, 1980.
35. Kofler, M.; Sommer, P.L.; Bollinger, H.R.; Schmidili, B.; Vecchi, M. Physiochemical properties and assay of the tocopherols. In *Vitamin and Hormones*; Harris, R.S., Wool, I.G., Marrian, G.F., Thimann, K.V., Eds.; Academic Press: New York, 1962; Vol. 20.
36. Schudel, P.; Mayer, H.; Isler, O. Tocopherols II: chemistry. In *The Vitamins*; Sebrell, W.H., Jr., Harris, R.S., Eds.; Academic Press: New York, 1972; Vol. V.
37. Duggan, D.E.; Bowman, R.L.; Brodie, B.B.; Udenfriend, S. A spectrophotofluorometric study of compounds of biological interest. Arch. Biochem. Biophys. **1957**, *68*, 1–14.
38. Netscher, T. Stereoisomers of tocopherols—syntheses and analytics. Chimia **1996**, *50*, 563–567.
39. Netscher, T. The synthesis and production of vitamin E. In *Lipid Synthesis and Manufacture*; Gunstone, F.D., Ed.; Sheffield Academic Press: Sheffield, England, 1999.
40. Bonrath, W.; Hass, A.; Hopmann, E.; Netscher, T.; Pauling, H.; Schager, F.; Wilderman, A. Synthesis of (all-rac)-α-tocopherol using fluorinated NH-acidic catalysts. Adv. Synthet. Catal. **2002**, *344*, 37–39.
41. Schuler, P. Natrual antioxidants exploited commercially. In *Food Antioxidants*; Hudson, B.J.F., Ed.; Elsevier Applied Science: New York, 1990.

42. Maza, A.; Ormsbee, R.A.; Strecker, L.R. Effects of deodorization and steam-refining parameters on finished oil quality. J. AOCS Int. **1992**, *69*, 1003–1008.
43. Ames, S.R. Tocopherols III: industrial preparations and production. In *The Vitamins*; Sebrell, W.H., Jr., Harris, R.S., Eds.; Acadmic Press: New York, 1972; Vol. V.
44. Mayer, H.; Schudel, P.; Regg, R.; Isler, O. Uber eine neue vitamin-e-synthese. Chimia **1962**, *16*, 367–369.
45. Mayer, H.; Schudel, P.; Regg, R.; Isler, O. Uber die chemie des vitamins. Die total synthese von (*2R*,4′R,8R)- und (*2S*,4′R,8′R)-α-tocophenol. Helv. Chim. Acta **1963**, *46*, 650–671.
46. Schudel, P.; Mayer, H.; Metzger, J.; Regg, R.; Isler, O. Uber die chemie des vitamins e .5. Die synthese von rac. All-*trans*-zeta1-und-epsilon-tocopherol. Helv. Chim. Acta **1963**, *46*, 2517–2526.
47. Mayer, H.; Schudel, P.; Regg, R.; Isler, O. Die absolute konfiguration des naturlichen alpha-tocopherols .4. Helv. Chim. Acta **1963**, *46*, 963–982.
48. The United States Pharmacopeia. *The United States Pharmacopeia, National Formulary, Rockville*; United States Pharmacopeial Convention: MD, 1980.
49. Eastman Chemical Company. Eastman Vitamin E TPCS NF. Publication EFC-226A, 1998.
50. Sokol, R.J.; Butler-Simon, N.; Conner, C.; Heubi, J.E.; Sinatra, F.R.; Suchy, F.J.; Heyman, M.B.; Perrault, J.; Rothbaum, R.J.; Levy, J.; Iannaccone, S.T.; Shneider, B.L.; Koch, T.K.; Narkewicz, M.R. Multicenter trial of *d*-alpha-tocopheryl polyethylene glycol-1000 succinate for treatment of vitamin E deficiency in children with chronic cholestasis. Gastroenterology **1993**, *104*, 1727–1735.
51. Bucke, C. The distribution and stability of alpha-tocopherol in subcellular fractions of broad bean leaves. Phytochemistry **1968**, *7*, 693–700.
52. Threlfall, D.R. The biosynthesis of vitamin E and K and related compounds. Vitam. Horm. **1971**, *29*, 153–200.
53. Green, J. The distribution of fat-soluble vitamins and their standardization and assay by biological methods. In *Fat Soluble Vitamins*; Morton, R.A., Ed.; Pergamon Press: Oxford, 1970; Vol. 9.
54. Janiszowska, W.; Korczak, G. The intracellular distribution of tocopherols in *Calendula officinalis* leaves. Phytochemistry **1980**, *19*, 1391–1392.
55. Janiszowska, W.; Korczak, G. Intracellular localization of tocopherol biosynthesis in *Calendula officinalis*. Phytochemistry **1987**, *26*, 1403–1407.
56. Hess, J.L. Vitamin E, α-tocopherol. In *Antioxidants in Higher Plants*; Alscher, R.G., Hess, J.L., Eds.; CRC Press: Boca Raton, 1993.
57. Glover, J. Biosynthesis of Vitamin E. In *Fat Soluble Vitamins*; Morton, R.A., Ed.; Pergamon Press: Oxford, 1970; Vol. 9.
58. Janiszowska, W.; Pennock, J.F. The biochemistry of vitamin E in plants. Vitamin. Horm. **1976**, *34*, 77–105.
59. Draper, H.H. Biogenesis. In *Vitamin E: A Comprehensive Treatise*; Machlin, L.J., Ed.; Marcel Dekker: New York, 1980.
60. Bramley, P.M.; Elmadfa, I.; Kafatos, A.; Kelly, F.J.; Manios, Y.; Roxborough, H.E.; Schuch, W.; Sheehy, P.J.A.; Wagner, K.H. Vitamin E. J. Sci. Food. Agric. **2000**, *80*, 913–938.

61. Norris, S.R.; Shen, X.; DellaPenna, D. Complementation of the Arabidopsis *pds 1* mutation with the gene encoding *p*-hydroxyphenylpyruvate dioxygenase. Plant Physiol. **1998**, *117*, 1317–1323.
62. Norris, S.R.; Barrette, T.R.; DellaPenna, D. Genetic dissection of carotenoid synthesis in *Arabidopsis* defines plastoquinone as an essential component of phytoene desaturation. Plant Cell **1995**, *7*, 2139–2149.
63. Garcia, I.; Rodgers, M.; Lenne, C.; Rolland, A.; Sailland, A.; Matringe, M. Subcellular localization and purification of a p-hydroxyphenylpyruvate dioxygenase from cultured carrot cells and characterization of the corresponding cDNA. Biochem. J. **1997**, *325*, 761–769.
64. Collakova, E.; DellaPenna, D. Isolation and functional analysis of homogentisate phytyltransferase from *Synechocystis* sp. PCC 6803 and Arabidopsis. Plant Physiol. **2001**, *127*, 1113–1124.
65. Schultze-Siebert, D.; Homeyer, U.; Soll, J.; Schultz, G. Synthesis of plastoquinone-9, $\alpha$-tocopherol and phylloquinone (vitamin $K_1$) and its integration in chloroplast carbon metabolism in higher plants. In *The Metabolism, Structure and Function of Plant Lipids*; Stumpf, P., Mudd, J., Eds.; Plenum Press: New York, 1987.
66. Oster, U.; Bauer, C.E.; Rudiger, W. Characterization of chlorophyll *a* and bacteriochlorophyll *a* synthesis by heterologous expression in *Escherichia coli*. J. Biol. Chem. **1997**, *272*, 9671–9676.
67. Shintani, D.K.; Cheng, Z.; DellaPenna, D. The role of 2-methyl-6-phytylbenzoquinone methyltransferase in determining tocopherol composition in *Synechocystic* sp. PCC6803. FEBS Lett. **2002**, *511*, 1–5.
68. Stocker, A.; Fretz, H.; Frick, H.; Ruttimann, A.; Woggon, W.-D. The substrate specificity of tocopherol cyclase. Bioorgan. Med. Chem. **1996**, *4*, 1129–1134.
69. Stocker, A.; Ruttimann, A.; Woggon, W.D. Identification of the tocopherol-cyclase in the blue-green algae *Anabaena variabilis* kutzing (Cyanobacteria). Helv. Chim. Acta **1993**, *76*, 1729–1738.
70. Stocker, A.; Netscher, T.; Ruttimann, A.; Muller, R.K.; Schneider, H.; Todaro, L.J.; Derungs, G.; Woggon, W.D. The reaction-mechanism of chromanol-ring formation catalyzed by tocopherol cyclase from *Anabaena variabilis* kutzing (Cyanobacteria). Helv. Chim. Acta **1994**, *77*, 1721–1737.
71. D'Harlingue, A.; Camara, B. Plastid enzymes of terpenoid biosynthesis: Purification and characterization of a gamma tocopherol methyltransferase. J. Biol. Chem. **1985**, *260*, 15200–15203.
72. Ishiko, H.; Shigeoka, S.; Nakano, Y, Mitsunaga T. Some properties of gamma tocopherol methyltransferase solubilized from spinach chloroplasts. Phytochemistry **1992**, *31*, 1499–1500.
73. Shigeoka, S.; Ishiko, H.; Nakano, Y. Isolation and properties of gamma tocopherol methyltransferase in *Euglena gracilis*. Biochim. Biophys. Acta **1992**, *1128*, 220–226.
74. Shintani, D.; DellaPenna, D. Elevating the vitamin E content of plants through metabolic engineering. Science **1998**, *282*, 2098–2071.
75. Koch, M.; Arango, Y.; Mock, H.P.; Heise, K.P. Factors influencing alpha-tocopherol synthesis in pepper fruits. J. Plant Physiol. **2002**, *159*, 1015–1019.

76. Grusak, M.A.; DellaPenna, D. Improving the nutrient composition of plants to enhance human nutrition and health. Annu. Rev. Plant Phys. **1999**, *50*, 133–161.
77. Hirschberg, J. Production of high-value compounds: carotenoids and vitamin E. Curr. Opin. Biotech. **1999**, *10*, 186–191.
78. DellaPenna, D. Nutritional genomics: manipulating plant micronutrients to improve human health. Science **1999**, *285*, 375–380.
79. McCoy, R.B.; King, M.M. Vitamin E: its role as a biological free radical scavenger and its relationship to the microsomal mixed-function oxidase system. In *Vitamin E: A Comprehensive Treatise*; Machlin, L.J., Ed.; Marcel Dekker: New York, 1980.
80. Burton, G.W. Vitamin E: molecular and biological function. Proc. Nutr. Soc. **1994**, *53*, 251–262.
81. Namki, M. Antioxidants/antimutagens in food. Crit. Rev. Food Sci. Nutr. **1990**, *29*, 273–300.
82. Halliwell, B. Antioxidants in human health and disease. Annu. Rev. Nutr. **1996**, *16*, 33–50.
83. del Rio, L.; Corpas, F.J.; Sandalio, L.M.; Palma, J.M.; Gomez, M.; Barroso, J.B. Reactive oxygen species, antioxidant systems and nitric oxide in peroxisomes. J. Exp. Botany **2002**, *53*, 1255–1272.
84. Thomas, J.A. Oxidative stress and oxidant defense. In *Modern Nutrition in Health and Disease*, 9th Ed.; Shills, M.E., Olson, J.A., Shike, M., Ross, A.C., Eds.; Williams & Wilkins: Baltimore, 1999.
85. Tappel, A.L. Will antioxidant nutrients slow aging processes? Geriatrics **1968**, *23*, 97–105.
86. McCay, P.B. Vitamin E: interactions with free radicals and ascorbate. Annu. Rev. Nutr. **1985**, *5*, 323–340.
87. Murphy, S.P. Dietary reference intakes of the U.S. and Canada: update on implications for nutrient databases. J. Food Comp. Anal. **2002**, *15*, 411–417.
88. Constantinescu, A.; Han, D.; Packer, L. Vitamin E recycling in human erythrocyte membranes. J. Biol. Chem. **1993**, *268*, 10906–10913.
89. Traber, M.G. Vitamin E. In *Modern Nutrition in Health and Disease*, 9th Ed.; Shills, M.E., Olson, J.A., Shike, M., Ross, A.C., Eds.; Williams & Wilkins: Baltimore, 1999.
90. Packer, L.; Weber, S.U.; Rimbach, G. Molecular aspects of $\alpha$-tocotrienol antioxidant action and cell signaling. J. Nutr. **2001**, *131*, 369S–373S.
91. Sies, H.; Stahl, W.; Sundquist, A.R. Antioxidant functions of vitamins: Vitamin E and C, beta-carotene and other carotenoids. Ann. NY Acad. Sci. **1992**, *669*, 7–20.
92. Machlin, L.J. Vitamin E. In *Handbook of Vitamins*; Machlin, L.J., Ed.; Marcel Dekker: New York, 1990.
93. Serbinova, E.; Kagen, V.; Han, D.; Packer, L. Free radical recycling and intramembrane mobility in the antioxidant properties of alpha-tocopherol and alpha-tocotrienol. Free Radic. Biol. Med. **1991**, *10*, 263–275.
94. Serbinova, E.; Packer, L. Antioxidant properties of $\alpha$-tocopherol and $\alpha$-tocotrienol. Methods Enzymol. **1994**, *234*, 354–367.
95. Theriault, A.; Chao, J.-T.; Wang, Q.; Gapor, A.; Adeli, K. Tocotrienol: a review of its therapeutic potential. Clin. Biochem. **1999**, *32*, 309–319.

96. Packer, L. Nutrition and biochemistry of the lipophilic antioxidants, vitamin E and carotenoids. In *Nutrition, Lipids, Health and Disease*; Ong, A.S.H., Niki, E., Packer, L., Eds.; American Oil Chemists Society: Champaign, IL, 1995.
97. Suzuki, Y.J.; Tsuchiya, M.; Wassall, S.R.; Choo, Y.M.; Govil, G.; Kagan, V.E.; Packer, L. Structural and dynamic membrane properties of $\alpha$-tocotrienol and $\alpha$-tocopherol: implication to the molecular mechanism of their antioxidant potency. Biochemistry **1993**, *32*, 10692–10699.
98. Qureshi, A.A.; Mo, H.; Packer, L.; Peterson, D.M. Isolation and identification of novel tocotrienols from rice bran with hypercholesterolemic, antioxidant, and antitumor properties. J. Agric. Food Chem. **2000**, *48*, 3130–3140.
99. Ricciarelli, R.; Zingg, J.-M.; Azzi, A. Vitamin E 80th anniversary: a double life, not only fighting radicals. IUBMB Life **2001**, *52*, 71–76.
100. Ricciarilli, R.; Zingg, J.-M.; Azzi, A. Vitamin E: protective role of a Janus molecule. FASEB J. **2001**, *15*, 2314–2325.
101. The 80th anniversity of vitamin E: beyond its antioxidant properties. Biol. Chem. **2002**, *383*, 457–465.
102. Rimbach, G.; Minihane, A.M.; Majewicz, J.; Fischer, A.; Pallauf, J.; Virgli, F.; Weinberg, P.D. Regulation of cell signaling by vitamin E. Proc. Nutr. Soc. **2002**, *61*, 415–425.
103. Brigelius-Flohé, R.; Kelly, F.J.; Salonen, J.T.; Neuzil, J.; Zingg, J.M.; Azzi, A. The European perspective on vitamin E: current knowledge and future research. Am. J. Clin. Nutr. **2002**, *76*, 703–716.
104. Gopalakrishna, R.; Gundimeda, U. Antioxidant regulation of protein kinase C in cancer prevention. J. Nutr. **2002**, *132*, 3819S–3823S.
105. Ricciarelli, R.; Tasinato, A.; Clement, S.; Ozer, N.K.; Boscoboinik, D.; Azzi, A. Alpha-tocopherol specifically inactivates cellular protein kinase C alpha by changing its phosphorylation state. Biochem. J. **1998**, *334*, 243–249.
106. Hendrich, S.; Lee, K.W.; Xu, X.; Wang, H.J.; Murphy, P.A. Defining food components as new nutrients. J. Nutr. **1994**, *124*, S1789–S1792.
107. Qureshi, A.A.; Burger, W.B.; Peterson, D.M.; Elson, C.E. The structure of an inhibitor of cholesterol biosynthesis isolated from barley. J. Biol. Chem. **1986**, *261*, 10544–10550.
108. Qureshi, A.A.; Qureshi, N.; Wright, J.J.; Shen, Z.; Kramer, G.; Gapor, A.; Chong, Y.H.; DeWitt, G.; Ong, A.; Peterson, D.M.; Bradlow, B.A. Lowering of serum cholesterol in hypercholesterolemic humans by tocotrienols (Palmvitee). Am. J. Clin. Nutr. **1991**, *53*, 10215–10265.
109. Qureshi, A.A.; Bradlow, B.A.; Brace, L.; Manganello, J.; Peterson, D.M.; Pearce, B.C.; Wright, J.J.; Gapor, A.; Elson, C.E. Response of hypercholesterolemic subjects to administration of tocotrienols. Lipids **1995**, *30*, 1171–1177.
110. Qureshi, A.A.; Qureshi, N.; Hasler-Rapacz, J.O.; Weber, F.E.; Chaudhary, V.; Crenshaw, T.D.; Gapor, A.; Ong, A.S.; Chong, Y.H.; Peterson, D.; Rapacz, R. Dietary tocotrienols reduce concentrations of plasma cholesterol, apolipoprotein B, thromboxane $B_2$, and platelet factor 4 in pigs with inherited hyperlipidemias. Am. J. Clin. Nutr. **1991**, *53*, 1042S–1046S.

111. Watkins, T.; Lenz, P.; Gapor, A.; Struck, M.; Tomeo, A.; Bierenbaum, M. $\gamma$-Tocotrienol as a hypocholesterolemic and antioxidant agent in rats fed atherogenic diets. Lipids **1993**, *28*, 1113–1118.
112. Qureshi, A.A.; Pearce, B.C.; Nor, R.M.; Gapor, A.; Peterson, D.M.; Elson, C.E. Dietary alpha-tocopherol attenuates the impact of gamma-tocotrienol on hepatic 3-hydroxy-3-methylglutaryl coenzyme A reductase activity in chickens. J. Nutr. **1996**, *126*, 389–394.
113. Parker, R.A.; Pearce, B.C.; Clark, R.W.; Gordon, D.A.; Wright, J.J. Tocotrienols regulate cholesterol production in mammalian cells by post transcriptional suppression of 3-hydroxy-3-methylglutaryl-coenzyme A reductase. J. Biol. Chem. **1993**, *268*, 11230–11238.
114. Goldstein, J.L.; Brown, M.S. Regulation of the mevalonate pathway. Nature **1990**, *343*, 425–430.
115. Correll, C.C.; Ng, L.; Edwards, P.A. Identification of farnesol as the non-sterol derivative of mevalonic acid required for the accelerated degradation of 3-hydroxy-3-methylglutaryl-coenzyme A reductase. J. Biol. Chem. **1994**, *269*, 17390–17393.
116. Qureshi, A.A.; Bradlow, B.A.; Salser, W.A.; Brace, L.D. Novel tocotrienols of rice bran modulate cardiovascular disease risk parameters of hypercholesterolemic humans. J. Nutr. Biochem. **1997**, *8*, 290–298.
117. Qureshi, A.A.; Sami, S.A.; Salser, W.A.; Khan, F.A. Synergistic effect of tocotrienol rich fraction ($TRF_{25}$) of rice bran and lovastatin on lipid parameters in hypercholesterolemic humans. J. Nutr. Biochem. **2001**, *12*, 318–329.
118. Qureshi, A.A.; Sami, S.A.; Salser, W.A.; Khan, F.A. Dose-dependent suppression of serum cholesterol by tocotrienol-rich fraction ($TRF_{25}$) of rice bran in hypercholesterolemic humans. Atherosclerosis **2002**, *161*, 199–207.
119. Pearce, B.C.; Parker, R.A.; Deason, M.E.; Qureshi, A.A.; Wright, J.J.K. Hypocholesterolemic activity of synthetic and natural tocotrienols. J. Med. Chem. **1992**, *35*, 3595–3606.
120. Qureshi, A.A.; Lane, R.H.; Salses, A.W. Tocotrienols and tocopherol-like compounds and methods for their use. International Patent Application No. PCI/US92//0277, 1993.
121. Wahlqvist, M.L.; Krivokuca-Bogetic, Z.; Lo, C.S.; Hage, B.; Smith, R.; Lukito, W. Differential serum responses of tocopherols and tocotrienols during vitamin supplementation in hypercholesterolemic individuals without change in coronary risk factors. Nutr. Res. **1992**, *12*, S181–S201.
122. Mensink, R.P.; van Houwelingen, A.C.; Kromhout, D.; Hornstra, G. A vitamin E concentrate rich in tocotrienols had no effect on serum lipids, lipoproteins, or platelet function in men with mildly elevated serum lipid concentrations. Am. J. Clin. Nutr. **1999**, *69*, 213–219.
123. O'Byrne, D.; Grundy, S.; Packer, L.; Devaraj, S.; Baldenius, K.; Hoppe, P.P.; Kraemer, K.; Jialal, I.; Traber, M.G. Studies of LDL oxidation following $\alpha$-, $\gamma$- or $\delta$-tocotrienyl acetate supplementation of hypercholesterolemic humans. Free Rad. Biol. Med. **2000**, *29*, 834–845.
124. Kerckhoffs, D.; Brouns, F.; Hornstra, G.; Mensink, R.P. Effects on the human serum lipoprotein profile of $\beta$-glucan, soy-protein and isoflavones, plant sterols and stanols, garlic and tocotrienols. J. Nutr. **2002**, *132*, 2494–2505.

# 2

# Nutrition and Health Implications of Vitamin E

## 2.1. INTRODUCTION

With publication of the Dietary Reference Intakes (DRI) for vitamin E by the Food and Nutrition Board, National Institute of Medicine (1), recommended intakes for vitamin E now are based on the *2R*-stereoisomeric forms of $\alpha$-tocopherol ($\alpha$-T). Other forms including the *2S*-stereoisomers present in synthetic *all-rac*-$\alpha$-T preparations and other tocopherols and tocotrienols in foods do not contribute to the intake requirement. Although sound scientific evidence backs the decision of the Panel on Dietary Antioxidants and Related Compounds to consider only the *2R*-stereoisomers when setting optimal human intake recommendations, scientists involved with food science aspects of vitamin E must take a broader view because of the general antioxidant actions of the tocopherols and tocotrienols in foods. Likewise, food chemists and nutritionists involved in nutrient databank operations must decide on proper presentation of food composition data on vitamin E. Use of the milligram $\alpha$-tocopherol equivalent (mg $\alpha$-TE) has been discontinued in presentation of the United States Department of Agriculture databank.

## 2.2. VITAMIN E NUTRITION

Several reviews completed since 1998 cover newer aspects of vitamin E nutrition.(1,2,3,4) The in-depth and well-referenced DRI report (1) represents the best source for a current overview of factors affecting human requirements for vitamin E. Other highly informative publications include those by Traber (2), Frei and Traber (3), and Bramley et al. (4). All readers interested in vitamin E nutrition should access the chapter on vitamin E in the latest edition of *Modern Nutrition in Health and Disease* (2) written by Dr. Maret Traber. It is not the purpose of this chapter to cover all aspects of vitamin E nutrition; however, we do discuss various aspects of significance to those involved with food delivery systems. The immense body of scientific studies developed over the past decade shows that we are just beginning to understand the impact of vitamin E on human well-being.

### 2.2.1. Absorption, Transport, and Preferential Selectivity for α-Tocopherol

Quite recent knowledge about absorption and transport of vitamin E led to the decision by the Panel on Antioxidants and Related Compounds(1) to base the DRIs for vitamin E on the *2R*-stereoisomers of $\alpha$-T. The absorption and transport processes for vitamin E follow the sequence outlined:

1. Natural and synthetic forms of the tocopherols and tocotrienols are equally absorbed from the intestinal lumen in the form of mixed micelles (1,5–10). Micelle formation relies on proper fat digestion to yield free fatty acids and mono- and diglycerides that act as emulsifiers with the bile salts. Disturbances in pancreatic function or liver secretion of bile, therefore, decrease absorption of the tocopherols and tocotrienols (2).
2. After passage of the micelles into the intestinal mucosa, chylomicrons are synthesized from fatty acids, lysophospholipids, *sn*-2 monoacylglycerides, cholesterol, and other fat-soluble substances including the tocopherols and tocotrienols (11). The chylomicrons are lipoproteins designed to transport dietary lipids and lipid-soluble substances from the intestinal mucosa through the lymphatic system to the circulatory system.
3. In the blood, triaclyglycerol components of the chylomicrons are hydrolyzed by lipoprotein lipase with the formation of lipid-depleted chylomicron remnants. At this point, some of the circulating tocopherols and tocotrienols are transferred to tissue and to high-density lipoproteins (HDLs). Transfer from the HDL to other circulating lipoproteins then occurs (2,6,11).
4. The chylomicron remnants, containing most of the absorbed tocopherols and tocotrienols (2), are taken up by the liver. Triacylglycerols are synthesized and together with other fat-soluble components are formed into very-low-density lipoproteins (VLDLs)

that mediate the transport of lipid from the liver to the peripheral tissue through the circulatory system (12).

5. In the liver, *RRR*-$\alpha$-T is preferentially incorporated into nascent VLDL (13). After secretion of the VLDL into the circulatory system, $\alpha$-T is transferred to HDL and to other lipoproteins after delipidation of the VLDLs. The process selectively enriches plasma and, thus, tissue with $\alpha$-T. The overall process is depicted in Figure 2.1.

**2.2.1.1. Role of the Hepatic $\alpha$-Tocopherol Transfer Protein.** The preferential incorporation of $\alpha$-T into nascent VLDL in the liver is accomplished by action of the $\alpha$-tocopherol transfer protein ($\alpha$-TTP), which has been identified, isolated, and characterized from rat and human liver cytosol (14–18). In vitro, the purified $\alpha$-TPP transfers $\alpha$-T between liposomes and microsomes (15,19). However, the transfer of $\alpha$-T to nascent VLDL has not been demonstrated in vivo (2). Hosomi et al. (19) showed that the relative affinity of $\alpha$-TTP was greatest for *RRR*-$\alpha$-T when compared to other tocopherols, tocopheryl esters, and $\alpha$-tocotrienol ($\alpha$-T3). Calculated on the basis of degree of competition with *RRR*-$\alpha$-T, the relative affinities were *RRR*-$\alpha$-T $= 100$, *RRR*-$\beta$-T $= 38$, *RRR*-$\gamma$-T $= 9$, *RRR*-$\delta$-T $= 2$, $\alpha$-tocopheryl acetate $= 2$, $\alpha$-tocopheryl quinone $= 2$, *SRR*-$\alpha$-T $= 11$, and $\alpha$-T3 $= 12$.

It is evident that $\alpha$-TTP can discriminate between *RRR*-$\alpha$-T and other forms of vitamin E, most likely on the basis of the number and position of the methyl groups on the chromanol ring(4) and the stereoisomerism at the 2 carbon of the chromanol ring of $\alpha$-T. Hosomi et al. (19) concluded that the biological activity of various forms of vitamin E is dependent upon tissue delivery and that their affinities for $\alpha$-TPP limit secretion into lipoproteins and ultimate delivery to tissues. Affinity for the $\alpha$-TTP was, therefore, proposed as a major determinant of biological activity.

### 2.2.2. Biological Activity

Initial estimations of the biological activity of the tocopherols and some of the tocotrienols were established by the rat fetal resorption assay.(20,21) The classical approach follows the ability of vitamin E-deficient rats to maintain pregnancy. If vitamin E is not provided during the first 10–15 days after conception, the embryos die and are resorbed (22). Feeding of known levels of various vitamin E compounds and observation of their effects on fetal survival established relative biological activities. It has been assumed that values of biological activity determined with test animals directly apply to humans (23). However, with recognition of the selectivity for 2-R isomers of $\alpha$-T through action of the $\alpha$-TTP, human requirements are now established by using only the 2-R isomeric forms of $\alpha$-T (1). Since the Dietary Reference Intakes refer only to

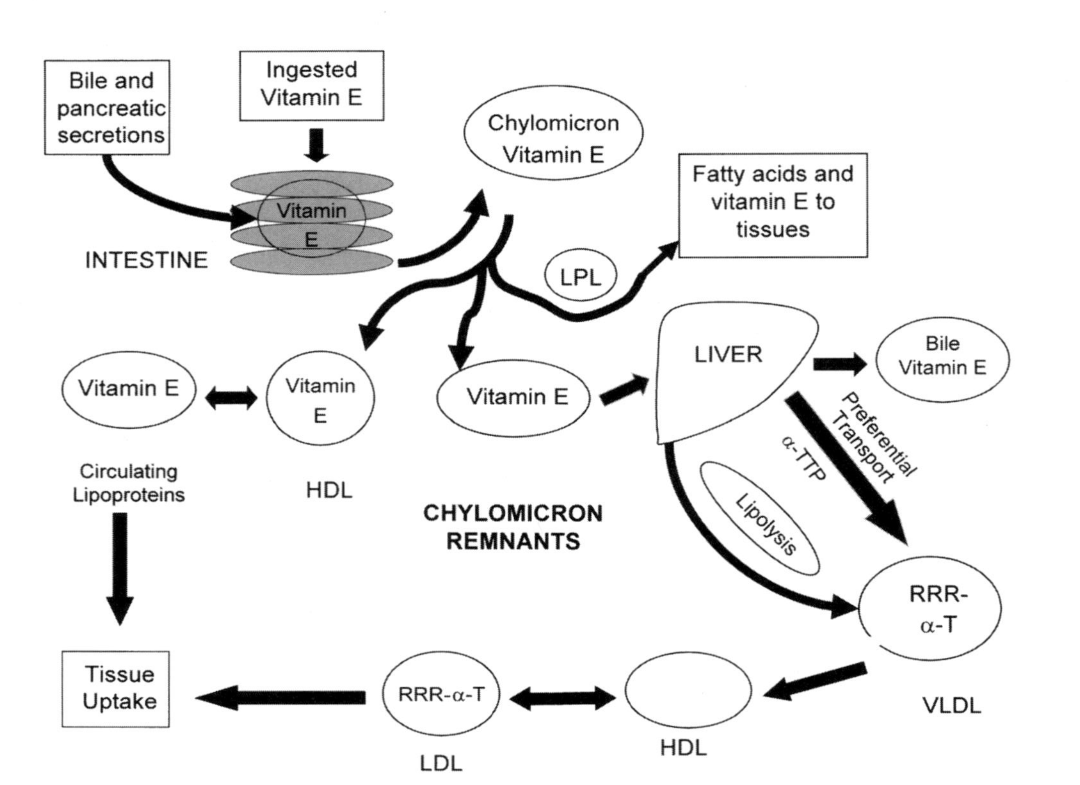


**FIGURE 2.1** Transport and delivery of vitamin E. LPL, lipoprotein lipase, $\alpha$-TTP, $\alpha$-tocopherol transport protein; LDL, low-density lipoprotein; HDL, high-density lipoprotein; VLDL, very-low-density lipoprotein. (Modified from Ref. 2.)

the 2-R isomers, confusion exists about currently used units to report vitamin E activity. Discussion follows on the various units used for vitamin E in foods and pharmaceuticals.

**2.2.2.1. International Units and United States Pharmacopeia Units and Conversion to α-Tocopherol (Milligrams).** An international unit (IU) of vitamin E was defined by the United States Pharmacopeia (USP) as 1 mg of *all-rac*-α-tocopheryl acetate on the basis of biological activity measured by the rat fetal resorption assay (24). Biological activities of tocopherols, tocotrienols, and synthetic forms of vitamin E are indicated in Table 2.1.(25,26) After 1980, the USP discontinued use of the IU and replaced it

**TABLE 2.1** Biological Activity of Natural and Synthetic Vitamin E Forms

| | Biological activity[a] | |
|---|---|---|
| Vitamin E forms | USP units (IU)/mg | Compared to *RRR*-α-T (%) |
| **Natural vitamin E (*RRR*-)** | | |
| α-Tocopherol | 1.49 | 100 |
| β-Tocopherol | 0.75 | 50 |
| γ-Tocopherol | 0.15 | 10 |
| δ-Tocopherol | 0.05 | 3 |
| α-Tocotrienol | 0.75 | 50 |
| β-Tocotrienol | 0.08 | 5 |
| γ-Tocotrienol | Not known | Not known |
| δ-Tocotrienol | Not known | Not known |
| **Synthetic** | | |
| *2R4′R8′R* α-Tocopherol | 1.49 | 100 |
| *2S4′R8′R* α-Tocopherol | 0.46 | 31 |
| *all-rac*-α-Tocopherol | 1.10 | 74 |
| *2R4′R8′S* α-Tocopherol | 1.34 | 90 |
| *2S4′R8′S* α-Tocopherol | 0.55 | 37 |
| *2R4′S8′S* α-Tocopherol | 1.09 | 73 |
| *2S4′S8′R* α-Tocopherol | 0.31 | 21 |
| *2R4′S8′R* α-Tocopherol | 0.85 | 57 |
| *2S4′S8′S* α-Tocopherol | 1.10 | 60 |
| *RRR*-α-Tocopheryl acetate | 1.36 | 91 |
| *RRR*-α-Tocopheryl acid succinate | 1.21 | 81 |
| *all-rac*-α-Tocopheryl acetate | 1.00 | 67 |
| *all-rac*-α-Tocopheryl acid succinate | 0.89 | 60 |

[a]USP, United States Pharmacopeia; IU, international unit; α-T, α-tocopherol.
*Source*: Modified from Refs. 25, 26.

with USP units derived from the same biological activity values as the IU (1). Therefore, 1 USP unit is defined as the activity of 1 mg of *all-rac*-$\alpha$-tocopheryl acetate, which equals the activity of 0.67 mg of *RRR*-$\alpha$-T or 0.74 mg of *RRR*-$\alpha$-tocopheryl acetate. In effect, the IU unit and the USP unit are equivalent (23). Biological activities relative to *RRR*-$\alpha$-T (100%) have been a convenient way to compare the different forms of vitamin E on a basis of IU or USP units and were used to calculate milligram $\alpha$-tocopherol equivalent (mg $\alpha$-TE) values for reporting vitamin E values. International units are still used in food fortification and labeling of supplements (1); however, use should be discontinued. Most applications in the Code of Federal Regulations (CFR) rely on the IU to specify regulatory statements pertaining to vitamin E. For example, IUs are used to specify the vitamin E content of infant formula (27). The USP units are commonly used by the pharmaceutical industry to label vitamin supplements (1).

The Institute of Medicine, Panel on Dietary Antioxidants and Related Compounds (1), recommended that USP units be redefined by USP to take into account the fact that *all-rac*-$\alpha$-T has only 50% of the activity of *RRR*-$\alpha$-T present in nature or with other 2*R*-isomers found in *all-rac*-$\alpha$-T preparations that are used for food fortification and in supplements (1). The selectivity for *RRR*-$\alpha$-T and other 2*R*-isomers of $\alpha$-T provided by $\alpha$-TTP and studies showing that 2*S*-isomers are not maintained by the human strongly support this approach to establishment of human requirements. Factors to convert USP units (IUs) to mg *RRR*-$\alpha$-T or other 2*R*-isomers of $\alpha$-T are given in Table 2.2. Derivation of the conversion factors given in Table 2.2 follows the general formula

$$\text{Molar conversion factor } (\mu\text{mol/IU}) = \frac{\text{USP conversion factor (mg/IU)} \times 1000\ (\mu\text{mol/mol})}{\text{molecular weight (mg/mol)}}$$

The formula for calculation for *RRR*-$\alpha$-tocopheryl acetate is

$$\begin{aligned}\text{Molar conversion factor } (\mu\text{mol/IU}) &= \frac{\text{USP conversion factor (mg/IU)} \times 1000\ (\mu\text{mol/mol})}{\text{molecular weight (mg/mol)}}\\ &= \frac{0.735\ (\text{mg/IU}) \times 1000\ (\mu\text{mol/mol})}{472\ (\text{mg/mol})}\\ &= 1.56\ (\mu\text{mol/IU})\end{aligned}$$

$$\alpha\text{-T conversion factor (mg/IU)} = \frac{\text{molar conversion factor } (\mu\text{mol/IU}) \times 430\ (\text{mg/mol})}{1000\ (\mu\text{mol/mol}) \times R}$$

**Table 2.2** Conversion Factors to Calculate α-Tocopherol from International Units or United States Pharmacopeia Units to Meet Dietary Reference Intakes for Vitamin E

| | USP units (IU)/mg[a] | mg/USP units (IU) | μmol/USP unit (IU) | α-Tocopherol mg/USP unit (IU) |
|---|---|---|---|---|
| **Natural vitamin E** | | | | |
| *RRR*-α-Tocopherol | 1.49 | 0.67 | 1.56 | 0.67 |
| *RRR*-α-Tocopheryl acetate | 1.36 | 0.74 | 1.56 | 0.67 |
| *RRR*-α-Tocopheryl acid succinate | 1.21 | 0.83 | 1.56 | 0.67 |
| **Synthetic vitamin E** | | | | |
| *all-rac*-α-Tocopherol | 1.10 | 0.91 | 2.12 | 0.45 |
| *all-rac*-α-Tocopheryl acetate | 1.00 | 1.00 | 2.12 | 0.45 |
| *all-rac*-α-Tocopheryl acid succinate | 0.89 | 1.12 | 2.12 | 0.45 |

[a]USP, United States Pharmacopeia; IU, international unit.
*Source*: Modified from Ref. 1.

where $R = 2$ for synthetic vitamin E and esters, $R = 1$ for natural vitamin E and esters.

So, the α-T conversion factor for *RRR*-α-tocopheryl acetate is determined as follows:

$$\alpha\text{-T conversion factor (mg/IU)} = \frac{\text{molar conversion factor } (\mu\text{mol/IU}) \times 430 \text{ (mg/mol)}}{1000\ (\mu\text{mol/mol}) \times R}$$

$$= \frac{1.56\ (\mu\text{mol/IU}) \times 430 \text{ (mg/mol)}}{1000\ (\mu\text{mol/mol}) \times 1}$$

$$= 0.67 \text{ (mg/IU)}$$

**2.2.2.2. Milligram α-Tocopherol Equivalents.** Milligram α-Tocopherol equivalents (mg αTEs) were defined for recommending dietary intakes of vitamin E on the basis of biological activity of tocopherols and tocotrienols determined by the rat fetal absorption test.(28–32) One milligram of α-TE is the activity of 1 mg of *RRR*-α-T. Total α-TEs (milligrams) of food containing only *RRR*-isomers are determined by multiplying the amount (milligrams) of α-T by

1.0, of $\beta$-T by 0.5, of $\gamma$-T by 0.1, of $\alpha$-T3 by 0.3, and of $\gamma$-T3 by 0.05. In fortified foods, the conversion factors for *all-rac*-$\alpha$-T and *all-rac*-$\alpha$-tocopheryl acetate are 0.74 and 0.67, respectively. Use of the $\alpha$-TE unit has been the accepted way of reporting vitamin E concentration in foods for approximately the past two decades. The Panel on Antioxidants and Related Compounds(1) determined from United States Department of Agriculture (USDA) food intake survey data that 80% of the mg $\alpha$-TE from foods arises from *RRR*-$\alpha$-T. Therefore, to convert mg $\alpha$-TE to mg *RRR*-$\alpha$-T, the conversion factor is 0.8.

The following conversions are fully explained in the Dietary Reference Intakes report:(1)

1. Milligrams (mg) of *RRR*-$\alpha$-T in a meal = mg of $\alpha$-TE $\times$ 0.8
2. Milligrams (mg) of *RRR*-$\alpha$-T in a food, fortified food, or multivitamin = IU (USP unit) of *RRR*-$\alpha$-T $\times$ 0.67 or IU (USP unit) of *all-rac*-$\alpha$-T $\times$ 0.45

Anytime both natural and synthetic forms of $\alpha$-T are present, analytical procedures must be capable of resolution of the specific compounds in order to apply the preceding formulas. Almost always in a fat-containing fortified food, both *RRR*-$\alpha$-T and *all-rac*-$\alpha$-tocopheryl acetate exist together.

### 2.2.3. Food Sources and Dietary Intakes

The Second National Health and Nutrition Examination Survey (NHANES II) has been extensively evaluated to determine dietary sources of vitamin E in the United States. Major food groups contribute the following percentages of total vitamin E: fats and oils, 20.2%; vegetables, 15.1%; meat, poultry, and fish, 12.6%; desserts, 9.9%; breakfast cereals, 9.3%; fruit, 5.3%; dairy products, 4.5%; mixed main dishes, 4.0%; nuts and seeds, 3.8%; soups, sauces, and gravies, 1.7% (1,33). Data in Table 2.3 reported as mg $\alpha$-TE show that fortified cereals are the most concentrated source of vitamin E in the U.S. diet. Other excellent sources are salad and cooking oils, instant breakfast and diet bars, mayonnaise and salad dressings, and peanuts and peanut butter. Figure 2.2 shows the distribution of vitamin E intakes for males and females reported as mg $\alpha$-TE. The distributions were thought to be skewed by a few individuals with very high intakes. According to these data, 69% of men and 80% of women are below the recommended allowance of 10 (men) and 8 (women) mg $\alpha$-TE per day (33).

Data collected from the Continuing Survey of Food Intakes by Individuals (CSFII, 1994) are listed in Table 2.4 (34). The tabulation shows that high-oil-content foods are major sources; cereals fortified with $\alpha$-tocopheryl acetate are also significant sources. Raw tomatoes and tomato products, because of high

**TABLE 2.3** Vitamin E Content in Usual Servings of Foods Reported by the Second National Health and Nutrition Examination Survey (1976–1980)

| Food group | Vitamin E/portion (mg α-TE)[a] | Vitamin E/100 g (mg α-TE) |
|---|---|---|
| Superfortifed cereals | 33.5 | 137.5 |
| Salad and cooking oils | 1.2 | 14.7 |
| Instant breakfast and diet bars | 4.3 | 12.8 |
| Mayonnaise and salad dressings | 1.3 | 11.3 |
| Peanuts and peanut butter | 1.6 | 8.0 |
| Salty snacks | 1.0 | 4.8 |
| Shellfish | 2.8 | 4.5 |
| Mustard and turnip greens, kale, and collards | 2.5 | 2.6 |
| Pies | 2.5 | 2.5 |
| Coleslaw and cabbage | 1.3 | 2.4 |
| Fried fish | 2.1 | 2.3 |
| Tuna, tuna salad, and tuna casserole | 1.3 | 2.1 |
| Spinach | 1.2 | 1.9 |
| French fries and fried potatoes | 1.9 | 1.5 |
| Fish, broiled, baked, or canned | 1.3 | 1.4 |
| Mixed dish with chicken | 1.5 | 1.2 |
| Pizza | 1.4 | 0.9 |
| Chili | 1.7 | 0.8 |
| Spaghetti with tomato sauce | 1.7 | 0.7 |
| Beef stew and pot pie | 1.4 | 0.4 |
| Melons | 1.2 | 0.4 |

[a]mg α-TE, milligram α-tocopherol equivalent.
*Source*: Modified from Ref. 33.

consumption, are significant sources of vitamin E in the U.S. diet. Data reported in the USDA Nutrient Database for Standard Reference, Release 16 (35), for selected foods are presented in Table 2.5. These foods represent the most concentrated vitamin E sources commonly consumed in the United States.

Using the CSFII and NHANES data as well as other studies, the DRI committee estimated the median daily intake of α-T from food and supplements at 9.8 mg for men and 6.8 mg for women (1). It was emphasized that data on vitamin E intake from food intake surveys may be low estimates as a result of potential for underreporting of energy and fat intake, problems with assessment of fats and oils added during food preparation, uncertainty about the types of fats added, and the variability of food composition tables. Plant oils that contain high levels of *RRR*-α-T include sunflower, cottonseed, peanut, wheat germ, rice bran, canola, palm, and safflower (36). These oils, therefore,

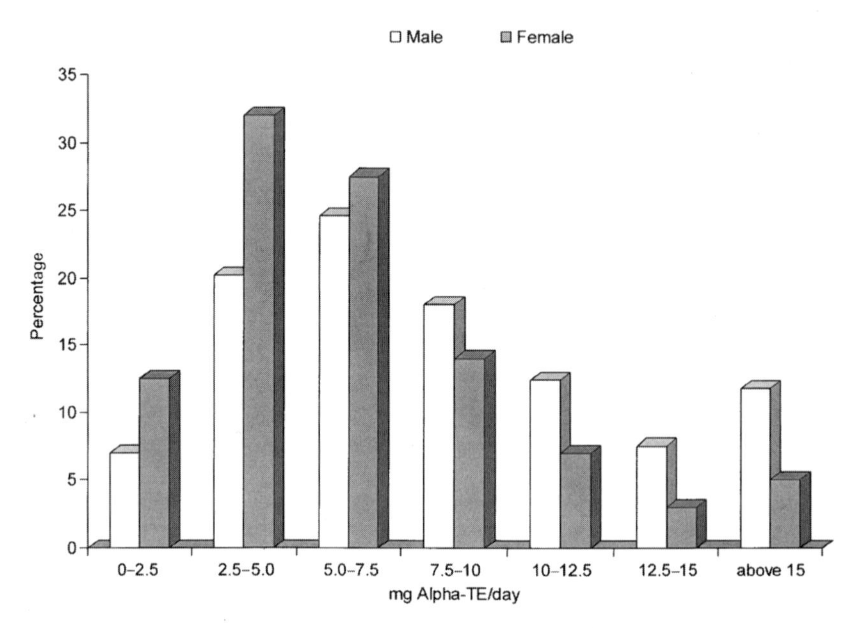


**FIGURE 2.2** Frequency distribution of vitamin E intakes for adults in the United States. Alpha-TE, $\alpha$-tocopherol equivalent. (Modified from Ref. 33.)

have more impact on $\alpha$-T intake than oils or fats with little $\alpha$-T such as lard, palm kernel, coconut, and butter.

## 2.2.4. Dietary Reference Intakes

The Institute of Medicine, Panel on Dietary Antioxidants and Related Compounds (1), considered hydrogen peroxide–induced hemolysis the best biomarker used in conjunction with plasma $\alpha$-T concentrations to estimate adult human requirements for $\alpha$-T. For adults, estimated average requirement (EAR) and recommended dietary allowance (RDA) were set at 12 and 15 mg, respectively. Complete DRI information is given in Table 2.6.

## 2.2.5. Vitamin E Deficiency

Vitamin E deficiency in humans is almost always due to factors other than dietary insufficiency. Deficiency results from genetic abnormalities in production of the $\alpha$-tocopherol transfer protein ($\alpha$-TTP), fat malabsorption syndromes, and protein-energy malnutrition (1). Fat malabsorption can be related to pancreatic and liver abnormalities that lower fat absorption,

**TABLE 2.4** Significant Sources of Vitamin E in the Diet in the United States

| | | % Vitamin E in U.S. diet[a] |
|---|---|---|
| 1 | Margarine, regular stick, 80% fat | 5.5 |
| 2 | Salad dressing, mayonnaise, soybean oil, with salt | 4.3 |
| 3 | Oil, soybean, salad, or cooking | 3.1 |
| 4 | Cereals, ready-to-eat, Total | 2.8 |
| 5 | Oil, corn, salad, or cooking | 2.7 |
| 6 | Shortening, composite, household | 2.5 |
| 7 | Salad dressing, Italian, commercial, regular, with salt | 2.4 |
| 8 | Peanut butter, smooth, with salt | 2.3 |
| 9 | Snacks, potato chips, plain, salted | 2.3 |
| 10 | Eggs, whole, raw, fresh, frozen | 2.0 |
| 11 | Sauce, pasta, spaghetti/marinara, ready-to-serve | 1.6 |
| 12 | Oil, canola | 1.4 |
| 13 | Tomato products, canned, sauce | 1.2 |
| 14 | Shortening, composite, institutional | 1.1 |
| 15 | Rolls, hamburger or hot dog, plain | 1.0 |
| 16 | Margarinelike spread, tub, composite, 60% fat, with salt | 1.0 |
| 17 | Milk, cow, whole, fluid, 3.3% fat | 1.0 |
| 18 | Oil, cottonseed, salad or cooking | 0.9 |
| 19 | Tomato products, canned, puree, without salt | 0.9 |
| 20 | Fast foods, chicken, breaded, fried, boneless, plain | 0.9 |
| 21 | Broccoli, cooked, boiled, drained | 0.9 |
| 22 | Tomatoes, red, ripe, raw | 0.7 |

[a]Calculated on the basis of milligram $\alpha$-tocopherol equivalent (mg $\alpha$-TE).
*Source*: Ref. 34.

abnormalities of the intestinal cells, length of the intestine, and defects in the synthesis or assembly of the chylomicrons (37). Genetic abnormalities in lipoprotein metabolism can produce low levels of chylomicrons, very-low-density lipoproteins (VLDLs) and low-density lipoprotein (LDL) that affect absorption and transport of vitamin E (37).

Abetalipoproteinemia is an autosomal recessive genetic disorder that leads to mutations in the microsomal triglyceride transfer protein (37–39). The disease is associated with ataxia and impaired intestinal absorption of lipids, vitamin E, and other fat-soluble vitamins except vitamin D, since the triglyceride transfer protein participates in the intracellular transport of lipids and other fat-soluble substances. Deficiency of vitamins E, A, and K results in clinical symptoms associated with abetalipoproteinemia. The microsomal triglyceride transfer protein is completely absent from the intestines of abetalipoproteinemia patients (40). Symptoms include steatorrhea with fat-engorged enterocytes,

**Table 2.5** α-Tocopherol Content of Foods

| NDB No.[a] | Description | Weight (g) | Common measure | Content/measure | mg/100 g |
|---|---|---|---|---|---|
| 8028 | Cereals ready-to-eat, Kellogg, Complete Wheat Bran Flakes | 29 | $\frac{3}{4}$ Cup | 26.9 | 92.7 |
| 8058 | Cereals ready-to-eat, Kellogg, Product 19 | 30 | 1 Cup | 20.1 | 67.1 |
| 8077 | Cereals ready-to-eat, General Mills, Whole Grain Total | 30 | $\frac{3}{4}$ Cup | 20.1 | 67.1 |
| 8246 | Cereals ready-to-eat, General Mills, Total Corn Flakes | 30 | 1 $\frac{1}{3}$ Cup | 20.1 | 67.1 |
| 4506 | Oil, vegetable, sunflower, linoleic (60% and over) | 13.6 | 1 Tbsp | 5.6 | 41.1 |
| 8247 | Cereals ready-to-eat, General Mills, Total Raisin Bran | 55 | 1 Cup | 20.3 | 36.9 |
| 4511 | Oil, vegetable safflower, salad or cooking, oleic, over 70% (primary safflower oil of commerce) | 13.6 | 1 Tbsp | 4.6 | 34.1 |
| 12061 | Nuts, almonds | 28.35 | 1 Oz (24 nuts) | 7.3 | 25.9 |
| 8067 | Cereals ready-to-eat, Kellogg, Special K | 31 | 1 Cup | 7.1 | 22.8 |
| 12537 | Seeds, sunflower seed kernels, dry roasted, with salt added | 32 | $\frac{1}{4}$ Cup | 6.8 | 21.3 |
| 12537 | Seeds, sunflower seed kernels, dry roasted, with salt added | 28.35 | 1 Oz | 6.0 | 21.3 |
| 4582 | Vegetable oil, canola | 14 | 1 Tbsp | 2.4 | 17.1 |
| 4042 | Oil, peanut, salad, or cooking | 13.5 | 1 Tbsp | 2.1 | 15.7 |
| 12120 | Nuts, hazelnuts, or filberts | 28.35 | 1 Oz | 4.3 | 15.0 |
| 4053 | Oil, olive, salad, or cooking | 13.5 | 1 Tbsp | 1.9 | 14.4 |
| 4518 | Oil, vegetable corn, salad, or cooking | 13.6 | 1 Tbsp | 1.9 | 14.3 |
| 4543 | Oil, soybean, salad, or cooking, (hydrogenated), and cottonseed | 13.6 | 1 Tbsp | 1.7 | 12.1 |
| 12635 | Nuts, mixed nuts, dry roasted, with peanuts, with salt added | 28.35 | 1 Oz | 3.1 | 10.9 |
| 12147 | Nuts, pine nuts, pignolia, dried | 28.35 | 1 Oz | 2.7 | 9.3 |
| 19811 | Snacks, potato chips, plain, unsalted | 28.35 | 1 Oz | 2.6 | 9.1 |
| 19411 | Snacks, potato chips, plain, salted | 28.35 | 1 Oz | 2.6 | 9.1 |

(*continued*)

**TABLE 2.5** *Continued*

| NDB No.[a] | Description | Weight (g) | Common measure | Content/ measure | mg/ 100 g |
|---|---|---|---|---|---|
| 16090 | Peanuts, all types, dry-roasted, with salt | 28.35 | 1 Oz (approx 28) | 2.2 | 7.8 |
| 16098 | Peanut butter, smooth | 28.35 | 1 Oz | 2.2 | 7.7 |
| 12637 | Nuts, mixed nuts, oil roasted, with peanuts, with salt added | 28.35 | 1 Oz | 2.0 | 7.2 |
| 12078 | Nuts, brazilnuts, dried, unblanched | 28.35 | 1 Oz (6–8 nuts) | 1.6 | 5.7 |
| 8219 | Cereals ready-to-eat, Quaker, Honey Nut Heaven | 49 | 1 Cup | 2.7 | 5.5 |
| 11578 | Vegetable juice cocktail, canned | 242 | 1 Cup | 12.1 | 5.0 |
| 11546 | Tomato products, canned, paste, without salt added | 262 | 1 Cup | 11.3 | 4.3 |
| 11464 | Spinach, frozen, chopped or leaf, cooked, boiled, drained, without salt | 190 | 1 Cup | 6.7 | 3.5 |
| 11208 | Dandelion greens, cooked, boiled, drained, without salt | 105 | 1 Cup | 3.6 | 3.4 |
| 11575 | Turnip greens, frozen, cooked, boiled, drained, without salt | 164 | 1 Cup | 4.4 | 2.7 |
| 18335 | Pie crust, standard-type, frozen, ready-to-bake, baked | 126 | 1 Pie shell | 3.3 | 2.6 |
| 18330 | Pie crust, cookie-type, prepared from recipe, graham cracker, baked | 239 | 1 Pie shell | 5.5 | 2.3 |
| 11549 | Tomato products, canned, sauce | 245 | 1 Cup | 5.1 | 2.1 |
| 11458 | Spinach, cooked, boiled, drained, without salt | 180 | 1 Cup | 3.7 | 2.1 |
| 6931 | Sauce, pasta, spaghetti/ marinara, ready-to-serve | 250 | 1 Cup | 5.1 | 2.0 |
| 11547 | Tomato products, canned, puree, without salt added | 250 | 1 Cup | 4.9 | 2.0 |
| 11461 | Spinach, canned, drained solids | 214 | 1 Cup | 4.2 | 1.9 |
| 11569 | Turnip greens, cooked, boiled, drained, without salt | 144 | 1 Cup | 2.7 | 1.9 |
| 15141 | Crustaceans, crab, blue, canned | 135 | 1 Cup | 2.5 | 1.8 |
| 11087 | Beet greens, cooked, boiled, drained, without salt | 144 | 1 Cup | 2.6 | 1.8 |
| 21024 | Fast foods, french toast sticks | 141 | 5 Sticks | 2.3 | 1.7 |

(*continued*)

**Table 2.5** *Continued*

| NDB No.[a] | Description | Weight (g) | Common measure | Content/ measure | mg/ 100 g |
|---|---|---|---|---|---|
| 21005 | Breakfast items, biscuit with egg and sausage | 180 | 1 Bisuit | 2.8 | 1.6 |
| 11821 | Peppers, sweet, red, raw | 149 | 1 Cup | 2.4 | 1.6 |
| 15071 | Fish, rockfish, Pacific, mixed species, cooked, dry heat | 149 | 1 Fillet | 2.3 | 1.6 |
| 21138 | Fast foods, potato, french fried in vegetable oil | 169 | 1 Large | 2.6 | 1.5 |
| 11093 | Broccoli, frozen, chopped, cooked, boiled, drained, without salt | 184 | 1 Cup | 2.4 | 1.3 |
| 11655 | Carrot juice, canned | 236 | 1 Cup | 2.7 | 1.2 |
| 11424 | Pumpkin, canned, without salt | 245 | 1 Cup | 2.6 | 1.1 |
| 11512 | Sweet potato, canned, vacuum pack | 255 | 1 Cup | 2.6 | 1.0 |
| 6559 | Soup, tomato, canned, prepared with equal volume water, commercial | 244 | 1 Cup | 2.3 | 1.0 |
| 11533 | Tomatoes, red, ripe, canned, stewed | 255 | 1 Cup | 2.1 | 0.8 |
| 22401 | Spaghetti with Meat Sauce, frozen entrée | 283 | 1 Package | 2.4 | 0.8 |
| 11531 | Tomatoes, red, ripe canned, whole, regular pack | 240 | 1 Cup | 1.7 | 0.7 |

[a]Nutrient Data Bank Number.
*Source*: Ref. 35.

absence of apolipoprotein B in the plasma, and absence of intestinal staining for apolipoprotein B in the intestine (38). Neurological symptoms including reflex changes, dyspraxia, and abnormal movements have been observed (38).

Friedreich's ataxia is an autosomal recessive disease characterized by cerebellar ataxia, dysarthria, sensory loss in the lower limbs, and other neurological symptoms (41,42). Early studies on Friedreich's ataxia identified a variant form characterized by normal fat absorption and very low levels of plasma vitamin E. Neurological symptoms were considered to be due to vitamin E deficiency (41,42). Homozygosity mapping showed that Friedreich's ataxia is characterized by defects at chromosome 9 (42), whereas the variant showed defects at chromosome 8 (43). With the specific differences noted at the chromosomal level, the newly recognized genetic defect was termed *familial isolated vitamin E deficiency* (43) or *ataxia with vitamin E deficiency* (AVED).

**TABLE 2.6** Dietary Reference Intake Values for the Vitamin E (Milligrams $\alpha$-Tocopherol/Day)

| Life stage group | EAR[a] | | RDA[b] | | AI[c] | | UL[d] Any form of supplementary $\alpha$-T (mg/day)[e] |
|---|---|---|---|---|---|---|---|
| | Male | Female | Male | Female | Male | Female | |
| 0–6 mo | | | | | 4.0 | 4.0 | |
| 7–12 mo | | | | | 5.0 | 5.0 | |
| 1–3 yr | 5 | 5 | 6 | 6 | | | 200 |
| 4–8 yr | 6 | 6 | 7 | 7 | | | 300 |
| 9–13 yr | 9 | 9 | 11 | 11 | | | 600 |
| 14–18 yr | 12 | 12 | 15 | 15 | | | 800 |
| 19–70 yr | 12 | 12 | 15 | 15 | | | 1000 |
| >70 yr | 12 | 12 | 15 | 15 | | | 1000 |
| Pregnancy | | | | | | | |
| 14–18 yr | | 12 | | 15 | | | 800 |
| 19–50 yr | | 12 | | 15 | | | 1000 |
| Lactation | | | | | | | |
| 14–18 yr | | 16 | | 19 | | | 800 |
| 19–50 yr | | 16 | | 19 | | | 1000 |

[a]EAR, estimated average requirement: the intake that meets the estimated nutrient needs of half of the individuals in a group.[b]RDA, recommended dietary allowance: the intake that meets the nutrient needs of almost all (97%–98%) of individuals in a group.[c]AI, adequate intake: the observed average or experimentally determined intake by a defined population or subgroup that appears to sustain a defined nutritional status, such a growth rate, normal circulating nutrient values, or other functional indicators of health. The AI is used if sufficient scientific evidence is not available to derive an EAR. The AI is not equivalent to an RDA.[d]UL, tolerable upper intake level.[e]$\alpha$-T, $\alpha$-tocopherol.
*Source*: Ref. 1.

Later work showed that AVED is an autosomal recessive neurodegenerative disease that leads to an impaired ability to incorporate *RRR*-$\alpha$-T into VLDL (44). Therefore, AVED was attributed to a defect in the $\alpha$-TTP gene (44). The primary cause of neurodegenerative symptoms in AVED patients is now known to be vitamin E deficiency due to the absence of a functioning $\alpha$-TTP (45,46) with inefficient transfer of *RRR*-$\alpha$-T from the liver and lack of recycling of plasma *RRR*-$\alpha$-T. Clinical symptoms include many neurological problems stemming from peripheral neuropathy with degeneration of the large-caliber axons in the sensory neurons (1). Common symptoms are ataxia, muscle weakness and hypertrophy, neurological abnormalities, reproductive disorders, and abnormalities of the liver, bone marrow, and brain (47). At the cellular level, increased oxidation can occur as a result of increased oxidative stress. The progression of vitamin E deficiency symptoms has been described as follows: hyporeflexia, ataxia, limitation in upward gaze, strabismus to long-tract defects, muscle weakness, visual field constriction, and centrocecal scotomata (38,48,49).

### 2.2.6. Toxicity of Vitamin E and the Tolerable Upper Intake Level

Vitamin E is one of the least toxic vitamins (50), and there is no evidence of side effects of consumption of vitamin E that occurs naturally in foods. Studies on toxicity are, therefore, limited to supplemental sources of vitamin E (1). Kappus and Diplock (51) reviewed the literature on vitamin E toxicity and concluded that humans show few side effects after supplemental doses below 2100 mg per day of tocopherol. Animal studies show that vitamin E is not mutagenic, carcinogenic, or teratogenic (52–54). Adults tolerate relatively high doses without significant toxicity; however, muscle weakness, fatigue, double vision, emotional disturbance, breast soreness, thrombophlebitis, nausea, diarrhea, and flatulence have been reported at tocopherol intakes at 1600–3000 mg/day (1,55–58).

It has been recognized that high intake of $\alpha$-T can cause hemorrhage, increase prothrombin time, and inhibit blood coagulation in animals (1). Such events have been observed in chicks(59) and rats,(52,60,61) but high doses of 500 mg/kg/day of *RRR*-$\alpha$-tocopheryl acetate were necessary to induce hemorrhagic events (1). Effects were reversible with administration of supplemental vitamin K.

Hemorrhagic toxicity in humans has been observed, but large clinical trials have yielded somewhat conflicting results. However, the DRI panel considered hemorrhagic effects as the best criterion to set the tolerable upper intake level (UL) for humans (1). In setting the UL, a lowest observed adverse effect level (LOAEL) of 500 mg/kg body weight/day for *all-rac*-$\alpha$-tocopheryl acetate was identified from the work of Wheldon et al. (60) on rats. An uncertainty factor (UF) for $\alpha$-T based on previous studies was calculated at 36 and used to convert the LOAEL to a no observed adverse effect level (NOAEL):

$$UL = \frac{LOAEL}{UF} = \frac{500\ \text{mg/day/kg}}{36} = 14\ \text{mg/day/kg}$$

$$14\ \text{mg/day/kg} \times 68.5\ \text{kg} \cong 1000\ \text{mg/day}$$

The great amount of uncertainty involved in the calculation led to establishment of the same UL for adult males and females (Table 2.6).

## 2.3. HEALTH IMPACTS OF VITAMIN E

It is generally accepted that oxidative damage at the cellular level is significant to the onset of chronic disease. Since vitamin E is the primary fat-soluble antioxidant in mammalian systems, a logical assumption is that supplementation of the human diet with vitamin E potentially could be significant in prevention and/ or slowing of the onset of various chronic disease states. This assumption taken together with increasing knowledge about the role vitamin E plays and potential roles other antioxidants available in the food supply might play produced an extremely large body of scientific literature on antioxidants and health. Unfortunately, the body of data does not provide for a clear conclusion on vitamin E and its overall worth when consumed at levels above the recommended dietary allowance (RDA). Diverse opinions about supplemental use of vitamin E remain. The fact remains that the Panel on Dietary Antioxidants and Related Compounds (1), when establishing the DRIs for vitamin E in 2000, concluded that clinical scientific evidence does not support supplemental usage of vitamin E. The literature appearing in nutrition and medical journals evaluating the impact of vitamin E supplementation in various diseases is, indeed, staggering in its quality and amount. In this section, some current views and experimental evidence on the value to human health of vitamin E at supplemental intake levels is presented.

### 2.3.1. Vitamin E and Aging

Aging is a normal process characterized by morphological and functional changes, most of which are degenerative, that occur as a living system grows older. The role of free radicals in the aging process and the ability of vitamin E to delay the overall process have been topics of intense investigation for decades. Harman, in a series of papers that began in 1956, presented and discussed the free radical theory on aging (62–68). This theory is based on the premise that aging is due to the accumulation of deteriorative changes resulting from free radical reactions at the cellular level that occur throughout the lifespan. Harman suggested that the functional life span could be increased by minimizing free radical events by keeping body weight low, by ingesting diets adequate in nutrients but containing minimal amounts of constituents that enhance free radical damage (copper, polyunsaturated fatty acids, etc.), and maintaining a diet high in antioxidants, including vitamin E (67).

Many theories on aging have been advanced and debated, and the free radical theory of aging continues to be prominent in such debates. Packer and Landvik (69) in 1989 stated, "Research has shown that free radical damage accumulates during the aging process, and evidence is increasing that lipid peroxidation may be an important factor in making aging the long and healthy process that it should be. Animal and human studies have demonstrated protective effects of vitamin E and other antioxidants on free radical reactions and peroxidative changes in the aging process." Likewise, Pryor (70) emphasized the potential of vitamin E and the need for continuing research with the following conclusion: "Although the current literature (up to 1989) gives good hope for a beneficial effect for vitamin E on the variety of pathologies, the data are not yet complete." Taking into account the conclusion of the DRI committee not to recommend supplementation, we are still at the stage of searching for scientific documentation that unequivocally proves the long-term benefits of increased intake of vitamin E. A general consensus is that a balanced diet, providing a goodly amount of many different antioxidants, is desirable for optimal health and, possibly, provides for increased longevity with increased maintenance of good functionality. However, the direct benefits of supplemental vitamin E to fighting specific disease states, as discussed in the following sections, are not clear and, in many instances, evidence of benefit seems to be less conclusive.

### 2.3.2. Vitamin E and Cardiovascular Disease

*Cardiovascular disease* (CVD) is a general term for diseases that affect the heart and/or blood vessels—coronary heart disease, stroke, peripheral vascular disease, and high blood pressure. Oxidation of low-density lipoprotein (LDL) is considered to be a major causative factor in development of CVD (1). As reviewed by the Panel on Dietary Antioxidants and Related Compounds (1), vitamin E has the following effects that may impact the in vivo development of CVD:

1. Inhibits LDL oxidation
2. Inhibits smooth muscle cell proliferation by inhibition of protein kinase C
3. Inhibits platelet adhesion, aggregation, and release reactions
4. Inhibits the generation of thrombin in the plasma that binds to platelet receptors, inducing aggregation
5. Decreases monocyte adhesion to the endothelium through down-regulation of expression of adhesion molecules
6. Decreases production of superoxide by monocytes
7. Increases synthesis of prostacyclin, which acts as a vascodilator and inhibitor of platelet aggregation
8. Upregulates expression of cytosolic phospholipase $A_2$ and cyclooxygenase
9. Inhibits the expression of intracellular and vascular cell adhesion molecules

Animal studies generally support the antioxidant hypothesis of atherosclerosis (1). However, review of large-scale epidemiological studies (Table 2.7) (71–78) and large-scale clinical intervention trials (Table 2.8) (79–83) by the DRI committee revealed many inconsistencies in end results provided by supplemental use of vitamin E. Therefore, supplemental vitamin E was not recommended for the general population as a means to prevent CVD.

Since publication of the DRI report, results of several large clinical intervention studies that support the DRI Panel conclusion have been published (Table 2.8). These include the Age-Related Cataract and Vision Loss Study (AREDS Report No. 9) (84), the Primary Prevention Project (PPP) (85), the MRC/BHF Heart Protection Study (HPS) (86), the Antioxidant Supplementation in Atherosclerosis Prevention Study (ASAP) (87–89), and the Secondary Prevention with Antioxidants of Cardiovascular Disease in Endstage Renal Disease (SPACE) (90). In each of these large-scale supplementation studies, no statistically significant effect of vitamin E in reducing risks of CVD was found (Table 2.8). Only the Antioxidant Supplementation in Atherosclerosis Prevention (ASAP) study reported that twice-daily doses of vitamin E (136 IU) when combined with slow-release vitamin C (250 mg) slowed atherosclerotic progression in hypercholesterolemic adults (87–89). The combined treatment had no effect on inflammatory events in healthy men with slight hypercholesterolemia (89). Regarding stroke, Yochum et al. (91) completed a prospective cohort study of 34,492 postmenopausal women to examine the association between antioxidant vitamin intakes and death of stroke. An inverse association was noted between death of stroke and vitamin E intake from food, but a protective effect for supplemental vitamin E, vitamin A, and carotenoids was not noted.

Adding further support to the DRI decision, Vivekananthan et al. (92) completed a metaanalysis of seven trials involving vitamin E supplementation and CVD: ATBC (79,80), CHAOS (81), GISSI (82), HOPE (83), AREDS (84), PPP (85), and HPS (86). Combined, the studies represented results from 81,788 subjects. Results (Figure 2.3) reported as odds ratios (95% confidence interval [CI]) showed that vitamin E supplementation did not decrease incidence of all-cause mortality, stroke, or risk of cardiovascular death. The authors concluded the following: "The lack of a salutary effect was consistently seen for various doses of vitamins in diverse populations. Our results, combined with the lack of mechanistic data for efficacy of vitamin E, do not support routine use of vitamin E."

Health claims for use on nutritional labels of conventional foods and supplements are of continuing concern and regulatory uncertainty for the U.S. Food and Drug Administration (FDA). In 1999, the U.S. Court of Appeals for the D.C. Circuit ruled in reference to dietary supplement labeling that the First Amendment does not permit FDA to reject health claims that FDA determines to

**TABLE 2.7** Vitamin E Intake and Cardiovascular Disease–Epidemiological Studies[a]

| Study | Subjects | Observations | Reference |
|---|---|---|---|
| Health Professionals Follow-Up Study | 39,910 Male health professionals free of CVD, high serum cholesterol level, and diabetes | No significant decrease in risk of CHD for total vitamin E intake and intake from supplements; however, though no proven causal relationship, association between high intake of vitamin E and lower CHD rate | 71 |
| Nurses Health Study | 87,245 Female nurses free from CVD and cancer | Women in the highest quintile of vitamin E intake had a relative risk of 0.66 compared to those in the lowest quintile; reduction in CHD risk was attributed to supplemental vitamin E intake; however, no proven causal relationship | 72 |
| Finnish Study of Antioxidant Vitamin Intake and Coronary Mortality | 2,748 Men and 2,385 women initially free from CHD | Significant inverse association between dietary intake of vitamin E and coronary mortality rate | 73 |
| Iowa Women's Health Study Dietary Antioxidant Vitamins and Death from CHD in Postmenopausal Women | 34,846 Postmenopausal women without CVD | Vitamin E intake from foods but not from supplements decreased CHD risk | 74 |

| Study | Subjects | Findings | Ref. |
|---|---|---|---|
| Established Populations for Epidemiological Studies of the Elderly | 11,178 Subjects 67–105 years old | Risks of all-cause mortality and CHD mortality were reduced by use of vitamin E supplements | 75 |
| Cholesterol Lowering Atherosclerosis Study (CLAS) | 162 Men treated with coronary bypass surgery were treated with colestipol niacin and advised to follow a cholesterol level–lowering diet or given only dietary advice | Combined data showed that vitamin E intakes were inversely correlated with progression of atherosclerosis in coronary and carotid arteries; within the drug treatment group, use of vitamin E supplements decreased coronary artery lesion development, but not in the placebo group; opposite results were found by using ultrasound measurements | 76–78 |
| Iowa Women's Health Study. Dietary Antioxidant Vitamins and Death from Stroke in Postmenopausal Women | 34,492 Postmenopausal women | Results suggested a protective effect of vitamin E from foods against death of stroke but not from supplemental vitamin E or other antioxidant vitamins | 91 |

[a]CVD, cardiovascular disease; CHD, coronary heart disease.

**TABLE 2.8** Vitamin E and Cardiovascular Disease—Intervention Studies[a]

| Study | Subjects | Dose | Observations | Reference |
|---|---|---|---|---|
| Alpha-Tocopherol, Beta-Carotene (ATBC) Cancer Prevention Study | 1,862 Men—all smokers | 50 mg *all-rac*-α-T acetate per day | No significant differences between the supplementation group and the placebo group in numbers of major coronary events over a median follow-up time of 5.3 yr | 79, 80 |
| Cambridge Heart Antioxidant Study (CHAOS) | 2,002 Patients with proven coronary atherosclerosis | 400 or 800 IU *RRR*-α-T per day | α-T Significantly reduced the risk of cardiovascular death and nonfatal MI | 81 |
| Gruppo Italiano per lo Studio della Sopravvivenza nell'Infarcto Micardico (GISSI) Prevention Study | 11,324 Patients surviving recent MI | 1 g daily of n-3 PUFA and 300 mg *all-rac*-α-T | n-3 Supplementation but not α-T significantly lowered risk of cardiovascular death, nonfatal MI, and stroke | 82 |
| Heart Outcomes Prevention Evaluation Study (HOPE) | 2,545 Women and 6,996 men at high CVD risk | 400 IU per day of natural source vitamin E | Vitamin E had no effect on cardiovascular outcomes | 83 |
| Age-Related Eye Disease Study (AREDS) | 4,757 Subjects, most aged 55–80 yr | 400 IU of vitamin E, 500 mg vitamin C, 15 mg β-carotene, or 80 mg zinc oxide + 2 mg cupric oxide per day | No statistically significant effect of antioxidants on mortality rate | 84 |

| | | | | |
|---|---|---|---|---|
| Primary Prevention Project (PPP) | 4,495 Subjects at risk of having a cardiovascular event | 300 mg all-rac-$\alpha$-T or 100 mg enteric coated aspirin per day | Aspirin lowered the frequency of all endpoints, significantly for cardiovascular death and total cardiovascular death; vitamin E showed no effects | 85 |
| The Heart Protection Study (HPS) | 20,536 Adults with coronary disease | 600 mg $\alpha$-T, 250 mg vitamin C, 20 mg $\beta$-carotene per day | No significant reductions in 5-yr mortality rate or incidence of any type of vascular disease or other major outcome | 86 |
| The Antioxidant Supplementation in Atherosclerosis Prevention Study (ASAP) | 520 Adults | 91 mg RRR-$\alpha$-T, 250 mg vitamin C, or combination, twice daily | Combined supplementation retarded progression of carotid atherosclerosis at 3 years. Effects were confirmed at 6 years. There were no antiinflammatory effects | 87, 88, 89 |
| Secondary Prevention with Antioxidants of CVD in Endstage Renal Disease (SPACE) | 196 Hemodialysis patients with preexisting CVD | 800 IU of vitamin E per day for median 519 days | Vitamin E supplementation reduced CVD endpoints and myocardial infarction | 90 |

[a] $\alpha$-T, $\alpha$-tocopherol; IU, international unit; PUFA, polyunsaturated fatty acid; MI, myocardial infarction; CVD, cardiovascular disease.

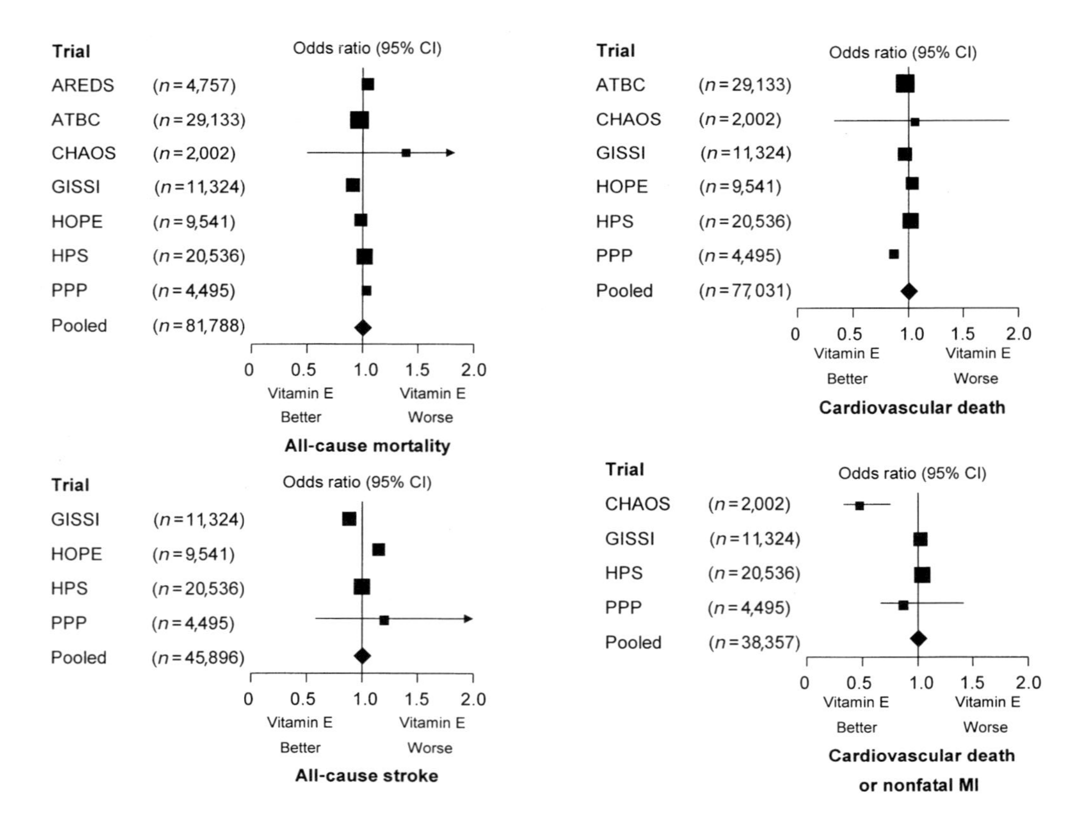


**FIGURE 2.3** Odds ratios for cardiovascular events for individuals treated with vitamin E or control therapy. CI, confidence interval; MI, myocardial infarction. (Modified from Ref. 92.)

be potentially misleading unless FDA also reasonably determines that no disclaimer would eliminate the potential deception. The court did not rule out FDA's discretion to claim it incurable by a disclaimer and ban it outright in cases in which evidence in support of the claim is outweighed by evidence against the claim. This court decision in response to *Pearson v. Shalala*, although not encompassing vitamin E and its relationship to CVD, led FDA to reconsider health claim petitions for consumption of antioxidant vitamins in relation to cancer, folic acid in relation to neural tube defects, fiber in relation to colorectal cancer, and omega-3 fatty acids in relation to coronary heart disease. The decision, in effect, initiated "qualified" health claims for dietary supplements as opposed to "unqualified" health claims, which must meet the Significant Scientific Agreement (SSA) standard set by Congress in the Nutrition Labeling and Education Act (NLEA) of 1990. The decision was based on a manufacturer's right to make statements about diet–health relationships when the science supporting the claim does not meet the SSA standard, provided that the claim about the relationship is stated or "qualified" in a way not misleading to consumers. Qualified health claims must, therefore, be accompanied by a disclaimer.

In order to improve information on food and supplement labels in the form of health claims and dietary guidance for consumers, FDA established the Task Force on Consumer Health Information for Better Nutrition Initiative. In its final report, issued July 10, 2003 (93), the Task Force set interim procedures that the FDA can use for qualified health claims in the labeling of conventional foods and supplements (94) and recommended that FDA promulgate regulations under notice-and-comment rulemaking pertinent to establishing qualified health claims. The interim procedure provides processes for filing qualified health claim petitions, prioritization for effective application of resources, opportunities for public comment, and methods to obtain third-party reviews of scientific data. On September 1, 2003, FDA began considering qualified health claims under its interim procedures (95).

In 2001, FDA was petitioned to authorize a health claim about the relationship between vitamin E dietary supplements and reduced risk of heart disease (96). Three proposed model claims were presented:

1. "As part of a healthy diet low in saturated fat and cholesterol, 400 IU/day of Vitamin E (*d*-$\alpha$-tocopherol or *dl*-$\alpha$-tocopherol) may reduce the risk of heart disease. Individuals who take anticoagulant medicine(s) should consult their physicians before taking supplemental Vitamin E."
2. "As part of a healthy diet low in saturated fat and cholesterol, 100–400 IU/day of natural Vitamin E (*d*-$\alpha$-tocopherol) may reduce the risk of heart disease. Individuals who take anticoagulant medicine(s) should consult their physicians before taking supplemental Vitamin E."

3. "As part of a healthy diet low in saturated fat and cholesterol, 200–800 IU/day of synthetic Vitamin E (*dl*-$\alpha$-tocopherol) may reduce the risk of heart disease. Individuals who take anticoagulant medicine(s) should consult their physicians before taking supplemental Vitamin E."

The Food and Drug Administration rejected the petition on the basis of not meeting the SSA standard (96). Subsequently, FDA reevaluated the petition according to the *Pearson v. Shalala* decision to determine whether or not to allow a qualified health claim. They concluded that

> there is no significant scientific agreement for a relationship between vitamin E supplements and CVD risk, and that the scientific evidence for a relationship is outweighed by the scientific evidence against the relationship. Should the scientific evidence change in the future, such that the agency would consider authorizing a health claim or exercising its enforcement discretion for a qualified health claim, FDA would consider potential safety concerns at that time. FDA does not intend to exercise enforcement discretion with respect to the use of a qualified health claim relating dietary supplement vitamin E intake and reduced risk of CVD (97).

With a relatively strong case emerging against the routine use of supplemental vitamin E as protection against CVD, it must be kept in mind that proper intake of $\alpha$-T throughout the life span is most likely significant to one's well-being. Also, proper intake is an elusive concept and subject to change as scientific data further document our requirements. Various interpretive articles including Keaney and coworkers (98), Traber (99), Dutta and Dutta (100), and Gey(101) explored the roles of vitamin E in broad perspectives. Significant to CVD, $\alpha$-T is now recognized as a controlling factor in the enhancement of the activity of nitric oxide in maintaining vascular homeostatsis, inhibition of superoxide production by monocytes and macrophages, and inhibition of platelet aggregation and smooth muscle proliferation through its inhibitory effect on protein kinase C. Future DRI recommendations will likely reflect revisions as this complicated area of human nutrition becomes better understood.

## 2.3.3. Vitamin E and Cancer

The many forms of cancer are characterized by uncontrolled growth and spread of abnormal cells, which, if not controlled, results in death. One mechanism of cancer onset that has received a great deal of scientific examination has been free radical damage to deoxyribonucleic acid (DNA) and the accumulation of unrepaired mutations as one ages (1). Much of the consumer's interest in antioxidants stems from the fact that dietary antioxidants, including vitamin E, may act as anticarcinogens through their ability to intercept and destroy free radicals. A diet high in fruits and vegetables is accepted as a means to lower cancer risks. However, the understanding of how specific components in the diet interact to lower cancer risk remains speculative (102–104). The U.S. Food and Drug Administration (FDA) excepted the association between high intake of fruits and vegetables and lowered cancer risks with an approved health claim for use on nutritional labels (105). The approved model claim statement is "Low fat diets rich in fruits and vegetables (foods that are low in fat and may contain dietary fiber, vitamin A, or vitamin C) may reduce the risk of some types of cancer, a disease with many factors. ——— (name of fruit or vegetable) is high in vitamin A and C, and it is a good source of dietary fiber." Vitamin E is not included in this statement since most fruits and vegetables are quite low in vitamin E content (see Chapter 8). However, the FDA did not approve a health claim to the effect that antioxidants in foods may lower the risk of cancer. This point was extensively debated. All interested in the history of antioxidant health claims should read Block's argument for an antioxidant health claim related to cancer risk (102). The *Pearson v. Shalala* court decision directed FDA to reconsider the health claim "Consumption of antioxidants may reduce the risk of certain kinds of cancer" for labeling use on dietary supplements. In reevaluation of the supporting data, FDA issued the conclusion that

> there is no significant scientific agreement for a relationship between antioxidant vitamins (i.e., vitamin C or vitamin E, alone or in combination) and certain kinds of cancer or of individual cancers (i.e., cancer of the bladder, breast, cervix, colon, and rectum, oral cavity/pharynx/esophagus, lung, prostate, pancreas, skin, stomach) and that the scientific evidence against a relationship outweighs the scientific evidence for a relationship. Therefore, FDA finds that health claims relating antioxidant vitamins (i.e., vitamin C or vitamin E, alone or in combination) and reduced risk of certain kinds of cancer or of individual cancers (i.e., cancer of the bladder, breast, cervix, colon and rectum, oral cavity/pharynx/esophagus, lung, prostate, pancreas, skin, stomach) are inherently misleading and cannot be made non-misleading with a disclaimer or other qualifying language (106).

This decision became the subject of a lawsuit (*Whitaker v. Thompson*) that challenged the FDA rejection of the health claim. In December 2002, the U.S. District Court of the District of Columbia found that the antioxidant claim was only potentially misleading and ordered FDA to permit the claim with a disclaimer. After the court's decision, the FDA issued on April 1, 2003, a letter(107) with three disclaimers to meet the court's criteria. The disclaimers to qualify the claim "Consumption of antioxidant vitamins may reduce the risk of certain kinds of cancer" are the following:

1. Some scientific evidence suggests that consumption of antioxidant vitamins may reduce the risk of certain forms of cancer. However, FDA has determined that this evidence is limited and not conclusive.
2. Some scientific evidence suggests that consumption of antioxidant vitamins may reduce the risk of certain forms of cancer. However, FDA does not endorse this claim because this evidence is limited and not conclusive.
3. FDA has determined that although some scientific evidence suggests that consumption of antioxidant vitamins may reduce the risk of certain forms of cancer, this evidence is limited and not conclusive.

FDA further stated:

> FDA intends to exercise its enforcement discretion with respect to antioxidant vitamin dietary supplements containing vitamin E and/or vitamin C when:
>
> 1. one of the above disclaimers is placed immediately adjacent to and directly beneath the antioxidant vitamin claim, with no intervening material, in the same size, typeface, and contrast as the claim itself; and
> 2. the supplement does not recommend or suggest in its labeling, or under ordinary conditions of use, a daily intake exceeding the Tolerable Upper Intake Level established by the Institute of Medicine (IOM) of 2000 mg per day for vitamin C and 1000 mg per day for vitamin E.

Whether or not the use of qualified health claims will be beneficial to the consumer remains to be seen. Since legal interpretations and scientifically based opinions can greatly differ, qualified health claims may have a greater chance of being a source of misinformation than of accurate information.

When establishing the DRIs for vitamin E, the Panel on Dietary Antioxidants and Related Compounds evaluated nine epidemiological studies (108–116) and nine intervention studies (79,117–124) published through 1998. The panel concluded that the studies did not provide consistent results and that the effect of vitamin E on cancer risk was less than the effect of vitamin E on cardiovascular risk. However, the panel emphasized that results obtained from the ATBC study (79,117) suggested that vitamin E supplements might lower risk of prostate cancer. Heinonen et al. (117) reported a 32% decrease in the incidence of prostate cancer in male smokers receiving 50 mg $\alpha$-T per day for clinical prostate cancer but not for latent cancer. Mortality rate of prostate cancer was 41% lower in the supplemental group. Since the supplementation time was 5–8 years, the conclusion was that long-term supplementation with $\alpha$-T substantially reduced prostate cancer incidence and mortality rates.

Since establishment of the DRIs, several large epidemiological studies have been published on bladder and urinary tract cancers (125–128), colorectal cancers (129–131), stomach and other gastric cancers (132), and prostate cancer (133) (Table 2.9). Most of these studies support the view of the Panel on Antioxidants and Related Compounds that evidence of a relationship between vitamin E intake and a decreased risk for most cancers is weak (1). In May 2001, the U.S. Food and Drug Administration provided an in-depth review of epidemiological and clinical studies completed through 2000, before the *Whitaker v. Thompson* suit and the U.S. District Court decision in December 2002 (106). The FDA, at that point in time, concluded that there was no significant scientific agreement for a relationship between antioxidant vitamins, including vitamin C and vitamin E, alone or in combination and certain cancers. This conclusion was somewhat negated by the court's direction to FDA to draft disclaimers for the health claim "Consumption of antioxidant vitamins may reduce the risk of certain kinds of cancers" for use on dietary supplements (107).

The Finnish data on male smokers (79,117) and the U.S. study on male health professionals (133), which suggested an inverse association between supplemental vitamin E and risk of fatal prostate cancer among current smokers or recent quitters, led the National Cancer Institute (NCI) to sponsor a large trial of the effects of selenium and vitamin E on prostate cancer. The Selenium and Vitamin E Cancer Prevention Trial (SELECT) is a randomized, prospective, double-blind study designed to show the effects of selenium and vitamin E alone and in combination on the incidence of prostate cancer (134–137). The study, initiated in 2001, will enroll 32,400 men and proceed through 2013. The supplement dosages include 400 mg *all-rac*-$\alpha$-tocopheryl acetate (400 IU) or 200 μg L-seleno-methionine or both or a placebo daily.

## 2.3.4. Vitamin E and Age-Related Eye Diseases

Cataract and age-related macular degeneration (AMD) represent the two most frequent disease states leading to vision loss worldwide. Both diseases usually occur in older adults. Oxidative stress with accumulation of free radical damage to the lens and retina has been considered causative to development of both cataract and AMD. Thus, the role of dietary and supplementary antioxidants, including vitamin E, $\beta$-carotene, other carotenoids, vitamin C, and selenium, in preventing or slowing such age-related eye diseases has been extensively investigated. The DRI panel(1) in 2000 noted the existence of nine epidemiological studies (138–146) and one clinical intervention study (147) relating vitamin E status and supplementation to risk of cataract. The

**TABLE 2.9** Recent Epidemiological and Intervention Studies on Vitamin E and Cancer Risk

| Study | Subjects | Observations | References |
|---|---|---|---|
| **Bladder and urinary tract cancer** | | | |
| Health Professionals Follow-Up Study | 47,909 Men followed since 1986 by use of a food frequency questionnaire | A statistically significant inverse relationship was found between vitamin E intake and bladder cancer risk | 125 |
| Alpha-Tocopherol, Beta-Carotene Cancer Prevention Study (ATBC), Finland | 29,133 Male smokers aged 50–69 yr receiving 50 mg $\alpha$-T daily or placebo for 5–8 yr | Long-term supplementation with (-T and (-carotene had no preventative effect on urinary tract cancers in middle-aged male smokers | 126 |
| Netherlands Cohort Study | Subcohort consisting of 3,500 subjects | Dietary and supplemental intake of vitamin A, vitamin C, vitamin E, folate, and most carotenoids was not associated with bladder cancer | 127 |
| Cancer Prevention Study II (CPSII) | 991,522 U.S. adults | Regular use of vitamin E supplements ($\geq$15 times per month) for $\geq$10 years was associated with a reduced risk of bladder cancer mortality; use for a shorter duration was not | 128 |
| **Colon cancer** | | | |
| Alpha-Tocopherol, Beta-Carotene Cancer Prevention Study (ATBC), Finland | 29,133 Male smokers aged 50–69 yr receiving 50 mg $\alpha$-T daily or placebo for 5–8 yr | No effect of vitamin E supplements on colorectal cancer incidence | 129 |

| | | | |
|---|---|---|---|
| Cancer Prevention Study II (CPSII) | 711,891 U.S. adults | No substantial effect was found for supplemented use of vitamin C or E on colorectal cancer | 130 |
| Nurses Health Study and Health Professionals Follow-Up Study | 87,998 Females and 47,344 males | Men with supplemental vitamin E intake of 300 IU/day or more may be at lower risk for colon cancer compared to that of "never" users. For women, there was no evidence of a vitamin E effect. Findings did not provide consistent support for an inverse association between supplemented vitamin E and colon cancer risk | 131 |
| Cancer Prevention Study II (CPSII) | 1,045,923 U.S. adults | Supplemental use of vitamin C, vitamin E, or multivitamins may not substantially reduce risk of stomach cancer in North America, where stomach cancer rates are low | 132 |
| **Prostate cancer** | | | |
| Health Professionals Follow-Up Study | 47,780 U.S. male health professionals | Supplemental vitamin E was not associated with prostate cancer risk. A suggestive inverse associate was apparent between supplemental vitamin E and risk of metastatic prostate cancer among current smokers and recent quitters. This finding was consistent with the Finnish trial among smokers (79,117) | 133 |

epidemiological studies were inconclusive, and the intervention study (147) showed no effect at 50 mg $\alpha$-T per day.

Several studies published since the DRI report was written are detailed in Table 2.10 (148–160). Of these, the Age-Related Eye Disease Study (AREDS) (155–157) and the Vitamin E, Cataract, and Age-Related Maculopathy Trial (VECAT) (158,159) have received considerable public and scientific coverage. Results from the AREDS study (Figure 2.4) showed zinc supplements or a mixture of zinc, vitamin E, vitamin C, and $\beta$-carotene significantly reduced the odds of development of AMD. The antioxidant supplement without the zinc did not significantly reduce the odds of development of advanced AMD. The strength of the data analysis led the researchers to recommend that "those with extensive intermediate size druzen, at least 1 druse, noncentral geographic atrophy in one or both eyes, and without contraindications such as smoking, should consider taking a supplement of antioxidants plus zinc such as that used in this study." In contrast, the AREDS study in the cataract arm (84) showed no effects of the high-dose antioxidant formulation on development and progression of cataract.

Earlier studies (161–163) associated eye health with diet. Results of the First National Health and Nutrition Examination Survey (NHANES I) showed that the frequency of consumption of fruits and vegetables, vitamin A, and ascorbic acid as well as other antioxidants was negatively correlated with AMD after adjustment for demographic and medical factors (161). They suggested that long-term antioxidant deficiency may be related to the development of the disease. The Eye Disease Care Control Study (EDCCS) included an ancillary study that associated dietary intake to risk of development of AMD in 876 individuals (162) and showed that only carotenoid intake was associated with lower incidence of AMD. Vitamin E and vitamin C intakes were not associated with lower risk. The following is the conclusion of the EDCCS study: "Increasing the consumption of foods rich in certain carotenoids, in particular dark green, leafy vegetables may decrease the risk of developing advanced or exudative AMD, the most visually disabling form of macular degeneration among older people. These findings support the need for further studies of the relationship."

Pertinent to cataract development, in the Beaver Dam Eye Study (163) intakes of foods and specific nutrients were evaluated for associations to development of cataract. In men, several nutrients, including vitamins E, A, and C, were associated with 40–50% reduced odds of cataract development. It was not possible from this study to differentiate the effects of specific nutrients or other food components. Association with intake of green vegetables was as strong as those found for individual nutrients. Taylor and Hobbs (164) in a review of nutritional influences on cataract development covering the literature through 2001 stated that it is "clear that oxidative stress is associated with compromises to the lens." The author's conclusions after review of epidemiological studies included the following: "The overall impression created by the data indicates that

**TABLE 2.10** Epidemiological and Intervention Studies on Age-Related Eye Diseases[a]

| Study | Subjects | Observations | References |
|---|---|---|---|
| **Epidemiological studies** | | | |
| **Cataract** | | | |
| Beaver Dam Eye Study | 400 Subjects randomly picked from the Beaver Dam Eye Study | Evaluation of serum carotenoid and tocopherol levels indicated a possible inverse association between cataract development and vitamin E. An association between cataract and serum carotenoids was not supported or ruled out | 148 |
| **Age-related macular degeneration (AMD)** | | | |
| Beaver Dam Eye Study | 1709 Subjects followed for 10 yr | No significant inverse associations were found between antioxidant intake or zinc intake and incidence of early age-related maculopathy. The study could not assess whether antioxidant intake was associated with early progression of age-related maculopathy | 149 |
| Pathologies Oculaires Liées à l'Age (POLA) | 2584 Subjects | Plasma $\alpha$-T levels showed a weak negative association with late AMD | 150 |

(*continued*)

TABLE 2.10 *Continued*

| Study | Subjects | Observations | References |
|---|---|---|---|
| **Intervention studies** | | | |
| **Cataract** | | | |
| Blue Mountains Eye Study | 2900 Subjects aged 49–97 yr | Higher intakes of protein, vitamin A, niacin, thiamin, and riboflavin and long-term use of supplements were associated with reduced prevalence of nuclear cataract. Vitamin E was not studied because of lack of data on the vitamin E content of foods consumed in Australia | 151, 152 |
| Age-Related Eye Disease Study (AREDS) | 4757 Subjects received daily doses of 500 mg vitamin C, 400 IU vitamin E, 15 mg $\beta$-carotene, or 80 mg Zn and 2 mg Cu, or antioxidants plus Zn or placebo | Use of a high-dose formulation of antioxidants in well-nourished older adults had no apparent effect on 7-yr risk of development or progression of age-related lens opacity or visual acuity loss | 84 |
| Madrid, Spain | 17 Patients with cataracts supplemented with 15 mg lutein, 100 mg $\alpha$-T or placebo, 3 times per week for up to 2 yr | Visual performance improved in the lutein group. A trend toward maintenance of visual acuity was noted in the $\alpha$-T group | 153 |

| | | | |
|---|---|---|---|
| **Age-related macular degeneration** | | | |
| ATBC Cancer Prevention Study | 941 Subjects at the end of the ATBC study (see Table 2.8) | No beneficial effect of long-term supplementation with $\alpha$-T or $\beta$-carotene on the occurrence of age-related maculopathy was found | 154 |
| Age-Related Eye Disease Study (AREDS) | Follow-up on 3640 subjects after >6 yr of oral doses of 500 mg vitamin C, 400 IU vitamin E, 15 mg $\beta$-carotene, or 80 mg Zn and 2 mg Cu, or antioxidants plus Zn or placebo | Zn and antioxidants plus Zn significantly reduced the odds of development of advanced age-related macular degeneration in subjects older than 55 yr of age | 155–157 |
| Vitamin E, Cataract, and Age-Related Maculopathy Trial (VECAT) | 1193 Subjects aged 50–80 yr given 500 IU vitamin E (335 mg) RRR-$\alpha$-T or placebo daily for 4 yr | Vitamin E supplementation did not influence the development and progression of age-related macular degeneration, visual acuity, or changes in visual function | 158–159 |
| Influence of Short Term Supplementation on Age-Related Maculopathy | 30 Patients with early age-related maculopathy were given 15 mg lutein, 20 mg vitamin E, and 18 mg nicotinamide or no treatment for 180 days | No evidence was shown for long-term benefit of antioxidants on age-related maculopathy. Results suggested that increasing the level of retinal antioxidants might influence early stages of the disease process as well as the normal aging process | 160 |

[a]IU, international unit; $\alpha$-T, $\alpha$-tocopherol.

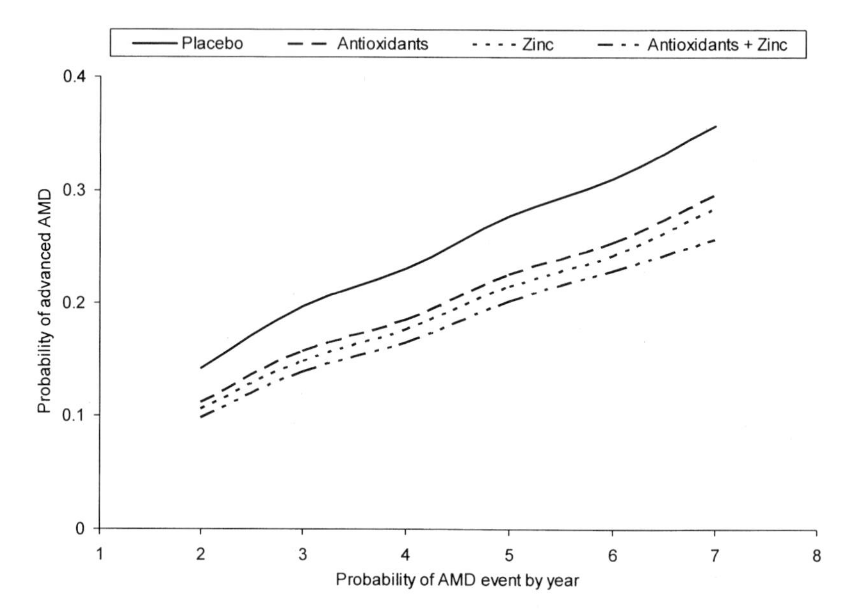


**FIGURE 2.4** Results of the Age-Related Eye Disease Study (AREDS). Probabilities of age-related molecular degeneration (AMD) of various treatments. (Modified from Ref. 155.)

nutrient intake is related to risk for cataract and that nutrition might be exploited to diminish risk for this debility." Evaluation of data specifically relating to vitamin E and cataract development provided "mixed" results.

## 2.3.5. Vitamin E and Other Diseases

**2.3.5.1. Neurodegenerative Diseases.** Neurodegenerative disease including Alzheimer's and Parkinson's disease are associated with aging, inflammatory processes, free radical damage, and other metabolic processes that influence well-being of the older population (165). Antioxidant intake has been postulated to influence onset and progression of many such disease states. Martin et al. (165) exhaustively reviewed the literature through 2000 on the roles of vitamins E and C on neurodegenerative disease and cognitive performance. Their general conclusion was that vitamin E and vitamin C have some protective effects on age-related deficits in behavioral function when vitamin intake is steady and started early in life. They further stated, "A rationale for possible clinical benefits of antioxidants for several degenerative conditions has arisen from the many years of basic science, including clinical and epidemiological studies. Substantial evidence implicates nutrition in the pathogenesis of neurodegenerative disease."

Since publication of the Martin et al. review (165), two significant epidemiological studies have been published on antioxidant intake and its relationship to Alzheimer's disease (166,167). Results of the Rotterdam Study(166) of 5395 subjects examined from 1990 to 1999 indicated that high dietary intake of vitamin E and vitamin C may lower the risk of Alzheimer's disease. In the highest tertile, subjects consumed $>15.5$ mg/day of vitamin E and $>133$ mg/day of vitamin C. $\beta$-Carotene and flavonoid intakes were not associated with decreased risk. Results of the Washington Heights–Inwood Columbia Aging Project involved 900 elderly subjects followed for 4 years. Over the study, Alzheimer's disease developed in 242. No association was found for intake of carotenoids, vitamin E, or vitamin C and Alzheimer's disease onset.

Tardive dyskinesia is characterized by excessive involuntary movement. Onset is common in individuals treated with antipsychotics. Its cause has been related to free radical damage associated with the treatment (168), and vitamin E has been used as a curative–preventative measure. Lohr et al. (168) reviewed the literature on oxidative mechanisms and tardive dyskinesia through 2001. Their conclusion was that vitamin E has limited use for treatment of the disease but that the area deserved further research.

**2.3.5.2. Inflammatory Disease.** Oxidative mechanisms are significant to the onset and progression of various inflammatory and autoimmune diseases including rheumatoid arthritis and systemic lupus erythematosus. In rheumatoid arthritis, antioxidants are thought to protect the tissue from damage by destroying reactive oxygen species produced by activated microphages, monocytes, and granulocytes and by suppressing the expression of cytokines and collagenase induced by tumor necrosis factor $\alpha$-9 (169). Antioxidant therapy has, therefore, been extensively studied as an alternative to accepted drug therapies (170). An extensive review of antioxidants and fatty acids in the amelioration of rheumatoid arthritis and related diseases indicated that combined supplementation with vitamin E and vitamin C is more effective than supplementation with either vitamin alone in prevention of inflammation associated with osteoarthritis (170). In the Iowa Women's Health Study supplemental vitamin E and vitamin C were inversely associated with rheumatoid arthritis. There was no association with total carotenoids, $\alpha$- or $\beta$-carotene, lycopene, or lutein/zeaxanthin. Inverse associations were noted for $\beta$-cryptoxanthin and supplemental zinc. Rennie et al. (171) in a general review of nutritional management of rheumatoid arthritis stated that dietary advice should be focused on a varied, balanced diet containing foods rich in antioxidants and adequate intake of iron, calcium, vitamin D, and water-soluble vitamins. Emphasis should be placed on increased intake of n-3 fatty acids.

### 2.3.6. Recent Recommendations on Vitamins and Chronic Disease Prevention

Fletcher and Fairfield (172,173) reviewed the use of vitamin supplements for chronic disease prevention and stated that suboptimal intake of some vitamins, at levels above those leading to classic vitamin deficiencies, can be risk factors for chronic diseases. They recommended that all adults take vitamin supplements tailored to their life situation and based on their doctor's advice. Specific responsibility was placed on the doctor to learn about their patients' use of vitamins to ensure proper supplement usage. Specific to vitamin E, recommendations for its use for reduction of prostate cancer were considered "premature." For use as a preventative against cardiovascular problems, the authors believed that the literature suggested that it might be useful in primary prevention when taken throughout long periods and that some subgroups of the population might benefit more that the general population.

Various recommendations about supplement use have been made by organizations associated with health care in the United States:

1. U.S. Preventative Services Task Force (174): Evidence is insufficient to recommend for or against the use of supplements of vitamins A, C, or E; multivitamins with folic acid; or antioxidant combinations for the prevention of cancer or cardiovascular disease.
2. American Academy of Family Physicians (175): The decision to provide special dietary intervention or nutrient supplementation must be on an individual basis using the family physician's best judgment based on evidence of benefit as well as lack of harmful effects.
3. American Heart Association (176): Vitamin or mineral substitutes are not a substitute for a balanced, nutritious diet that limits excess calories, saturated fat, trans fat, and dietary cholesterol. Scientific evidence does not suggest that consuming antioxidant vitamins can eliminate the need to reduce blood pressure, lower blood cholesterol level, or stop smoking.
4. American Cancer Society (177): Antioxidants are substances that protect the body's cells from damage caused by free radicals (by-products of the body's normal processes). Examples of antioxidants include vitamin C, vitamin E, $\beta$-carotene, and selenium. If you want to take in more antioxidants, health experts recommend eating a variety of fruits and vegetables, which are good sources of antioxidants. Taking large doses of antioxidant supplements is usually not recommended while undergoing chemotherapy and radiation therapy. Talk with your doctor to determine the best time to take antioxidant supplements.

## REFERENCES


1. Food and Nutrition Board. *Institute of Medicine. Dietary Reference Intakes for Vitamin C, Vitamin E, Selenium, and Carotenoids*; National Academy of Sciences Press: Washington, DC, 2000; 186–283.
2. Traber, M.G. Vitamin E. In *Modern Nutrition in Health and Disease*, 9th Ed.; Shils, M.E., Olson, J.A., Shike, M., Ross, A.C., Eds.; William and Wilkins: Baltimore, 1999; 347–362.
3. Frei, B.; Traber, M.G. The new US dietary reference intakes for vitamins C and E. Redox Report **2001**, *6*, 5–9.
4. Bramley, P.M.; Elmadfa, I.; Kafatos, A.; Kelly, F.J.; Manios, Y.; Roxborough, H.E.; Schuch, W.; Sheehy, P.J.A.; Wagner, K.H. Review vitamin E. J. Sci. Food. Agric. **2000**, *80*, 913–938.
5. Meydani, M.; Cohn, J.S.; Macauley, J.B.; McNamara, J.R.; Blumberg, J.B.; Schaefer, E.J. Postprandial changes in the plasma concentration of alpha- and gamma-tocopherol in human subjects fed a fat-rich meal supplemented with fat-soluble vitamins. J. Nutr. **1989**, *119*, 1252–1258.
6. Traber, M.G.; Kayden, H.J. Preferential incorporation of alpha-tocopherol vs. gamma-tocopherol in human lipoproteins. Am. J. Clin. Nutr. **1989**, *49*, 517–526.
7. Traber, M.G.; Burton, G.W.; Ingold, K.U.; Kayden, H.J. *RRR*- and *SRR*-alpha-tocopherols are secreted without discrimination in human chylomicrons, but *RRR*-alpha-tocopherol is preferentially secreted in very low density lipoproteins. J. Lipid Res. **1990**, *31*, 675–685.
8. Traber, M.G.; Burton, G.W.; Hughes, L.; Ingold, K.U.; Hidaka, H.; Malloy, M.; Kane, J.; Hyams, J.; Kayden, H.J. Discrimination between forms of vitamin E by humans with and without genetic abnormalities of lipoproteins metabolism. J. Lipid Res. **1992**, *33*, 1171–1182.
9. Traber, M.G.; Rader, D.; Acuff, R.; Brewer, H.B.; Kayden, H.J. Discrimination between *RRR*- and *all*-racemic-alpha-tocopherols labeled with deuterium by patients with abetalipoproteinemia. Atherosclerosis **1994**, *108*, 27–37.
10. Kiyose, C.; Muramatsu, R.; Fujiyama-Fujiwara, Y.; Ueda, T.; Igarashi, O. Biodiscrimination of alpha-tocopherol stereoisomers during intestinal absorption. Lipids **1995**, *30*, 1015–1018.
11. Traber, M.G.; Lane, J.C.; Lagmay, N.R.; Kayden, H.J. Studies on the transfer of tocopherols between lipoproteins. Lipids **1992**, *27*, 657–663.
12. Lichtenstein, A.H.; Jones, P.J.H. Lipids: Absorption and Transport. In *Modern Nutrition in Health and Disease*, 8th Ed.; Bowman, B.A., Russell, R.M., Eds.; ILSI Press: Washington, DC, 2001; 92–103.
13. Traber, M.G.; Rudel, L.L.; Burton, G.W.; Hughes, L.; Ingold, K.U.; Kayden, H.J. Nascent VLDL from liver perfusions of cynomolgus monkeys are preferentially enriched in *RRR*- compared with *SRR*-alpha-tocopherol: studies using deuterated tocopherols. J. Lipid Res. **1990**, *31*, 687–694.
14. Catignani, G.L.; Bieri, J.G. Rat liver alpha-tocopherol binding protein. Biochim. Biophys Acta **1977**, *497*, 349–357.
15. Sato, Y.; Hayiwara, K.; Arai, H.; Inoue, K. Purification and characterization of the alpha-tocopherol transfer protein from rat liver. FEBS Lett. **1991**, *288*, 41–45.

16. Yoshida, H.; Yusin, M.; Ren, I.; Kuhlenkamp, J.; Hirano, T.; Stolz, A.; Kaplowitz, N. Identification, purification and immunochemical characterization of a tocopherol-binding protein in rat liver cytosol. J. Lipid Res. **1992**, *33*, 343–350.
17. Kuhlenkamp, J.; Ronk, M.; Yusin, M.; Stolz, A.; Kaplowitz, N. Identification and purification of a human liver cytosolic tocopherol binding protein. Protein Expr. Purif. **1993**, *4*, 382–389.
18. Arita, M.; Sato, Y.; Miyata, A.; Tanabe, T.; Takahashi, E.; Kayden, H.; Arai, H.; Inoue, K. Human alpha-tocopherol transfer protein: cDNA cloning, expression, and chromosomal localization. Biochem. 1995 J. *306*, 437–443.
19. Hosomi, A.; Arita, M.; Sato, Y.; Kiyose, C.; Ueda, T.; Igarashi, O.; Arai, H.; Inoue, K. Affinity for alpha-tocopherol transfer protein as a determinant of the biological activities of vitamin E analogs. FEBS Lett. **1997**, *409*, 105–108.
20. Carpenter, D.L.; Slover, H.T. Lipid composition of selected margarines. JAOCS **1973**, *50*, 372–376.
21. Weiser, H.; Vecchi, M. Stereoisomers of alpha-tocopheryl acetate: Characterization of the samples by physico-chemical methods and determination of biological activities in the rat resorption-gestation test. Int. J. Vitam. Nutr. Res. **1981**, *51*, 100–113.
22. Friedrich, W. Vitamin E. In *Vitamins*; Walter de Gruyter: New York, 1988; 215–283.
23. National Research Council. *Recommended Dietary Allowances*, 10th Ed.; National Academy Press: Washington, DC, 1989; 99–100.
24. United States Pharmacopeial Convention. *U.S. Pharmacopeia National Formulory. USP 25/NF20. Nutritional Supplements, Official Monographs*; United States Pharmacopeial Convention: Rockville, MD, 2002.
25. Pryor, W.A. *Vitamin E Abstracts*; VERIS, The Vitamin E Research and Information Service: LaGrange, IL: 1995; VII pp.
26. Eitenmiller, R.R.; Landen, W.O., Jr. Vitamin E. In *Vitamin Analysis for the Health and Food Sciences*; CRC Press: Boca Raton, 1998; 109–148.
27. 21 CFR 107. Infant Formula.
28. Bieri, J.G.; Evarts, R.P. Tocopherols and fatty acids in American diets: The recommended allowance for vitamin E. J. Am. Diet. Assoc. **1973**, *62*, 147–151.
29. Bieri, J.G.; Evarts, R.P. Gamma-tocopherol: Metabolism, biological activity and significance in human vitamin E nutrition. Am. J. Clin. Nutr. **1974**, *27*, 980–986.
30. McLaughlin, J.; Weihrauch, J. Vitamin E content of foods. J. Am. Diet. Assoc. **1979**, *75*, 647–665.
31. National Research Council. *Recommended Dietary Allowances*, 9th Ed.; National Academy of Sciences: Washington, DC, 1980; 64 pp.
32. Murphy, S.P. Dietary reference intakes for the U.S. and Canada: Update on implications for nutrient databases. J. Food Compos. Anal. **2002**, *15*, 411–417.
33. Murphy, S.P.; Subar, A.F.; Block, G. Vitamin E intakes and sources in the United States. Am. J. Clin. Nutr. **1990**, *52*, 361–367.
34. Haytowitz, D. USDA Nutrient Data Laboratory, Personal communication, 2003.
35. United States Department of Agriculture, Agricultural Research Service. USDA Nutrient Database for Standard Reference, Release 16, Nutrient Data Laboratory

Home Page. http://www.nal.usda.gov/fnic/foodcomp. Nutrient Data Laboratory, USDA: Riverdale, MD, 2003.
36. Eitenmiller, R.R. Vitamin E content of fats and oils—nutritional implications. Food Technol. **1997**, *51*, 78–81.
37. Rader, D.J.; Brewer, H.B. Abetalipoproteinemia—new insights into lipoprotein assembly and vitamin E metabolism from a rare genetic disease. JAMA **1993**, *270*, 865–869.
38. Gordon, N. Hereditary vitamin E deficiency. Dev. Med. Child Neurol. **2001**, *43*, 133–135.
39. Wetterau, J.R.; Aggerbeck, L.P.; Laplaud, P.M.; McLean, L.R. Structural properties of the microsomal triglyceride-transfer protein complex. Biochemistry **1991**, *30*, 4406–4412.
40. Wetterau, J.R.; Aggerbeck, L.P.; Bouma, M.E.; Eisenberg, C.; Munck, A.; Hermier, M.; Schmitz, J.; Gay, G.; Rader, D.J.; Gregg, R.E. Absence of microsomal triglyceride transfer protein in individuals with abetalipoproteinemia. Science **1992**, *258*, 999–1001.
41. Stumpf, D.A.; Sokol, R.; Bettis, D.; Neville, H.; Ringel, S.; Angelini, C.; Bell, R. Friedreich's disease. V. Variant form with vitamin E deficiency and normal fat absorption. Neurology **1987**, *37*, 68–74.
42. Hamida, M.B.; Belal, S.; Sirugo, G.; Hamida, C.B.; Panayides, K.; Ionannou, P.; Beckmann, J.; Mandel, J.L.; Hentati, F.; Koenig, M.; Middleton, L. Friedreich's ataxia phenotype not linked to chromosome 9 and associated with selective autosomal recessive vitamin E deficiency in two inbred Tunisian families. Neurology **1993**, *43*, 2179–2183.
43. Hamida, C.B.; Doerflinger, N.; Belal, S.; Linder, C.; Reutenauer, L.; Dib, C.; Gyapay, G.; Vignal, A.; Le Paslier, L.; Cohen, D.; Pandolfo, M.; Mokini, V.; Novelli, G.; Hentati, F.; Hamida, M.B.; Mandel, J.-L.; Koenig, M. Localization of Friedreich ataxia phenotype with selective vitamin E deficiency to chromosome 8q by homozygosity mapping. Nat. Genet. **1993**, *5*, 195–200.
44. Ouahchi, K.; Arita, M.; Kayden, H.; Hentati, F.; Hamida, M.B.; Sokol, R.; Arai, H.; Inoue, K.; Mandel, J.-L.; Koenig, M. Ataxia with isolated vitamin E deficiency is caused by mutations in the $\alpha$-tocopherol transfer protein. Nat. Genet. **1995**, *9*, 141–145.
45. Cavalier, L.; Ouahchi, K.; Kayden, H.J.; Di Donato, S.; Reutenauer, L.; Mandel, J.-L.; Koenig, M. Ataxia with isolated vitamin E deficiency: heterogeneity of mutations and phenotypic variability in a large number of families. Am. J. Hum. Genet. **1998**, *62*, 301–310.
46. Feki, M.; Belal, S.; Feki, H.; Souissi, M.; Frih-Ayed, M.; Kaabachi, N.; Hentati, F.; Hamida, M.B.; Mebazaa, A. Serum vitamin E and lipid-adjusted vitamin E assessment in Friedreich ataxia phenotype patients and unaffected family members. Clin. Chem. **2002**, *48*, 577–579.
47. Olsen, R.E.; Munson, P.L. Fat-soluble vitamins. In *Principles of Pharmacology*; Munson, P.L., Mueller, R.A., Breese, G.R., Eds.; Chapman and Hall: New York, 1994; 927–947.

48. Tanyel, M.C.M.; Mancano, L.D. Neurological findings in vitamin E deficiency. Am. Fam. Physician **1997**, *55*, 197–201.
49. McCarron, M.O.; Russell, A.J.C; Metcalfe, R.A.; Deysilva, R. Chronic vitamin E deficiency causing spinocerebellar degeneration, peripheral neuropathy and centrocecal scotomata. Nutrition **1999**, *15*, 217–219.
50. Tappel, A.L. Vitamin E. In *The Vitamins: Fundamental Aspects in Nutrition and Health*; Combs, G.F., Ed.; Academic Press: California, 1992; 179–203.
51. Kappus, H.; Diplock, A.T. Tolerance and safety of vitamin E: a toxicological position report. Free Radic. Biol. Med. **1992**, *13*, 55–74.
52. Abdo, K.M.; Rao, G.; Montgomery, C.A.; Dinowitz, M.; Kanagalingam, K. Thirteen week toxicity study of d-alpha-tocopheryl acetate (vitamin E) in Fischer 344 rats. Food Chem. Toxicol. **1986**, *24*, 1043–1050.
53. Dysmsza, H.A.; Park, J. Excess dietary vitamin E in rats. Fed. Am. Soc. Exp. Biol. **1975**, *34*, 912–916.
54. Krasavage, W.J.; Terhaar, C.J. d-alpha-Tocopheryl poly(ethylene glycol) 1000 succinate: acute toxicity, subchronic feeding, reproduction, and teratologic studies in the rat. J. Agric. Food Chem. **1977**, *25*, 273–278.
55. Anderson, T.W.; Reid, D.B. A double-blind trial of vitamin E in angina pectoris. Am. J. Clin. Nutr. **1974**, *27*, 1174–1178.
56. Tsai, A.C.; Kelley, J.J.; Peng, B.; Cook, N. Study on the effect of megavitamin E supplementation in man. Am. J. Clin. Nutr. **1978**, *31*, 831–837.
57. Bendich, A.; Machlin, L.J. Safety of oral intake of vitamin E. Am. J. Clin. Nutr. **1998**, *48*, 612–619.
58. Machlin, L.J. Use and safety of elevated dosages of vitamin E in adults. Int. J. Vitam. Nutr. Res. **1989**, *30*, 56–68.
59. March, B.E.; Wong, E.; Seier, L.; Sim, J.; Biely, J. Hypervitaminosis E in the chick. J. Nutr. **1973**, *103*, 371–377.
60. Wheldon, G.H.; Bhatt, A.; Keller, P.; Hummler, H. *d,l*-Alpha-tocopheryl acetate (vitamin E): long-term toxicity and carcinogenicity study in rats. Int. J. Vitam. Nutr. Res. **1983**, *53*, 287–296.
61. Takahashi, O.; Ichikawa, H.; Sasaki, M. Hemorrhagic toxicity of d-alpha-tocopherol in the rat. Toxicology **1990**, *63*, 157–165.
62. Harman, D. Aging: a theory based on free radical and radiation chemistry. Gerontology **1956**, *11*, 298–300.
63. Harman, D. Role of free radicals in mutation, cancer, aging, and the maintenance of life. Radiat. Res. **1962**, *16*, 753–763.
64. Harman, D. The biological clock: the mitochondria? J. Am. Geriatr. Soc. **1972**, *20*, 145–147.
65. Harman, D. The aging process. Proc. Natl. Acad. Sci. USA **1981**, *78*, 7124–7128.
66. Harman, D. Free radical theory of aging: History. In *Free Radicals and Aging*; Emerit, I., Chance, B., Eds.; Birkhauser: Basel, 1992; 1–10.
67. Harman, D. Free-radical theory of aging: increasing the functional life span. Ann. NY Acad. Sci. **1994**, *717*, 1–15.
68. Harman, D. Free radical theory of aging: Alzheimers disease pathogenesis. Age **1995**, *18*, 97–119.

69. Packer, L.; Landvik, S. Vitamin E: introduction to biochemistry and health benefits. In *Vitamin E Biochemistry and Health Implications*; Diplock, A.T., Machlin, L.J., Packer, L., Pryor, W.A., Eds.; Ann. NY Acad. Sci. **1989**, *570*, 1–6.
70. Pryor, W.A. Vitamin E: the status of current research and suggestions for future studies. In *Vitamin E Biochemistry and Health Implications*; Diplock, A.T., Machlin, L.J., Packer, L., Pryor, W.A., Eds.; Ann. NY Acad. Sci. **1989**, *570*, 400–405.
71. Rimm, E.B.; Stampfer, M.J.; Ascherio, A.; Giovannucci, E.; Colditz, G.A.; Willett, W.C. Vitamin E consumption and the risk of coronary heart disease in men. N. Engl. J. Med. **1993**, *328*, 1450–1456.
72. Stampfer, M.J.; Hennekens, C.H.; Manson, J.E.; Colditz, G.A.; Rosner, B.; Willett, W.C. Vitamin E consumption and the risk of coronary disease in women. N. Engl. J. Med. **1993**, *328*, 1444–1449.
73. Knekt, P.; Reunanen, A.; Jarvinen, R.; Seppanen, R.; Heliovaara, M.; Aromaa, A. Antioxidant vitamin intake and coronary mortality in the longitudinal population study. Am. J. Epidemiol. **1994**, *139*, 1180–1189.
74. Kushi, L.H.; Folsom, A.R.; Prineas, R.J.; Mink, P.J.; Wu, Y.; Bostick, R.M. Dietary antioxidant vitamins and death from coronary heart disease in postmenopausal women. N. Engl. J. Med. **1996**, *334*, 1156–1162.
75. Losonczy, K.G.; Harris, T.B.; Havlik, R.J. Vitamin E and vitamin C supplement use and the risk of all-cause and coronary heart disease mortality in older persons: the established populations for epidemiologic studies of the elderly. Am. J. Clin. Nutr. **1996**, *64*, 190–196.
76. Azen, S.P.; Mack, W.J.; Cashin-Hemphill, L.; Labree, L.; Shircore, A.M.; Selzer, R.H.; Blankenhorn, D.H.; Hodis, H.N. Progression of coronary artery disease predicts clinical coronary events: long-term follow-up from the cholesterol lowering Atheroclerosis study. Circulation **1996**, *93*, 34–41.
77. Azen, S.P.; Qian, D.; Mack, W.J.; Sevanian, A.; Selzer, R.H.; Liu, C.R.; Liu, C.H.; Hodis, H.N. Effect of supplementary antioxidant vitamin intake on carotid arterial wall intima-media thickness in a controlled clinical trial of cholesterol lowering. Circulation **1996**, *94*, 2369–2372.
78. Hodis, H.N.; Mack, W.J.; Laßree, L.; Cashin-Hemphill, L.; Sevanian, A.; Johnson, R.; Azen, S.P. Serial coronary angiographic evidence that antioxidant vitamin intake reduces progression of coronary artery atherosclerosis. JAMA **1995**, *273*, 1849–1854.
79. The Alpha-Tocopherol, Beta Carotene cancer prevention study group: the effect of vitamin E and beta carotene on the incidence of lung cancer and other cancers in male smokers. N. Engl. J. Med. **1994**, *330*, 1029–1035.
80. Rapola, J.M.; Virtamo, J.; Ripatti, S.; Huttunen, J.K.; Albanes, D.; Taylor, P.R.; Heinonen, O.P. Randomized trial of alpha-tocopherol and beta-carotene supplements on incidence of major coronary events in men with previous myocardial infarction. Lancet **1997**, *349*, 1715–1720.
81. Stephens, N.G.; Parsons, A.; Schofield, P.M.; Kelly, F.; Cheeseman, K.; Mitchinson, M.J.; Brown, M.J. Randomized controlled trial of vitamin E in patients with coronary disease: Cambridge heart antioxidant study (CHAOS). Lancet **1996**, *347*, 781–786.

82. GISSI—Prevenzione Investigators. Dietary supplementation with n-3 polyunsaturated fatty acids and vitamin E after myocardial infarction: results of the GISSI—Prevenzione Trial. Lancet **1999**, *354*, 447–455.
83. The Heart Outcomes Prevention Evaluation Study Investigators. Vitamin E supplementation and cardiovascular events in high risk patients. N. Engl. J. Med. **2000**, *342*, 154–160.
84. Age-Related Eye Disease Study Research Group. A randomized, placebo-controlled, clinical trial of high-dose supplementation with vitamins C and E and beta carotene for age-related cataract and vision loss: AREDS report No. 9. Arch. Ophthalmol. **2001**, *119*, 1439–1452.
85. Collaborative Group of the Primary Prevention Project (PPP). Low dose aspirin and vitamin E in people at cardiovascular risk: a randomized trial in general practice. Lancet **2001**, *357*, 89–95.
86. Heart Protection Study Collaborative Group, MRC/BHF. Heart Protection Study of antioxidant vitamin supplementation in 20,536 high-risk individuals: a randomized placebo-controlled trial. Lancet **2002**, *360*, 23–33.
87. Salonen, J.T.; Nyyssönen, K.; Salonen, R., et al. Antioxidant supplementation in atherosclerosis prevention (ASAP) study: a randomized trial of the effect of vitamins E and C on 3-year progression of carotid atherosclerosis. J. Intern. Med. **2000**, *248*, 377–386.
88. Salonen, R.M.; Nyyssonen, K.; Kaikkonen, J.; Porkkala-Sarataho, E.; Voutilainen, S.; Rissanen, T.H.; Tuomainen, T.P.; Valkonen, V.P.; Ristonmaa, U.; Lakka, H.M.; Vanharanta, M.; Salonen, J.T.; Poulsen, H.E. Six-year effect of combined vitamin C and E supplementation on atherosclerotic progression: the antioxidant supplementation in atherosclerosis prevention (ASAP) Study. Circulation **2003**, *107*, 947–953.
89. Bruunsgaard, H.; Poulsen, H.E.; Pedersen, B.K.; Nyyssonen, K.; Kaikkonen, J.; Salonen, J.T. Long-term combined supplementation with $\alpha$-tocopherol and vitamin C have no detectable anti-inflammatory effects in healthy men. J. Nutr. **2003**, *133*, 1170–1173.
90. Boaz, M.; Smetana, S.; Weinstein, T.; Matas, Z.; Gafter, U.; Laina, A.; Knecht, A.; Weissgarten, Y.; Brunner, D.; Fainaru, M.; Green, M.S. Secondary prevention with antioxidants of cardiovascular disease in endstage renal disease (SPACE): randomized, placebo-controlled trial. Lancet **2000**, *356*, 1213–1218.
91. Yochum, L.A.; Folsom, A.R.; Kushi, L.H. Intake of antioxidant vitamins and risk of death from stroke in postmenopausal women. Am. J. Clin. Nutr. **2000**, *72*, 476–483.
92. Vivekananthan, D.P.; Penn, M.S.; Sapp, S.K.; Hsu, A.; Topol, E.J. Use of antioxidant vitamins for the prevention of cardiovascular disease: meta-analysis of randomized trials. Lancet **2003**, *361*, 2017–2023.
93. FDA/CFSAN. Consumer Health Information for Better Nutrition Initiative: Task Force Final Report, July 10, 2003. http://www.cpsan.fda.gov/~dms/nuttftoc.html.
94. FDA/CFSAN. Consumer Health Information for Better Nutrition Initiative: Task Force Final Report, Attachment E—Interim Procedures for Qualified Health Claims. Guidance: Interim Procedures for Qualified Health Claims in the Labeling

of Conventional Human Food and Human Dietary Supplements, July 10, 2003. http://www.cfsan.fda.gov/~dms/nuttftoc.html.
95. FDA/CFSAN. FDA's Implementation of "Qualified Health Claims": Questions and Answers, August 27, 2003. http://www.cfsan.fda.gov/~dms/labqhcqa.html.
96. FDA/CFSAN. Response to Health Claim Petition Regarding Dietary Supplements of Vitamin E and Reduced Risk of Heart Disease. Docket No. 99P-4375. January 11, 2001. http://www.cfsan.fda.gov/~dms/nuttftoc.html.
97. FDA/CFSAN. Letter Regarding Dietary Supplement Health Claim for Vitamin E and Heart Disease. Docket No. 99P-4375, February 9, 2001. http://www.dfsan.fda.gov/~dms/nuttftoc.html.
98. Keaney, J.F., Jr, Simon, D.I.; Freedman, J.E. Vitamin E and vascular homeostasis: implications for atherosclerosis. FASEB J. **1999**, *13*, 965–976.
99. Traber, M.G. Does vitamin E decrease heart attack risk? Summary and implications with respect to dietary recommendations. J. Nutr. **2001**, *131*, 395S–397S.
100. Dutta, A.; Dutta, S.K. Vitamin E and its role in the prevention of atherosclerosis and carcinogenesis: a review. J. Am. Coll. Nutr. **2003**, *22*, 258–268.
101. Gey, K.F. Vitamin E plus C and interacting conutrients required for optimal health. Biofactors **1998**, *7*, 113–174.
102. Block, G. The data support a role for antioxidants in reducing cancer risk. Nutr. Rev. **1992**, *50*, 207–213.
103. Byers, T.; Guerrero, N. Epidemiologic evidence for vitamin C and vitamin E in cancer prevention. Am. J. Clin. Nutr. **1995**, *62*, 13855–13925.
104. Tzonou, A.; Signorello, L.B.; Lagiou, P.; Wuu, J.; Trichopoulos, D.; Trichopoulou, A. Diet and cancer of the prostate: a case-control study in Greece. Int. J. Cancer **1999**, *80*, 704–708.
105. 21CFR 101.78. Fruits and vegetables and cancer.
106. FDA/CFSAN. Letter Regarding Dietary Supplement Health Claim for Antioxidant Vitamins and Certain Cancers. May 4, 2001. Docket No. 91N-0101. http://www.cfsan.fda.gov/~dms/nuttftoc.html.
107. FDA/CFSAN. Letter Regarding Dietary Supplement Health Claim for Antioxidant Vitamins and Risk of Certain Cancers. April 1, 2003. http://www.cfsan.fda.gov/~dms/nuttftoc.html.
108. Yong, L.C.; Brown, C.C; Schatzkin, A.; Dresser, C.M.; Slesinski, M.J.; Cox, C.S.; Taylor, P.R. Intake of vitamins E, C, and A and risk of lung cancer: the NHANES I epidemiologic followup study. Am. J. Epidemiol. **1997**, *146*, 231–243.
109. Comstock, G.W.; Alberg, A.J.; Huang, H.Y.; Wu, K.; Burke, A.E.; Hoffman, S.C.; Norkus, E.P.; Gross, M.; Cutler, R.G.; Morris, J.S.; Spate, V.L.; Helzlsouer, K.J. The risk of developing lung cancer associated with antioxidants in the blood: ascorbic acid, carotenoids, alpha-tocopherol, selenium, and total peroxyl radical absorbing capacity. Cancer Epidemiol. Biomarker Prev. **1997**, *6*, 907–916.
110. Verhoeven, D.T.; Assen, N.; Goldbohm, R.A.; Dorant, E.; van t'Veer, P.; Sturmans, F.; Hermus, R.J. van den Brandt, P.A. Vitamins C and E, retinol, beta-carotene and dietary fiber in relation to breast cancer risk: a prospective cohort study. Br. J. Cancer **1997**, *75*, 149–155.

111. Eichholzer, M.; Stahelin, H.B.; Gey, K.F.; Ludin, E.; Bernasconi, F. Prediction of male cancer mortality by plasma levels of interacting vitamins: 17 Year followup of the prospective Basel study. Int. J. Cancer **1996**, *66*, 145–150.
112. van t'Veer, P.; Strain, J.J; Fernandez-Crehuet, J.; Martin, B.C.; Thamm, M.; Kardinal, A.F.; Kohlmeirer, L.; Huttunen, J.K.; Martin-Moreno, J.M.; Kok, F.J. Tissue antioxidants and postmenopausal breast cancer: the European community multicentre study on antioxidants, myocardial infarction and cancer of the breast (EURAMIC). Cancer Epidem. Biomar. **1996**, *5*, 441–447.
113. Dorgan, J.F.; Sowell, A.; Swanson, C.A.; Potischman, N.; Miller, R.; Schussler, N.; Stephenson, H.E. Jr. Relationships of serum carotenoids, retinol, alpha-tocopherol, and selenium with breast cancer risk: results from a prospective study in Columbia, Missouri (United States). Cancer Cause Control **1998**, *9*, 89–97.
114. Comstock, G.W.; Bush, T.L.; Helzlsouer, K. Serum retinol, beta-carotene, vitamin E, and selenium as related to subsequent cancer of specific sites. Am. J. Epidemiol. **1992**, *135*, 115–121.
115. Andersson, S.O.; Wolk, A.; Bergstrom, R.; Giovannucci, E.; Lindgren, C.; Baron, J.; Adami, H.O. Energy nutrient intake and prostate cancer risk: a population-based case-control study in Sweden. Int. J. Cancer **1996**, *68*, 716–722.
116. Knekt, P.; Aromaa, A.; Maatela, J.; Aaran, R.K.; Nikkari, T.; Hakama, M.; Hokulinen, T.; Peto, R.; Saxen, E.; Teppo, L. Serum vitamin E and risk of cancer among Finnish men during a 10-year follow-up. Am. J. Epidemiol. **1988**, *127*, 28–41.
117. Hainonen, O.P.; Albanes, D.; Virtamo, J.; Taylor, P.R.; Huttunen, J.K.; Hartman, A.M.; Haapakoski, J.; Malila, N.; Rautalahti, M.; Ripatti, S.; Mäenpää, H.; Teerenhovi, L.; Koss, L.; Virolainen, M.; Edwards, B.K. Prostate cancer and supplementation with alpha-tocopherol and beta-carotene: Incidence and mortality in a controlled trial. J. Natl. Cancer Inst. **1998**, *90*, 440–446.
118. London, R.S.; Sundaram, G.S.; Murphy, L.; Manimekalai, S.; Reynolds, M.; Goldstein, P.J. The effect of vitamin E on mammary dysplasia: a double-blind study. Obstet. Gynecol. **1985**, *65*, 104–106.
119. Ernster, V.L.; Goodson, W.H.; Hunt, T.K.; Petrakis, N.L.; Sickles, E.A.; Miike, R. Vitamin E and benign breast "disease": A double-blind, randomized clinical trial. Surgery **1985**, *97*, 490–494.
120. Chen, L.H.; Boissonnaeault, G.A.; Glauert, H.P. Vitamin C, vitamin E and cancer. Anticancer Res. **1998**, *8*, 739–748.
121. Decrosse, J.J.; Miller, H.H.; Lesser, M.L. Effect of wheat fiber and vitamins C and E on rectal polyps in patients with familial adenomatous polyposis. J. Natl. Cancer Inst. **1989**, *81*, 1290–1297.
122. Greenberg, E.R.; Baron, J.A.; Tosteson, T.D.; Freeman, D.H.; Beck, G.J.; Bond, J.H.; Colacchio, T.A.; Coller, J.A.; Frankl, H.D.; Haile, R.W.; Mandel, J.S.; Nierenberg, D.W.; Rothstein, R.; Snover, D.C.; Stevens, M.M.; Summers, R.W.; van Stolk, R.U. A clinical trial of antioxidant vitamins to prevent colorectal adenoma. N. Engl. J. Med. **1994**, *331*, 141–147.
123. Hofstad, B.; Almendingen, K.; Vatn, M.; Andersen, S.; Owen, R.; Larsen, S.; Osnes, M. Growth and recurrence of colorectal polyps: a double-blind 3-year intervention with calcium and antioxidants. Digestion **1998**, *59*, 148–156.

124. McKeown-Eyssen, G.; Holloway, C.; Jazmaji, V.; Bright-See, E.; Dion, P.; Bruce, W.R. A randomized trial of vitamins C and E in the prevention of recurrence of colorectal polyps. Cancer Res. **1988**, *48*, 4701–4705.
125. Michaud, D.S.; Spiegelman, D.; Clinton, S.K.; Rimm, E.B.; Willett, W.C.; Giovannucci, E. Prospective study of dietary supplements, macronutrients, micronutrients, and risk of bladder cancer in US men. Am. J. Epidemiol. **2000**, *152*, 1145–1153.
126. Virtamo, J.; Edwards, B.K.; Virtanen, M.; Taylor, P.R.; Malila, N.; Albanes, D.; Huttunen, J.K.; Hartman, A.M.; Hietanen, P.; Mäenpää, H.; Koss, L.; Nordling, S.; Heinonen, O.P. Effects of supplemental alpha-tocopherol and beta-carotene on urinary tract cancer: incidence and mortality in a controlled trial (Finland). Cancer Cause Control **2000**, *11*, 933–939.
127. Zeegers, M.P.A.; Goldbohm, R.A.; van den Brandt, P.A. Are retinol, vitamin C, vitamin E, folate and carotenoids intake associated with bladder cancer risk? Results from the Netherlands cohort study. Br. J. Cancer **2001**, *85*, 977–983.
128. Jacobs, E.J.; Henion, A.K.; Briggs, P.J.; Connell, C.J.; McCullough, M.L.; Jonas, C.R.; Rodriguez, C.; Calle, E.E.; Thun, M.J. Vitamin C and vitamin E supplement use and bladder cancer mortality in a large cohort of US men and women. Am. J. Epidemiol. **2002**, *156*, 1002–1010.
129. Albanes, D.; Malila, N.; Taylor, P.R.; Huttunen, J.K.; Virtamo, J.; Edwards, B.K.; Rautalahti, M.; Hartman, A.M.; Barrett, M.J.; Pietinen, P.; Hartman, T.J.; Sipponen, P.; Lewin, K.; Teerenhovi, L.; Hietanen, P.; Tangrea, J.A.; Virtanen, M.; Heinonen, O.P. Effects of supplemental alpha-tocopherol and beta-carotene on colorectal cancer: Results from a controlled trial (Finland). Cancer Cause Control **2000**, *11*, 197–205.
130. Jacobs, E.J.; Connell, C.J.; Patel, A.V.; Chao, A.; Rodriguez, C.; Seymour, J.; McCullough, M.L.; Calle, E.E.; Thun, M.J. Vitamin C and vitamin E supplement use and colorectal cancer mortality in a large American cancer society cohort. Cancer Epidem. Biomar. **2001**, *10*, 17–23.
131. Wu, K.; Willett, W.C.; Chan, J.M.; Fuchs, C.S.; Colditz, G.A.; Rimm, E.B.; Giovannucci, E.L. A prospective study on supplemental vitamin E intake and risk of colon cancer in women and men. Cancer Epidem. Biomar. **2002**, *11*, 1298–1304.
132. Jacobs, E.J.; Connell, C.J.; McCullough, M.L.; Chao, A.; Jonas, C.R.; Rodriguez, C.; Calle, E.E.; Thun, M.J. Vitamin C, vitamin E, and multivitamin supplement use and stomach cancer mortality in the cancer prevention study II Cohort. Cancer Epidem. Biomar. **2002**, *11*, 35–41.
133. Chan, J.M.; Stampfer, M.J.; Ma, J.; Rimm, E.B.; Willett, W.C.; Giovannucci, E.L. Supplemental vitamin E intake and prostate cancer risk in a large cohort of men in the United States. Cancer Epidem. Biomar. **1999**, *8*, 893–899.
134. Moyad, M.A. Selenium and vitamin E supplements for prostate cancer: evidence or embellishment? Urology **2002**, *59*, 9–19.
135. Cook, E.D. Selenium and vitamin E cancer prevention trial—this one's for us. J. Natl. Med. Assoc. **2002**, *94*, 856–858.
136. Klein, E.A.; Lippman, S.M.; Thompson, I.M.; Goodman, P.J.; Albanes, D.; Taylor, P.R.; Coltman, C. The selenium and vitamin E cancer prevention trial. World J. Urol. **2003**, *21*, 21–27.

137. Klein, E.A.; Thompson, I.M.; Lippman, S.M.; Goodman, J.P.; Albanes, D.; Taylor, P.R.; Coltman, C. SELECT: the selenium and vitamin E cancer prevention trial. Urol Oncol-Semin. O. I. **2003**, *21*, 59–65.
138. Mohan, M.; Sperduto, R.; Angra, S.; Milton, R.; Mathur, R.; Underwood, B.; Jaffery, N.; Pandya, C.; Chhabra, V.; Vajpayee, R.B.; Kalra, V.K.; Sharma, Y.R.; India-US case-control study of age-related cataracts. Arch. Ophthalmol. **1989**, *107*, 670–676.
139. Robertson, J.M.c.D.; Donner, A.P.; Trevithick, J.R. Vitamin E intake and risk for cataracts in humans. Ann. NY Acad. Sci. **1989**, *570*, 372–382.
140. Jacques, P.F.; Chylack, L.T., Jr. Epidemiologic evidence of a role for the antioxidant vitamins and carotenoids in cataract prevention. Am. J. Clin. Nutr. **1991**, *53*, 352S–355S.
141. Leske, M.C.; Chylack, L.T., Jr, Wu, S.Y. The lens opacities case-control study—risk factors for cataract. Arch. Ophthalmol. **1991**, *109*, 244–251.
142. Hankinson, S.E.; Stampfer, M.J.; Seddon, J.M.; Colditz, G.A.; Rosner, B.; Speizer, F.E.; Willett, W.C. Nutrient intake and cataract extraction in women: a prospective study. Br. Med. J. **1992**, *305*, 335–339.
143. Vitale, S.; West, S.; Hallfrisch, J.; Alston, C.; Wang, F.; Moorman, C.; Muller, D.; Singh, V.; Taylor, H.R. Plasma antioxidants and risk of cortical and nuclear cataract. Epidemiology **1993**, *4*, 195–203.
144. Knekt, P.; Heliovaara, M.; Rissanen, A.; Aromaa, A.; Aaran, R.K. Serum antioxidant vitamins and risk of cataract. Br. Med. J. **1992**, *305*, 1392–1394.
145. Mares-Perlman, J.A.; Klein, B.K.; Klein, R.; Ritter, L.L. Relation between lens opacities and vitamin and mineral supplement use. Ophthalmology **1994**, *101*, 315–325.
146. Mares-Perlman, J.A.; Brady, W.E.; Klein, R.; Klein, B.K.; Palta, M.; Bowen, P.; Stacewicz-sapuntzakis, M. Serum levels of carotenoids and tocopherols in people with age-related maculopathy. Invest. Ophthalmol. Vis. Sci. **1994**, *35*, 2004–2004.
147. Teikari, J.M.; Rautalahti, M.; Haukka, J.; Jarvinen, P.; Harman, A.M.; Virtamo, J.; Albanes, D.; Heinonen, O. Incidence of cataract operations in Finnish male smokers unaffected by alpha tocopherol or beta carotene supplements. J. Epidemiol. Community Health **1998**, *52*, 468–472.
148. Lyle, B.J.; Mares-Perlman, J.A.; Klein, B.E.K.; Klein, R.; Palta, M.; Bowen, P.E.; Greger, J.L. Serum carotenoids and tocopherols and incidence of age-related nuclear cataract. Am. J. Clin. Nutr. **1999**, *69*, 272–277.
149. VandenLangenberg, G.M.; Mares-Perlman, J.A.; Klein, R.; Klein, B.E.K.; Brady, W.E.; Palta, M. Associations between antioxidant and zinc intake and the 5-year incidence of early age-related maculopathy in the Beaver Dam eye study. Am. J. Epidemiol. **1998**, *148*, 204–214.
150. Delcourt, C.; Cristol, J.-P.; Tessier, F.; Léger, C.L.; Descomps, B.; Papoz, L.; POLA Study Group. Age-related macular degeneration and antioxidant status in the POLA Study. Arch. Ophthalmol. **1999**, *117*, 1384–1390.
151. Cumming, R.G.; Mitchell, P.; Smith, W. Diet and cataract—the blue mountains eye study. Ophthalmology **2000**, *107*, 450–456.
152. Kuzniarz, M.; Mitchell, P.; Cumming, R.G.; Flood, V.M. Use of vitamin supplements and cataract: the blue mountains eye study. Am. J. Epidemiol. **2001**, *132*, 19–26.

153. Olmedilla, B.; Granado, F.; Blanco, I.; Vaquero, M. Lutein, but not α-tocopherol, supplementation improves visual function in patients with age-related cataracts: A 2-y double-blind, placebo-controlled pilot study. Nutrition **2003**, *19*, 21–24.
154. Teikari, J.M.; Laatikainen, L.; Virtamo, J.; Haukka, J.; Rautalahti, M.; Liesto, K.; Albanes, D.; Taylor, P.; Heinonen, O.P. Six-year supplementation with alpha-tocopherol and beta-carotene and age-related maculopathy. Acta Ophthalmol. Scand. **1998**, *76*, 224–229.
155. Age-Related Eye Disease Study Research Group. A randomized, placebo-controlled, clinical trial of high-dose supplementation with vitamins C and E, beta carotene, zinc for age-related macular degeneration and vision loss. Arch. Ophthalmol. **2001**, *119*, 1417–1436.
156. Hammond, B.R.; Johnson, M.A. The age-related eye disease study (AREDS). Nutr. Rev. **2002**, *60*, 283–288.
157. Gaynes, B.I. AREDS misses on safety. Arch. Ophthalmol. **2003**, *121*, 416–417.
158. Taylor, H.R.; Tikellis, G.; Robman, L.D.; McCarty, C.A.; McNeil, J.J. Vitamin E supplementation and macular degeneration: randomized controlled trial. Br. Med. J. **2002**, *325*, 11–14.
159. Hall, N.F. Prevention of age related macular degeneration. Br. Med. J. *325*, 1–2.
160. Falsini, B.; Piccardi, M.; Iarossi, G.; Fadda, A.; Merendino, E.; Valentini, P. Influence of short-term antioxidant supplementation on macular function in age-related maculopathy. Ophthalmology **2003**, *110*, 51–61.
161. Goldberg, J.; Flowerdew, G.; Smith, E.; Brody, J.A.; Tso, M.O.M. Factors associated with age-related macular degeneration. Am. J. Epidemiol. **1988**, *128*, 700–710.
162. Seddon, J.M.; Ajani, U.A.; Sperduto, R.D.; Hiller, R.; Blair, N.; Burton, T.C.; Farber, M.D.; Gragoudas, E.S.; Haller, J.; Miller, D.T.; Yannuzzi, L.A.; Willett, W. Dietary carotenoids, vitamins A, C, and E, and advanced age-related macular degeneration. JAMA **1994**, *272*, 1413–1420.
163. Mares-Perlman, J.A.; Brady, W.E.; Klein, B.E.K.; Klein, R.; Haus, G.J.; Palta, M.; Ritter, L.L.; Shoff, S.M. Diet and nuclear lens opacities. Am. J. Epidemiol. **1995**, *141*, 322–334.
164. Taylor, A.; Hobbs, M. 2001 assessment of nutritional influences on risk for cataract. Nutrition **2001**, *17*, 845–857.
165. Martin, A.; Youdim, K.; Szprengiel, A.; Shukitt-Hale, B.; Joseph, J. Roles of vitamins E and C on neurodegenerative diseases and cognitive performance. Nutr. Rev. **2002**, *60*, 308–326.
166. Engelhart, M.J.; Geerlings, M.I.; Ruitenberg, A.; van Swieten, J.C.; Hofman, A.; Witteman, J.C.M.; Breteler, M.M.B. Dietary intake of antioxidants and risk of Alzheimer disease. JAMA **2002**, *287*, 3223–3229.
167. Luchsinger, J.A.; Tang, M.-X.; Shea, S.; Mayeux, R. Antioxidant vitamin intake and risk of Alzheimer Disease. Arch. Neurol. **2003**, *60*, 203–208.
168. Lohr, J.B.; Kuczenski, R.; Niculescu, A.B. Oxidative mechanisms and tardive dyskinesia. CNS Drugs **2003**, *17*, 47–62.
169. Cerhan, J.R.; Saag, K.G.; Merlino, L.A.; Mikuls, T.R.; Criswell, L.A. Antioxidant micronutrients and risk of rheumatoid arthritis in a cohort of older women. Am. J. Epidemiol. **2003**, *157*, 345–354.

170. Darlington, L.G.; Stone, T.W. Antioxidants and fatty acids in the amelioration of rheumatoid arthritis and related disorders. Br. J. Nutr. **2001**, *85*, 251–269.
171. Rennie, K.L.; Hughes, J.; Lang, R.; Jebb, S.A. Nutritional management of rheumatoid arthritis: a review of the evidence. J. Hum. Nutr. Dietet **2003**, *16*, 97–109.
172. Fairfield, K.M.; Fletcher, R.H. Vitamins for chronic disease prevention in adults. J. Am. Med. Assoc. **2002**, *287*, 3116–3126.
173. Fletcher R.H.; Fairfield, K.M. Vitamins for chronic disease prevention in adults. JAMA **2002**, *287*, 3127–3129.
174. U.S. Preventive Service Task Force. Routine vitamin supplementation to prevent cancer and cardiovascular disease: recommendations and rationale. Ann. Intern. Med. **2003**, *139*, 51–55.
175. American Academy of Family Physicians. AAFP Clinical Recommendations, Vitamin. http://www.aafp.org/x2590.xml, 2003.
176. American Heart Association. Vitamin and mineral supplements. http://www.americanheart.org/presenter.jhtml?identifier=4788, 2003.
177. American Cancer Society. Effects of supplements on cancer treatment. http://www.cancer.org/docroot/MBC/MBC_6_1_DietarySupplements.asp, 2003.

# 3

# Oxidation and the Role of Vitamin E as an Antioxidant in Foods

## 3.1. INTRODUCTION

Lipid oxidation is a degradative free radical reaction that causes loss of shelf life, palatability, functionality, and nutritional quality of oils, fats, and foods containing unsaturated lipids (1). Moreover, there is growing interest in the problem of lipid oxidation as related to health status. Lipid oxidation in vivo is believed to play an important etiological role in coronary heart disease, atherosclerosis, cancer, the aging process, and many disease states (2,3). Therefore, ingestion of foods containing oxidized lipids is of concern since the products of lipid oxidation may promote in vivo oxidation.

Vitamin E compounds (tocopherols and tocotrienols) are well recognized for their effective inhibition of lipid oxidation in foods and biological systems, and their mechanism as antioxidants is also well understood. It is widely accepted that the antioxidant activity of the tocopherols and tocotrienols is mainly due to their ability to donate their phenolic hydrogens to lipid free radicals. Lesser impact is achieved through singlet oxygen quenching. Extensive research that has occurred over many decades has identified natural antioxidants, led to the availability of many excellent synthetic antioxidants, and provided in-depth understanding of mechanisms of antioxidant action. Recent reviews of food antioxidants include Reische et al. (1), Frankel (2), Jadhav et al. (3), Nawar (4), Shahidi and Naczk(5) Decker (6,7), McClements and Decker (8), Kamal-Eldin and Appelqvist (9), Erickson (10) and Morrissey et al. (11). One of the most useful reviews, which specifically deals with the antioxidant properties of tocopherols and tocotrienols with emphasis on reaction mechanisms, was prepared by Kamal-Eldin and Appelqvist (9).

## 3.2. LIPID OXIDATION

Initiation of autoxidation occurs when an $\alpha$-methylenic hydrogen molecule is abstracted from an unsaturated fatty acid by exposure of lipids to catalysts such as light, heat, ionizing radiation, or metal ions or through the action of lipoxygenase to form a lipid (alkyl) radical (R·) (Eq. 1) (1,5).

$$RH \longrightarrow R\cdot + H\cdot \quad (1)$$

The high reactivity of lipid radicals with triplet oxygen leads to the rapid formation of a peroxy radical (ROO·) in a propagation reaction (Eq. 2).

$$R\cdot + O_2 \longrightarrow ROO\cdot + H\cdot \quad (2)$$

Peroxy radicals react with unsaturated fatty acids to form a hydroperoxide and a new unstable lipid radical (Eq. 3). This lipid radical then reacts with oxygen to produce another peroxy radical, resulting in a self-catalyzing oxidative mechanism (Eq. 4), hence, the name *autoxidation*. The formation of the alkyl free radical (R·) represents a significant self-propagating reactant for the autocatalytic chain reaction.

$$ROO\cdot + RH \longrightarrow ROOH + R\cdot \quad (3)$$

$$R\cdot + O_2 \longrightarrow ROO\cdot + H\cdot \quad (4)$$

Hydroperoxides are unstable to chemical and environmental conditions and can break down to produce radicals that further accelerate propagation reactions. These reactions are typically referred to as *branching steps* or *secondary decomposition reactions* (Eqs. 5 and 6). The decomposition of the hydroperoxide is often homolytic in its progression, rapidly occurring at elevated temperatures.

$$ROOH \longrightarrow RO\cdot + OH \quad (5)$$

$$RO\cdot + RH \longrightarrow ROH + R\cdot \quad (6)$$

Secondary decomposition products are responsible for causing rancid off-flavors as well as providing reactants that result in a complex interaction with other substances. The overall effects are reduced shelf life, oxidized off-flavor, and lower nutritional value of foods containing oxidizing lipid systems (1,5,12).

## 3.3. ANTIOXIDANTS

Antioxidants delay the onset of oxidation or slow the rate at which it proceeds. These substances can occur as natural constituents of foods, be intentionally added as a natural or synthetic antioxidant, or, as is the case for Maillard reaction products, be formed during processing (1). Their role is not to enhance or improve the quality of foods but to maintain food quality and extend shelf life by preventing or delaying oxidation of labile fatty acids and lipid-soluble components (1,12). The schematic presented in Figure 3.1 is an overview of lipid oxidation in food and the interaction of antioxidants (1).

### 3.3.1. Primary and Secondary Antioxidants

Antioxidants may be classified as primary antioxidants and secondary antioxidants on the basis of their function. Some antioxidants show more than one mechanism of activity and are often referred to as *multiple-function antioxidants* (1). Primary, or chain-breaking, antioxidants are free radical acceptors that delay or inhibit the initiation step or interrupt the propagation step of autoxidation by donating a hydrogen to a radical originating in the food. At this point, alkyl and peroxy radicals are converted to more stable, nonradical products by hydrogen atoms donated by the antioxidant. The antioxidant radicals (A·) that are produced at this stage are more stable and less readily available to promote further autoxidation. As hydrogen donors, primary antioxidants have higher affinities for peroxy radicals than unsaturated fatty acids (6). Therefore, free radicals formed during the propagation steps of autoxidation are scavenged by the primary antioxidants (Eqs. 7 and 8). Antioxidants may also interact directly with lipid radicals (Eq. 9).

$$\mathrm{ROO\cdot + AH \longrightarrow ROOH + A\cdot} \tag{7}$$

$$\mathrm{RO\cdot + AH \longrightarrow ROH + A\cdot} \tag{8}$$

$$\mathrm{R\cdot + AH \longrightarrow RH + A\cdot} \tag{9}$$

The antioxidant radical produced by hydrogen donation has a very low reactivity with lipids. This low reactivity reduces the rate of propagation, since reaction of the antioxidant radical with oxygen or lipids is very slow compared to the reactivity of the lipid free radicals (1). Factors influencing free radical scavenging of phenolic antioxidants include the following (5,6):

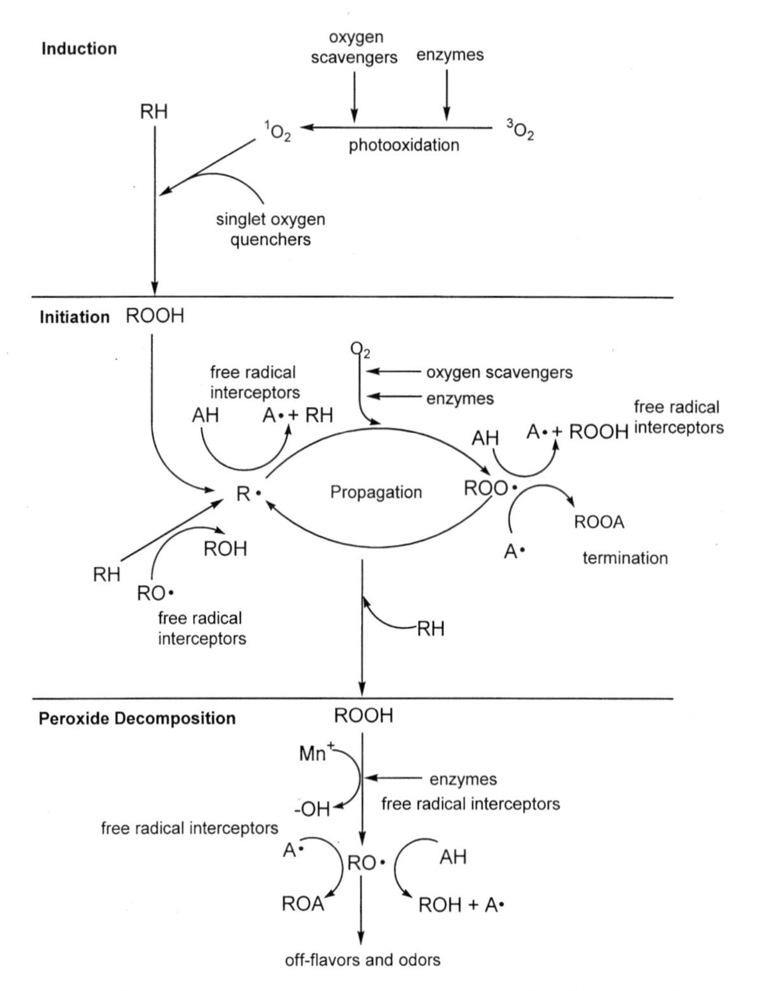


**FIGURE 3.1** Overview of lipid oxidation in food. (Modified from Ref. 1.)

1. Antioxidants primarily react with peroxy radicals that are present in higher concentration than other radical species. Peroxy radicals react more readily with low-energy hydrogens of the antioxidant because of their lower energy when compared to other radicals.
2. Antioxidants do not compete effectively with radicals significant to the initiation stage of the reaction (R·, ·OH).
3. Antioxidant efficiency depends on the ability of the free radical scavenger to donate hydrogen to the free radical.

4. The hydrogen bond energy of the antioxidant influences its ability to donate hydrogen. As the bond energy of the antioxidant decreases, its ability to transfer hydrogen to the free radical increases.
5. The ability of an antioxidant to donate hydrogen can be predicted from standard one-electron reduction potentials. Compounds with lower reduction potentials than the reduction potential of a free radical can donate hydrogen to the free radical. The reduction potential ($E^{0'}$) of $\alpha$-tocopherol ($\alpha$-T) is 500 mV compared to 1000 mV for the peroxy radical; therefore, $\alpha$-T can donate hydrogen to the free radical.
6. The most efficient antioxidants form low-energy free radicals produced by resonance delocalization of the unpaired electrons throughout the phenolic ring. Resonance stabilization of the $\alpha$-T radical system is depicted in Figure 3.2.
7. Good antioxidants do not produce radicals that react rapidly with oxygen to form peroxides.
8. Substitution of the phenol ring influences the effectiveness of the antioxidant.
   a. Alkyl groups in the ortho and para positions increase the reactivity of the hydroxyl hydrogen with lipid radicals.
   b. Bulky substitutions at the ortho position increase the stability of phenoxy radicals.
   c. A second hydroxy group at the ortho or para position stabilizes the phenoxy radical through an intramolecular hydrogen bond.

Antioxidant radicals are capable of participating in termination reactions with peroxy (Eq. 10), oxy (Eq. 11), and other lipid radicals as well as with other antioxidant free radicals (Eq. 12). The formation of antioxidant dimers is possible in fats and oils, indicting that phenolic antioxidant radicals readily undergo termination reactions.

$$\mathrm{ROO\cdot} + \mathrm{A\cdot} \longrightarrow \mathrm{ROOA} \tag{10}$$

$$\mathrm{RO\cdot} + \mathrm{A\cdot} \longrightarrow \mathrm{ROA} \tag{11}$$

$$\mathrm{A\cdot} + \mathrm{A\cdot} \longrightarrow \mathrm{AA} \tag{12}$$

Termination reactions effectively stop the autocatalytic free radical chain mechanism as long as the antioxidant remains active. However, termination reactions involving antioxidant radicals decrease the antioxidant concentration, since the products cannot be recycled back to the active antioxidant form. Antioxidant capacity of tocopherol dimers and trimers is largely unstudied.

Before initiation of autoxidation, there must be an induction period in which antioxidants are consumed and free radicals are generated. Therefore,

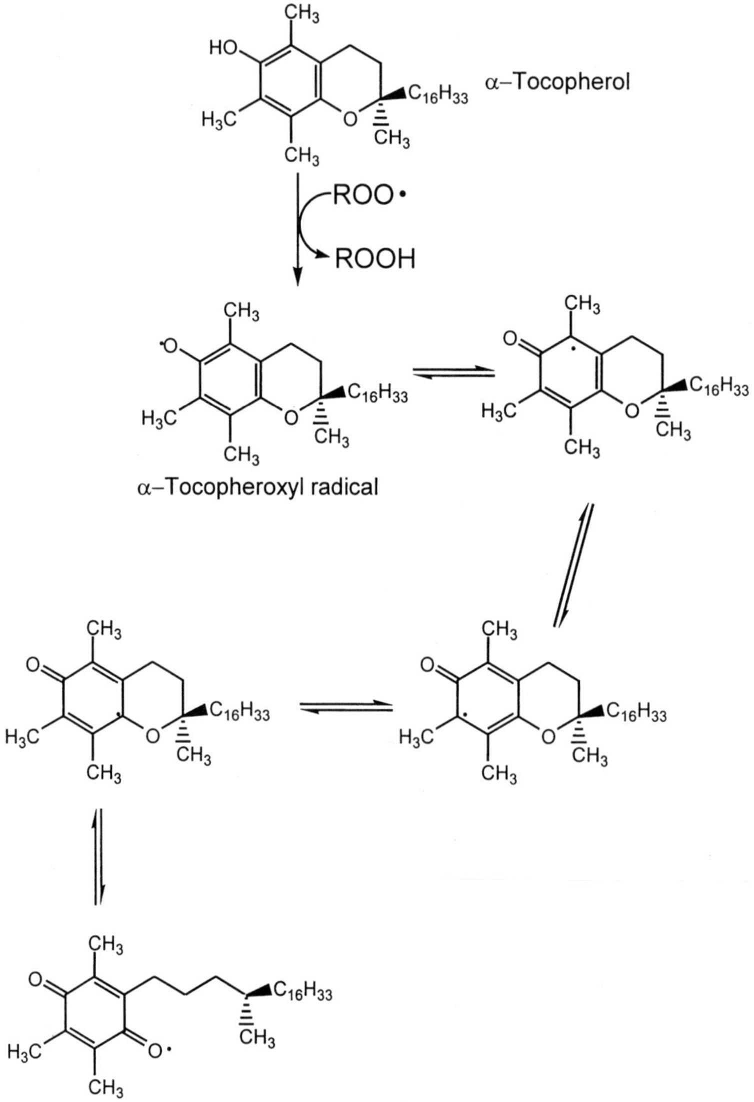

**FIGURE 3.2** Resonance stabilization of $\alpha$-tocopherol. (Modified from Refs. 4 and 6.)

primary antioxidants are most effective if they are present during the induction and initiation stages of oxidation before propagation.

The most commonly used primary antioxidants in foods are synthetic compounds as a result of their cost, availability, and reactivity. Examples of important primary phenolic antioxidants include butylated hydroxyanisole (BHA), butylated hydroxytoluene (BHT), propyl gallate (PG), ethoxyquin, and tertiary butylhydroquinone (TBHQ) (Figure 3.3). Tocopherols are the most commonly used natural primary antioxidants.

Secondary, or preventive, antioxidants act through numerous possible mechanisms. They can chelate prooxidant metals and deactivate them, replenish hydrogen to primary antioxidants, inactivate hydroperoxides to nonradical species, quench singlet oxygen, absorb ultraviolet radiation, or act as oxygen scavengers. These antioxidants are often referred to as *synergists* because they promote the antioxidant activity of primary antioxidants. Citric acid, ascorbic

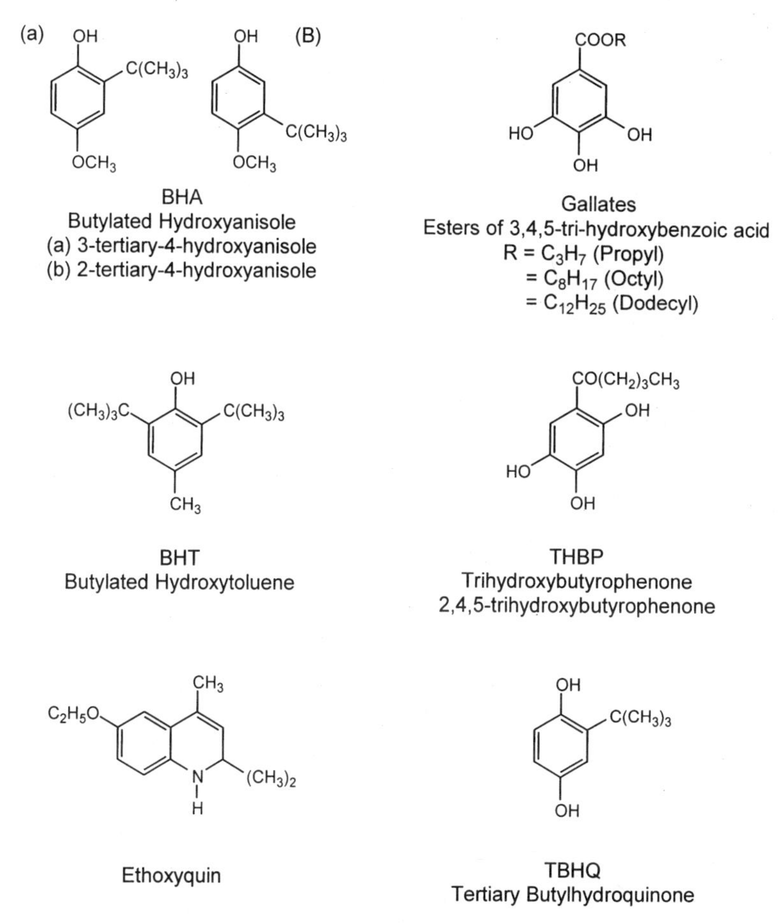


**FIGURE 3.3** Structures of commonly used synthetic antioxidants.

acid, ascorbyl palmitate, lecithin, and tartaric acid are good examples of synergists (1). Natural secondary antioxidants such as the carotenoids often possess excellent singlet oxygen–quenching properties (Figure 3.4). Chemical and physical factors participating in control of oxidation of foods and other biological systems are summarized in Table 3.1 (7).

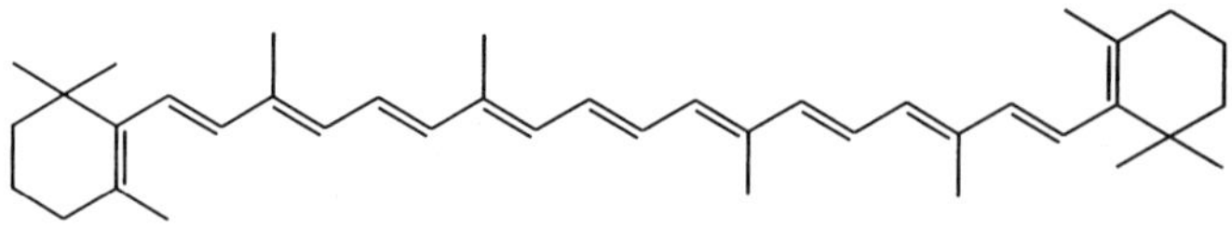

β-Carotene

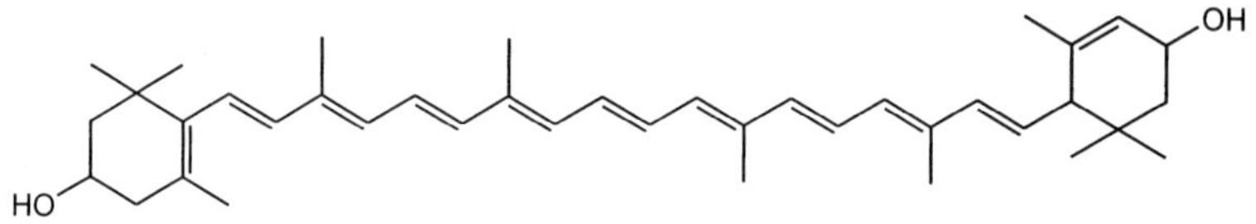

Lutein

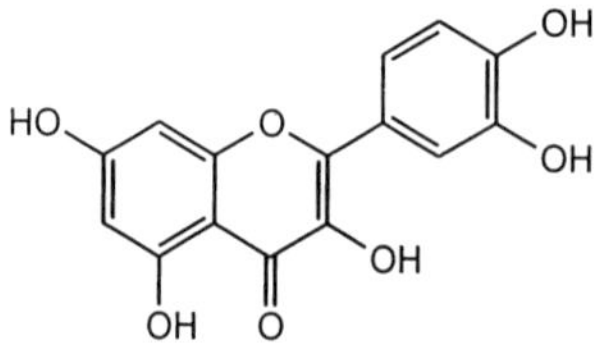

Quercetin Flavonols

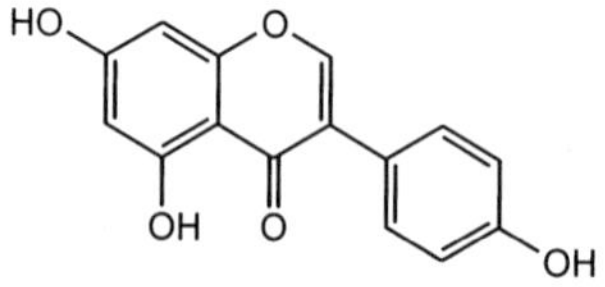

Genistein Isoflavones

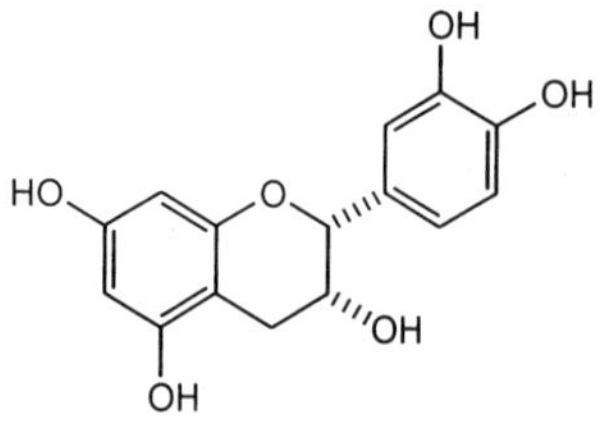

Epicatechin

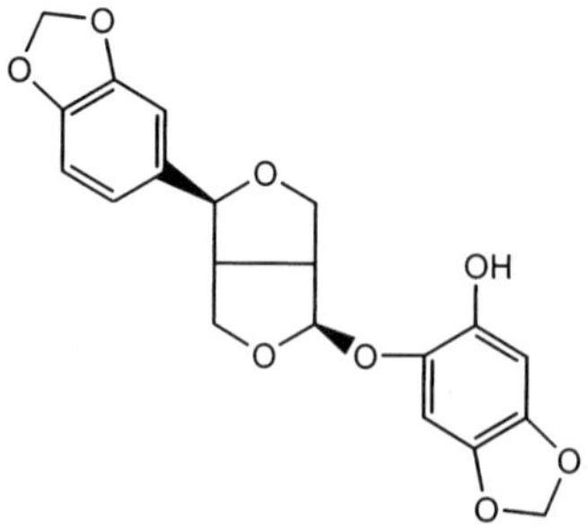

Sesaminol

**FIGURE 3.4** Structures of commonly occurring compounds with secondary antioxidant capacity.

**TABLE 3.1** Factors Involved in the Oxidative Stability of Foods Providing Control Points for Antioxidants

| Chemical |
| --- |
| Control of free radicals |
| Control of lipid oxidation catalysts |
| Prooxidant metals |
| Singlet oxygen |
| Lipoxygenase |
| Inactivation of oxidation intermediates |
| Superoxide anion |
| Peroxides |
| Photoactivated sensitizer |
| Alterations in lipid oxidation breakdown products |
| Antioxidant interactions |
| **Physical** |
| Interfacial charges of dispersed lipids |
| Inhibition of oxygen diffusion |
| Metal chelation |
| Physical state of the lipid |
| Liquid |
| Crystals |

*Source*: Modified from Ref. 7.

### 3.3.2. Vitamin E as an Antioxidant

The effectiveness of vitamin E as an antioxidant in a specific matrix is difficult to predict from published studies because of the variation in experimental conditions used to conduct such research. Studies often apply to oxidation in model systems and/or to specific food matrices under highly variable environmental and chemical conditions. Adding complexity to the interpretation of results, methods of determining antioxidant action are quite diverse in what is measured and how the experimental results are reported. It is often difficult to compare results from investigation to investigation, even if the same matrix is studied. The relative antioxidant activities of the tocopherols in vivo are $\alpha$-T > $\beta$-T > $\gamma$-T > $\delta$-T; however, relative antioxidant activities in model and food systems are variable (9). Conditions influenced by experimental design, chemical properties of the food matrix, and environmental factors all interact to add to the complexity of oxidation events and to the variability noted for antioxidant efficiencies of the tocopherols and tocotrienols. Factors that influence the antioxidant activity of the various forms of vitamin E are discussed in the following sections of the chapter.

**3.3.2.1. Structural Requirements and Tocopherol Reactions During Lipid Oxidation.** Unsubstituted phenols are inactive as hydrogen donors; thus, the hydroxyl group at position 6 of the chromanol ring provides the hydrogen for donation to lipid free radicals (Figure 3.2). Because of this simple structural requirement, formation of the ester bond at the position 6 hydroxyl eliminates the antioxidant activity of $\alpha$-T when converted to $\alpha$-tocopheryl acetate. Variation in relative antioxidant efficiencies of tocopherols and tocotrienols is related to the presence and stereochemical characteristics of electron-releasing substituents in the ortho- and/or para-position to the hydroxyl substituent (position 6) (9,13). Kamal-Eldin and Appelqvist (9) summarized the following antioxidant characteristics of tocopherols and tocotrienols:

1. Chromanols are believed to be the most efficient natural lipid antioxidants. The phytyl tails provide excellent lipid solubility.
2. Peroxy radicals react with tocopherols many times faster than with acyl lipids. Therefore, one tocopherol molecule can protect many magnitude greater numbers of polyunsaturated fatty acid molecules.
3. Antioxidants must form radicals that are not reactive with stable molecules such as molecular oxygen, lipids, and lipid peroxides. Their reactive capability should be limited to donation of hydrogens to radicals and to termination reactions.
4. The chromanol ring is stabilized by resonance delocalization of the chromanoxyl radical at position 6 after donation of the phenolic hydrogen (Figure 3.2).
5. The delocalization of the unpaired electrons induces radical sites on the ortho- and para-positions relative to the hydroxyl group (Figure 3.2).
6. Electron-releasing groups at the ortho- and/or para-position to the hydroxyl at position 6 increase the electron density of the active centers. This effect facilitates homolytic fission of the O—H bond, increases the stability of the phenoxyl radical, and improves the statistical chances for reaction with peroxy radicals (9,14,15).
7. $\alpha$-T, because of the presence of two ortho-methyl groups, is expected to be a better antioxidant than $\beta$-, $\gamma$-, and $\delta$-T.
8. Carbon-centered alkyl radicals have more affinity for the phenoxyl oxygen, whereas oxygen-centered radicals prefer to add to an ortho- or para-position of the phenoxyl radical. Substitution at the ortho-position 5 accounts for the differences in antioxidant activity noted between $\alpha$- and $\beta$-T and $\gamma$- and $\delta$-T.
9. The ortho-position 7 is sterically hindered. Therefore, ortho-position 5 is the primary site for radical–radical (termination) reactions.

10. Peroxy radicals oxidize $\alpha$-T primarily to 8a-peroxy-tocopherone, which degrades to $\alpha$-tocopherylquinone (Figure 3.5).

**3.3.2.2. $\alpha$-Tocopherol Reactions.** Pathways for the interaction of $\alpha$-T in an autoxidizing lipid system as presented by Kamal-Eldin and Appelqvist (9) are shown in Figures 3.5 and 3.6. Some routes for $\gamma$-T are presented in Figure 3.7 (16–18). Antioxidant action for $\alpha$-T proceeds through the following steps (9,19–22).

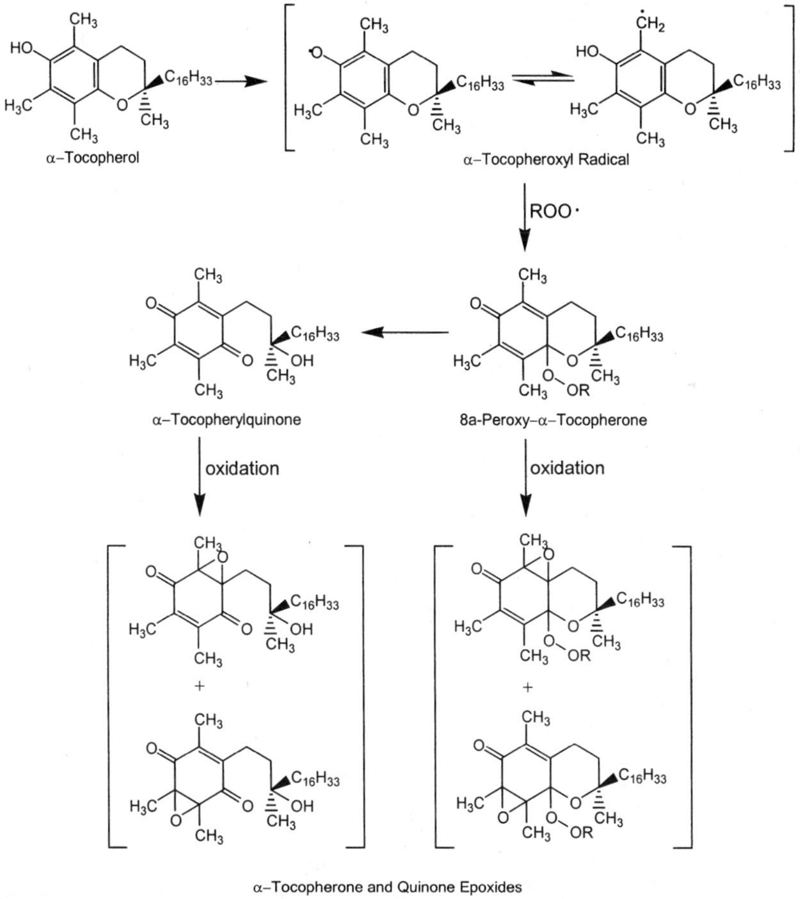

$CH_3$ HO $H_3C$ O $C_{16}H_{33}$ $CH_3$ $CH_3$
α–Tocopherol

•O $CH_3$ $H_3C$ O $C_{16}H_{33}$ $CH_3$ $CH_3$ ⇌ HO $\dot{C}H_2$ $H_3C$ O $C_{16}H_{33}$ $CH_3$ $CH_3$
α–Tocopheroxyl Radical

ROO·

O $CH_3$ $H_3C$ O $C_{16}H_{33}$ $CH_3$ O OR $CH_3$
8a-Peroxy–α–Tocopherone

O $CH_3$ $H_3C$ O $C_{16}H_{33}$ OH $CH_3$ $CH_3$
α–Tocopherylquinone

oxidation

oxidation

O $CH_3$ O $H_3C$ O $C_{16}H_{33}$ OH $CH_3$ $CH_3$ + O $CH_3$ $H_3C$ O O $C_{16}H_{33}$ OH $CH_3$ $CH_3$

O $CH_3$ O $H_3C$ O $C_{16}H_{33}$ $CH_3$ O OR $CH_3$ + O $CH_3$ $H_3C$ O O $C_{16}H_{33}$ $CH_3$ O OR $CH_3$

α–Tocopherone and Quinone Epoxides

**FIGURE 3.5** Formation of 8a-peroxy-$\alpha$-tocopherones, $\alpha$-tocopherylquinone, tocopherone, and quinone epoxides. (Modified from Ref. 9.)

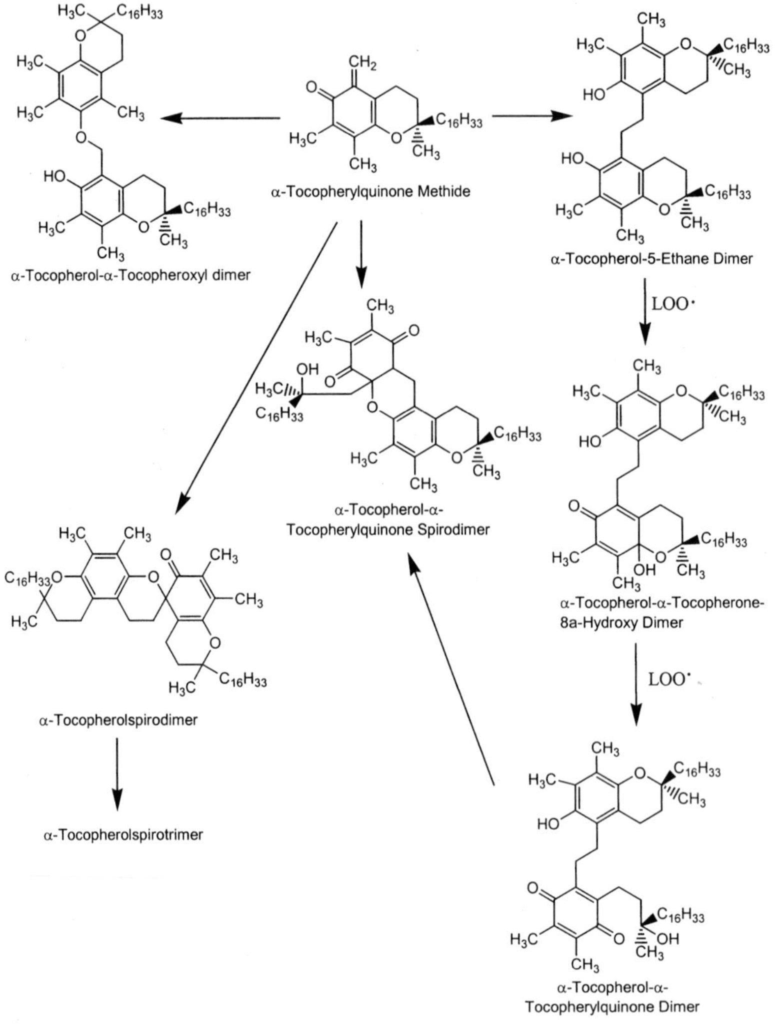

**FIGURE 3.6** Formation of dimers and trimers from $\alpha$-tocopherylquinone methide intermediate. (Modified from Ref. 9.)

1. $\alpha$-T reacts with peroxyl radicals with the formation of hydroperoxides and the $\alpha$-tocopheroxyl radical, which is resonance stabilized.
2. The $\alpha$-tocopheroxyl radical forms 8a-substituted tocopherones through peroxyl addition at C-8a, yielding 8a-(peroxy)-tocopherones or 8a-(hydroxy)-tocopherones through electron transfer and hydrolysis (Figure 3.5).

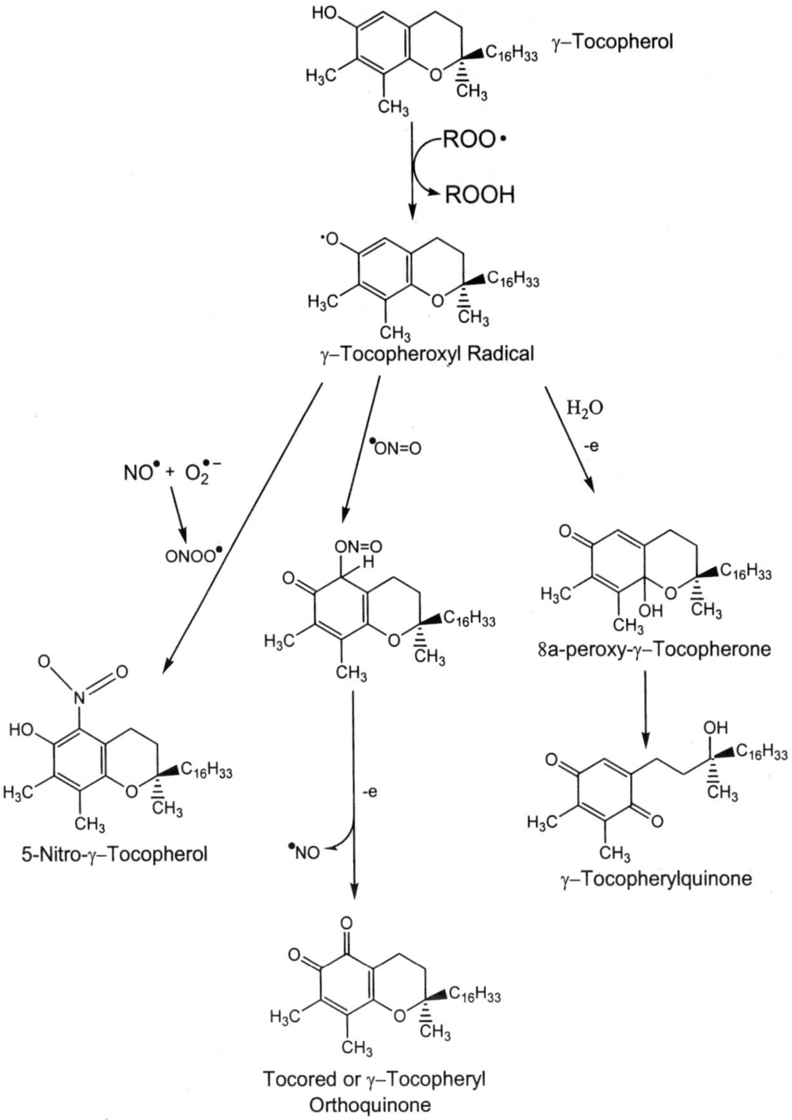

**FIGURE 3.7** γ-Tocopherol reactions with oxygen radicals and nitrogen oxide species. (Modified from Refs. 16 and 17.)

3. The tocopherones yield $\alpha$-tocopherylquinone through hydrolysis and rearrangement.
4. The tocopheroxyl radical dimerizes through the tocopherol-5-ethane dimer (Figure 3.6).
5. Further reactions yield various dimers, trimers, spirodimers, spirotrimers, and epoxides.
6. Tocotrienols are thought to yield radicals and polymers similar to their respective tocopherols.

**3.3.2.3. $\gamma$-Tocopherol Reactions.** Excellent studies by Ishikawa and Yuki(23) and Ishikawa(24) characterized dimerization of the tocopherols through synergistic reaction with trimethylamine oxide (TMAO). Reaction products of $\gamma$-T in the presence of TMAO during autoxidation of methyl linoleate were $\gamma$-T diphenyl ether dimer and $\gamma$-T biphenyl dimers. Interconversion of the $\gamma$-T dimers and $\gamma$-T occurred during autoxidation. All tocopheryl dimers were antioxidants (23). Structures of some $\gamma$-T dimers are illustrated in Figure 3.8.

$\gamma$-Tocopherol can donate protons to peroxy radicals with formation of the $\gamma$-tocopheroxyl radical (Figure 3.7). Further oxidation yields $\gamma$-tocopheryl quinone and $\gamma$-tocopheryl orthoquinone in a manner similar to oxidation of $\alpha$-T. Because of the absence of a methyl group at C-5 of the chromanol ring, $\gamma$-T is less capable of donating hydrogen to free radicals than $\alpha$-T. It, therefore, is a less effective chain-breaking antioxidant than $\alpha$-T in most oxidizing lipid systems. The lack of substitution at C-5 gives $\gamma$-T the ability to trap lipophilic reactive nitrogen species at the C-5 position. It is established that $\gamma$-T detoxifies nitrogen dioxide more effectively than $\alpha$-T and probably complements the action of $\alpha$-T in this respect (16–18). Further, $\gamma$-T undergoes nitrogenation by peroxynitrite, which is formed by the reaction of nitric oxide with superoxide (25,26).

$$NO\cdot + O_2\cdot^- \longrightarrow ONOO^-$$

$\gamma$-Tocopherol is thus converted to the stable 5-nitro-$\gamma$-T (Figure 3.7). In this capacity, $\gamma$-T acts as a nucleophilic trap for peroxynitrite, which is considered to be a significant mutagenic oxidant and nitrating species (25). Peroxynitrite is known to be highly reactive with various biologically significant cellular components including amino acids, glutathione, sulfhydryls, low-density lipoproteins, deoxyribonucleic acids (DNA), liposomes, and microsomes (25–27). Because peroxynitrite is believed to be an important etiological factor in various chronic disease states, the role of $\gamma$-T as a detoxifying agent is receiving increased attention.

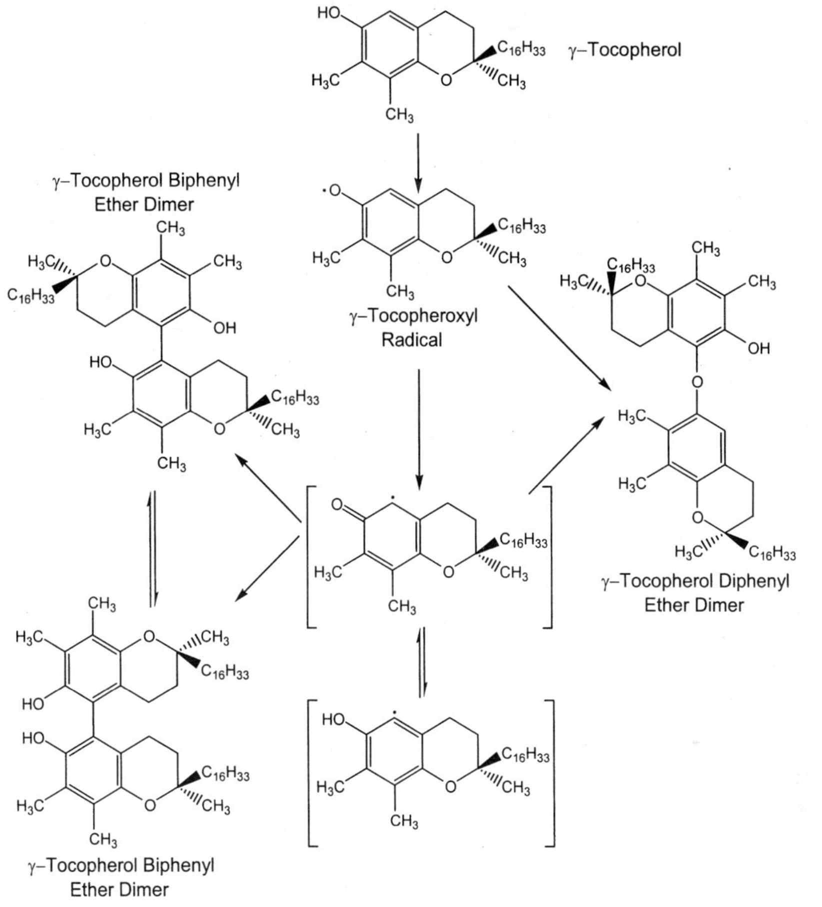

**FIGURE 3.8** Structures of γ-tocopherol dimers. (Modified from Refs. 23 and 24.)

Since 5-nitro-γ-T is a stable compound, it has been suggested as a biomarker for the presence of lipid-soluble electrophiles such as reactive nitrogen species (25). Brannan and Decker (27) examined the potential use of 5-nitro-γ-T as a lipid phase, peroxynitrite biomarker for lipid oxidation to measure or detect oxidative changes in muscle foods. Since 5-nitro-γ-T is present at low levels in fresh muscle, is easily and rapidly produced, is stable, and is easily quantified, it would be an ideal biomarker of lipid oxidation in meat and meat products. However, Brannen and Decker (27) found very low yields of 5-nitro-γ-T under various model system conditions. They concluded that 5-nitro-γ-T was not useful to confirm the presence of peroxynitrite in muscle foods.

**3.3.2.4. Prooxidant or Inversion Effects.** Many earlier studies completed in model systems, edible oils, fats, and food matrices showed that tocopherols are prooxidative above concentrations that provide antioxidant protection (28–39). More recently, studies completed with pure triacylglycerols have indicated that the tocopherols are not prooxidants but may act synergistically with prooxidants already in the system (9,40–45).

Research by Huang et al. (34), Cillard et al. (28,29), and Jung and Min (39) is representative of the demonstration of prooxidation effects produced by high levels of tocopherols in edible oils. Huang et al. (34) used bulk corn oil stripped of natural tocopherols to show the effect of known levels of $\alpha$- and $\gamma$-T on hydroperoxide formation. $\alpha$-Tocopherol had maximal antioxidant activity at 100 ppm and at 250–500 ppm in 10% oil-in-water emulsions, whereas $\gamma$-T showed maximal antioxidant activity at 250–500 ppm in bulk oil with no difference in activity between 250 and 1000 ppm. $\alpha$-Tocopherol started showing prooxidant activity at 250 ppm in bulk oil and at 500 ppm in emulsions. $\gamma$-T did not have prooxidant activity in either bulk oil or emulsions. Both $\alpha$- and $\gamma$-T inhibited hexanal formation as the antioxidant concentration and length of oxidation time increased. This observation indicated that the ability of tocopherols to inhibit formation of secondary degradation reactions is an important attribute and that property, in some cases, could be as significant as the inhibition of hydroperoxide formation to food quality. Cillard and Cillard (36) reported that at 0.05 mole of tocopherol per mole of linoleic acid, $\alpha$-T was a prooxidant. Under similar conditions, $\delta$- and $\gamma$-T maintained antioxidant capacity at this concentration level. The antioxidant and prooxidant effects, therefore, depend on tocopherol concentration and on the specific tocopherols present in the system. The work by Cillard and Cillard(36) is historically significant in that they were among the first to follow tocopherol degradation during autoxidation by LC. During the oxidation of linoleic acid in aqueous solution, the rate of tocopherol loss was $\alpha$-T $>$ $\gamma$-T $>$ $\delta$-T. Cillard et al. (28,29) also reported that $\alpha$-T was a prooxidant during autoxidation of linoleic acid in an aqueous medium at pH 6.9 at a concentration of $1.25 \times 10^{-4}$ M. The linoleic acid autoxidation rate was followed by using spectrophotometric measurement of conjugated dienes and GC determination of unoxidized linoleic acid. The addition of $\alpha$-T to the linoleic acid model system increased the rate of formation of conjugated dienes and the rate of loss of linoleic acid, especially during the first 4 days of autoxidation (Figures 3.9 and 3.10). $\alpha$-Tocopherol was rapidly destroyed during the prooxidant reaction. These observations agreed with those of Bazin et al. (37) and Husain et al. (38) who reported that $\alpha$-T exhibited prooxidant activity at concentrations of $1.25 \times 10^{-4}$ M and $1.25 \times 10^{-5}$ M. However, the prooxidant behavior of $\alpha$-T was unaffected by surfactants used in the aqueous system or by the presence of different salts (30).

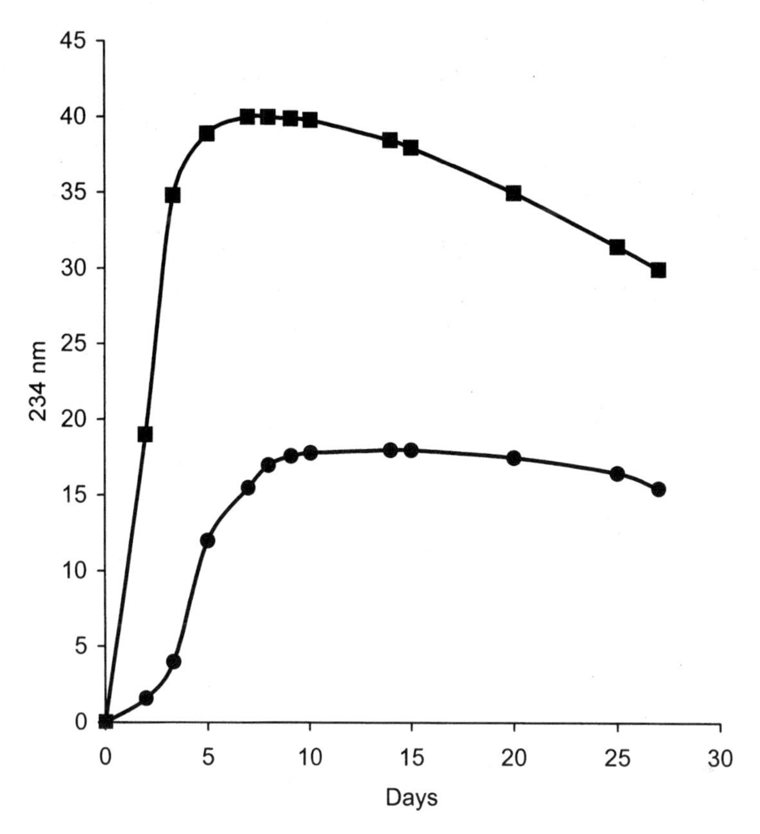


**FIGURE 3.9** Conjugated diene measurement during linoleic acid autoxidation in aqueous medium, ●, Linoleic acid without $\alpha$-tocopherol; ■, linoleic acid with $\alpha$-tocopherol ($5 \times 10^{-2}$ M). (Modified from Ref. 28.)

The effects of 0, 100, 250, 500, and 1000 ppm of $\alpha$-, $\gamma$-, and $\delta$-T on the oxidative stability of purified soybean oil stored in the dark at 55°C are listed in Table 3.2 (39). The oxidation was measured by peroxide value and headspace oxygen consumption. The peroxide value of oil containing 100 ppm $\alpha$-T was lower than that of the control. Peroxide values increased as the $\alpha$-T concentration increased from 100 to 250, 500, and 1000 ppm (Table 3.2.). As the concentration of $\gamma$-T increased from 0 to 100 and 250 ppm, peroxide values decreased. Peroxide values decreased progressively as concentration of $\delta$-T increased from 0 to 100, 250, and 500 ppm. The tocopherols showed significant prooxidant effects at higher concentrations of 100, 250, and 500 ppm of $\alpha$-, $\gamma$-, and $\delta$-T, respectively. The optimal concentration of the tocopherols for the oxidative stability of

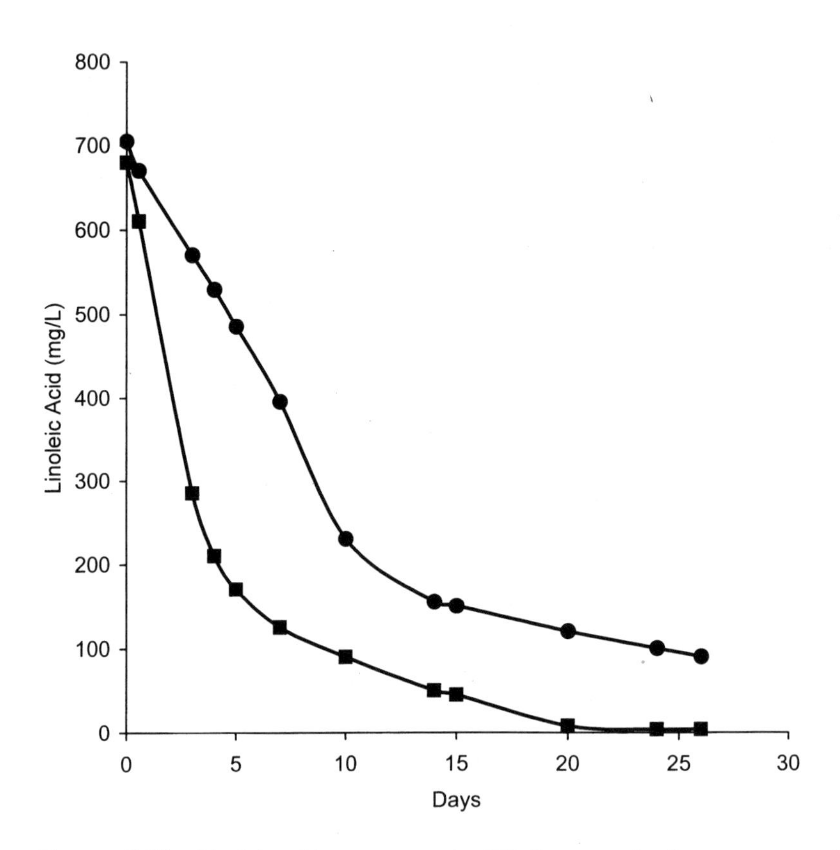


**FIGURE 3.10** Linoleic acid measurement by GC after extraction from aqueous medium and methylation. ●, Linoleic acid without $\alpha$-tocopherol; ■, linoleic acid with $\alpha$-tocopherol ($5 \times 10^{-2}$ M). (Modified from Ref. 28.)

soybean oil was related to the oxidative stability of each tocopherol. The lower the specific oxidative stability of the specific tocopherol, the lower the optimal concentration required for that tocopherol for maximal oxidative stability of the oil. This research is often cited as a practical guide for usage levels for oxidation control by natural tocopherols. In general, the antioxidant efficacy decreases with increasing concentrations and reaches a point at which where an apparent prooxidant effect occurs.

Kamal-Eldin and Appelqvist (9) concluded from their work and prior research by others that the tocopherols are not prooxidants but, at high concentrations, act as prooxidant synergists with prooxidants already in the system (transition metals, preformed hydroperoxides, various reactive oxygen species, heme proteins, and other photosensitizers). The overall effect was explained as follows: "Each antioxidant/substrate combination has critical

**TABLE 3.2** The Effect of Tocopherols on Peroxides in Purified Soybean Oil During Dark Storage at 55°C

| | Peroxide value (mEq/kg oil) | | | | | |
|---|---|---|---|---|---|---|
| | 1 Day | 2 Day | 3 Day | 4 Day | 5 Day | 6 Day |
| α-Tocopherol (ppm) | | | | | | |
| 0 | 10.4 | 24.4 | 36.7 | 51.3 | 60.9 | 70.3 |
| 100 | 8.2 | 21.8 | 32.9 | 47.8 | 56.8 | 66.6 |
| 250 | 9.1 | 25.1 | 38.1 | 53.8 | 62.9 | 73.1 |
| 500 | 11.1 | 29.7 | 43.6 | 60.6 | 71.0 | 80.8 |
| 1000 | 17.9 | 44.4 | 55.2 | 71.0 | 79.4 | 87.8 |
| γ-Tocopherol (ppm) | | | | | | |
| 0 | 10.4 | 24.4 | 36.7 | 51.3 | 60.9 | 70.3 |
| 100 | 9.2 | 23.1 | 35.9 | 49.1 | 59.0 | 68.7 |
| 250 | 8.3 | 23.3 | 33.4 | 48.2 | 58.2 | 67.7 |
| 500 | 8.1 | 23.6 | 35.9 | 52.1 | 62.0 | 73.2 |
| 1000 | 12.4 | 32.1 | 45.1 | 60.4 | 70.7 | 78.5 |
| δ-Tocopherol (ppm) | | | | | | |
| 0 | 10.4 | 24.4 | 36.7 | 51.3 | 60.9 | 70.3 |
| 100 | 9.2 | 22.4 | 35.4 | 49.2 | 59.1 | 68.8 |
| 250 | 7.6 | 21.1 | 31.5 | 46.4 | 55.6 | 64.9 |
| 500 | 7.1 | 21.0 | 31.8 | 46.7 | 56.2 | 66.2 |
| 1000 | 10.4 | 26.7 | 40.3 | 54.8 | 65.8 | 72.5 |

*Source*: Modified from Ref. 39.

concentration ratios for maximum stability. Below these critical concentration ratios, inhibition (of oxidation) is below optimum and above which the antioxidant may invert their effects and synergize the present prooxidants."

Recent studies on purified edible oil triacylglycerols support the inversion of antioxidant activity phenomenon. Research on pure triacylglycerols from sunflower, butter oil, rapeseed, and fish oil, containing no prooxidants, indicates that α- and γ-T do not exhibit prooxidant effects (40–45). Representative of this research, Kulås and Ackman (43,44) compared formation of hydroperoxides in menhaden oil and in purified menhaden triacylglycerols. At α-T concentration ≥250 ppm, α-T was a prooxidant in the unpurified oil but inhibited hydroperoxide formation at all levels in the purified triacylglycerols. Fuster et al. (40) purified sunflower oil triacylglycerols to the extent that tocopherols were not detectable by LC. The stability of the purified triacylglycerols was studied at concentrations of α- and γ-T from 1 to 200 ppm at 55°C. Both tocopherols reduced peroxide value by more than 90% at levels >20 ppm. $\alpha$-Tocopherol had greater antioxidant ability than $\gamma$-T at concentrations $\leq$40 ppm. However, at levels >200 ppm, $\gamma$-T showed better activity than $\alpha$-T. Neither tocopherol acted as a prooxidant at concentrations up to 2000 ppm. A protection factor (PF) (Figure 3.11) was calculated to demonstrate tocopherol concentration effects on oxidative stability of the sunflower triacylglycerols.

$$PF = (PV_{\mathrm{CONTROL}} - PV_{\mathrm{SAMPLE}})/PV_{\mathrm{CONTROL}}$$

## 3.4. ANTIOXIDANT ACTIONS OF VITAMIN E

### 3.4.1. Model Systems

Use of model systems consisting of free fatty acids, fatty acid methyl esters, or purified triacylglycerol substrates has been the predominant approach to the study of factors influencing the antioxidant activity of vitamin E. Such research

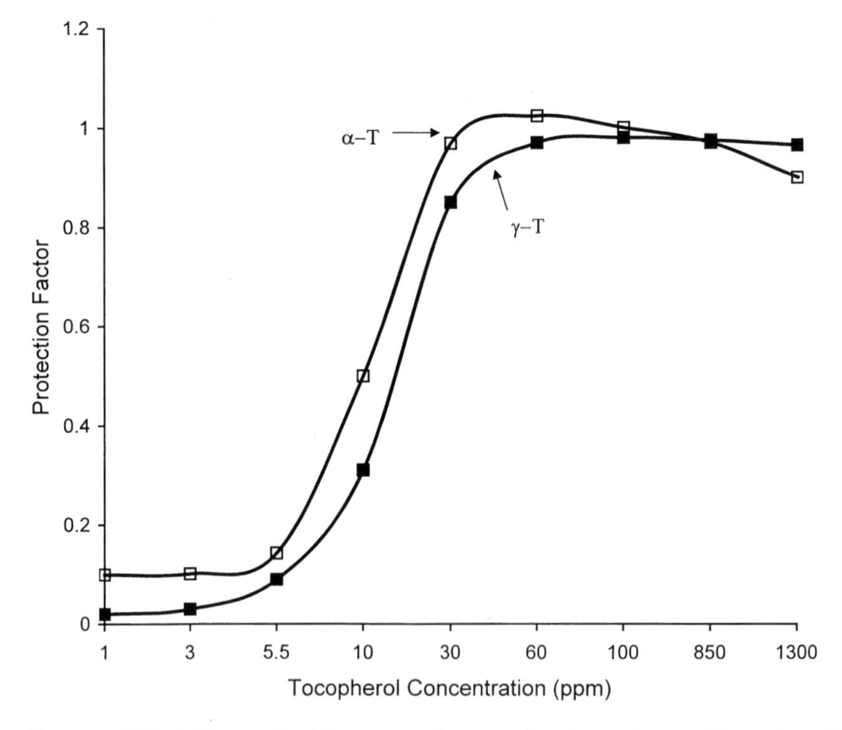


**FIGURE 3.11** Effects of adding $\alpha$- and $\gamma$-tocopherol on the stability of purified sunflower oil. Peroxide value (PV) was measured, and a protection factor was calculated as $PF$ (protection factor) $= (PV_{\mathrm{control}} - PV_{\mathrm{sample}})/PV_{\mathrm{control}}$. $\alpha$-T, $\alpha$-tocopherol; $\gamma$-T, $\gamma$-tocopherol. (Modified from Ref. 40.)

was initiated shortly after the discovery of the tocopherols and led to the understanding of the mechanism of lipid oxidation, the interaction of antioxidants, and the nutritional and technological significance of vitamin E. Use of simple substrate model systems eliminates the interaction of vitamin E with other natural antioxidants and prooxidants that exist in more complex fats and oils, in raw or processed foods, or in vivo. Model system research summarized in Table 3.3. includes both historically significant and more recent studies that have led to increased knowledge about the action of vitamin E in foods.

Advances attributable to model system studies include delineation of the following:

1. Differences in antioxidant efficiencies of the tocopherols and tocotrienols (40,45–56)
2. Temperature effects on oxidation mechanisms and effectiveness of different antioxidants (33,36,46,47,53–58,64)
3. The mechanism of autoxidation (29,31–33,38,50,61,63,64)
4. The role of photocatalysis as an initiator of autoxidation and the ability of vitamin E to quench singlet oxygen (57,60,62,65)
5. Inversion of antioxidant activity (28,29,32,33,37,38)
6. The synergistic effects of food compounds with vitamin E (29,37,38,47–49,59,61,65,66)

### 3.4.2. Fats and Oils

In general, the addition of vitamin E to fats and oils depends on the level of natural antioxidants in the refined product and the intended use of the oil. Refined, bleached, and deodorized (RBD) vegetable oils seldom require addition of antioxidants because of the high residual amounts of vitamin E after the refining process. Added vitamin E in some edible oils could easily increase concentrations sufficiently to produce inversion of antioxidant activity. Animal fats, as opposed to vegetable oils, have little naturally occurring vitamin E and require stabilization with antioxidants. Buck (67) reviewed the chemical characteristics and practical applications of antioxidant usage in fats and oils. Guidelines for antioxidant usage in both animal and vegetable fats and oils given by Buck (67) include the following:

1. Because of low levels of natural antioxidants, addition of antioxidants is commonly required to increase shelf life of the fats and the processed foods containing these as ingredients.
2. Antioxidant activity in animal fats and oils is generally TBHQ > propyl gallate > BHA > BHT > tocopherols.
3. Addition of acid synergists with primary antioxidants to animal fats increases oxidative stability.
4. Addition of antioxidants to vegetable oils increases oxidative stability.

**TABLE 3.3** Summaries of Research on the Antioxidant Activity of Tocopherols and Tocotrienols in Model Systems, Fats and Oils, and Foods[a]

| Research area | Vitamin E forms | Amount | Substrates | Cofactors | Measurements | Observations | Ref. |
|---|---|---|---|---|---|---|---|
| **Model systems** | | | | | | | |
| Relative antioxidant activity of α-, β-, and γ-T at various temperatures | α-, β-, γ-T | — | β-Carotene, ethyl oleate | Gossypol | β-Carotene loss, PV | α-, β-, and γ-T: equal antioxidant activity at low temperature; γ-T more active than α-T with lard at 90°C; antioxidant activity increase in the order of δ- > γ- > β- > α-T | 1944, 48 |
| Comparison of the antioxidant activity of tocopherols | α-, β-, γ-, δ-T | 0.0025%, 0.005%, 0.01% | Lard ester, methyl linoleate | None | PV | Tocopherols not protective in presence of light; in methyl linoleate at 50°C, antioxidant activity increase in the order γ- > δ- > β- > α-T | 1959, 46 |
| Antioxidant activities of the tocopherols in distilled methyl esters of edible oils | α-, β-, γ-, δ-T | 0.01% | Distilled methyl esters of cottonseed, linseed, and cod liver oil fatty acids | None | PV | γ-T Better antioxidant than α-T | 1960, 47 |
| Synergistic antioxidant activity of nucleic acids with tocopherol | α-, γ-, δ-T | $3.76 \times 10^{-6}$ M | Methyl linoleate | Nucleic acids | PV | Nucleic acids synergestic with tocopherols | 1977, 49 |
| Quenching effect of α-, γ-, and δ-T on the methylene blue sensitized photo-oxidation of methyl linoleate | α-, γ-, δ-T | $10^{-3}$ M | Methyl linoleate | None | GC | α-T Better inhibitor of photo induced oxidation than other tocopherols | 1974, 62 |
| Effect of experimental factors on the prooxidant effect of α-T during the autoxidation of linoleic acid | α-T | $1.25 \times 10^{-4}$–$5.0 \times 10^{-2}$ M | Linoleic acid | Surfactant, salts | Conjugated dienes, GC | α-T Prooxidant under all conditions at concentration $\geq 1.25 \times 10^{-3}$ mole per mole linoleic acid | 1980, 28 |

| | | | | | | | |
|---|---|---|---|---|---|---|---|
| Inhibitory effect of vitamin E on singlet oxygen–initiated photooxidation of methyl linoleate | $\alpha$-, $\gamma$-, $\delta$-T | 1.0 M% | Methyl linoleate | $\beta$-Carotene | HPLC | Greatest inhibitory effect on singlet oxygen–initiated photoxidation shown by $\delta$-T | 1980, 57 |
| Prooxidant effect of $\alpha$-T | $\alpha$-T | $\alpha$-T | Linoleic acid | None | Conjugated dienes, GC | $\alpha$-T A prooxidant | 1980, 29 |
| Prooxidant effect of tocopherols | $\alpha$-, $\gamma$-, $\delta$-T | $2.5 \times 10^{-3}$ and $5.0 \times 10^{-2}$ mole per mole linoleic acid | Linoleic acid | None | GC | $\alpha$-T A prooxidant at $2.5 \times 10^{-3}$ and $5.0 \times 10^{-2}$ mole per mole linoleic acid; $\gamma$- and $\delta$-T antioxidants at same concentrations | 1980, 36 |
| Effects of $\alpha$-T on distribution of end products formed from methyl linolenate and methyl linoleate during autoxidation | $\alpha$-T | 0.05%, 0.5%, 5% | Methyl linolenate, methyl linoleate | None | PV, conjugated dienes, HPLC | 0.05% $\alpha$-T inhibition of oxidation; prooxidant effect shown at higher concentrations; trans, trans isomers and only cis, trans formed at high $\alpha$-T concentrations | 1981, 30 |
| Effect of $\alpha$-T on autoxidation rate of arachidonic acid in aqueous medium and effect of some synergists on antioxidant activity of $\alpha$-T | $\alpha$-T | $1.25 \times 10^{-6}$, $1.25 \times 10^{-5}$, $1.25 \times 10^{-4}$ M | Arachidonic acid | Cysteine, nucleic acid | Conjugated dienes | $\alpha$-T A prooxidant at $1.25 \times 10^{-4}$ M and $1.25 \times 10^{-5}$ M; prooxidant activity of $\alpha$-T reduced by cysteine | 1984, 37 |
| Effect of $\alpha$-, $\gamma$-, and $\delta$-T on autoxidation of linoleic acid | $\alpha$-, $\gamma$-, $\delta$-T | 0.038%, 0.38%, 3.8% for $\alpha$-T; 3.8% for $\gamma$- and $\delta$-T | Linoleic acid | None | HPLC | Prooxidant effect of $\alpha$-T demonstrated at high concentrations; distribution of cis, trans hydroperoxide geometric isomers modified by tocopherols | 1984, 31 |
| Inhibition of oxidation of methyl linoleate in solution by vitamin E and vitamin C | $\alpha$-T | 0.273 mM, 0.595 mM | Methyl linoleate | Ascorbic acid | Oxygen uptake | Vitamin C synergistic with $\alpha$-T | 1984, 59 |

*(continued)*

**TABLE 3.3** *Continued*

| Research area | Vitamin E forms | Amount | Substrates | Cofactors | Measurements | Observations | Ref. |
|---|---|---|---|---|---|---|---|
| Effect of α-T during autoxidation of methyl linoleate in bulk phase without external initiator | α-T | 0.1%, 1.0% | Methyl linoleate | Ascorbyl palmitate | HPLC | α-T A prooxidant at 0.1% and 1% concentrations; prooxidant effect suppressed by ascorbyl palmitate | 1986, 32 |
| Antioxidant activities of α-, β-, γ-, and δ-T in oxidation of methyl linoleate | α-, β-, γ-, δ-T | 0.2–0.3 mM | Methyl linoleate | None | Oxygen uptake | Antioxidant activity increased in the order α- > β- > γ- > δ-T | 1986, 50 |
| MDA production during prooxidant effect of α-T on linoleic and archidonic acids | α-T | $1.25 \times 10^{-4}$ M | Linoleic, arachidonic acid | None | Conjugated dienes, HPLC | Prooxidant effect of α-T greater with linoleic acid than arachidonic acid | 1987, 38 |
| Abilities of α-T, β-carotene, and retinol to inhibit adriamycin-dependent microsomal lipid peroxidation in air and at low oxygen partial pressures | α-T | 0–100 nM/mg Microsomal protein | Liver microsomes | β-Carotene, retinol | TBARS | α-T And β-carotene inhibition oxidation at ≥50 nM/g microsomal protein; β-carotene more effective than α-T at low $O_2$ pressure; α-T more effective in aerobic conditions | 1988, 66 |
| Interaction betwen β-carotene and α-T in membrane system | α-T | 6.0, 6.5 nM/mg Protein | Microsomal membrane | β-Carotene | Malondialdehyde | β-Carotene synergistic with α-T | 1992, 61 |
| Effects of γ-T at concentrations <50 μg/g | γ-T | <50 μg/g | TAG isolated from rapeseed and butter oil | — | PV, AnV | Low levels of γ-T effective as antioxidants | 1997, 52 |
| Effects of α- and γ-T on autoxidation in oil-in-water emulsions | α-, γ-T | 1.5–300 μg/g | 10% Oil-in-water emulsions of rapeseed oil triacylglycerols | β-Carotene | PV, hexanal | At 1.5 μg/g γ-T better antioxidant than α-T; β-carotene, at 2.0 μg/g, synergistic with α-T; no synergism between β-carotene and γ-T, α- and γ-T protection of β-carotene in fat emulsions | 1997, 80 |

| | | | | | | | |
|---|---|---|---|---|---|---|---|
| Antioxidant effects of $\alpha$- and $\gamma$-T on autooxidation of purified sunflower oil | $\alpha$-, $\gamma$-T | 20–200 ppm | Purified sunflower and rapeseed oils | $FeSO_4$ | PV | Both tocopherols: reduction of PV by 90% when present at concentrations $>20$ ppm; $\alpha$-T better antioxidant than $\gamma$-T at $<40$ ppm, but worse at $>200$ ppm; no prooxidant effect of $\alpha$- and $\gamma$-T up to 2000 ppm and no synergistic effect of $\alpha$- and $\gamma$-T observed; increase in amount of $\alpha$- and $\gamma$-T destroyed caused by addition of $FeSO_4$ | 1998, 40 |
| Interactions of carotenoids and $\gamma$-T on hydroperoxide formation | $\gamma$-T | 10, 15 $\mu$g/g | TAC purified from low–erucic acid rapeseed oil | Carotenoids, lutein | PV | $\gamma$-T inhibition of hydroxide formation; prooxidant effect of carotenoids inhibited by adding $\gamma$-T; combination of lutein and $\gamma$-T more effective than $\gamma$-T in inhibiting hydroperoxide formation of TAC | 1996, 106 |
| Influence of tocopherols on TAG at 180°C up to 10 h | $\alpha$-, $\beta$-, $\gamma$-, $\delta$-T | 200–250 mg/kg | Triolein, trilinolein | — | HPLC, HPSEC, GC | $\alpha$-T Loss rapid and independent of TAG unsaturation; $\delta$-T most stable; polymeric TG formation decrease with addition of tocopherols | 1999, 56 |
| Antipolymerization effect of $\alpha$- and $\gamma$-T in purified high-oleic sunflower TAG at 180°C | $\alpha$-, $\gamma$-T | | Purified TAG | Stripped TAG | HPLC, HPSEC, GC | $\alpha$- and $\gamma$-T Inhibition of TAG polymerization until almost totally consumed | 1998, 55 |
| **Fats and oils** | | | | | | | |
| Antioxidant activity of tocopherols | $\alpha$-, $\beta$-, $\gamma$-T | 0.01%–0.2% | Lard, oleo oil, esters of cottonseed oil | None | Oxygen absorption | Antioxidant activity increase in the order $\alpha$- $>$ $\beta$- $>$ $\gamma$-T; no antioxidant activity of esters | 1937, 54 |

*(continued)*

**TABLE 3.3** *Continued*

| Research area | Vitamin E forms | Amount | Substrates | Cofactors | Measurements | Observations | Ref. |
|---|---|---|---|---|---|---|---|
| Antioxidant activity of α-, γ-, and δ-T and of unsubstituted tocol and 5, 7-dimethyl tocol | α-, β-, δ-T | 0.25–7.5 μm/200 mg Substrate | Purified menhaden oil, squalene | Unsubstituted tocol, 5,7-dimethyl tocol | Weight gain, PV | γ-T Better antioxidant than α- and δ-T; no temperature effect | 1968, 70 |
| Antioxidant effectiveness of α-, γ-, and δ-T during oxidation of lard | α-, γ-, δ-T | 0–650 μg/g | Lard | None | Oxygen uptake | Antioxidant activity increased in the order α- > γ- > δ-T; activity decreased with increasing concentration; above 250 ppm no antioxidant activity increase | 1968, 83 |
| Antioxidant activity of tocopherols | α-, γ-T | 0.02%–0.2% | Animal fat, vegetable oil, oleic and linoleic acids | Ascorbyl palmitate, BHA, BHT, PG | PV | γ-T More active than α-T in animal fats; γ-T activity in animal fat increase with concentration increased; tocopherols more active in oleic acid than BHT; low antioxidant activity of tocopherols added to vegetable oils | 1974, 58 |
| Oxidative stability of natural tocopherols and tocotrienols in corn and soybean oil and to evaluate antioxidant activity of individual tocopherols in stripped corn oil | α-, β-, γ-, δ-T | 0.02% | Corn and soybean oils, stripped corn oil | None | PV | Antioxidant activity increase in the order γ- > δ- > β- > α-T at 200 ppm in stripped corn oil; vitamin E loss more rapid in corn oil than in soybean oil | 1974, 69 |
| Effects of α-, γ-, and δ-T on oxidative stability of purified soybean oil | α-, γ-, δ-T | 0–1000 ppm | Purified soybean oil | None | PV, headspace oxygen | Optimal concentrations for antioxidant activity: 100, 250 and 500 ppm for α-, γ-, and δ-T, respectively | 1990, 39 |

| | | | | | | | |
|---|---|---|---|---|---|---|---|
| Effect of temperature on antioxidative action of α-T and ferulic acid in lipid oxidation | α-T | 0.2–2.0 g/kg | Purified lard | Ferulic acid | PV | Prooxidant effect of increasing α-T levels greater at lower temperatures; antioxidant effect of α-T increase at elevated temperatures | 1992, 64 |
| Effect of lipophilic and hydrophilic antioxidants on oxidation of tocopherol-stripped corn oil | α-T | 100, 500 ppm | Tocopherol-stripped corn oil in bulk and in oil-in-water emulsion | Ascorbyl palmitate, ascorbic acid, Trolox | Conjugated dienes, hexanal | Lipophilic antioxidants (α-T, ascorbyl palmitate) most effective in oil-in-water emulsions; hydrophilic antioxidants (Trolox, ascorbic acid) more active in bulk oil | 1994, 77 |
| Effectiveness of individual tocopherols and their mixtures in inhibiting formation and decomposition of hydroperoxides in bulk corn oil stripped of natural tocopherols | γ-, δ-T, mixture of α- and γ-T | 100–5000 ppm | Tocopherol-stripped corn oil | None | Hydroperoxides, hexanal | δ-T Inhibition of formation and decomposition of hydroperoxides at 200 ppm; γ-T prooxidant at 5000 ppm but still inhibited hydroperoxide decomposition; hexanal formation inhibited by α- and γ-T mixtures at all concentration levels | 1995, 45 |
| Effectiveness of α-T and Trolox in corn oil emulsified with nonionic Tween 20 at different pH at 60°C | α-T | 130, 150 ppm | Corn oil (bulk and emulsified) | Trolox | Conjugated dienes, hydroperoxides, hexanal | Antioxidant activity of α-T increased in emulsions with increasing pH; α-T more effective than Trolox in inhibiting hexanal formation | 1996, 35 |
| Antioxidant effectiveness of α-T and its water-soluble analog, Trolox, in different lipid systems | α-T | 150, 300 μM | Linoleic acid, corn oil, methyl linoleate | Trolox | Conjugated dienes, hydroperoxides, hexanal | In bulk and emulsified linoleic acid, better antioxidant activity of Trolox than of α-T; in bulk corn oil Trolox superior to α-T with opposite effects noted in emulsified corn oil | 1996, 72 |

(*continued*)

**TABLE 3.3** *Continued*

| Research area | Vitamin E forms | Amount | Substrates | Cofactors | Measurements | Observations | Ref. |
|---|---|---|---|---|---|---|---|
| Antioxidant properties of α-T, γ/δ-T, and δ-T concentrate alone and in combination with ascorbyl palmitate and lecithin on oxidative stability of fish oil | α-T, γ/δ-T, δ-T | 0.2%–2.0% | Fish oil refined from menhaden and Chilean fish oils | Ascorbyl palmitate, lecithin | PV | Antioxidant activity increase in order $\delta > \gamma/\delta > \alpha$-T at 2% concentration; lecithin synergistic with tocopherols | 1998, 101 |
| Effect of tocopherols to inhibit oxidation of olive and linseed oil at 120°C | α-, γ-, δ-T | α-T: 10–200 mg/100 g, γ-T: 10–800 mg/100 g, δ-T: 10–100 mg/100 g | Olive and linseed oils | — | Rancimat, HPLC | γ- and δ-T and mixture improvement of stability of olive but not of linseed oil, >100 mg γ-T/100 g prooxidative | 2000, 74 |
| Effect of tocopherols and tocotrienols as antioxidants in coconut fat at 60 and 160°C | α-, γ-, δ-T, α-, β-, γ-, δ-T3 | 0.01%–0.5% for T, 0.01%–0.1% for T3 | Coconut fat | — | HPLC, PV | α- and β-T3 and α-T least effective antioxidants; γ- and δ-T3 more effective than γ- and δ-T | 2001, 75 |
| Effect of tocopherols on frying stability of regular and modified canola oils at 175°C for 72 h | α-, γ-T | 468–801 mg/kg total tocopherols | Regular, high oleic–low-linolenic, low-linolenic–high-oleic | — | HPLC, PV, GC | Regular canola oil half-life for total tocopherol >72 h; in modified oils tocopherol half-life 3–6 h | 2001, 76 |
| **Food** | | | | | | | |
| Antioxidant effectiveness during storage of ground beef | α-T | 0.005% | Ground beef | Ascorbic acid, L-ascorbyl stearate, citric acid | PV | All antioxidants except ascorbic acid: slight effect in decreasing rate of lipid and heme oxidations compared to untreated samples; definite prooxidant action of ascorbic acid | 1975, 85 |

| | | | | | | | |
|---|---|---|---|---|---|---|---|
| Antioxidant effect of $\alpha$-T in cooked or uncooked fresh ground pork | $\alpha$-T | 100, 200 ppm | Cooked or uncooked ground pork | None | TBA | Oxidation slowed by $\alpha$-T in cooked ground pork stored at either 4°C, or −20°C and in cooked samples refrigerated for 12 d | 1986, 87 |
| Effects of antioxidants in combination with irradiation on lipid peroxidation and lipolysis in ground chicken | $\alpha$-T | 0.01% | Minced chicken meat | BHT | TBA, carbonyl content, FFA content | Inhibition of oxidative rancidity by addition of $\alpha$-T or BHT; meat treated with antioxidants before irradiation; lower TBA values than in untreated irradiated products | 1998, 90 |
| Effects of exogenous vitamin E and ascorbic acid on pigment and lipid stability in raw ground beef | $\alpha$-T | 6 mg/kg tissue | Raw ground beef | Ascorbic acid | TBA, metmyoglobin | $\alpha$-T and ascorbic acid inhibition of oxidation of lipids and meat pigments; ascorbic acid synergistic with $\alpha$-T | 1991, 86 |
| Effects of tocopherols and ascorbyl palmitate in cooked, minced turkey on lipid oxidation | Mixture | 200 ppm | Cooked minced turkey, modified atmosphere packaging | Ascorbyl palmitate | TBARS | Significant reduction of lipid oxidation by tocopherols; synergism between tocopherol and ascorbyl palmitate observed; synergism dependent on $O_2$ availability | 1994, 91 |
| Effect of natural tocopherols extracted from soybean oil on oxidation of turkey meat | Mixture | 50–150 ppm | Cooked, minced turkey meat | Ascorbyl palmitate | TBARS | Tocopherol reduction of maximal level of TBARS; rate constant for development of TBARS reduced more by ascorbyl palmitate | 1996, 89 |
| Antioxidative activity of $\alpha$- and $\delta$-T | $\alpha$-, $\delta$-T, and mixture | 50, 100, 200 ppm | Minced turkey meat ball | Ascorbyl palmitate | Hexanal by GC, TBARS | Antioxidant activity of $\alpha$- and $\delta$-T equal and greater than that of ascorbyl palmitate; at 100 ppm, antioxidant activity of $\alpha$- and $\delta$-T enhanced by ascorbyl palmitate | 1996, 88 |

*(continued)*

**TABLE 3.3** *Continued*

| Research area | Vitamin E forms | Amount | Substrates | Cofactors | Measurements | Observations | Ref. |
|---|---|---|---|---|---|---|---|
| Effects of mixed tocopherols on lipid oxidation | Mixture | 200 ppm | Cooked beef patties | $\beta$-Carotene | TBARS, volatile compounds | Mixed tocopherol reduction of TBARS values; similar results for tocopherol with $\beta$-carotene; no difference between tocopherol and tocopherol + $\beta$-carotene; no antioxidant activity of $\beta$-carotene alone | 1997, 84 |
| Antioxidant efficacy of $\alpha$-T in retarding lipid oxidation reactions catalyzed by $Cu^{2+}$ | $\alpha$-T | 0.1%, 5% | Flour–lipid dough system | MRP | TBARS | Similar antioxidant activity of $\alpha$-T and Glu-Lys MRP; $\alpha$-T superior to Fru-Lys MRP; MRP not synergistic or antagonistic with $\alpha$-T | 1998, 82 |
| Effects of $\gamma$-T on stability of potato chips fried in triolein at 190°C | $\gamma$-T | 0, 100, 400 ppm | Potatoes | — | HPLC, volatiles by MS, sensory | $\gamma$-T inhibition of oxidation at all levels of retention in frying oil; nonanal formation decreased during storage at 60°C | 2003, 92 |

[a] $\alpha$-T, $\alpha$-tocopherol; HPLC, high-performance liquid chromatography; GC, gas chromatography; BHA, butylated hydroxyanisole; BHT, butylated hydroxytoluene; MDA, malondialdehyde; TAG, triacylglyceride; HPSEC, high performance size-exclusion chromatography; AnV, p-anisidine value; TG, triglyceride; MRP, Maillard reaction products; MS, mass spectrometry; PG, propyl gallate; FFA, free fatty acids.

5. Antioxidant activity in vegetable oils is generally TBHQ > propyl gallate > BHT > BHA.
6. Vitamin E is usually not used in vegetable oils when regulations permit use of more effective synthetic antioxidants.

Effectiveness of various antioxidant treatments for stability of soybean oil and lard is indicated in Figure 3.12.

Widely varying studies have defined the antioxidant activities of the tocopherols in fats and oils under many different experimental conditions. Some of these studies, summarized in Table 3.3, provide the following conclusions applicable to the antioxidant activity of vitamin E:

1. Antioxidant activity of specific tocopherols and tocotrienols varies with the type of fat or oil (45–51,68–73).
2. Antioxidant activity varies with the state of the fat (34,35,71,77–82).
3. Temperature effects can be substantial. Antioxidant efficiencies of the tocopherols change at varying temperatures. Activity cannot be extrapolated from cold or ambient to what occurs at frying temperatures (47,48,69,71,92).

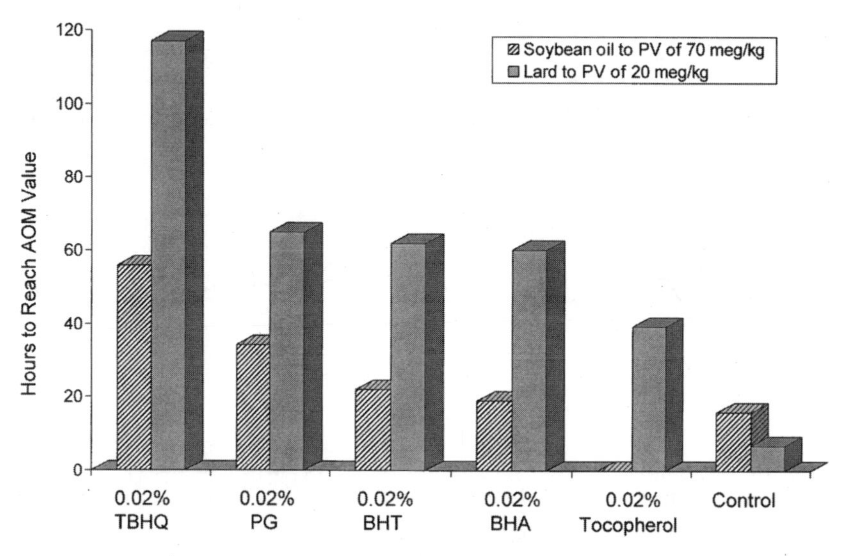


**FIGURE 3.12** Effects of various antioxidants on the stability of soybean oil and lard as measured by the active oxygen method (AOM). TBHQ, tertiary butyl hydtoquinone; PG, propyl gallate; BHT, butylated hydroxy toluene; BHA, butylated hydroxy anisole. (Modified from Ref. 67.)

4. Concentration effects are of significant practical concern, since inversion of antioxidant activity usually occurs at concentrations above 500 ppm (28,29,34,35,39,51,83).
5. The presence of other natural antioxidants in complex foods can act synergistically with vitamin E (57,61,66,78,80,84,86,89,91).

As early as 1937, Olcott and Emerson(54) showed that the tocopherols were effective antioxidants in lard and oleo oil at concentrations of 0.01%–0.20%. They demonstrated that the antioxidant activities differ, that $\gamma$-T has the strongest activity ($\gamma$-T > $\beta$-T > $\alpha$-T), and that the esters are inactive. Later research by Olcott and van der Veer (70) and Parkhurst et al. (83) further established that $\gamma$- and $\delta$-T were more effective antioxidants than $\alpha$-T in fat under the specific conditions of their research. Both of these studies used tocopherol stripped fats and oils (lard and menhaden oil). Parkhurst et al. (83) clearly established that antioxidant activity decreased at increasing concentrations once maximal inhibition of autoxidation was achieved. Each tocopherol had limited increased activity above 250 ppm (Figure 3.13). Olcott and van der Veer (70)

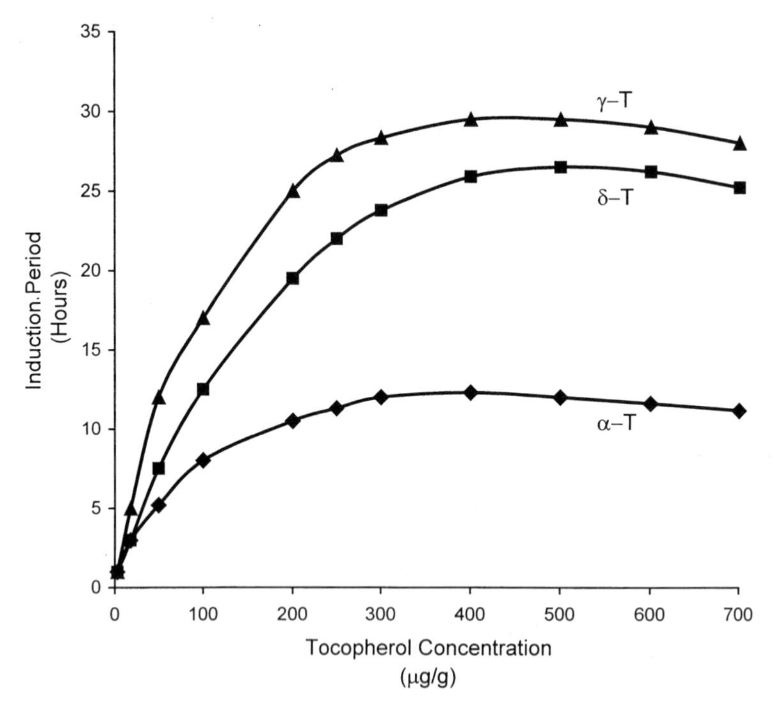


**FIGURE 3.13** Induction period vs. tocopherol concentration in lard at 97°C. $\gamma$-T, $\gamma$-tocopherol; $\delta$-T, $\delta$-tocopherol; $\alpha$-T, $\alpha$-tocopherol. (Modified from Ref. 83.)

were the first to establish clearly that the hydrogen on position 5 of the chromanol ring in $\gamma$- and $\delta$-T was significant to antioxidant activity.

Chow and Draper (69) found that vitamin E oxidation and peroxide formation occurred more rapidly in corn oil than in soybean oil, and that differences could not be explained in terms of differences in the vitamin E and fatty acid content of these oils. When corn and soybean oils were heated to 70°C with vigorous agitation, the rates of $\alpha$-T and $\alpha$-T3 losses were greater than the rates of $\gamma$-T and $\gamma$-T3 losses. In soybean oil, $\gamma$-T was destroyed faster than $\delta$-T. In corn oil stripped of naturally occurring tocopherols, the antioxidant activity of tocopherols added back at 0.02% was in the order of $\gamma$-T > $\delta$-T > $\beta$-T > $\alpha$-T. The rates of losses for $\gamma$- and $\delta$-T in soybean oil did not agree with their relative antioxidant activities at similar concentrations in corn oil. This work led to the significant understanding that total vitamin E concentration in an oil is not a foolproof indicator of oil stability. Further, stability of different oils can be greatly affected by natural antioxidants and synergists other than vitamin E and by the presence of prooxidants.

### 3.4.3. Foods

Maintenance of food quality for extended shelf life requires the use of antioxidants. Although synthetic antioxidants are more commonly used in foods because of availability, cost, and activity considerations, use of natural vitamin E preparations has dramatically increased over the past two decades. The growth of the natural vitamin E market with respect to food antioxidant activity is directly linked to the consumer's positive perception of natural food ingredients compared to synthetic ingredients and to the significant advances in nutrition knowledge about benefits of tocopherols and tocotrienols in the human diet. Increased demand has led to increased production of natural vitamin E for use in foods and to increased cost. Studies summarized in Table 3.3 show the effectiveness of tocopherols as antioxidants under widely varying conditions.

As discussed in Chapter 4, supplementation of $\alpha$-T to animal rations increases $\alpha$-T concentration in vivo and increases oxidative stability of fresh and processed meats. Further, tocopherols are known to reduce warmed-over flavor (WOF) in cooked meat products. Research has shown the practicality of using tocopherols in processed meats as the primary antioxidant. Representative studies summarized in Table 3.3 include ground beef,(84–86) ground pork (87), and ground chicken and turkey (88–91). Lee and Lillard(84) added a mixed tocopherol concentrate containing 12.0% $\alpha$-T, 1.4% $\beta$-T, 57.4% $\gamma$-T, and 29.2% $\delta$-T to ground beef. Cooked hamburger patties were stored at 4°C for 5 days and lipid oxidation was measured by thiobarbituric acid–reactive substance (TBARS) and by the concentration of hexanal in the headspace. At 200 ppm, the

**TABLE 3.4** Thiobarbituric Acid Reactive Substances and Headspace Hexanal Peak Areas in Freshly Cooked or Reheated 2- and 5-Day Stored Beef Patties at 4°C ± 1°C

| | | Storage (days) | | |
|---|---|---|---|---|
| Treatment | Measurement | 0 | 2 | 5 |
| Control | TBARS | 0.65 | 5.57 | 7.15 |
| | Hexanal | ND[a] | 55.21 | 97.83 |
| 200 ppm Tocopherol mixture | TBARS | 0.54 | 2.41 | 2.79 |
| | Hexanal | ND | 19.31 | 26.24 |

[a]Not detectable; TBARS, thiobarbituric acid reactive substance.
*Source*: Modified from Ref. 84.

mixed tocopherol preparation dramatically reduced TBARS and hexanal formation (Table 3.4.). A high correlation was found between hexanal, an indicator of WOF, and TBARS. $\beta$-Carotene when added to the ground beef at 200 and 400 ppm did not inhibit oxidation or formation of WOF. The effectiveness of tocopherols as inhibitors of oxidation and formation of WOF in cooked meats has been documented in several studies with meat products produced from red meat and poultry (84–91). Effective levels for $\alpha$-T range from 50 to 200 ppm. $\alpha$-T at 100 ppm inhibited lipid oxidation in irradiated ground chicken during chilled storage (90). The addition of antioxidants before irradiation was synergistic in decreasing the level of free fatty acids. $\alpha$-Tocopherol and BHT were the most effective antioxidants, as measured by thiobarbituric acid (TBA), carbonyl levels, and sensory evaluation (Table 3.5.).

**TABLE 3.5** Thiobarbituric Acid Values and Carbonyl Content of Treated Minced Chicken Meat During Storage at 0°C–3°C

| | | Storage (week) | | | | |
|---|---|---|---|---|---|---|
| Treatment | Measurement | 0 | 1 | 2 | 3 | 4 |
| Control | TBA[a] | 0.67 | 0.81 | 1.34 | 1.46 | 2.47 |
| | Carbonyl content[b] | 0.60 | 0.78 | 1.89 | 2.35 | 2.89 |
| Control + $\alpha$-T | TBA | 0.30 | 0.40 | 0.68 | 1.06 | 1.27 |
| | Carbonyl content | 0.14 | 0.35 | 0.46 | 0.53 | 0.64 |
| Irradiated | TBA | 0.82 | 1.02 | 2.86 | 4.03 | 4.34 |
| | Carbonyl content | 1.17 | 1.99 | 2.35 | 3.14 | 3.64 |
| Irradiated + $\alpha$-T | TBA | 0.38 | 0.46 | 0.98 | 1.65 | 2.60 |
| | Carbonyl content | 0.24 | 0.49 | 0.60 | 0.71 | 0.85 |

[a]TBA, thiobarbituric acid; $\alpha$-T, $\alpha$-tocopherol.
[b]umoles/g meat
*Source*: Modified from Ref. 90.

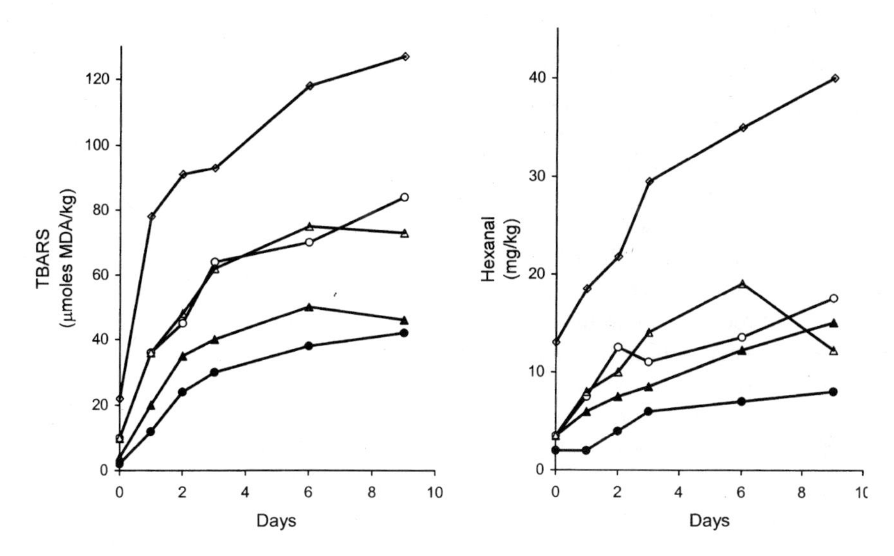


**FIGURE 3.14** The effects of *RRR*-$\alpha$-tocopherol and *RRR*-$\delta$-tocopherol added individually or in combination with ascorbyl palmitate (AP) to cooked turkey meat balls based on measurement of (A) thiobarbituric acid–reactive substance and (B) hexanal in headspace. ○, 100 ppm $\alpha$-T; △, 100 ppm $\delta$-T; •, 100 ppm $\alpha$-T + 200 ppm AP; ▲, 100 ppm $\delta$-tocopherol + 200 ppm; ◇, control batch without antioxidants added. TBARS, thiobarbituric acid–reactive substance; MDA malondialdehyde, (Modified from Ref. 88.)

Addition of mixed tocopherols from soybean oil improved the oxidative stability of cooked, minced turkey meat (88–89). At 50, 100, and 150 ppm, the mixed tocopherol reduced TBARS and the rate constant for TBARS development significantly. RRR $\alpha$-T and RRR $\delta$-T, when added individually, reduced TBARS values and hexanal headspace concentration. Without added ascorbyl palmitate, $\alpha$- and $\delta$-T had similar antioxidant activity. In the presence of ascorbyl palmitate (200 ppm), $\alpha$-T produced on additional decrease in hexanal formation (Figure 3.14).

## 3.4.4. Regulation for Application of Vitamin E

Various forms of vitamin E are classified as generally recognized as safe (GRAS) when used in accordance with good manufacturing practices by the United States Food and Drug Administration in the Code of Federal Regulations (CFR) (93). Specific sections of the CFR pertaining to vitamin E include the following:

21 CFR 182.3890
Product—Tocopherols
Usage—Chemical preservative
Conditions—GRAS
21 CFR 182.8890
Product—Tocopherols
Usage—Nutrient
Conditions—GRAS
21 CFR 107.100
Product—Vitamin E
Usage—Infant formula specification
Conditions—Must contain 0.7 IU/100 kilocalories
21 CFR 184.1890
Product—*RRR*-α-tocopherol and *all-rac*-α-tocopherol
Usage—Inhibitors of nitrosamine formation for use in pumping bacon
Conditions—Good manufacturing practices (GMP)
9 CFR 424.21
Product—Tocopherols
Usage—Rendered animal fat or a combination of such fat and vegetable fat
Conditions—0.03%. A 30% concentration of tocopherols in vegetable oils shall be used when added as an antioxidant to products designated as "lard" or "rendered pork fat"
9 CFR 424.21
Product—Tocopherols
Usage—Dry sausage, semidry sausage, dried meats, uncooked or cooked fresh sausage made with beef and/or pork, uncooked or cooked Italian sausage products, uncooked or cooked meatballs, uncooked or cooked meat pizza toppings, brown and serve sausages, pregrilled beef patties, and restructured meats
Conditions—Not to exceed 0.03% based on fat content. Not used in combination with other antioxidants
9 CFR 424.21
Product—Tocopherols
Usage—Various poultry products
Conditions—0.03% based on fat content (0.02% in combination with any other antioxidant for use in poultry, except TBHQ, based or fat content)

## 3.5. TOCOPHEROL INTERACTIONS

Because of the complexity of food systems, tocopherols, other antioxidants, and synergists can interact to produce multimechanistic barriers to lipid oxidation.

The role of vitamin E together with other antioxidants and/or synergists is well recognized in controlling oxidative stress in mammalian and plant systems. Such interactions with tocopherols and tocotrienols play a significant role in controlling oxidative events in natural and processed foods. Kamal-Eldin and Appelquist(9) specified four potential mechanisms that can produce synergistic antioxidant effects in oxidizing lipids:

1. A tocopherol sparing effect when vitamin E is present with another antioxidant, which can be a free radical interceptor or singlet oxygen quencher
2. A tocopherol regeneration system that can regenerate the tocopherols from tocopheroxyl radicals to restore the antioxidant activity
3. The presence of trace metal chelators that remove heavy metal catalysts from the system
4. The presence of microemulsions formed by phospholipids that concentrate the tocopherols with the phenolic group positioned near the polar region where lipid radicals are concentrated

### 3.5.1. Tocopherols and Ascorbic Acid

Interaction of vitamin E and ascorbic acid regenerates vitamin E in autoxidizing lipid systems (Chapter 2). Since Tappel (94) first proposed the significance of the interaction to living systems, much research has clearly defined the understanding of the event and its significance. Barclay et al. (95,96) and Niki et al. (97) were among the first researchers to demonstrate the interaction and propose mechanisms that suggested donation of a hydrogen atom by ascorbic acid to tocopheroxyl radicals to regenerate vitamin E. Location of the tocopheroxyl radical in the micelle near the aqueous phase interface and proper alignment of ascorbic acid in the aqueous phase were essential to regeneration. Niki (98), in an early review, proposed the diagram shown in Figure 3.15 to demonstrate regeneration of vitamin E by ascorbic acid. Buettner (99) presented the diagram shown in Figure 3.16 to explain lipid oxidation at the membrane level. The events occur in the following sequence:

1. Initiation of autoxidation by an oxidizing radical (R·, RO·, ROO·)
2. Oxygenation to form a peroxy radical with conjugation of the unconjugated fatty acid chain
3. Partitioning of the peroxy radical to the water–membrane interface, placing it in proximity to the tocopherol
4. Conversion of the peroxy radical to lipid hydroperoxide with formation of the tocopheroxyl radical
5. Recycling of the tocopheroxyl radical by ascorbate to tocopherol, readying the ascorbate radical for recycling by various enzyme systems

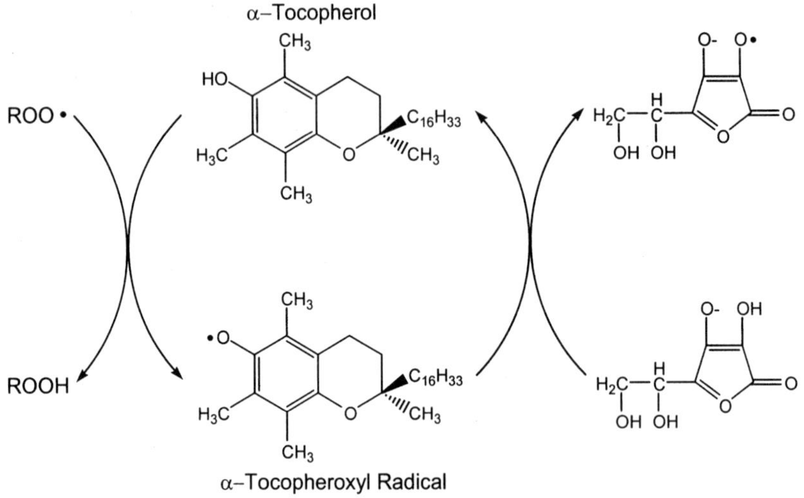

α–Tocopherol

ROO•

ROOH

α–Tocopheroxyl Radical

**FIGURE 3.15** Regeneration of $\alpha$-tocopherol from the $\alpha$-tocopheroxyl radical by ascorbic acid. (Modified from Ref. 99.)

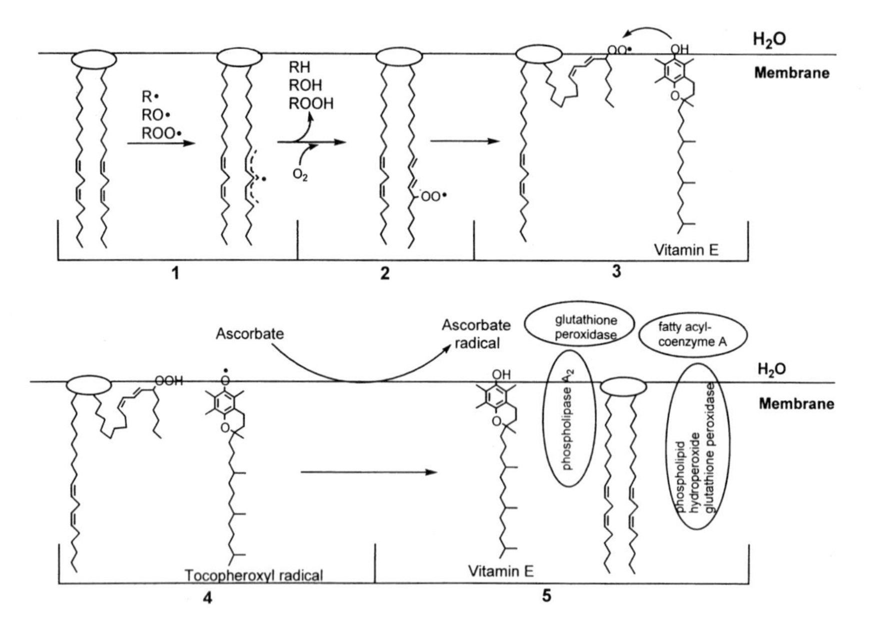


**FIGURE 3.16** Representation of the positions of $\alpha$-tocopherol and ascorbic acid at the membrane–water interface. (Modified from Ref. 99.)

The preceding discussion pertains to the role of vitamin E and ascorbic acid at the cellular membrane level only in living systems; however, regeneration of vitamin E by vitamin C bears much practical significance to control of autoxidation in food commodities and processed foods. Synergistic activity of vitamin E and ascorbic acid as antioxidants in animal and vegetable fats and oils was observed before interactions in cellular membranes (100). Since early observations in foods, a great number of literature citations indicate the usefulness of ascorbic acid or ascorbyl palmitate in multicomponent antioxidant preparations. Representative of such work, Hamilton et al. (101) found that maximal antioxidant effect occurred with 2% $\delta$-T, 0.1% ascorbyl palmitate, and 0.5% lecithin in refined Chilean fish oil stored at 20°C under air (Figure 3.17). However, delay in oxidation as measured by PV did not improve flavor stability of the oil. Yi et al. (78) had previously reported that at 0.01%–0.02% ascorbic acid was required in refined sardine oil to obtain synergism with $\delta$-T.

### 3.5.2. Tocopherols and Carotenoids

Carotenoids act as antioxidants by quenching singlet oxygen and scavenging radicals.(102–104)

$$^1O_2 + \text{Carotenoid} \rightarrow {}^3O_2 + {}^3\text{Carotenoid}$$

$$\text{ROO}\cdot + \text{Carotenoid} \rightarrow \text{ROOH} + \text{Carotenoid}\cdot$$

$$\text{Carotenoid}\cdot + O_2 \leftrightarrows \text{Carotenoid} - \text{OO}\cdot$$

Carotenoids synergistically act with vitamin E and ascorbic acid (104). A regeneration cycle, similar to that thought to be operative with vitamin E and ascorbic acid, has been postulated for regeneration of the tocopheroxyl radical by interaction with carotenoids (Figure 3.18) (105). Synergistic inhibition of lipid oxidation in rat liver microsomes has been documented (61).

In foods, carotenoids are added after other processing to enhance color (105). Inherent susceptibility to oxidation can limit their usage. Additionally, carotenoids are prooxidants under various environmental conditions. Haila et al. (106) studied interactions of several carotenoids including lutein, lycopene, $\beta$-carotene, and annatto with $\gamma$-T in triacylglycerides prepared from low–erucic acid rapeseed oil. Lutein, lycopene, and $\beta$-carotene were prooxidants, and annatto and $\gamma$-T inhibited formation of hydroperoxides. Addition of $\gamma$-T inhibited the prooxidant effect of the carotenoids and color changes. A combination of lutein and $\gamma$-T was synergistic in the inhibition of oxidation. The authors thought that $\gamma$-T retarded formation of carotenoid radicals and further degradation products. Elimination of color loss and the prooxidant effect were achieved at a $\gamma$-T concentration of 3 $\mu$g/g.

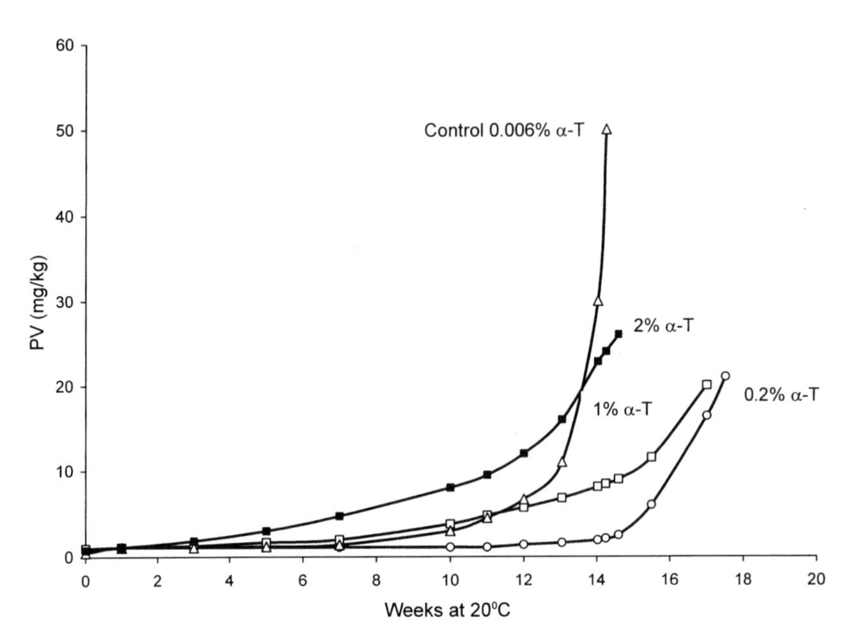


**FIGURE 3.17** The effect of $\alpha$-tocopherol ($\alpha$-T) on peroxidation in air of Chilean fish oil that contained lecithin (0.5%) and ascorbyl palmitate (0.1%) at 20°C. PV, peroxide value. (Modified from Ref. 101.)

Lee and Lillard (84) determined effectiveness of a tocopherol mixture and $\beta$-carotene in preventing lipid oxidation in cooked beef patties. Ground meat was treated with one of the following: 200 ppm of $\beta$-carotene, 400 ppm of $\beta$-carotene, 200 ppm of spray-dried mixed tocopherol concentrate, or a mixture of $\beta$-carotene and tocopherol concentrate (each 200 ppm). The tocopherol mixture reduced TBARS values, but $\beta$-carotene alone at both 200 and 400 ppm had no antioxidant activity. The mixture of tocopherols and $\beta$-carotene reduced TBARS values, but there was no significant difference between the tocopherol and

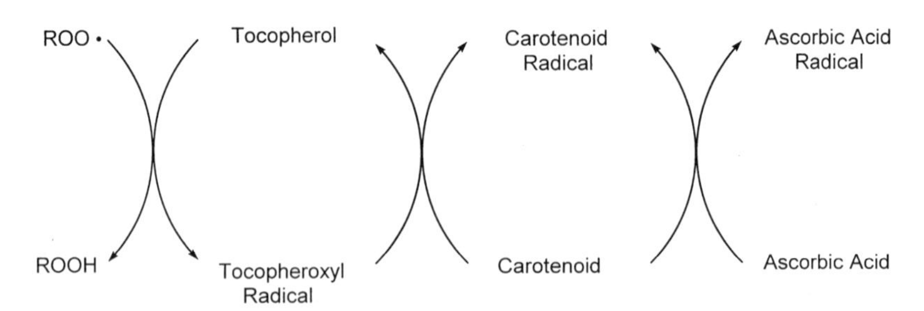


**FIGURE 3.18** Interaction of tocopherols, carotenoids, and ascorbic acid. (Modified from Ref. 105.)

tocopherol–$\beta$-carotene treatment. They concluded that synergistic antioxidant activity between the tocopherol isomers and $\beta$-carotene could not be determined. Heinonen et al. (80) reported a synergistic effect of $\alpha$-T and $\beta$-carotene on oxidation of 10% oil-in-water emulsions of rapeseed oil. In this system, $\alpha$-T (1.5 μg/g) showed antioxidant activity, inhibiting both the formation and decomposition of lipid hydroperxoides. At concentrations of 0.45, 2, and 20 μg/g, $\beta$-carotene acted as a prooxidant, in terms of the formation of lipid hydroperoxides, hexanal, or 2-heptanal. However, the combination of $\beta$-carotene and $\alpha$-T was significantly better in retarding oxidation than $\alpha$-T alone.

## REFERENCES


1. Reische, D.W.; Lillard, D.A.; Eitenmiller, R.R. Antioxidants. In *Foods Lipids: Chemistry, Nutrition and Biotechnology*; Akoh, C.C., Min, D.B., Eds.; Marcel Dekker: New York, 2002.
2. Frankel, E.N. Antioxidants in lipid foods and their impact on food quality. Food. Chem. **1996**, *57*, 51–55.
3. Jadhav, S.J.; Nimbalkar, S.S.; Kulkarni, A.D.; Madhavi, D.L. Lipid oxidation in biological and food systems. In *Food Antioxidants: Technological, Toxicological, and Health Perspectives*; Madhavi, D.L., Deshpande, S.S., Salunkhe, D.K., Eds.; Marcel Dekker: New York, 1996.
4. Nawar, W.W. Lipids. In *Food Chemistry*, 3rd Ed.; Fennema, O.R., Ed.; Marcel Dekker: New York, 1996.
5. Shahidi, F.; Naczk, M. Antioxidant properties of food phenolics. In *Food Phenolics: Sources, Chemistry, Effects, Applications*; Technomic Publishing: Lancaster, PA, 1995.
6. Decker, E.A. Antioxidant mechanisms. In *Food Lipids: Chemistry, Nutrition and Biotechnology*, 2nd Ed.; Akoh, C.C., Min, D.B., Eds.; Marcel Dekker: New York, 2002.
7. Decker, E.A. Strategies for manipulating the prooxidative/antioxidative balance of foods to maximize oxidative stability. Trends Food Sc. **1998**, *9*, 241–248.
8. McClements, D.J.; Decker, E.A. Lipid oxidation in oil-in-water emulsions: impact of molecular environment on chemical reactions in heterogeneous food systems. J. Food Sci. **2000**, *65*, 1270–1280.
9. Kamal-Eldin, A.; Appelqvist, L. The chemistry and antioxidant properties of tocopherols and tocotrienols. Lipids **1996**, *31*, 671–701.
10. Erickson, M.C. Lipid oxidation of muscle foods. In *Food Lipids: Chemistry, Nutrition and Biotechnology*, 2nd Ed.; Akoh, C.C., Min, D.B., Eds.; Marcel Dekker: New York, 2002.
11. Morrissey, P.A.; Kerry, J.P.; Galvin, K. Lipid oxidation in muscle food. In *Freshness and Shelf Life of Foods*; Cadwaller, K.R., Weenen, H., Eds.; ACS symposium series 836; American Chemical Society: Washington, DC, 2003.
12. Labuza, T.P. Kinetics of lipid oxidation in foods. Crit. Rev. Food Technol. **1971**, *2*, 355–405.

13. Burton, G.W.; Doba, T.; Gabe, E.J.; Hughes, L.; Lee, F.L.; Prasad, L.; Ingold, K.U. Autooxidation of biological molecules. 4. Maximizing the antioxidant activity of phenols. J. Am. Chem. Soc. **1985**, *107*, 7053–7065.
14. Pokorny, J. Major factors affecting the autoxidation of lipids. In *Autoxidation of Unsaturated Lipids*; Chan, H.W.S., Ed.; Academic Press: London, 1987.
15. Cort, W.M. Hemoglobin peroxidation test screens antioxidants. Food Technol. **1974**, *10*, 60–66.
16. Cooney, R.V.; Franke, A.A.; Harwood, P.J.; Hatch-Pigott, V.; Custer, L.J.; Mordan, L.J. $\gamma$-Tocopherol detoxification of nitrogen dioxide: superiority to $\alpha$-tocopherol. Proc. Natl. Acad. Sci. **1993**, *90*, 1771–1775.
17. Cooney, R.V.; Harwood, P.J.; Franke, A.A.; Narala, K.; Sundstrom, A.-K.; Benggen, P.; Mordan, L.J. Products of $\gamma$-tocopherol reaction with $NO_2$ and their formation in rat insulinoma (RINm 5F) cells. Free Radic. Biol. Med. **1995**, *19*, 259–264.
18. Jiang, Q.; Christen, S.; Shigenaga, M.K.; Ames, B.N. $\gamma$-Tocopherol, the major form of vitamin E in the US diet, deserves more attention. Am. J. Clin. Nutr. **2001**, *74*, 714–722.
19. Winterle, J.; Dulin, D.; Mill, T. Products and stoichiometry of reaction of vitamin E with alkylperoxy radicals. J. Org. Chem. **1984**, *49*, 491–495.
20. Yamauchi, R.; Matsui, T.; Kato, K.; Ueno, Y. Reaction products of $\alpha$-tocopherol with methyl linoleate–peroxyl radicals. Lipids **1990**, *25*, 152–158.
21. Liebler, D.C.; Burr, J.A. Oxidation of vitamin E during iron-catalyzed lipid peroxidation: evidence for electron-transfer reactions of the tocopheroxyl radical. Biochemistry **1992**, *31*, 8278–8284.
22. Liebler, D.C.; Burr, J.A. Antioxidant stoichiometry and the oxidative fate of vitamin E in peroxyl radical scavenging reactions. Lipids **1995**, *30*, 789–793.
23. Ishikawa, Y.; Yuki, E. Reaction products from various tocopherols with trimethylamine oxide and their antioxidative activities. Agric. Biol. Chem. **1975**, *39*, 851–857.
24. Ishikawa, Y. Effects of amino compounds on the formation of $\gamma$-tocopherol reducing dimers in autooxidizing linoleate. JAOCS **1982**, *59*, 505–510.
25. Christen, S.; Woodall, A.A.; Shigenaga, M.K.; Souyhwell-Keely, P.T.; Duncan, M.W.; Ames, B.A. $\gamma$-Tocopherol traps mutagenic electrophiles such as $NO_x$ and complements $\alpha$-tocopherol: physiological implications. Proc. Natl. Acad. Sci. USA **1997**, *94*, 3217–3222.
26. Goss, S.P.A.; Hogg, N.; Kalyanaraman, B. The effect of $\alpha$-tocopherol on the nitration of $\gamma$-tocopherol by peroxynitrite. Arch. Biochem. Biophys **1999**, *363*, 333–340.
27. Brannan, R.G.; Decker, E.A. Degradation of $\gamma$ -and $\alpha$-tocopherol and formation of 5-nitro-$\gamma$-tocopherol induced by peroxynitrite in liposomes and skeletal muscle. Meat Sci. **2002**, *64*, 149–156.
28. Cillard, J.; Cillard, P.; Cormier, M.; Girre, L. $\alpha$-Tocopherol prooxidant effect in aqueous media: increased autoxidation rate of linoleic acid. JAOCS **1980**, *57*, 252–255.
29. Cillard, J.; Cillard, P.; Cormier, M. Effect of experimental factors on the prooxidant behavior of $\alpha$-tocopherol. JAOCS **1980**, *57*, 255–261.

30. Peers, K.E.; Coxon, D.T.; Chan, H.W.S. Autoxidation of methyl linolenate and methyl linoleate: the effect of $\alpha$-tocopherol. J. Sci. Food Agric. **1981**, *32*, 898–904.
31. Koskas, J.P.; Cillard, J.; Cillard, P. Autooxidation of linoleic acid and behavior of its hydroperoxides with and without tocopherols. JAOCS **1984**, *61*, 1466–1469.
32. Terao, J.; Matsushita, S. The peroxidizing effect of $\alpha$-tocopherol on autoxidation of methyl linoleate in bulk phase. Lipids **1986**, *21*, 255–260.
33. Takahashi, M.; Yoshikawa, Y.; Niki, E. Oxidation of lipids. XVII. Crossover effect of tocopherols in the spontaneous oxidation of methyl linoleate. Bull. Chem. Soc. Jpn **1989**, *62*, 1885–1890.
34. Huang, S.W.; Fankel, E.N.; German, J.B. Antioxidant activity of $\alpha$- and $\gamma$-tocpherols in bulk oils and in oil-in-water emulsions. J. Agric. Food Chem. **1994**, *42*, 2108–2114.
35. Huang, S.-W.; Hopia, A.; Schwarz, K.; Frankel, E.N.; German, J.B. Antioxidant activity of $\alpha$-tocopherol and Trolox in different lipid substrates: Bulk oils vs oil-in-water emulsions. J. Agric. Food Chem. **1996**, *44*, 444–452.
36. Cillard, J.; Cillard, P. Behavior of alpha, gamma, and delta tocopherols with linoleic acid in aqueous media. JAOCS **1980**, *57*, 39–42.
37. Bazin, B.; Cillard, J.; Koskas, J.P.; Cillard, P. Arachidonic acid autoxidation in an aqueous media: effect of $\alpha$-tocopherol, cysteine and nucleic acids. JAOCS **1984**, *61*, 1212–1215.
38. Husain, S.R.; Cillard, J.; Cillard, P. $\alpha$-Tocopherol prooxidant effect and malondialdehyde production. JAOCS **1987**, *64*, 109–113.
39. Jung, M.Y.; Min, D.B. Effects of $\alpha$-, $\gamma$-, and $\delta$-tocopherols on oxidative stability of soybean oil. J. Food Sci. **1990**, *55*, 1464–1465.
40. Fuster, M.D.; Lampi, A.M.; Hopia, A.; Kamal-Eldin, A. Effects of $\alpha$- and $\gamma$-tocopherols on the autoxidation of purified sunflower triacylglycerols. Lipids **1998**, *33*, 715–722.
41. Lampi, A.-M.; Piironen, V. $\alpha$- and $\gamma$-Tocopherols as efficient antioxidants in butter oil triacylglycerols. Fett./Lipid. **1998**, *100*, 292–295.
42. Lampi, A.-M.; Kataja, L.; Kamal-Eldin, A.; Piironen, V. Antioxidant activities of $\alpha$- and $\gamma$-tocopherols in the oxidation of rapeseed oil triacylglycerols. JAOCS **1999**, *76*, 749–755.
43. Kulås, E.; Ackman, R.G. Protection of $\alpha$-tocopherol in nonpurified and purified fish oil. JAOCS **2001**, *78*, 197–203.
44. Kulås, E.; Ackman, R.G. Properties of $\alpha$-, $\gamma$-, and $\delta$-tocopherol in purified fish oil triacylglycerols. JAOCS **2001**, *78*, 361–367.
45. Huang, S.W.; Frankel, E.N.; German, J.B. Effects of individual tocopherols and tocopherol mixtures on the oxidative stability of corn oil triglycerides. J. Agric. Food Chem. **1995**, *43*, 2345–2350.
46. Lea, C.H.; Ward, R.J. Relative antioxidant activity of the seven tocopherols. J. Sci. Food Agric. **1959**, *10*, 537–548.
47. Lea, C.H. On the antioxidant activities of the tocopherols. II. Influence of substrate, temperature and level of oxidation. J. Sci. Food Agric. **1960**, *11*, 212–218.
48. Hove, E.L.; Hove, Z. The effect of temperature on the relative antioxidant activity of $\alpha$-, $\beta$-, and $\gamma$-tocopherols and of gossypol. J. Biol. Chem. **1944**, *156*, 623–632.

49. Ikeda, N.; Fukuzumi, K. Synergistic antioxidant effect of nucleic acids and tocopherols. JAOCS **1977**, *54*, 360–366.
50. Niki, E.; Tsuchiya, J.; Yoshikawa, Y.; Yamamoto, Y.; Kamiya, Y. Oxidation of lipids. XIII. Antioxidant activities of $\alpha$-, $\beta$-, $\gamma$-, and $\delta$-tocopherols. Bull. Chem. Soc. Jpn **1986**, *59*, 497–501.
51. Warner, K. Effects of adding various tocopherol ratios on the stability of purified vegetable oils. INFORM **1993**, *4*, 529.
52. Lampi, A.M.; Hopia, A.I.; Piironen, V.I. Antioxidant activity of minor amounts of $\gamma$-tocopherol in natural triacylglycerols. JAOCS **1997**, *74*, 549–555.
53. Ohkatsu, Y.; Kajiyana, T.; Arai, Y. Antioxidant activities of tocopherols. Polym. Degrad. Stabil. **2001**, *72*, 303–311.
54. Olcott, H.S.; Emerson, O.H. Antioxidants and the autoxidation of fats. IX. The antioxidant properties of the tocopherols. J. Am. Chem. Soc. **1937**, *59*, 1008–1009.
55. Lampi, A.J.; Kamal-Eldin, A. Effect of $\alpha$- and $\gamma$-tocopherols on thermal polymerization of purified high-oleic sunflower triacylglycerols. JAOCS **1998**, *75*, 1699–1703.
56. Barrera-Arellano, D.; Ruiz-Méndez, V.; Márquez Ruiz, G.; Dobarganes, C. Loss of tocopherols and formation of degradation compounds in triacylglycerol model systems heated at high temperature. J. Sci. Food Agric. **1999**, *79*, 1923–1928.
57. Terao, J.; Yamauchi, R.; Murakami, H.; Matsushita, S. Inhibitory effects of tocopherols and $\beta$-carotene on singlet oxygen–initiated photooxidation of methyl linoleate and soybean oil. J. Food Process Preserv. **1980**, *4*, 79–93.
58. Cort, W.M. Antioxidant activity of tocopherols, ascorbyl palmitate, and ascorbic acid and their mode of action. JAOCS **1974**, *51*, 321–325.
59. Niki, E.; Saito, M.; Kawakami, A.; Kamiya, Y. Inhibition of oxidation of methyl linoleate by vitamin E and vitamin C. J. Biol. Chem. **1984**, *259*, 4177–4182.
60. Yamauchi, R.; Matsushita, S. Quenching effect of tocopherols on the methyl linoleate photooxidation and their oxidation products. Agric. Biol. Chem. **1977**, *41*, 1425–1430.
61. Palozza, P.; Krinsky, N.I. $\beta$-Carotene and $\alpha$-tocopherol are synergistic antioxidants. Arch. Biochem. Biophys **1992**, *297*, 184–187.
62. Fahrenholtz, S.R.; Doleiden, F.H.; Trozzolo, A.M.; Lamola, A.A. On the quenching of singlet oxygen by $\alpha$-tocopherol. Photochem. Photobiol. **1974**, *20*, 505–509.
63. Mäkinen, M.; Kamal-Eldin, A.; Lampi, M.-M.; Hopia, A. Effects of $\alpha$- and $\gamma$-tocopherols on formation of hydroperoxides and two decomposition products from methyl linoleate. JAOCS **2000**, *77*, 801–806.
64. Marinova, E.M.; Yanishlieva, N.V. Effect of temperature on the antioxidative action of inhibitors in lipid autoxidation. J. Sci. Food Agric. **1992**, *60*, 313–318.
65. Grams, G.W.; Eskins, K. Dye-sensitized photooxidation of tocopherols: correlation between singlet oxygen reactivity and vitamin E activity. Biochemistry **1972**, *11*, 606–608.
66. Vile, G.F.; Winterbourn, C.C. Inhibition of adriamycin-promoted microsomal lipid peroxidation by $\beta$-carotene, $\alpha$-tocopherol and retinol at high and low oxygen partial pressures. FEBS Lett. **1988**, *238*, 353–356.

67. Buck, D.F. Antioxidants. In *Food Additive User's Handbook*; Smith, J., Ed.; Blackie: London, 1991.
68. Lea, C.H. Antioxidants in dry fat systems. I. Influence of the fatty acid composition of the substrate. J. Sci. Food Agric. **1960**, *11*, 143–150.
69. Chow, C.K.; Draper, H.H. Oxidative stability and antioxidant activity of the tocopherols in corn and soybean oils. Int. J. Vitamin. Nutr. Res. **1974**, *44*, 396–403.
70. Olcott, H.S.; van der Veer, J. Comparison of antioxidant activities of tocol and its methyl derivatives. Lipids **1968**, *3*, 331–334.
71. Yuki, E.; Ishikawa, Y. Tocopherol contents of nine vegetable frying oils and their changes under simulated deep-fat frying conditions. J. Am. Oil Chem. Soc. **1976**, *53*, 673–676.
72. Huang, S.W.; Hopia, A.; Schwarz, K.; Frankel, E.N.; German, J.B. Antioxidant activity of $\alpha$-tocopherol and Trolox in different lipid substrates: Bulk oils vs oil-in-water emulsions. J. Agric. Food Chem. **1996**, *44*, 444–452.
73. Kovats, T.K.; Berndorfer-Kraszner, E. On the antioxidative mechanism of alpha-, beta-, gamma-, and delta-tocopherols in lard. Nahrung **1968**, *12*, 407–414.
74. Wagner, K.-Heinz; Elmadfa, I. Effects of tocopherols and their mixtures on the oxidative stability of olive oil and linseed oil under heating. Eur. J. Lipid Sci. Technol. **2000**, *102*, 624–629.
75. Wagner, K.-Heinz; Wotruba, F.; Elmadfa, I. Antioxidative potential of tocotrienols and tocopherols in coconut fat at different oxidation temperatures. Eur. J. Lipid Sci. Technol. **2001**, *103*, 746–751.
76. Normand, L.; Eskin, N.A.M.; Przybylski, R. Effect of tocopherols on the frying stability of regular and modified canola oils. JAOCS **2001**, *78*, 369–373.
77. Frankel, E.N.; Huang, S.W.; Kanner, J.; German, J.B. Interfacial phenomena in the evaluation of antioxidants: bulk oils vs emulsions. J. Agric. Food Chem. **1994**, *42*, 1054–1059.
78. Yi, O.S.; Han, D.; Shin, H.K. Synergistic antioxidative effects of tocopherol and ascorbic acid in fish oil/lecithin/water system. J. Am. Oil Chem. Soc. **1991**, *68*, 881–883.
79. Riisom, T.; Sims, R.J.; Fioriti, J.A. Effect of amino acids on the autoxidation of safflower oil in emulsions. J. Am. Oil Chem. Soc. **1980**, *57*, 354–359.
80. Heinonen, M.; Haila, K.; Lampi, A.M.; Piironen, V. Inhibition of oxidation in 10% oil-in-water emulsions by $\beta$-carotene with $\alpha$- and $\gamma$-tocopherols. J. Am. Oil Chem. Soc. **1997**, *74*, 1047–1052.
81. Huang, S.W.; Frankel, E.N.; Schwarz, K.; German, J.B. Effect of pH on antioxidant activity of $\alpha$-tocopherol and Trolox in oil-in-water emulsions. J. Agric. Food Chem. **1996**, *44*, 2496–2502.
82. Wijewickreme, A.N.; Kitts, D.D. Oxidative reactions of model Maillard reaction products and $\alpha$-tocopherol in a flour–lipid mixture. J. Food Sci. **1998**, *63*, 466–471.
83. Parkhurst, R.M.; Skinner, W.A.; Sturm, P.A. The effect of various concentrations of tocopherols and tocopherol mixtures on the oxidative stabilities of a sample of lard. J. Am. Oil Chem. Soc. **1968**, *45*, 641–642.
84. Lee, K.T.; Lillard, D.A. Effects of tocopherols and $\beta$-carotene on beef patties oxidation. J. Food Lipids **1997**, *4*, 261–268.

85. Benedict, R.C.; Strange, E.D.; Swift, C.E. Effect of lipid antioxidants on the stability of meat during storage. J. Agric. Food Chem. **1975**, *23*, 167–173.
86. Mitsumoto, M.; Faustman, C.; Cassens, R.G.; Arnold, R.N.; Schaefer, D.M.; Scheller, K.K. Vitamins E and C improve pigment and lipid stability in ground beef. J. Food Sci. **1991**, *56*, 194–197.
87. Whang, K.; Aberle, E.D.; Judge, M.D.; Peng, I.C. Antioxidative activity of $\alpha$-tocopherol in cooked and uncooked ground pork. Meat Sci. **1986**, *17*, 235–249.
88. Bruun-Jensen, L.; Skovgaard, I.M.; Skibsted, L.H. The antioxidant activity of *RRR*-$\alpha$-tocopherol vs *RRR*-$\delta$-tocopherol in combination with ascorbyl palmitate in cooked, minced turkey. Food Chem. **1996**, *56*, 347–354.
89. Bruun-Jensen, L.; Skovgaard, I.M.; Madson, E.A.; Skibsted, L.H.; Bertelsen, G. The combined effect of tocopherols, L-ascorbyl palmitate and L-ascorbic acid on the development of warmed-over flavour in cooked, minced turkey. Food Chem. **1996**, *55*, 41–47.
90. Kanatt, S.R.; Paul, P.; D'Souza, S.F.; Thomas, P. Lipid peroxidation in chicken meat during chilled storage as affected by antioxidants combined with low-dose gamma irradiation. J. Food Sci. **1998**, *63*, 198–200.
91. Bruun-Jensen, L.; Skovgaard, I.M.; Skibsted, L.H.; Bertelsen, G. Antioxidant synergism between tocopherols and ascorbyl palmitate in cooked, minced turkey. Z. Lebensm. Unters Forsch. **1994**, *199*, 210–213.
92. Warner, K.; Neff, W.E.; Eller, F.J. Enhancing quality and oxidative stability of aged fried food with $\gamma$-tocopherol. J. Agric. Food Chem. **2003**, *51*, 623–627.
93. Office of the Federal Register, National Archives and Records. Code of Federal Regulations. 9 CFR 424.21, 21 CFR 104.100, 21 CFR184.1890, 21 CFR182.3890, 21 CFR 182.8890. Administration. U.S. Government Printing Office: Washington, DC, 2003.
94. Tappel, A.L. Will antioxidant nutrients slow aging processes? Geriatrics **1968**, *23*, 97–105.
95. Barclay, L.R.C.; Locke, S.J.; MacNeil, J.M. The autoxidation of unsaturated lipids in micelles: synergism of inhibitors vitamins C and E. Can. J. Chem. **1983**, *61*, 1288–1290.
96. Barclay, L.R.C.; Locke, S.J.; MacNeil, J.M. Autooxidation in micelles: synergism of vitamin C with lipid-soluble vitamin E and water-soluble Trolox. Can. J. Chem. **1985**, *63*, 366–374.
97. Niki, E.; Saito, T.; Kawakami, A.; Kamiya, Y. Inhibition of oxidation of methyl linoleate in solution by vitamin E and vitamin C. J. Biol. Chem. **1984**, *259*, 4177–4182.
98. Niki, E. Interaction of ascorbate and $\alpha$-tocopherol. Ann. N Y Acad. Sci. **1987**, *498*, 186–199.
99. Buettner, G.R. The pecking order of free radicals and antioxidants: lipid peroxidation, $\alpha$-tocopherol, and ascorbate. Arch. Biochem. Biophys. **1993**, *300*, 535–543.
100. Golumbic, C.; Mattill, H.A. Antioxidants and the autoxidation of fats. XIII. The antioxigenic action of ascorbic acid is associated with tocopherols, hydroquinones and related compounds. J. Am. Chem. Soc. **1941**, *63*, 1279–1280.

101. Hamilton, R.J.; Kalu, C.; McNeill, G.P.; Padley, F.B.; Pierce, J.H. Effects of tocopherols, ascorbyl palmitate, and lecithin on autoxidation of fish oil. JAOCS **1998**, *75*, 813–822.
102. Krinsky, N.I. The antioxidant and biological properties of the carotenoids. Ann. N Y Acad. Sci. **1998**, *854*, 443–447.
103. Young, A.J.; Lowe, G.M. Antioxidant and prooxidant properties of carotenoids. Arch. Biochem. Biophys. **2001**, *385*, 20–27.
104. Burton, G.W. Antioxidant action of carotenoids. J. Nutr. **1989**, *119*, 109–111.
105. Böhm, F.; Edge, R.; Land, E.J.; McGarvey, D.J.; Truscott, T.G. Carotenoids enhance vitamin E antioxidant efficiency. J. Am. Chem. Soc. **1997**, *119*, 621–622.
106. Haila, K.M.; Lievonen, S.M.; Heinonen, M.I. Effects of lutein, lycopene, annatto, and $\gamma$-tocopherol on autoxidation of triglycerides. J. Agric. Food Chem. **1996**, *44*, 2096–2100.

# 4

# Dietary Vitamin E Supplementation for Improvement of Oxidative Stability of Muscle Foods, Milk, and Eggs

## 4.1. INTRODUCTION

Animals cannot synthesize vitamin E, and, therefore, the levels of vitamin E in animal tissues vary according to the dietary intake of the vitamin. $\alpha$-Tocopheryl acetate ($\alpha$-TAC) is widely used for dietary supplementation by the animal and poultry feed industries because the ester form is more stable to oxidation than the corresponding alcohol form. Muscle levels of $\alpha$-tocopherol ($\alpha$-T) are increased by dietary supplementation and, in turn, increase oxidative stability of the muscle, meat products, milk, and eggs during processing and refrigerated or frozen storage. Additionally, such products then become a more significant source of $\alpha$-T to the consumer.

Oxidation of lipids is a major cause of deterioration in the quality of muscle foods that affects many quality characteristics, including flavor, color, texture, nutritional value, and safety. The rate and extent of lipid oxidation are influenced by several factors, e.g., the balance between antioxidant and prooxidant levels, the content and fatty acid composition of muscle fat, the degree of mechanical processing, the methods of packaging, and storage conditions (1). Supplementation of poultry, animal, and fish diets with vitamin E is a highly effective method to delay lipid oxidation of meats and meat products during processing, storage, and retail display. Several recent reviews on this topic include Jensen and associates (1), Frigg and associates (2), Morrissey and associates (3), Buckley and associates (4), Liu and associates (5), Sheehy and associates (6), Faustman and associates (7) and Morrissey and associates (8). This chapter focuses on the effects of vitamin E supplementation of poultry, animal, and fish diets as a means to increase the $\alpha$-T levels in food products to improve quality through retardation of oxidation, improve other quality factors, and increase availability of $\alpha$-T to the consumer.

## 4.2. BROILERS

As early as 1948, Kummerow and colleagues (9) showed that the stability of turkey skin as measured by peroxide value over an 18-month storage period at $-13^{\circ}C$ increased when the birds were fed a tocopherol concentrate. Early work with broilers proved that supplementation of poultry diets with vitamin E increased the $\alpha$-T concentration in carcass fat, muscle, plasma, and various organs and increased oxidative stability of adipose tissue and muscle (10–17). More recent research on feeding supplemental levels of vitamin E to broilers is discussed in the following sections and summarized in Table 4.1.

### 4.2.1. Vitamin E Supplementation and Tissue Levels

Bartov and Bornstein (18–19) found that the $\alpha$-T levels in plasma, liver, and adipose tissue of broilers markedly increased as dietary $\alpha$-TAC increased. Also, content of $\alpha$-T in abdominal fat increased as the duration of $\alpha$-TAC supplementation increased. In 1991, Sheehy and coworkers (20) investigated the effect of feeding $\alpha$-T on the concentrations of $\alpha$-T in various tissues of chicks. One-day-old male ISA Brown chicks were fed a vitamin E–deficient corn–soy-based starter diet or that diet supplemented with *all-rac*-$\alpha$-TAC to concentrations of 25, 65, and 180 mg $\alpha$-T/kg diet for 24 days. Concentrations of $\alpha$-T in plasma, liver, lung, heart, and thigh muscle increased as the dietary content increased. Concentrations of $\alpha$-T in tissues responded to dietary intake in the order of heart $\approx$ lung $>$ liver $>$ thigh muscle $>$ brain. Also, a linear relationship existed between the concentration of $\alpha$-T in the diet and the tissue levels of $\alpha$-T. $\alpha$-T deposition did not reach saturation in tissues with dietary $\alpha$-T content up to 180 mg/kg diet. Morrissey and associates (21) fed broilers 200 mg $\alpha$-TAC/kg diet for 5 weeks before slaughter. The basal diet contained 30 mg $\alpha$-TAC/kg diet. They found increased $\alpha$-T content in plasma and all tissues studied.

**TABLE 4.1** Selected Summaries of Research Supplementing Chicken Rations with Vitamin E[a]

| Research topic | Vitamin E forms | Amount per kg feed | Cofactor | Observations | Ref. |
|---|---|---|---|---|---|
| Feeding of $\alpha$-TAC, ethoxyquin, and BHT and rancidity development in prefried, frozen broiler parts | $\alpha$-TAC | 11, 22, 220 IU | Ethoxyquin, BHT | $\alpha$-TAC/kg fed for 36 days pre slaughter decreased TBA; feeding BHT diet did not significantly reduce rancidity development; 0.04% ethoxyquin reduced TBA | 1972, 25 |
| Dietary fat and $\alpha$-TAC supplement effects on the tissue concentration of $\alpha$-T and the stability of carcass fat and meat of broilers | $\alpha$-TAC | 0–60 mg | Dietary fat | Plasma, liver, and adipose tissue $\alpha$-T level increased markedly as dietary vitamin E levels rose; stability of abdominal fat and meat was little affected by the degree of saturation of carcass fat in the absence of dietary vitamin E; dietary vitamin E significantly improved stability | 1977, 18 |
| $\alpha$-TAC, BHT, and ethoxyquin and the stability of abdominal fat and muscle tissue of broilers having carcass fat of different degrees of saturation | $\alpha$-TAC | 10–30 mg | BHT, ethoxyquin | $\alpha$-TAC and ethoxyquin markedly improved oxidative stability; BHT improved fat stability only | 1977, 26 |
| Stability of carcass fat and meat of broilers as a function of duration of feeding $\alpha$-TAC or ethoxyquin in diets containing unsaturated or saturated fat supplements | $\alpha$-TAC | 40 mg | Ethoxyquin, length of supplement | $\alpha$-T content of abdominal fat and fat stability increased as a function of the duration of $\alpha$-TAC feeding | 1978, 19 |

| | | | | | |
|---|---|---|---|---|---|
| BHT, ethoxyquin, Endox-50, α-TAC, and vitamin E status on the stability of carcass tissues of broilers possessing saturated or unsaturated carcass fat | α-TAC | 10, 30 mg | BHT, ethoxyquin | Ethoxyquin, BHT, and Endox-50 consistently increased α-T levels in carcass fat of birds fed diets with or without α-TAC supplementation; stability of abdominal fat and thigh meat increased with the combination of ethoxyquin and α-TAC | 1981, 46 |
| Oxidized oil and dietary antioxidant supplementation and the antioxidant concentration in the subcellular membranes of broiler meat, and the influence of three dietary treatments on the oxidative stability of membrane-bound lipids | α-TAC | 200 mg | Oxidized oil | Oxidized oil in broiler diets induced rapid oxidation of the membrane-bound lipids and decreased their stability to MetMb-hydrogen peroxide–catalyzed peroxidation; supplementation of the broiler diets with α-TAC increased the α-T level in the microsomal and soluble protein fraction of the white meat; the increased α-T level stabilized the membrane-bound lipids | 1989, 29 |

(*continued*)

**Table 4.1** *Continued*

| Research topic | Vitamin E forms | Amount per kg feed | Cofactor | Observations | Ref. |
|---|---|---|---|---|---|
| Oxidized oil, fatty acid composition of muscle lipids, and oxidative stability of broiler meat as influenced by dietary BHA/BHT and $\alpha$-TAC supplementation | $\alpha$-TAC | 200 mg | BHA, BHT, oxidized oil | Oxidized oil reduced broiler body and carcass weights; $\alpha$-TAC and BHA/BHT supplementation improved growth; feeding oxidized oil to broilers resulted in meat that underwent rapid oxidative changes during refrigerated and frozen storage; dietary $\alpha$-TAC and BHA/BHT increased $\alpha$-T and BHA/BHT concentrations in meat and significantly improved oxidative stability | 1989, 43 |
| Response of neutral lipids and phospholipids in dark and white meats of broilers to dietary oils and to $\alpha$-TAC supplementation and influence on oxidative stability of meat | $\alpha$-TAC | 100 mg | Dietary oils | Coconut, olive, and linseed oil significantly affected fatty acid composition of neutral lipids and, to a lesser extent, fatty acid composition of phospholipids; meat from broilers fed olive oil or coconut oil was consistently more stable than meat from the linseed oil group; dietary supplementation with $\alpha$-TAC significantly improved oxidative stability | 1989, 38 |

| | | | | | |
|---|---|---|---|---|---|
| Dietary oils and α-TAC supplementation and fatty acid composition and stability of membrane lipids of broiler muscles | α-TAC | 100 mg | Dietary oils | Fatty acid composition of both neutral lipids and phospholipids of mitochondria and microsomes was influenced by dietary oil composition; supplementation with α-TAC increased α-T level in microsomal membranes; in dark meats oxidation in microsomes and mitochondria was dependent on fatty acid composition of membrane lipids, and, to a lesser extent, on α-T content | 1990, 39 |
| Feeding α-TAC and the concentrations of α-T in various chicken tissues | α-TAC | 250, 650, 1800 mg | | Tissue α-T concentrations responded to dietary intake in the order heart = lung > liver > thigh muscle > brain | 1991, 20 |
| High concentrations of vitamin E fed during different age periods and growth, performance, and meat stability of 7-wk-old broiler chicks | α-TAC | 100, 150 mg | | Food intake, weight gain, and food efficiency were not significantly affected by α-TAC supplementation; stability of meat of birds fed vitamin E was significantly higher than that of birds that did not receive additional vitamin E | 1992, 31 |

(*continued*)

**TABLE 4.1** *Continued*

| Research topic | Vitamin E forms | Amount per kg feed | Cofactor | Observations | Ref. |
|---|---|---|---|---|---|
| Feeding fresh, heated, or α-TAC-supplemented heated vegetable oils and growth and α-T status of chicks, fatty acid composition, and oxidative stability of muscle lipids | α-TAC | 50 mg | Oxidized oil | Plasma α-T level was significantly correlated with α-T concentrations in thigh and breast muscle; fatty acid profiles of muscle lipids reflected dietary fatty acid composition; consumption of heated sunflower and linseed oil reduced α-T status, altered fatty acid composition of muscle lipids, and increased susceptibility to lipid oxidation; supplementation of diets containing heated oils with α-TAC resulted in some alleviation of effects | 1993, 42 |
| Effect of feeding diets containing fresh or heated sunflower oil (HSO), with or without α-TAC, on α-T concentrations and fatty acid composition of chick tissues and stability of these tissues against Fe-ascorbate-induced lipid oxidation | α-TAC | α-T difference between heated and fresh oil | Oxidized oil | α-T in tissues of chicks fed HSO and HSO supplemented with α-TAC (HSE) was significantly lower than that of chicks fed on fresh sunflower oil; supplementation with α-TAC reduced susceptibility to lipid oxidation | 1994, 44 |

| | | | | | |
|---|---|---|---|---|---|
| Antioxidant role of all-rac-α-TAC and a mixture of natural source RRR-α-, γ-, and δ-TAC | α-TAC, natural source TAC | 100, 500 mg | — | No differences between the supplemented groups were observed with respect to weight gain, feed consumption, packed cell volume, etc; increasing levels of α-, γ-, and δ-T were found in blood plasma with increasing dietary levels of these tocopherols; mixture of natural source RRR-α-, γ-, and δ-TAC was an efficient in protecting live chickens as α-TAC | 1995, 32 |
| Oxidative stability of broiler muscle and effect of using either synthetic α-TAC or mixture of natural source RRR-α-, γ-, and δ-T for vitamin E supplementation | α-TAC, natural source TAC | 100, 500 mg | — | Dietary vitamin E resulted in improved oxidative stability of broiler muscle; supplementation of broiler feed with 100 mg α-TAC improved stability of precooked broiler breast and precooked thigh muscles during chill storage; mixed tocopherol source was less effective in protecting broiler muscles than the synthetic α-TAC | 1995, 33 |

(continued)

**TABLE 4.1** *Continued*

| Research topic | Vitamin E forms | Amount per kg feed | Cofactor | Observations | Ref. |
|---|---|---|---|---|---|
| Dietary vitamin E and oxidative and sensory qualities of different parts (leg and breast) of chicken meat | $\alpha$-TAC | 200 mg | — | Muscle $\alpha$-T levels of supplemented group were 6- to 7-fold higher than those of group on control diet; $\alpha$-TAC supplementation increased oxidative stability | 1996, 27 |
| Dietary $\alpha$-TAC, $\alpha$-T status of plasma and tissues, and rate of iron-ascorbate-induced lipid peroxidation | $\alpha$-TAC | 200 mg | — | Supplementation with $\alpha$-TAC for up to 4 wk pre slaughter resulted in significant reductions in lipid oxidation and increased $\alpha$-T level in plasma and all tissues | 1997, 21 |
| Combined effect of vitamin A and E and oxidative stability of drumstick meat of broilers | $\alpha$-TAC | 150 mg | Vitamin A (retinyl acetate) | TBARS values were very low and not significantly affected by dietary vitamin A and E or their combinations; TBARS values in the meat of birds fed on the vitamin E–free diets were markedly increased, resulting in a significant difference from vitamin E supplementation; vitamin A alone or in combination with vitamin E did not affect TBARS values | 1997, 47 |

| | | | | | |
|---|---|---|---|---|---|
| Oxidized dietary sunflower oil, dietary $\alpha$-TAC supplementation, and $\alpha$-T concentrations in broiler muscle; storage stability of refrigerated, cooked, minced muscle | $\alpha$-TAC | 30 and 200 mg | Oxidized oil | Oxidized oil increased oxidation in raw and cooked muscle and reduced oxidative stability during storage; supplementation with $\alpha$-TAC improved stability of muscle; oxidative stability increased as muscle $\alpha$-T increased | 1997, 45 |
| n-3 Fatty acid enrichment of poultry meat and extension of shelf life through dietary tocopherol supplementation | Not specified | 100 IU | n-3 Fatty acid | n-3 Fatty acid levels of breast and thigh muscles were significantly elevated by feeding linseed oil; $\alpha$-T contents and oxidative stability of breast and thigh muscles were significantly increased by vitamin E supplementation | 1997, 40 |
| Oxidative stability of membrane fractions of broiler dark and white meat | $\alpha$-TAC | 20, 200 mg | Dietary fat | Concentrations of $\alpha$-T in membrane of breast and thigh muscles were significantly influenced by $\alpha$-T level in feed; deposition of $\alpha$-T was not influenced by type of oil in feed, except in mitochondrial fraction of breast, oxidative stability of membrane fractions tended to increase with increasing concentration of $\alpha$-T | 1997, 30 |

*(continued)*

**Table 4.1** *Continued*

| Research topic | Vitamin E forms | Amount per kg feed | Cofactor | Observations | Ref. |
|---|---|---|---|---|---|
| Dietary $\alpha$-TAC supplementation, gamma-irradiation, and $\alpha$-T retention and lipid oxidation in cooked, minced chicken | $\alpha$-TAC | 100, 200, 400 mg | Irradiation | $\alpha$-T concentrations increased with increasing dietary supplementation; concentration of $\alpha$-T decreased during storage, but retention was not affected by irradiation; levels of TBARS and COPs during storage were reduced by dietary $\alpha$-TAC supplementation | 1998, 48 |
| Effect of dietary MUFA composition and $\alpha$-TAC supplementation on quality attributes in chicken products after refrigerated and frozen storage | $\alpha$-TAC | 200 mg | Dietary fat | Supplemental $\alpha$-T increased $\alpha$-T content of muscles; dietary fat did not influence drip loss in thawed breast fillets during refrigerated storage, but supplemental $\alpha$-T reduced drip loss; TBARS and WOF development were reduced by supplemental $\alpha$-T; storage stability was not adversely affected by dietary fat | 1998, 49 |
| Dietary $\alpha$-TAC supplementation and COPs generation in processed chicken during refrigerated storage | $\alpha$-TAC | 20, 200, 800 mg | — | Dietary supplementation at 200 and 800 mg $\alpha$-TAC/kg significantly increased $\alpha$-T concentrations in cooked muscle and decreased TBARS and cholesterol oxidation during storage | 1998, 22 |

| | | | | | |
|---|---|---|---|---|---|
| Dietary fat and supplementation of $\alpha$-TAC or $\beta$-carotene and vitamin E content and lipid oxidation in raw, cooked, and chilled-stored broiler leg meat | $\alpha$-TAC | 200 mg | $\beta$-Carotene | $\alpha$-TAC supplementation increased $\alpha$-T tissue levels and reduced lipid oxidation; oxidative stability of leg meat tended to decrease with dietary sunflower oil; effects of $\beta$-carotene on $\alpha$-T levels and oxidative stability depended on dietary fat and its concentration in feed; $\beta$-carotene at 15 ppm acted as antioxidant in fresh and cooked meat from sunflower and olive oil trials; in stored meat, $\beta$-carotene at 50 ppm increased TBARS level | 1999, 23 |
| Postslaughter addition of carnosine to meat from $\alpha$-TAC, supplemented birds in the presence of salt and its effects on cholesterol oxidation | $\alpha$-TAC | 200 mg | Carnosine, salt | Salt accelerated lipid and cholesterol oxidation after cooking and refrigerated storage; carnosine inhibited lipid and cholesterol oxidation in salted patties; dietary $\alpha$-TAC reduced lipid and cholesterol oxidation in salted patties; the combination of carnosine and dietary $\alpha$-TAC resulted in greatest lipid and cholesterol stability in salted meat | 1999, 35 |

(*continued*)

**TABLE 4.1** *Continued*

| Research topic | Vitamin E forms | Amount per kg feed | Cofactor | Observations | Ref. |
|---|---|---|---|---|---|
| Occurrence of PSE in chicken as affected by vitamin E | α-TAC | 150 IU to 200 IU | | Dietary supplementation inhibited PSE in heat stressed chicks | 2001, 34 |
| α-TAC supplementation, dietary fat, ascorbic acid, and oxidative stability | α-TAC, ascorbic acid | 0, 225 mg | Fat source | α-TAC provided excellent protection against oxidation | 2001, 36 |
| α-TAC supplementation, dietary fat, ascorbic acid, and oxidative stability | α-TAC, ascorbic acid | 0, 225 mg | Fat source | α-TAC decreased cholesterol oxidation in raw and cooked dark meat | 2001, 37 |
| High levels of α-TAC supplementation and α-T deposition | α-TAC | 0, 100, 1000, 10,000, 20,000 mg | | α-T increased at all levels of supplementation in eggs, liver, and muscle; α-T transfer decreased at higher dosages, but highest α-T concentrations resulted from the 20,000-mg level | 2002, 154 |

[a] α-TAC, α-tocopherol acetate; BHT, butylated hydroxytoluene; TBA, thiobarbituric acid; α-T, α-tocopherol; MetMb, metmyoglobin; BHA, butylated hydroxyanisole; HSE, heated sunflower oil supplemented with α-TAC; HSO, heated sunflower oil; TBARS, thiobarbituric acid–reactive substance; MUFA, monounsaturated fatty acid; WOF, warmed-over flavor; COP, cholesterol oxidation products; PSE, pale, soft, exudative.

The order was heart > lung > liver > thigh muscle > breast muscle > brain, an order very similar to the results reported by Sheehy and colleagues (20). The duration of supplementation time required to approach saturation differed from tissue to tissue (Figure 4.1). Saturation levels of $\alpha$-T were reached at 1 week for liver and plasma, 3 weeks for heart, lung, and thigh muscle, and 4 weeks for breast muscle. Both Sheehy and coworkers (20) and Morrissey and associates (21) suggested that the low concentrations of $\alpha$-T in brain tissue were due to either poor tissue uptake or high turnover. A higher amount of $\alpha$-T in lung and heart is required to protect these tissues against the high oxygen tension and freshly oxygenated blood (21). In order to optimize $\alpha$-T levels in muscle and retard oxidation, a supplemental dietary level of 200 mg $\alpha$-TAC/kg diet was recommended to be fed at least 4 weeks before slaughter.

Other research confirmed that dietary supplementation of broiler diets with $\alpha$-TAC increased $\alpha$-T levels in cooked muscle and in raw, cooked, and stored chicken meat (22,23). $\alpha$-T concentrations in breast and thigh muscle increased 4.1- and 2.0-fold with supplementation of 200 mg $\alpha$-TAC/kg feed and 10- and 4.7-fold with supplementation of 800 mg/kg feed, respectively (22). The 200- and 800-mg supplemental levels significantly decreased formation of cholesterol oxidation products in breast and thighs stored at 4°C. A diet supplemented at the

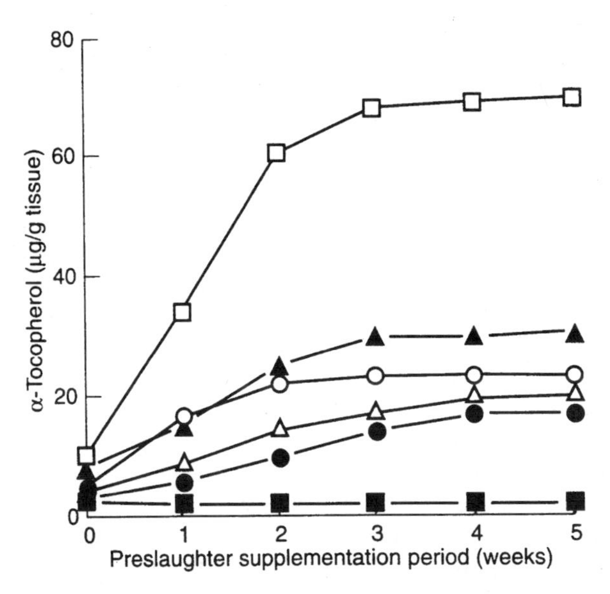


**FIGURE 4.1** $\alpha$-Tocopherol concentrations in heart, (□), liver (○), lung (▲), brain (■), thigh (△), and breast (●) muscle of chicks fed a basal diet up to slaughter at 6 weeks, or chicks fed an $\alpha$-TAC-supplemented diet for 1 to 5 weeks. $\alpha$-TAC, $\alpha$-tocopherol acetate. (From Ref. 21.)

200-mg $\alpha$-TAC/kg level increased $\alpha$-T in broiler tissue four- to seven-fold compared to that of a control diet (23).

### 4.2.2. Effect of Dietary Vitamin E on Oxidative Stability

The primary objective of supplementation of broiler diets with vitamin E is to prevent and/or delay lipid oxidation in fresh or processed products. Positive effects include prevention or delay of rancidity in uncooked meats and warmed-over flavor in cooked meats, cholesterol oxidation in processed and stored poultry products, and color deterioration and drip loss in fresh meats. Increased incorporation of $\alpha$-T into membranes presents a first-line defense mechanism against the initiation of oxidation of the unsaturated lipids present in the membrane and the negative effects oxidation has on quality (5,24)

One of the earliest studies showing the ability of dietary vitamin E to improve oxidative stability in broiler meat was by Webb and colleagues in 1972 (25). They investigated the effects of feeding $\alpha$-TAC at concentrations of 11 (7.4 mg $\alpha$-T), 22 (14.8 mg $\alpha$-T), and 220 IU (147.8 mg $\alpha$-T)/kg feed for 36 days along with ethoxyquin (EQ) and butylated hydroxytoluene (BHT) on rancidity development in broiler meat. Feeding 11 or 22 IU/kg feed for 36 days or feeding 220 IU/kg feed for 12 days held thiobarbituric acid (TBA) numbers below those of the control. Feeding BHT at 0.01%, 0.02%, or 0.04% of the diet did not significantly reduce rancidity development, but 0.04% EQ reduced TBA numbers. Bartov and Bornstein (26) also studied the effect of vitamin E, BHT, and EQ on the stability of abdominal fat and muscle tissue of broilers. Supplementation of $\alpha$-TAC at 10 and 20 mg/kg diet for about 30 days improved the stability of abdominal fat and thigh and breast muscle in terms of TBA numbers. Effects of various dietary supplementation approaches on the quality of frozen chicken meat evaluated by sensory as well as by instrumental techniques using gas chromatograph–mass spectrometry (GC–MS) showed significant effects on off-flavor scores (27). Samples from vitamin E-supplemented birds had a fresher flavor when compared to the control samples. Analysis of the constituents in the aroma concentrates of meats from control and supplemented birds indicated that levels of aldehydes, which are markers for rancid flavor of meats, were much higher in the control samples when compared to the supplemented samples. The muscles from chickens fed a basal diet were more susceptible to induced oxidation than the muscles from chickens fed a supplemented diet, including a finisher diet, containing 200 mg $\alpha$-TAC/kg. Oxidative changes of dark meat (leg) from the control group were much more extensive than those of white meat (breast) from the same control group even though $\alpha$-T level of leg muscle was higher than that of breast muscle. This result confirmed previous findings that lipid peroxidation rate was higher in microsomes from dark muscle tissue of broilers when compared to white muscle microsomes (28,29). The higher oxidation rate in dark broiler meat is due to higher total lipid content compared to that of white meat. Lauridsen and coworkers (30) also found that oxidative changes were much more extensive in subcellular membranes isolated from thigh muscles compared to membranes from breast muscles.

Bartov and Frigg (31) determined the effect of feeding pattern of vitamin E on the performance and the oxidative stability of the drumstick meat of 7-week-old broiler chicks. They evaluated the five feeding treatments listed in Table 4.2. Food intake, weight gain, and food efficiency were not significantly affected by the vitamin E feeding pattern. The TBA values were significantly negatively correlated with the amount of vitamin E consumed during induced oxidation of the tissue by incubation in a water bath at 37°C for 1 h under constant shaking (Table 4.2). The oxidative stability of the meat of birds fed the various combinations of vitamin E (treatments 3, 4, and 5) was significantly higher than that of birds that did not receive additional vitamin E (treatment 1). The muscle of birds that received vitamin E continuously (treatment 2) showed the best oxidative stability.

Synthetic $\alpha$-TAC is as effective as a mixture of natural sources of *RRR*-$\alpha$-, $\gamma$-, and $\delta$-TAC for dietary vitamin E supplementation in protecting the live chicken (32,33). Blood analyses including packed cell volume and in vitro hemolysis to indicate erythrocyte fragility and plasma enzyme levels, including those of aspartate aminotransferase, creatine kinase, and glutathione peroxidase, showed only small differences between control chicks and groups supplemented with vitamin E, either natural or synthetic. Excretion of ethane and pentane was not evident, confirming minimal in vivo peroxidation and oxidative stress in the live birds. A mixture of natural source *RRR*-$\alpha$-, $\gamma$-, and $\delta$-TAC was as efficient as *all-rac* $\alpha$-T at levels of 100 or 500 mg/kg feed. Vitamin E supplementation at these levels also protects heat stressed birds from development of pale, soft, exudative (PSE) meat (34).

Supplementation above the basal diet level that contained 72 mg/kg $\alpha$-T from natural ingredients and a supplementation rate of 46 mg *all-rac*-$\alpha$-TAC/kg feed had little effect on the oxidative stability of raw, chilled, or frozen muscles. Addition of 100 mg of either mixed natural source TAC or *all-rac*-$\alpha$-TAC increased oxidative stability of precooked muscles over those of the control (33) (Figure 4.2). Increasing the supplementation rate from 100 to 500 mg/kg feed of *all-rac*-$\alpha$-TAC did not significantly improve oxidative stability of the precooked muscle; however, addition of 500 mg/kg of natural source mixed tocopherols did slightly improve oxidative stability from the 100-mg/kg rate. The study conclusively showed that the mixture of natural source *RRR*-tocopherols was less effective on a weight basis when compared to the *all-rac*-$\alpha$-T, confirming the role of $\alpha$-T as an antioxidant in chicken muscles. A supplementation of 200 mg/kg

**TABLE 4.2** Effect of Dietary Vitamin E Concentration and the Age Period of Its Supplementation on the Plasma α-Tocopherol Level and on the Meat Stability of Broiler Chicks[a]

| Treatment | Vitamin E added (mg/kg) | Age of vitamin E feeding (wk) | Vitamin E consumed (mg/chick)[b] | Plasma α-T (mg/L) | TBA values[c] | |
|---|---|---|---|---|---|---|
| | | | | | Initial | After incubation[d] |
| 1 | None | 0–7 | 129 | 6.4 | 0.37 | 6.71 |
| 2 | 100 | 0–7 | 558 | 25.1 | 0.22 | 1.15 |
| 3 | 150 | 0–3 | 259 | 8.6 | 0.22 | 4.30 |
| 4 | 150 | 0–3 | | | | |
| | 100 | 6–7 | 357 | 22.9 | 0.21 | 3.13 |
| 5 | 100 | 5–7 | 317 | 23.2 | 0.19 | 3.77 |

*Source*: Modified from Ref. 31

[a]Means of ± standard error of 12 birds (three of each of the four replicates). TBA, thiobarbituric acid; α-T, α-tocopherol.
[b]Data based on the analyzed values of the diets and amount of food intake.
[c]Expressed as milligrams sodium salt of malonaldehyde *bis*-bisulfite per kilogram meat.
[d]In water bath at 37°C for 1 h under constant shaking.

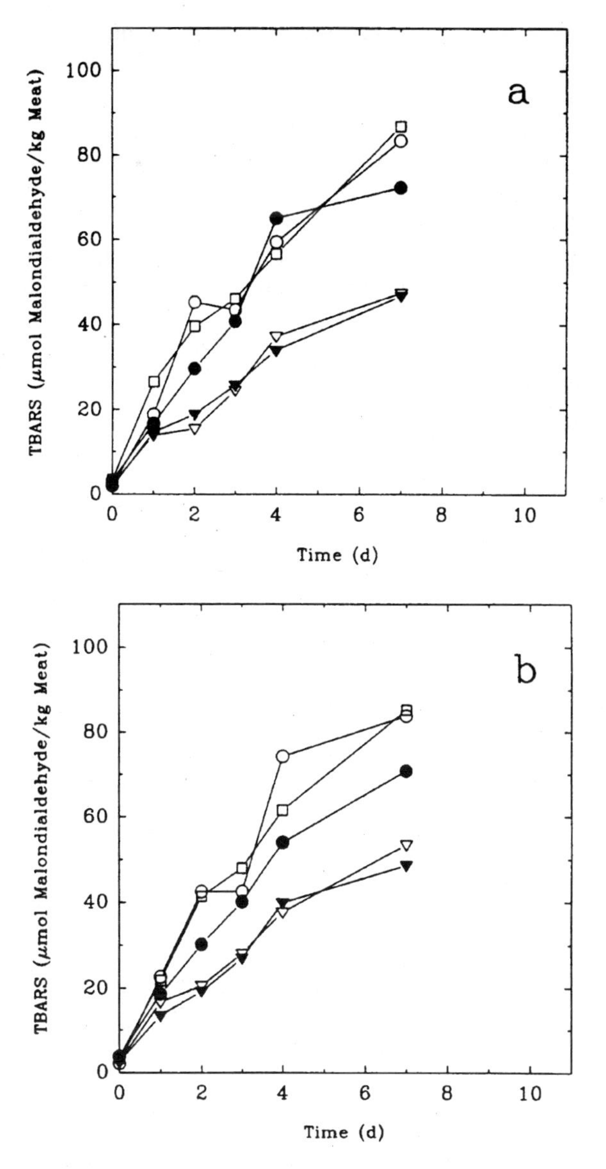


**FIGURE 4.2** Progression in oxidation in precooked, chill stored (a) breast muscle and (b) thigh muscle from broilers fed basal feed (□), basal feed supplemented with 100 mg mixture of natural source RRR-$\alpha$-, $\gamma$-, $\delta$-TAC/kg feed (○), basal feed supplemented with 100 mg all-rac-$\alpha$-TAC/kg feed (▽), basal feed supplemented with 500 mg mixture of natural source RRR-$\alpha$-, $\gamma$-, $\delta$-tocopheryl acetate/kg feed (▼). $\alpha$-TAC, $\alpha$-tocopherol acetate; TBARS, thiobarbituric acid–reactive subtance. (From Ref. 33.)

with *all-rac-α*-TAC to give a final feed content approximating 200 mg/kg α-T was recommended (33). This level was thought to be sufficient to protect precooked broiler meat during chill storage and processing.

Since chicken dark meat tends to be oxidized more rapidly than breast meat, the effect of supplemental vitamin E on the stability of processed and/or frozen dark meat products is significant. Research published in 1999 and 2001 (35–37) indicated that dark meat from vitamin E–supplemented birds is significantly more stable than that from nonsupplemented birds during frozen storage. Also, α-TAC at 200 mg/kg counteracts the prooxidant effect of NaCl in salted products (Figure 4.3) (35).

## 4.2.3. Effect of Dietary Fat and Vitamin E on Lipid Oxidation

Oils and other fats are commonly added to broiler diets to meet high energy demand of the fast growing broilers and to improve the efficiency of feed utilization. Since dietary recommendations for humans stress intake of low levels of saturated fats, research has focused on the production of chicken meat with modified fatty acid profiles. However, as the degree of unsaturation of the muscle lipid increases, the oxidative stability of the muscle decreases. This relationship presents a need to adjust the antioxidant capacity of the muscle to compensate for the higher muscle levels of unsaturated fatty acids. Increased antioxidant capacity can be easily

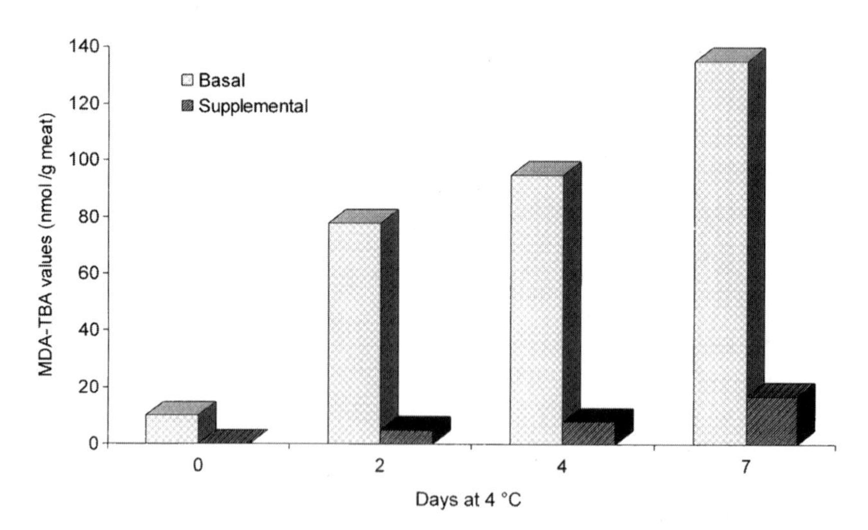


**FIGURE 4.3** Effect of 1% salt on the oxidative stability of refrigerated, cooked thigh patties from broilers fed 30 mg/kg or 200-mg/kg diet α-TAC. α-TAC, α-tocopherol acetate; MDA-TBA, malonaldehyde-thiobarbitaric acid values. (Modified from Ref. 35.)

achieved by dietary vitamin E supplementation. $\alpha$-Tocopherol from the supplementation incorporates into membrane-bound phospholipids, acting as an antioxidant (24) where oxidative changes are initiated in meat and meat products.

**4.2.3.1. Fat Composition.** Significant research has determined the influence of dietary fat supplementation on fatty acid composition of carcass fat and on the oxidative stability of the fat and meat of the chicken. Evaluation of the effect of different oils (coconut, olive, linseed, and partially hydrogenated soybean oils) on lipid composition of the neutral lipids and the phospholipids of white and dark broiler meat showed that different oils significantly affected the fatty acid composition of the neutral lipid and, to a lesser extent, the fatty acid composition of the phospholipids (Table 4.3) (38). The modified fatty acid composition, in turn, influenced the oxidative stability of the meat during refrigerated (4°C) and frozen (−20°C) storage (Table 4.4). The neutral lipids from broilers fed linseed oil contained a much higher amount of linolenic acid (C18:3) than the lipids from other broiler groups, and the neutral lipids from broilers fed coconut oil showed much higher levels of C12:0 and C14:0. $\alpha$-Tocopherol supplementation had no effect on the fatty acid composition of the neutral lipids. The meats from the broilers fed linseed oil had higher thiobarbituric acid–reactive substance (TBARS) numbers than the corresponding samples from the control group fed partially hydrogenated soybean oil (HSBO). These higher numbers were reflective of the higher polyunsaturated fatty acid (PUFA) concentrations in both the neutral lipids and the phospholipids from the broilers fed the linseed oil diet. On the other hand, the meat samples from the group fed coconut oil showed smaller PUFA contents and were more stable to oxidation than the samples from the HSBO-fed group. This observation agrees with the results of Asghar et al. (39). Meat from broilers fed linseed oil contained relatively high amounts of C18:3, C22:5$\omega$3, and C22:6. The meat from broilers fed coconut oil contained higher amounts of C12:0 and C14:0.

Nam et al (40). investigated the influence of dietary linseed oil and vitamin E on fatty acid composition, $\alpha$-T content, and lipid peroxidation of breast and thigh muscles in broiler chicks. The broilers were fed 10% linseed oil and 10% linseed oil containing 100 IU vitamin E (67.1 mg $\alpha$-T/kg feed). Linseed oil supplementation significantly reduced saturated fatty acid (SFA) levels in both breast and thigh muscles, and $\alpha$-T contents and oxidative stability of breast and thigh muscles were significantly increased by vitamin E supplementation. Feeding olive oil compared to feeding tallow resulted in approximately a twofold increase in the monounsaturated fatty acid (MUFA)/saturated fatty acid (SFA) ratio (41). Vitamin E supplementation increased $\alpha$-T content of the muscles and oxidative stability of minced thigh meat patties during refrigerated (4°) and frozen (−20°C) storage, confirming prior observations that changes in the fatty acid composition of the membrane-bound lipids and/or the supplementation of

**TABLE 4.3** Percentage Fatty Acid Composition of Neutral Lipids and Phospholipids Isolated from Dark Meat of Broilers Fed Different Dietary Oils and $\alpha$-Tocopherol

| Fatty acid | Coconut oil | Olive oil | Linseed oil | HSBO + $\alpha$-T[a] | HSBO |
|---|---|---|---|---|---|
| C12 : 0 | 11.1 (0.9)[b] | – (–) | – (–) | – (–) | – (–) |
| C14 : 0 | 7.3 (1.9) | 0.3 (–) | 0.4 (–) | 0.5 (–) | 0.4 (–) |
| C16 : 0 | 19.7 (15.7) | 17.4 (16.3) | 17.3 (16.3) | 18.1 (16.9) | 18.4 (16.5) |
| C16 : 1 | 4.0 (0.9) | 4.0 (0.8) | 4.4 (1.1) | 4.4 (0.8) | 4.9 (0.8) |
| C18 : 0 | 6.4 (14.2) | 3.7 (12.4) | 4.6 (13.0) | 4.7 (12.5) | 4.5 (13.1) |
| C18 : 1 | 31.4 (15.7) | 49.4 (20.0) | 28.5 (16.3) | 33.6 (15.6) | 33.8 (15.9) |
| C18 : 2 | 14.1 (17.2) | 18.7 (15.0) | 17.9 (15.2) | 28.9 (20.2) | 30.5 (19.1) |
| C18 : 3 | 1.9 (4.5) | 1.9 (5.0) | 23.7 (5.1) | 3.4 (5.4) | 3.7 (7.2) |
| C22 : 4 | 0.6 (2.9) | 1.0 (4.3) | 0.3 (1.9) | 0.3 (2.5) | 0.3 (1.5) |
| C22 : 5$\omega$6 | 0.1 (1.3) | 0.2 (1.6) | 0.2 (0.6) | 0.2 (0.6) | 0.3 (1.3) |
| C22 : 5$\omega$3 | 0.5 (1.4) | 1.0 (1.7) | 0.8 (5.3) | 0.4 (2.8) | 0.6 (1.6) |
| C22 : 6 | 0.2 (1.7) | 0.1 (1.6) | 0.4 (5.1) | 0.2 (1.8) | 0.3 (1.7) |

[a]HSBO, hydrogenated soybean oil; $\alpha$-T, $\alpha$-tocopherol.
[b]The values in parentheses represent the percentage fatty acid in phospholipids.
*Source*: Modified from Ref. 38.

**TABLE 4.4** Thiobarbituric Acid–Reactive Substance Numbers of Dark Meat Stored at 4°C and −20°C from Broilers Fed Dietary Oils and α-Tocopherol[a]

| Time of storage | Coconut oil | Olive oil | Linseed oil | HSBO + α-T[a] | HSBO |
|---|---|---|---|---|---|
| Storage at 4°C | | | | | |
| 2 days | 0.19 | 0.15 | 1.40 | 0.08 | 0.19 |
| 3 days | 0.68 | 0.53 | 2.28 | 0.27 | 0.49 |
| 4 days | 1.14 | 0.68 | 3.98 | 0.30 | 1.40 |
| 6 days | 1.47 | 1.29 | 4.70 | 0.49 | 1.56 |
| Storage at −20°C | | | | | |
| 2 days | 0.19 | 0.15 | 1.40 | 0.08 | 0.19 |
| 2 months | 0.84 | 0.78 | 3.31 | 0.42 | 1.13 |
| 6 months | 1.38 | 1.24 | 4.36 | 0.78 | 1.43 |

[a]Milligrams malonaldehyde per kilogram meat; HSBO, hydrogenated soybean oil.
[b]α-T, α-tocopherol.
*Source*: Modified from Ref. 38.

α-T through feeding can be helpful to increase the stability of the membrane-bound lipids and, in turn, stabilize the meat during storage.

#### 4.2.3.2. Quality of Dietary Fat.

Oxidized fats or abused fats from frying operations or by-products such as distillation residues from edible oil refining processes are often used for animal feeding. The consumption of the abused fats from the ration is low and not believed harmful (3). However, there is a concern that feeding the abused fats may cause various types and degrees of abnormalities including low growth rate, vitamin E deficiency, and nutritional encephalopathy (42,49). In general, feeding oxidized oil to chicken results in a reduced concentration of α-T in muscle tissues. As a consequence, the susceptibility of the muscle tissue to oxidation is increased. This effect can be alleviated by dietary vitamin E supplementation.

Investigations on the effects of feeding fresh, heated, or α-TAC-supplemented heated vegetable oils show effects on growth, α-T status, fatty acid composition, and oxidative stability of muscle lipids (42). Diets containing 80 g/kg fresh sunflower oil (FSO), fresh linseed oil (FLO), heated sunflower oil (HSO), heated linseed oil (HLO), α-TAC-supplemented (50 mg/kg), heated sunflower oil (HSE), or α-TAC-supplemented (50 mg/kg), heated linseed oil (HLE) produced a slight, but not significant depression in body weight in chicks compared to those FSO. Growth was significantly depressed by feeding HLO and HLE compared to feeding FLO. Other studies also reported that oxidized oil caused a significant reduction in broiler body and carcass weights, suggesting that oxidation impaired the nutritional value of the oil and, in turn, the efficiency of nutrient utilization (43,44).

Evaluation of the effects of feeding diets with various fresh or heated oils on $\alpha$-T concentrations in plasma and muscle of broilers showed that the $\alpha$-T concentrations in plasma, thigh, and breast muscle from chicks fed FSO or FLO were significantly greater than those from chicks fed HSO or HLO (42). Concentrations of $\alpha$-T from the chicks fed HSE or HLE were significantly higher than those from chicks given HSO and HLO. Levels of $\alpha$-T were significantly lower in chicks fed heated oils compared to those of chicks given fresh oil even though $\alpha$-T supplementation compensated for the difference between the fresh and heated oil. The work suggested that certain oxidation products in heated oils may be absorbed and destroy $\alpha$-T in the tissues; therefore, higher levels of $\alpha$-T are needed in the diet. In plasma TBARS were significantly elevated in chicks fed on HSO and HSE compared to TBARS in FSO-fed chicks. A similar trend was observed in chicks fed the corresponding linseed oil diet. After incubation of thigh and breast muscle homogenates with iron ascorbate to induce oxidation, the muscles from HSO group was most susceptible to peroxidation, followed by that of the HSE group. The muscles from chicks fed FSO showed the greatest oxidative stability (Figure 4.4). These results agree with the earlier findings (29) that oxidized oil in broiler diets induced rapid oxidation of membrane-

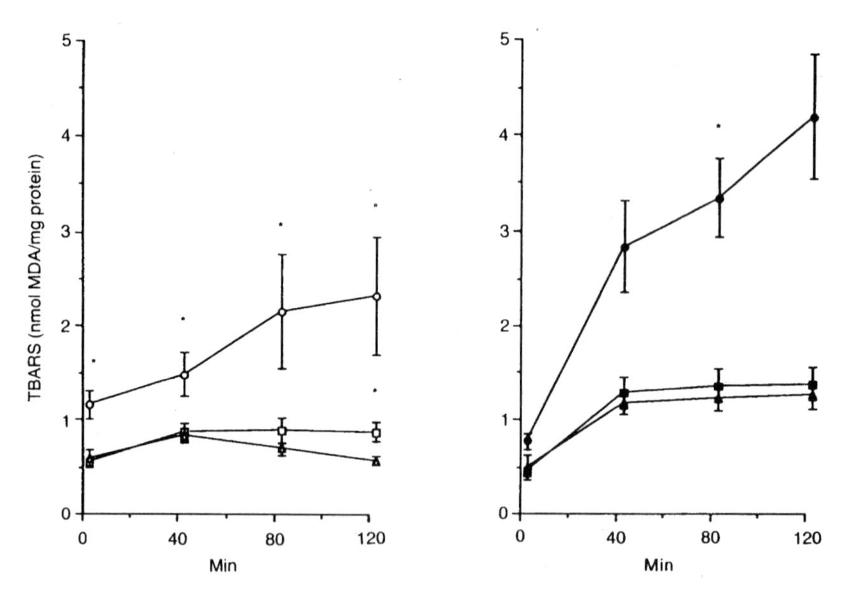


**FIGURE 4.4** Iron ascorbate–induced lipid peroxidation in breast muscle of chicks fed on diets containing fresh sunflower oil (FSO) (△), fresh linseed oil (FLO) (▲), heated sunflower oil (HSO) (○), heated linseed oil (HLO) (●), heated $\alpha$-TAC-supplemented sunflower oil (HSE) (□), or heated $\alpha$-TAC-supplemented linseed oil (HLE) (■). $^*p < 0.05$ versus FSO or FLO group. MDA, malondialdehyde; TBARS, thiobarbituric acid–reactive substances. (From Ref. 42.)

bound lipids, but supplementation of the broiler diet with $\alpha$-T stabilized the membrane-bound lipid against oxidation. Studies on the effects of oxidized dietary sunflower oil and $\alpha$-TAC supplementation on $\alpha$-T concentrations in broiler muscle and storage stability of refrigerated, cooked, minced muscle showed similar results (45). Feeding oxidized oil resulted in reduced muscle $\alpha$-T concentrations, increased oxidation in raw and cooked muscle, and reduced oxidative stability of the muscle during refrigerated and frozen storage. Supplementation with 200–400 mg/kg $\alpha$-TAC improved the stability of the muscle, stability increased as muscle $\alpha$-T concentration increased (Table 4.5).

The overall body of literature clearly shows that the consumption of abused and/or oxidized oil by chicks depresses growth, reduces $\alpha$-T level in plasma and muscles, and alters fatty acid composition with concomitant decreased oxidative stability of the muscle during storage. Such adverse effects can be at least partially overcome by the supplementation of diets with vitamin E.

## 4.3. TURKEY

Turkey muscle and further processed products from turkey are more susceptible to the development of rancidity and/or warmed-over flavor during storage as a result of higher concentrations of PUFA compared to those of chicken. Vitamin E supplementation in diets increases tissue tocopherol levels, resulting in retardation of the onset of rancidity in a fashion similar to that previously discussed for broilers. Research showing the effects of dietary vitamin E supplementation in turkey diets is summarized in Table 4.6.

**TABLE 4.5** Lipid Oxidation in Raw and Cooked Minced Breast and Thigh Muscle from Broilers Fed on Diets Containing Fresh Sunflower Oil and 30 (FS30) or 200 (FS200) mg $\alpha$-Tocopheryl Acetate/kg or Oxidized Sunflower Oil and 0 (OS0), 30 (OS30), or 200 (OS200) mg $\alpha$-Tocopheryl Acetate/kg

| | Thiobarbituric acid–reactive substances (mg malonaldehyde/kg meat)[a] | | | |
|---|---|---|---|---|
| | Breast | | Thigh | |
| Group | Raw | Cooked | Raw | Cooked |
| FS30 | 0.20a[b] | 0.47a | 0.37a | 2.14a |
| FS200 | 0.14a | 0.46a | 0.16b | 1.30b |
| OS0 | 1.71c | 6.79c | 2.28d | 14.96d |
| OS30 | 0.26b | 2.20b | 0.62c | 4.41c |
| OS200 | 0.17a | 0.47a | 0.34a | 1.94a |

[a]Values are means of six analyses performed in duplicate.
[b]Values in the same column that are followed by the same letter are not significantly different ($P < 0.05$).
*Source*: Modified from Ref. 45.

**Table 4.6** Selected Summaries of Research Supplementing Turkey Rations with Vitamin E[a]

| Research topic | Vitamin E forms | Amount | Cofactor | Observations | Ref. |
|---|---|---|---|---|---|
| Tocopherol supplementation and the α-T and peroxide content of tissues | Mixed tocopherols | 4.0, 4.2 mg/Bird | — | Liver concentration was increased 6 times; that of other tissues was doubled; peroxide development decreased during storage of fat of treated birds parallel with increase in α-T content | 1947, 50 |
| α-TAC supplementation and the stability of precooked frozen turkey and of mechanically deboned turkey | α-TAC | 10, 100 mg/lb Feed | — | Injected vitamin E (10 and 100 IU) and oral treatment (100 IU) resulted in lower TBA values; panelists preferred the meat from turkeys supplemented with 100 IU oral | 1972, 57 |
| Method and level of tocopherol supplementation in stabilizing turkey lipids | α-TAC | 10, 100 mg/lb Feed | — | Tocopherol supplementation, oral or injected, reduced rate of lipid oxidation during cooking | 1972, 58 |
| Feeding of vitamin E at low levels and flavor of cooked turkey meat after periods of short and extended frozen storage | α-TAC | 22 mg/kg | Fish meal | TBA numbers for meat from 0% and 2.5% fish meal diet were lower than numbers from 10% fish meal diet; including 22 IU vitamin E of diet in 10% fish meal diet significantly reduced TBA numbers | 1973, 59 |

| | | | | | |
|---|---|---|---|---|---|
| Dietary concentration of vitamin E and tissue concentration and rancidity development during storage of uncooked birds; optimal levels of supplementation | α-T | 20–240 mg/kg Feed for chicken, 100–400 mg/kg for turkey | — | In broilers, all supplemental levels of vitamin E delayed onset of rancidity; 40 IU/kg fed for 8 wk or 160 IU/kg fed for 5 d produced optimal TBA value effect; in turkey, all supplemental levels delayed onset of rancidity; 200 IU/kg fed for 4 wk or 400 IU/kg fed for 3 wk yielded optimal TBA value effects | 1975, 56 |
| Effects of increased dietary vitamin E level and period of its supplementation on stability and sensory quality of different parts of turkey meat | α-TAC | 45 mg/kg Diet | — | Increasing vitamin E supplement from 5 to 45 mg/kg diet improved stability of breast meat; sensory evaluation of meat did not show that increased dietary vitamin E level improved quality of breast and thigh meat | 1983, 60 |
| Effects of dietary fat supplements with different degrees of fatty acid saturation and addition of vitamin E on simultaneous oxidative and hydrolytic changes in turkey meat during frozen storage | α-TAC | 60 mg/kg | Dietary fat | Fatty acid composition of muscle TG was significantly affected by the dietary fat; that of phospholipids was influenced only slightly by different diets; both oxidative and lipolytic changes were greater in leg muscle than in breast muscle; high dietary tocopherol levels resulted in decreased oxidation on storage of meat tissues, as did feeding of more saturated fat diet | 1983, 64 |

*(continued)*

**Table 4.6** *Continued*

| Research topic | Vitamin E forms | Amount | Cofactor | Observations | Ref. |
| --- | --- | --- | --- | --- | --- |
| Effect of dietary concentration of α-TAC on tocopherol tissue deposition and oxidative stability of uncooked turkey tissue during nonfrozen and frozen storage; effect of air and $N_2$ atmospheres on storage stability of turkey tissues | α-TAC | 1.63–275 mg/kg feed | — | As dietary levels increase d, α-T deposition for breast, thigh, and composite increased but not for skin and fat; overall TBA values were significantly lowered by treatment (varying amount of α-TAC) and storage time but not storage atmosphere | 1984, 51 |
| Combined effect of excess Fe, supplied either in diet or by injection, and various levels of dietary vitamin E on oxidative stability of thigh muscle of turkeys | α-TAC | 0, 28, 150 mg/kg | Fe | No interaction was observed between Fe and vitamin E treatments and TBARS values | 1996, 65 |

| | | | | | |
|---|---|---|---|---|---|
| Efficacy of two dietary sources and an injectable form of vitamin E to improve vitamin E status of poults | d-α-TAC, d-α-T | 12, 80, 150 IU/kg diet | — | Concentration, source, or route of vitamin administration did not affect growth parameters, plasma creatine kinase, plasma TG, or liver lipid peroxidation; plasma, RBC, and liver α-T levels decreased from hatching to 14 d of age in poults fed either source of vitamin E; use of 80 or 150 IU of dietary vitamin E (either source) reduced extent of depletion of α-T at all ages and reduced susceptibility of RBC to hemolysis; there was no effect of source of dietary vitamin E on concentration of α-T in plasma, RBC, or liver or on RBC hemolysis | 1996, 66 |
| Effect of feeding high concentrations of α-T to turkey for a long period on oxidative stability of raw and cooked turkey burgers during storage | α-TAC | 300, 600 mg/kg | — | Dietary supplementation with α-TAC significantly reduced TBARS numbers in both raw and cooked burgers during refrigerated and frozen storage | 1996, 52 |

(*continued*)

**TABLE 4.6** *Continued*

| Research topic | Vitamin E forms | Amount | Cofactor | Observations | Ref. |
|---|---|---|---|---|---|
| Effect of feeding supplemental vitamin E on oxidative stability, quality, and color of turkey breast tissues | α-TAC | 5×, 10×, 25× NRC diet | — | TBA values were inversely related to dietary vitamin E levels; no differences in TBA values for the 5×, 10×, 25× NRC diet; mean color scores increased with increased dietary vitamin E levels | 1997, 61 |
| Effect of dietary vitamin E supplementation on storage stability of irradiated raw turkey meat as related to packaging and off-flavor development in irradiated raw turkey meat | α-TAC | 200, 400, 600 IU/kg diet | Packaging | Dietary α-TAC at >200 IU/kg decreased lipid oxidation and reduced total volatiles of raw turkey patties after 7 d of storage; antioxidant effects of dietary α-T were more notable when patties were loosely packaged than when vacuum-packaged | 1997, 63 |
| Effect of dietary fat together with tocopherol on lipid and protein oxidation during refrigerated storage of turkey muscle | α-TAC | 400 ppm | Dietary fat | Vitamin E supplementation delayed lipid oxidation for any dietary fat source; no positive effect on color stability was noted; muscle of supplemented turkey fed tallow had higher vitamin E content than muscle of those fed rapeseed or soy oil | 1998, 54 |

| | | | | | |
|---|---|---|---|---|---|
| Dietary vitamin E supplementation and the storage stability of irradiated cooked turkey meat with different packaging | α-TAC | 25–600 IU/kg | Packaging | TBARS values gradually decreased as dietary α-TAC increased and >200-IU treatments were helpful in maintaining low TBARS values in irradiated breast and leg meat patties; with vacuum packaging, irradiated cooked breast patties oxidized more than nonirradiated patties, but prooxidant effect of irradiation in cooked leg meat was not consistent; volatiles were highly correlated with TBARS values | 1998, 62 |
| Reducing residual nitrite levels in cooked turkey ham and cooked cured turkey patties produced from meat containing high and low levels of dietary α-TAC | α-TAC | 600 mg/kg feed | Nitrite | Dietary supplementation resulted in significant increase in α-T levels in meat; dietary supplementation with α-TAC (60 and 120 mg/kg feed) significantly improved oxidative and color stability of all low-nitrite products produced when compared to that of nonsupplemented controls | 1998, 53 |

(*continued*)

**Table 4.6** *Continued*

| Research topic | Vitamin E forms | Amount | Cofactor | Observations | Ref. |
|---|---|---|---|---|---|
| Fat source and vitamin E supplementation on the antioxidant status of turkey muscles | α-TAC | 200 ppm | Unsaturated fat | Feeding rapeseed oil increased antioxidant enzyme activities and glutathione peroxidase concentration; dietary soy oil increased glutathione peroxidase activity compared to that for other dietary fat sources; with tallow, most antioxidant enzyme activities were lower than with rapeseed or soy oil; for any feeding mode, vitamin E supplementation did not affect antioxidant enzyme activities and glutathione concentration | 1999, 55 |

[a] α-T, α-tocopherol; α-TAC, α-tocopherol acetate; TBA, thiobarbituric acid; TG, triglyceride, TBARS, thiobarbituric acid–reactive substance; RBC, red blood cell; NRC, National Research Council; d-α-TAC, *RRR*-α-tocophenol acetate; d-α-T, *RRR*-α-tocophenol.

### 4.3.1. Vitamin E Supplementation and Tissue Levels

It is well demonstrated that dietary vitamin E supplementation increases α-T concentration in turkey tissues. In 1947, Criddle and Morgan (50) found that the α-T level in liver was increased six times after feeding of 32.9 g mixed tocopherols per bird during 21 days of feeding. α-Tocopherol concentrations in other tissues increased twofold. Peroxide development in the fat of the vitamin E–treated birds during storage decreased as the α-T content of the tissues increased. Significant increases of α-T levels in breast, thigh, and tissue composites were found as dietary α-TAC levels increased (51). However, no significant differences were noted for skin and subcutaneous fat levels. α-Tocopherol levels of burgers from turkeys fed on the supplemental diets (300 and 600 mg α-TAC/kg for 21 weeks) were greater than those from turkeys fed on the basal diets (30 mg α-TAC/kg) for both fresh and cooked samples (Table 4.7) (52). α-Tocopherol levels in tissues from birds fed a diet containing 600 mg α-TAC/kg feed significantly increased compared to those from birds fed the basal diet (20 mg α-TAC/kg feed) (53).

Variations occur in tocopherol deposition among tissue types (51). The α-T levels in thigh tissue were significantly higher than in breast tissue in all treatments. Sheldon (51) postulated that a greater amount of α-T is deposited in thigh tissue than in breast tissue because the more highly developed vascular system of the thigh tissue provides for greater tocopherol deposition than possible in other tissues. Other studies confirmed the variations in α-T deposition among various tissues (54,55). Vitamin E contents in sartorius muscle (thigh) were higher than in pectoralis major (breast) (55). These results were similar to those noted by Morrissey and coworkers (21), who found higher vitamin E level in thigh muscle than in breast muscle in broilers. Mercier and associates (54) also pointed out that the accumulation of vitamin E in turkey is low compared to that in broilers. α-Tocopherol levels in turkey liver and breast muscle were considerably lower than those in broilers after supplementing the same

**TABLE 4.7** Effect of Dietary Vitamin E Fed to Turkeys for 21 Weeks on α-Tocopherol Contents of Burgers Made from Breast Muscle

| Supplementation level[a] | α-Tocopherol (μg/g) | |
|---|---|---|
| | Raw burgers | Cooked burgers |
| 30 | 0.58a[b] | 0.64a |
| 300 | 3.56b | 3.29b |
| 600 | 5.67c | 5.60c |

[a]Milligrams α-TAC/kg feed. α-T, α-tocopherol acetate.
[b]Within columns, numbers having different letters are significantly different to at least $P < 0.01$.
*Source*: Modified from Ref. 52.

amount of vitamin E for similar feeding periods (Table 4.8) (56). In addition, the time required to reach a plateau in response to dietary vitamin E supplementation is longer for turkeys than for broilers. Approximately 13 weeks is required to reach the plateau for thigh and breast muscle in turkeys fed 300 and 600 mg $\alpha$-TAC/kg (52), whereas 1 to 4 weeks is required for $\alpha$-T to plateau in various tissues, including liver, lung, heart, thigh, and breast muscle, in broilers fed 200 mg $\alpha$-TAC/kg (20). Therefore, higher levels of $\alpha$-T and longer periods of supplementation are required to optimize tissue concentration in turkey compared to broilers (52).

### 4.3.2. Effect of Dietary Vitamin E on Oxidative Stability

Early studies showing the ability of dietary vitamin E to improve oxidative stability in turkey meat include Criddle and Morgan (50), Webb and colleagues (57–59). and Marusich and coworkers (56). These studies showed that increasing vitamin E content in diets improved the oxidative stability of the turkey meat as measured by peroxide development and increases in TBA values during storage.

The effects of increased dietary vitamin E and the length of the period of its supplementation on the stability and the sensory quality of different turkey tissues have been thoroughly investigated. Inverse correlations usually exist between TBA numbers and tocopherol levels in breast and thigh meat (51,60). Dietary supplementation with $\alpha$-TAC (300 and 600 mg/kg feed) significantly reduced TBARS values in both raw and cooked burgers during refrigerated and frozen storage (Figure 4.5) (52). The mean values of $\alpha$-T in raw and cooked burgers stored at 4°C did not change during storage, whereas the mean values of $\alpha$-T decreased in both raw and cooked burgers during frozen storage (Figure 4.6). Supplementation of diets with 300 mg $\alpha$-TAC/kg feed as an effective dietary concentration for turkeys when fed from day 1 to slaughter (21 weeks) has been recommended (52). These results are consistent with other reports by Sheldon

**TABLE 4.8** Liver and Breast Muscle Concentration of $\alpha$-Tocopherol in Chickens and Turkeys

| | | Tissue $\alpha$-tocopherol (mg/100 g tissue, weeks) | | | | | |
|---|---|---|---|---|---|---|---|
| | | Liver | | | Breast muscle | | |
| Species | Vitamin E supplement (IU/kg feed) | 4 | 6 | 8 | 4 | 6 | 8 |
| Chicken | 40 | 2.98 | 2.78 | 2.51 | 0.43 | 0.47 | 0.50 |
| Turkey | 37 | 0.60 | 0.63 | 0.59 | 0.14 | 0.13 | 0.14 |

*Source*: Modified from Ref. 56.

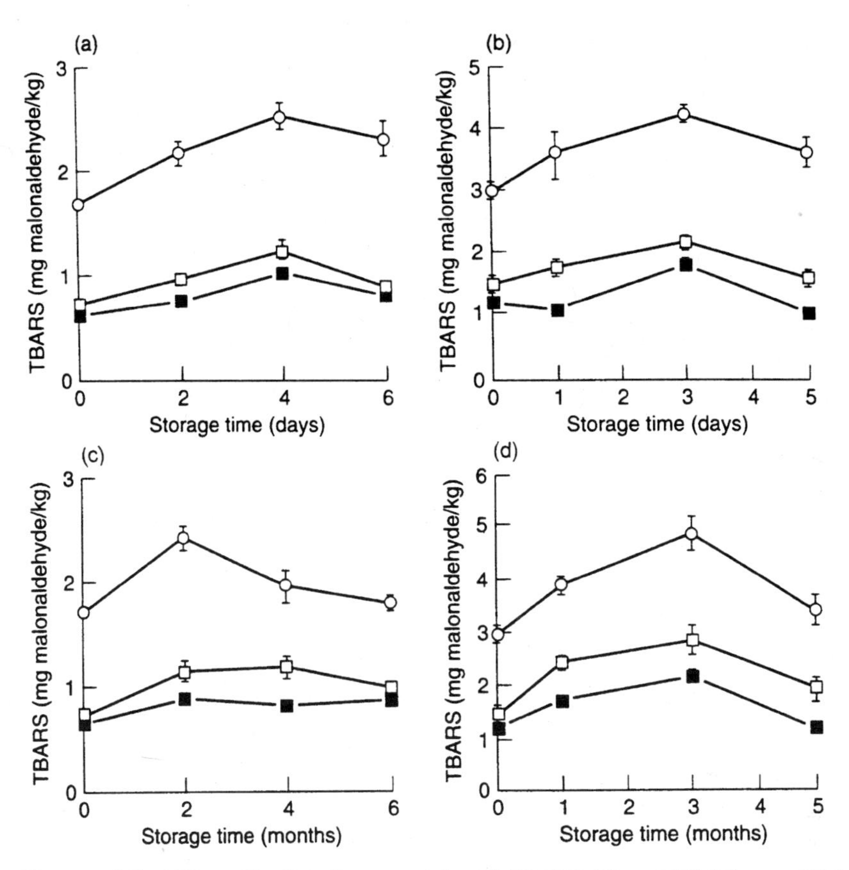


**FIGURE 4.5** Effect of feeding diets containing 20 (○), 300 (□), and 600 (■) mg $\alpha$-TAC/kg on the oxidative stability of (a) raw and (b) cooked turkey burgers during refrigerated storage and (c) raw and (d) cooked turkey burgers during frozen (−20°C) storage. TAC, $\alpha$-tocopherol acetate; TBARS, thiobarbituric acid–reactive substance. (From Ref. 52.)

and associates (61) and Walsh and colleagues (53). Vitamin E supplementation (600 mg $\alpha$-TAC/kg feed for 147 days) significantly reduced TBARS numbers and increased the stability of meat color and intensity measured by Hunter a values (a measure of red color intensity) in turkey hams and patties produced from supplemented meat during storage at 4°C (53).

Ahn et al (62). determined the effects of dietary vitamin E supplementation on the oxidative stability and development of volatiles in irradiated cooked turkey meat (leg and breast) with different packaging during storage at 4°C. Turkeys were fed diets containing from 25 to 100 mg $\alpha$-TAC/kg feed up to 105 days of age. At 105 days, the turkeys were randomly assigned diets containing

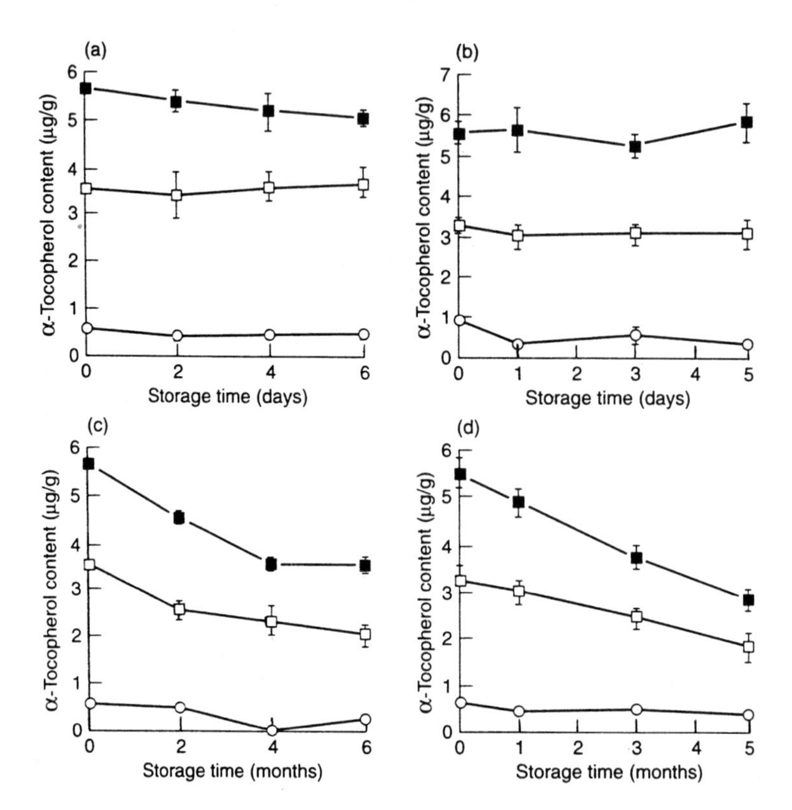


**FIGURE 4.6** Changes in $\alpha$-T content (μg/g) of burgers from turkeys supplemented with 20 (○), 300 (□), or 600 (■) mg $\alpha$-TAC/kg diet during storage. (a) raw muscle stored at 4°C, (b) cooked muscle stored at 4°C, (c) raw muscle stored at −20°C, (d) cooked muscle stored at −20°C. (From Ref. 52.)

200, 400, and 600 mg $\alpha$-TAC/kg feed to increase tissue vitamin E content in the short term from 105 to 122 days. Turkeys fed 25 mg $\alpha$-TAC/kg feed from 1 to 122 days were used as a control. The TBARS values gradually decreased as the dietary $\alpha$-TAC level increased (Table 4.9). Total volatiles were highly correlated with lipid oxidation of the meat measured by TBARS. These results confirm earlier findings by Sheldon (51) and Ahn et al. (63), who reported that production of total volatiles in turkey meat was reduced by dietary vitamin E supplementation. The TBARS values of leg meat were much higher than those of the breast, probably because of higher fat content in leg meat than in breast meat, even though the $\alpha$-T levels in leg muscles are higher than those in breast. The amount of $\alpha$-TAC (100 mg $\alpha$-TAC/kg feed) was not enough to control lipid oxidation of the cooked meat stored under aerobic conditions. A combination of

**TABLE 4.9** Effect of Dietary Vitamin E and Storage Time at 4% on the Thiobarbituric Acid–Reactive Substance Values of Vacuum-Packaged Turkey Breast and Leg Meat Patties

| Dietary vitamin E (IU/kg feed) | Day 0 | | Day 3 | | Day 7 | |
|---|---|---|---|---|---|---|
| | Breast | Leg | Breast | Leg | Breast | Leg |
| | (mg Malonaldehyde/kg meat) | | | | | |
| 25 | 1.23 | 2.85 | 1.16 | 3.24 | 1.18 | 3.99 |
| 200 | 0.64 | 2.02 | 0.71 | 1.83 | 0.84 | 3.43 |
| 400 | 0.52 | 2.02 | 0.35 | 1.54 | 0.64 | 2.96 |
| 600 | 0.44 | 1.68 | 0.31 | 1.23 | 0.58 | 2.77 |

*Source*: Modified from Ref. 62.

dietary $\alpha$-TAC and vacuum packaging could be a good strategy to minimize oxidation of the cooked meat (62).

### 4.3.3. Effect of Dietary Fat and Vitamin E on Lipid Oxidation

Sklan et al (64). determined the effects of dietary fat supplements (tallow and soybean oil) and vitamin E supplementation on the oxidative and hydrolytic changes in turkey meat during frozen storage. Turkeys were fed commercial diets until they were 15 weeks old. The birds were then randomly divided into three groups fed diets containing either beef tallow, soybean oil, or soybean oil with an additional 60 mg $\alpha$-TAC/kg feed for 9 weeks before slaughter. Triglyceride levels in both breast and thigh muscle reflected the dietary fatty acid composition, whereas fatty acid composition of phospholipids was less influenced by the diet (Table 4.10). These observations follow those reported for broilers (38). The meat from the turkeys fed soybean oil had significantly greater levels of conjugated oxidation products, oxodienes, and hydroxydienes than meat from turkeys fed other diets. Oxidative changes in the meat during storage were affected by initial PUFA levels in the tissues and by $\alpha$-T levels. Oxidation rates were influenced by lipolysis rates and indicated an interaction between lipolysis and oxidation in the development of deterioration of turkey during frozen storage.

Investigation of the effect of dietary fat and $\alpha$-TAC supplementation on lipid and protein oxidation during refrigerated storage of turkey muscle showed that muscles of supplemented turkeys fed more saturated tallow had a higher $\alpha$-T content than those fed rapeseed or soybean oil (54). However, there was no effect on vitamin E deposition in broiler meats when effects of dietary oils of coconut, olive, or linseed were compared (38,39). More unsaturated oils such as rapeseed

**TABLE 4.10** Fatty Acid Composition of Breast and Leg Muscle Triglycerides and Phospholipids of Turkey Fed Diets A (Tallow), B (Soybean Oil), or C (Soybean Oil + Tocopherol)[a]

| | | Percentage | | | | |
|---|---|---|---|---|---|---|
| | | 16:0 | 18:0 | 18:1 | 18:2 | 20:4 |
| Diet A | | | | | | |
| Breast | TG | 37.5 | 9.1 | 32.0 | 14.5 | — |
| | PL | 28.5 | 25.6 | 30.0 | 11.0 | 4.0 |
| Leg | TG | 36.0 | 13.4 | 30.5 | 14.3 | — |
| | PL | 25.1 | 28.9 | 23.7 | 17.4 | 4.7 |
| Diet B | | | | | | |
| Breast | TG | 31.4 | 9.2 | 29.6 | 26.0 | — |
| | PL | 29.5 | 27.8 | 20.4 | 14.3 | 7.0 |
| Leg | TG | 32.2 | 9.3 | 30.0 | 25.5 | — |
| | PL | 27.5 | 37.5 | 11.0 | 17.8 | 5.4 |
| Diet C | | | | | | |
| Breast | TG | 28.3 | 9.5 | 27.7 | 30.3 | — |
| | PL | 27.0 | 27.0 | 26.1 | 15.6 | 4.1 |
| Leg | TG | 31.0 | 10.1 | 29.0 | 27.5 | — |
| | PL | 19.3 | 37.0 | 15.7 | 20.2 | 7.8 |

[a]TG, triglyceride; PL, phospholipid.
*Source*: Modified from Ref. 64.

and soybean oil compared to tallow in the diet induced greater oxidation and/or destruction of the additional, supplemental vitamin E (54). Vitamin E supplementation decreased TBARS values compared to control values for all dietary fats (Figure 4.7). The $\alpha$-T content of muscles was negatively correlated with TBARS values.

## 4.4 PORK

Dietary supplementation with $\alpha$-T improves the oxidative stability of pork by increasing the endogenous vitamin E level. In addition, dietary vitamin E supplementation is closely associated with an improvement in some other meat qualities, including color, drip loss, and cholesterol oxidation of the pork during storage or retail display. The effects of dietary vitamin E supplementation to pigs on the oxidative and storage stability and on the other quality parameters of pork and pork products are discussed in the following section and summarized in Table 4.11.

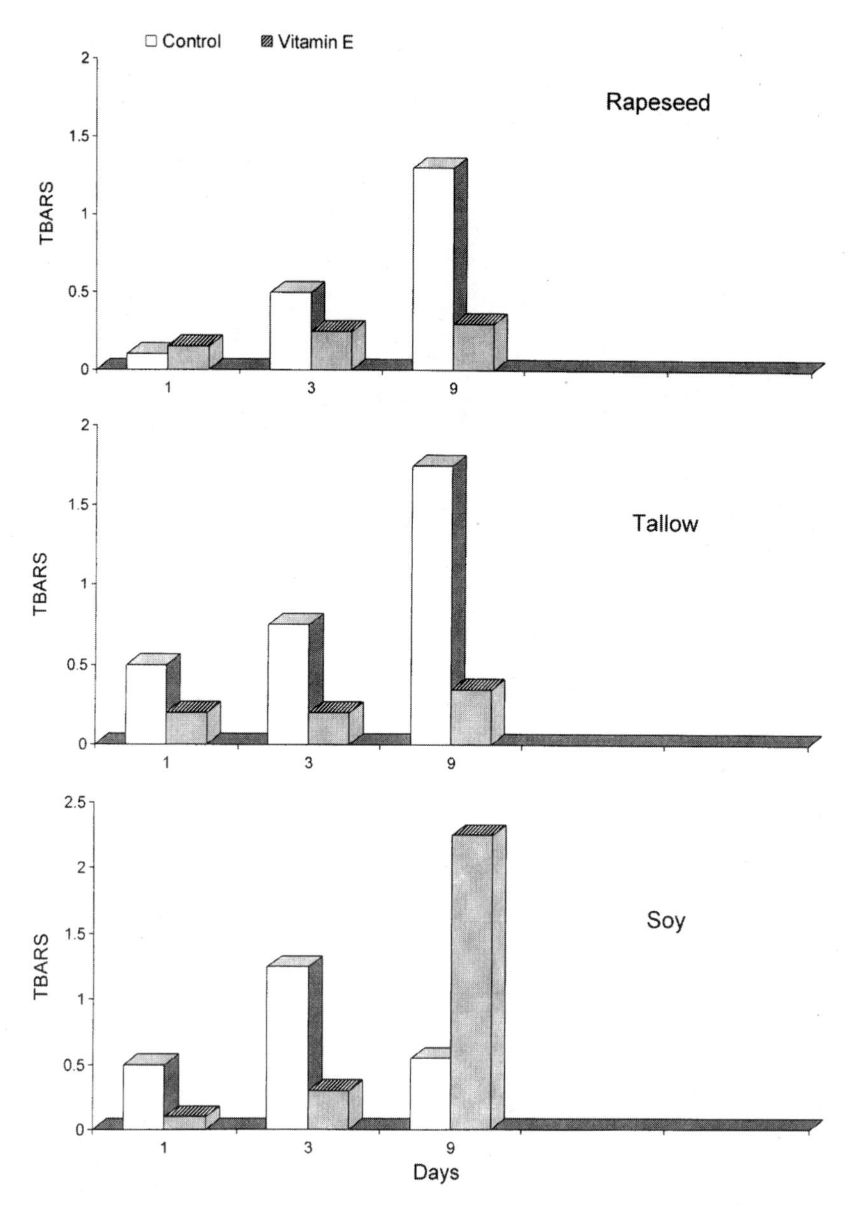


**FIGURE 4.7** Mean TBARS values, for 1, 3, or 9 days of storage (mg MDA/kg feed) in control and supplemented m. sartorius from turkeys fed different fats. α-T, α-tocopherol; α-TAC, α-tocopherol acetate; TBARS, thiobarbituric acid–reactive substance; MDA, malondialdehyde. (Modified from Ref. 54.)

**TABLE 4.11** Selected Summaries of Research Supplementing Pig Rations with Vitamin E[a]

| Research topic | Vitamin E forms | Amount per kg food | Cofactor | Observations | Ref. |
|---|---|---|---|---|---|
| Dietary supplements of copper and vitamin E and growth composition and stability of depot fat | $\alpha$-T | 22, 44, 88 IU | Copper | Copper and vitamin E did not affect growth rate or feed efficiency; supplemental copper significantly decreased melting point of depot fat by increasing proportions of unsaturated fatty acids; supplementation improved oxidative stability of depot fat from copper-fed pigs | 1973, 105 |
| Antioxidant status of pigs fed vitamin E–supplemented diets and erythrocyte lipid peroxidation | $\alpha$-TAC | 0, 10, 30 mg | Fresh or oxidized fat | Erythrocyte lipid peroxidation decreased and blood $\alpha$-T level increased with vitamin E supplementation | 1983, 106 |
| Dietary tocopherol, oxidized oil, and oxidative stability of membranal lipids and pork products during refrigerated and frozen storage | $\alpha$-TAC | 200 mg | Oxidized oil, salt | Membrane-bound $\alpha$-T stabilized membranal lipids and reduced lipid oxidation in pork chops and patties; oxidized dietary oil decreased stability of both membranal lipids and pork products; addition of salt to pork patties accelerated oxidation when patties were stored under fluorescent light and in darkness | 1989, 94 |
| $\alpha$-T supplementation and oxidative stability of raw and cooked muscle, membranal lipids, and rendered fat | $\alpha$-TAC | 200 mg | | $\alpha$-TAC supplementation increased $\alpha$-T level in plasma and muscle; oxidative stability of raw and cooked meat and membrane-bound lipids increased | 1990, 67 |

| | | | | | |
|---|---|---|---|---|---|
| Tissue levels of α-T and susceptibility of tissue lipids to oxidation | α-TAC | 200 mg | None | α-TAC supplementation increased tissue α-T level and reduced iron-induced lipid oxidation; oxidative stability of raw and cooked porcine muscle was improved | 1990, 68 |
| Vitamin E supplementation and subcellular deposition of α-T in muscle and quality | α-TAC | 10, 100, 200 IU | Level of vitamin E | α-T in adipose tissue, LD, mitochondrial, and microsomal fractions of muscle significantly increased with increasing levels of dietary vitamin E; oxidative stability of membranes increased | 1991, 73 |
| Oxidized dietary lipid and cholesterol oxidation in pork | α-TAC | 0, 100, 200 mg | Oxidized lipid | Oxidation decreased with dietary α-T supplementation; rate of formation of lipid and cholesterol oxidation products was low in raw samples compared to that in cooked samples | 1992, 95 |
| Dietary fat, fatty acid profiles, and susceptibility to lipid oxidation | α-TAC | 10, 50 mg | Dietary fat | α-T levels were higher in plasma, muscle, and adipose tissues in pigs receiving α-TAC compared to a basal diet; α-TAC supplementation significantly increased oxidative stability; higher C18 : 2/C18 : 1 ratios led to increased oxidation rates | 1992, 69 |
| Oxidized lipid or α-TAC in pig diets and free radical production in microsomal membrane fractions; lipid oxidation in pork chops during refrigerated storage | α-TAC | 200 mg | Oxidized lipid | Free radical production and lipid oxidation were significantly lower in muscle microsomes from pigs fed α-TAC; susceptibility of pork lipids to oxidation during refrigerated storage was significantly lower in chops from pigs fed supplemented diet | 1993, 96 |

(*continued*)

**TABLE 4.11** *Continued*

| Research topic | Vitamin E forms | Amount per kg food | Cofactor | Observations | Ref. |
|---|---|---|---|---|---|
| Oxidized dietary lipid and vitamin E and fluidity of muscle microsomal membranes | $\alpha$-TAC | 200 mg | Corn oil | Microsomes from pigs fed $\alpha$-TAC were significantly less susceptible to $FeCl_2$-induced lipid oxidation and to changes in membrane fluidity compared to muscle microsomes from pigs fed basal diet | 1994, 103 |
| Dietary fat quality and $\alpha$-T and color stability; relationship between lipid oxidation and color deterioration | $\alpha$-TAC | 10, 100, 200 mg | Oxidized oil | Lipid oxidation and surface redness were significantly influenced by dietary $\alpha$-TAC levels but not by degree of oxidation of dietary corn oil | 1994, 97 |
| Vitamin E and meat quality | $\alpha$-TAC | 500, 1000 mg | | $\alpha$-TAC supplementation reduced drip loss in unfrozen LT; 1000 mg reduced excess release of $Ca^{2+}$ and prevented formation of PSE; erythrocyte fragility and phospholipase $A_2$ activity of pig were significantly reduced by vitamin E addition | 1995, 102 |
| Dietary vitamin E and discoloration rate of pork bone and muscle | $\alpha$-TAC | 198, 297 mg | Lighting, modified atmosphere | Lipid oxidation was increased by modified atmosphere packaging, but detrimental effect was offset by $\alpha$-TAC supplementation; higher supplementation levels improved bone color stability regardless of packaging atmosphere or lightning conditions | 1995, 98 |

| | | | | |
|---|---|---|---|---|
| Supplemental vitamin E, lipid oxidation, shelf life, and sensory characteristic of precooked pork oxidation was lower in vitamin E–supplemented chops and roasts; off-flavor intensity scores were more acceptable and storage/cooking losses were lower for vitamin E–supplemented animals | Not 1995, 107 | specified | 100 mg | Lipid |
| $\alpha$-T stability and lipid oxidation during storage of meat | $\alpha$-TAC | 200 mg | $\alpha$-T was higher in muscle and adipose tissue from supplemented group; TBARS values were lower in muscles from supplemented group than those from control; $\alpha$-T in muscle tissue did not change during storage; in adipose tissue $\alpha$-T concentration decreased with lipid oxidation | 1995, 70 |
| $\alpha$-TAC supplementation, oxidative stability, and sensory quality of pork | $\alpha$-TAC | 60, 200 mg | $\alpha$-TAC-supplemented samples were lighter and more red, tasted fresher, and were more tender and juicy; $\alpha$-TAC supplementation increased oxidative stability | 1996, 99 |

*(continued)*

**TABLE 4.11** *Continued*

| Research topic | Vitamin E forms | Amount per kg food | Cofactor | Observations | Ref. |
|---|---|---|---|---|---|
| Vitamin E supplementation, growth, slaughter characteristics, and quality characteristics of fresh pork stored for extended periods then displayed under retail conditions | α-TAC | 100 mg | | Growth traits, slaughter characteristics, and proximate composition did not differ between dietary treatment groups; α-T concentrations were greater and TBA values were lower during extended retail display for supplemented animals; color, sensory characteristics, total plate counts, pH, purge, and drip and cook losses were not influenced by vitamin E supplementation | 1996, 104 |
| α-TAC and ascorbic acid supplementation and vitamin retention after heating of liver or chops | α-TAC | 200 mg | Ascorbic acid | α-T and ascorbic acid supplementation increased liver α-T level; α-T retention during heating was not affected | 1996, 108 |
| Supplemental α-TAC, vitamin E deposition, and meat quality | α-TAC | 100, 200, 700 mg | | α-T in LD and PM were linearly related to logarithm of dietary vitamin E supplementation in both raw and cooked meat; dietary α-TAC supplementation significantly reduced lipid oxidation; 100 mg α-TAC/kg feed resulted in sufficient α-T levels in muscles to ensure minimal drip loss and optimal color stability | 1997, 75 |

| | | | | | |
|---|---|---|---|---|---|
| Vitamin E, subcellular deposition of α-T in muscle, and oxidative stability | α-TAC | 30, 200, 1000 mg/kg diet | | α-T level in muscle, mitochondria, and microsome increased with increasing levels of dietary vitamin E; differences in α-T concentration in subcellular fractions and intact muscle resulted in enhanced stability of membranes and tissue | 1997, 74 |
| Vitamin E, and sensory and keeping quality of cured cooked hams | α-TAC | 200 mg | — | α-T levels were 5-fold higher in cured and cooked hams produced from supplemented animals; after 16 d of storage, sensory panel detected significant preference (95%) for the hams produced from pigs fed supplemented diet | 1997, 77 |
| Dietary fat, fatty acids, vitamin E, and lipid oxidation | α-TAC | 1000 mg/Head/day | Oilseed | Fatty acid pattern in diet influenced fatty acid pattern of back fat; vitamin E supplementation stabilized fat with increased PUFA | 1997, 86 |
| Vitamin E, color stability, and lipid oxidation | — | 200 IU | — | Meat from supplemented pigs was more resistant to lipid oxidation; effects on color stability were variable | 1998, 79 |
| Feeding diets with full-fat rapeseed with or without supplemental α-TAC and lipid oxidation | α-TAC | 200 mg | None | α-TAC supplementation reduced muscle drip loss, increased tissue α-T concentration, and reduced susceptibility of fat to oxidation | 1998, 109 |

*(continued)*

**Table 4.11** *Continued*

| Research topic | Vitamin E forms | Amount per kg food | Cofactor | Observations | Ref. |
|---|---|---|---|---|---|
| Vitamin E supplementation, performance, and fresh pork quality | $\alpha$-TAC | 200 mg | | Dietary $\alpha$-TAC had no effect on performance or meat quality traits; vitamin E levels were five times higher in muscles of supplemented group; vitamin E treatment reduced TBA values, particularly after frozen storage | 1998, 100 |
| Vitamin E, oleic acid, copper intake, and quality of fresh and cooked pork chop | $\alpha$-TAC | 100 and 200 mg | Oleic acid, copper | $\alpha$-T levels were higher with oleic acid and vitamin supplementation; color stability was increased; oxidative stability was not affected by increasing $\alpha$-T | 1998, 91 |
| Dietary rapeseed oil, $CuSO_4$, and vitamin E meat quality | $\alpha$-TAC | 100, 200 mg | Rapeseed oil, copper sulfate | Supplementation of rapeseed oil diets with vitamin E significantly decreased lipid oxidation | 1998, 90 |
| Vitamin E and color stability of pasteurized ham | $\alpha$-TAC | 200 IU | Packaging | Redness component of vacuum-packaged ham prepared from vitamin E–supplemented pigs was more stable | 1998, 101 |
| Rapeseed oil with or without added vitamin E and development of WOF in precooked pork patties | $\alpha$-TAC | 200 mg | Rapeseed oil | Rapeseed oil increased content of MUFA and PUFA and reduced amount of SFA in products; level of vitamin E in noncooked patties increased with $\alpha$-TAC supplementation; supplementation effectively counteracted effects of rapeseed oil on lipid oxidation | 1998, 87 |

| | | | | | |
|---|---|---|---|---|---|
| Dietary vitamin E and oxidative stability of pork chops and sausages | α-TAC | 100, 200 mg | Copper, rapeseed oil | Rapeseed oil in diets increased amount of MUFA and PUFA; vitamin E significantly increased oxidative stability of pork chops and decreased adverse effect of rapeseed oil on oxidative stability | 1998, 92 |
| Approaches to inhibition of lipid oxidation | α-TAC | 500 mg | Vitamin E level, cooking condition, packaging | Significant two-way and three-way interactions were observed among effects of muscle α-T levels, cooking conditions, and packaging on lipid oxidation | 1998, 71 |
| Vitamin E and nitrite levels in cooked ham and bacon | α-TAC | 500 mg | Nitrite | α-TAC supplementation improved oxidative stability of low-nitrite products and improved color | 1998, 80 |
| Vitamin E, copper with rapeseed oil and effects on lipid oxidation | α-TAC | 100, 200 mg | Copper, rapeseed oil | Muscle α-T concentrations increased with increasing vitamin E level; antioxidative status was higher in PM than in LD; susceptibility to lipid oxidation was reduced in LD with increasing dietary vitamin E level and in PM with increasing dietary copper level | 1999, 93 |

(*continued*)

**TABLE 4.11** *Continued*

| Research topic | Vitamin E forms | Amount per kg food | Cofactor | Observations | Ref. |
|---|---|---|---|---|---|
| Increasing muscular content of vitamin E and color intensity and stability | α-TAC | 100, 200 mg | Sunflower oil, copper | Increased dietary vitamin E level increased α-T concentrations in muscles; color measures of fresh chops, green hams, and matured hams did not reveal significant differences among groups | 1999, 110 |
| α-TAC supplementation, α-T in dry cured hams and oxidative stability | α-TAC | 200 mg | — | α-T concentrations in thigh muscle, unprocessed thighs, and final products were higher in pigs fed supplemented diet than in those fed basal diet; hams from pigs fed basal diet oxidized more rapidly; no effect on color | 1999, 78 |
| α-TAC supplementation and oxidative stability of Italian hams | α-TAC | 100–200 mg | Oleic acid | Lipid and cholesterol oxidation were slightly inhibited by α-TAC supplementation | 2000, 82 |

| | | | | | |
|---|---|---|---|---|---|
| $\alpha$-TAC supplementation and oxidative stability of bacon | $\alpha$-TAC | 10, 200 mg | Fish meal, wood and liquid smoke | 200 mg $\alpha$-TAC/kg reduced lipid oxidation; combination of lipid and wood smoke also decreased oxidation | 2002, 84 |
| $\alpha$-TAC supplementation and lipid and cholesterol oxidation in cooked pork with elevated n-3 fatty acids | $\alpha$-TAC | 200 mg | Dietary oils | $\alpha$-TAC supplementation reduced lipid and cholesterol oxidation in cooked pork from all dietary groups | 2001, 85 |
| $\alpha$-TAC supplementation effects on quality with MUFA and PUFA diets | $\alpha$-TAC | 200 mg | MUFA, PUFA | $\alpha$-TAC supplementation increased tissue $\alpha$-T level and decreased oxidation in dry-cured hams from animals fed elevated levels of MUFA and PUFA | 2003, 72 |
| $\alpha$-TAC supplementation and fresh pork quality | $\alpha$-TAC | 12–351 IU | Vacuum packaging | $\alpha$-TAC supplementation did not improve fresh pork quality; improved oxidative stability was noted in vacuum-packaged chops during case display over 8 d | 2003, 111 |

[a] $\alpha$-T, $\alpha$-tocopherol; $\alpha$-TAC, $\alpha$-tocopherol acetate; LD,M. longissimus dorsi; LT, M. longissimus thoracis; PSE, pale, soft, exudative; TBARS, thiobarbituric acid–reactive substance; TBA, thiobarbituric acid; PM, M. psoas major; PUFA, polyunsaturated fatty acid; WOF, warmed-over flavor; MUFA, monounsaturated fatty acid; SFA, saturated fatty acid.

### 4.4.1. Vitamin E Supplementation and Tissue Levels

The effects of feeding pigs supplemental α-TAC and the deposition of α-T in plasma and muscle have been extensively studied. In pigs fed diets containing 200 mg α-TAC/kg feed for 2 weeks before slaughter, the mean α-T level in plasma and muscle increased from 2.4 to 6.0 μg/mL and from 3.2 to 7.0 μg/g, respectively (67). This report is in agreement with the results reported in other studies (68–72). The α-T level in plasma increased from 2.03 to 5.48 μg/mL by increasing the dietary α-T level to 159.1 mg α-TAC/kg feed. The α-T levels in tissue samples taken from pigs fed the supplemented diet were found to be two- or threefold higher in lung, heart, kidney, and muscle (Table 4.12) (68). The α-T content of adipose tissue (milligrams per kilogram [mg/kg] of tissue) from pigs fed 200 mg α-TAC/kg feed was 20.3 compared to 12.0 for unsupplemented pigs (70). A linear decrease in α-T content of the adipose tissue occurred during 14 days of storage at 4°C. The α-T content of muscle tissue from the supplemented group was higher than that from the control group and did not change during the storage period (70).

Levels of α-tocopherol in adipose tissue, *M. longissimus dorsi* (LD) muscle, and mitochondrial and microsomal fractions of the muscle significantly increased with increasing levels of dietary vitamin E (73). The greatest amount of α-T was present in the mitochondria, followed by the microsomes. α-Tocopherol in the intact tissues and subcellular fractions significantly increased with the level of α-TAC supplementation in the diet (74). This observation agrees with later

**TABLE 4.12** α-Tocopherol Content of Plasma and Tissue Samples of Pigs Fed Basal and α-Tocopherol Acetate–Supplemented Diets

| | Dietary treatment[a] | |
|---|---|---|
| Sample | Basal | Supplemented |
| Plasma α-tocopherol (μg/mL plasma) | 2.0 | 5.5[b] |
| Tissue α-tocopherol (ng/mg protein) | | |
| Lung | 25.3 | 71.4[c] |
| Liver | 39.2 | 98.7[b] |
| Heart | 27.4 | 79.9[b] |
| Kidney | 10.3 | 28.3[b] |
| Muscle | 7.6 | 21.8[b] |
| Muscle mitochondria | 45.3 | 124.2[b] |
| Muscle microsomes | 62.4 | 164.8[b] |

[a]Mean values of six analyses performed in duplicate.
[b]α-Tocopherol levels differ significantly ($p < 0.01$) from basal group levels.
[c]α-Tocopherol levels differ significantly ($p < 0.05$) from basal group levels.
*Source*: Modified from Ref. 68.

research that showed that α-T concentrations in muscles were significantly increased by increasing the concentration of α-TAC of the diet (75,76).

Increased α-T level has been noted in processed products from vitamin E–supplemented pigs (77,78) α-Tocopherol levels in cured cooked hams of pigs fed the control diet and the supplemented diet (200 mg α-TAC/kg feed) increased from 0.54 to 2.87 μg/g of muscle tissue, respectively. The α-T levels of the fresh meat from the control and supplemented groups were 1.3 and 6.7 μg/g of tissue, respectively (77). α-T concentrations in thigh muscle, unprocessed thighs, and final products (dry-cured ham) were higher in pigs fed 200 mg α-TAC/kg feed than in those fed basal diet (10 mg α-TAC/kg feed) (78).

### 4.4.2. Effect of Dietary Vitamin E on Oxidative Stability

It is well known that the rate and extent of lipid oxidation in meats and meat products depend on the concentration of α-T in the tissues (4). Jensen and coworkers (75) studied the effect of feeding supplemental levels of α-TAC on its deposition in two porcine muscles, LD and *M. psoas major* (PM), and the effect on lipid oxidation of raw and cooked meats. Pigs were fed 100, 200, and 700 mg α-TAC/kg feed. Muscle α-T levels of the two muscles were linearly related to the logarithm of dietary vitamin E supplementation in both raw and cooked meat. The oxidative stability of lipids in LD and PM muscles and cooked meat during chill storage at 4°C was positively correlated to the levels of dietary α-TAC and to the concentration of endogenous α-T. Similar results were also presented by others in evaluation of the effect of three levels of dietary vitamin E in the diet of pigs on the oxidative stability of meats (73,74). Pork chops from the pigs fed 100 and 200 IU/kg feed had significantly lower TBARS values than those from the control pigs (10 IU/kg feed) when exposed to fluorescent light at 4°C for 10 days (Table 4.13) (73). Porcine mitochondria, microsomes, and intact tissue from the pigs fed the higher levels of α-TAC (200 and 1000 mg α-TAC/kg feed) had significantly lower TBARS values than those from the control group fed 30 mg α-TAC/kg feed (Figure 4.8) (74). The TBARS values of the samples from the pigs fed 1000 mg α-TAC/kg feed were consistently lower than those from the pigs fed 200 mg α-TAC/kg feed. Improvement of oxidative stability of minced pork (79), cured and dry-cured ham (72,77,78,80,81) cured pork sausage (82), restructured pork (83), bacon (84), and cooked pork (71,85) was noted with α-TAC supplementation.

Evaluation of the effect of feeding high levels of vitamin E on oxidative stability and sensory quality of cured and cooked hams showed that 200 mg/kg feed inhibited oxidation (77). The GC-MS analyses of the volatile compounds of the cooked hams stored at 6°C for 3 weeks and −18°C for 3 months indicated

**Table 4.13** Influence of Dietary Vitamin E Supplementation on the Oxidative Stability (Thiobarbituric Acid–Reactive Substance, mg Malonaldehyde/kg Sample) of Pork Chops and Ground Pork Stored at 4°C Under Fluorescent Light

| Storage (days) | Vitamin E supplementation (mg/kg feed)[a] | | |
|---|---|---|---|
| | 10 | 100 | 200 |
| | | Pork chops | |
| 0 | 0.28a | 0.27a | 0.27a |
| 3 | 1.54a | 0.56b | 0.35b |
| 6 | 2.96a | 0.94b | 0.58b |
| 10 | 5.17a | 2.96ab | 1.33b |
| | | Ground pork | |
| 1 | 1.34a | 0.36b | 0.22b |
| 4 | 3.49a | 1.13b | 0.41c |
| 8 | 5.38a | 3.27b | 1.59c |

[a]The values in the table are the group mean; in a row mean values that have the same letter are not significantly different ($p > 0.05$).
*Source*: Modified from Ref. 73.

higher concentrations of the aldehydes and sulfur components in the control samples when compared to the supplemented samples for both storage conditions (Figure 4.9) (77).

Walsh and associates (80) investigated the effect of reducing residual nitrite levels on the oxidative stability of cured pork products (bacon and ham) manufactured from meat containing high and low levels of dietary $\alpha$-TAC. Sodium nitrite is used in the preparation of cured meat products to kill bacteria, to form pink color of cured meat, and to maintain meat flavor by acting as an antioxidant. However, it is desirable to reduce the level of nitrite in cured meat products because of its implications for nitrosamine formation, a known carcinogen. Dietary supplementation (500 mg $\alpha$-TAC/kg feed) in combination with 100 mg residual nitrite/kg meat in bacon and ham retarded lipid oxidation during refrigerated storage for 8 weeks. The bacon and hams processed from the meat of the control group (10 mg $\alpha$-TAC/kg feed) containing 100 mg residual nitrite/kg meat had similar TBARS numbers to those produced from supplemented vitamin E meat containing 50 mg residual nitrite/kg meat. Therefore, dietary vitamin E supplementation may be used to reduce the level of nitrite in cured pork products. Use of pork muscle from animals supplemented with the 410 mg $\alpha$-T/kg ration to produce a cured pork sausage did not have an effect on TBARS development during storage under various conditions compared to that of control sausage (82). However, the authors attributed the lack of an increase in antioxidant effect to the strong antioxidant capacity of

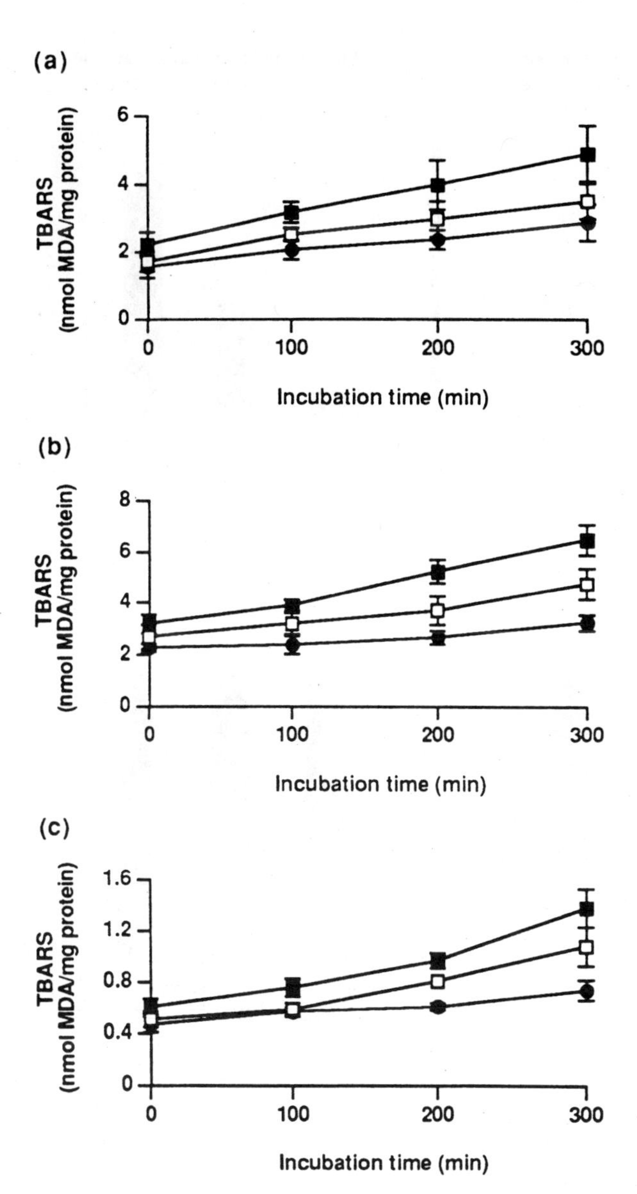


**FIGURE 4.8** Effect of feeding diets containing 30 (■), 200 (□), and 1000 (●) mg $\alpha$-TAC/kg on iron-induced lipid oxidation of porcine (a) mitochondria, (b) microsomes, and (c) intact tissue. $\alpha$-TAC, $\alpha$-tocopherol acetate; TBARS, thiobarbituric acid–reactive subtance. (From Ref. 74.)

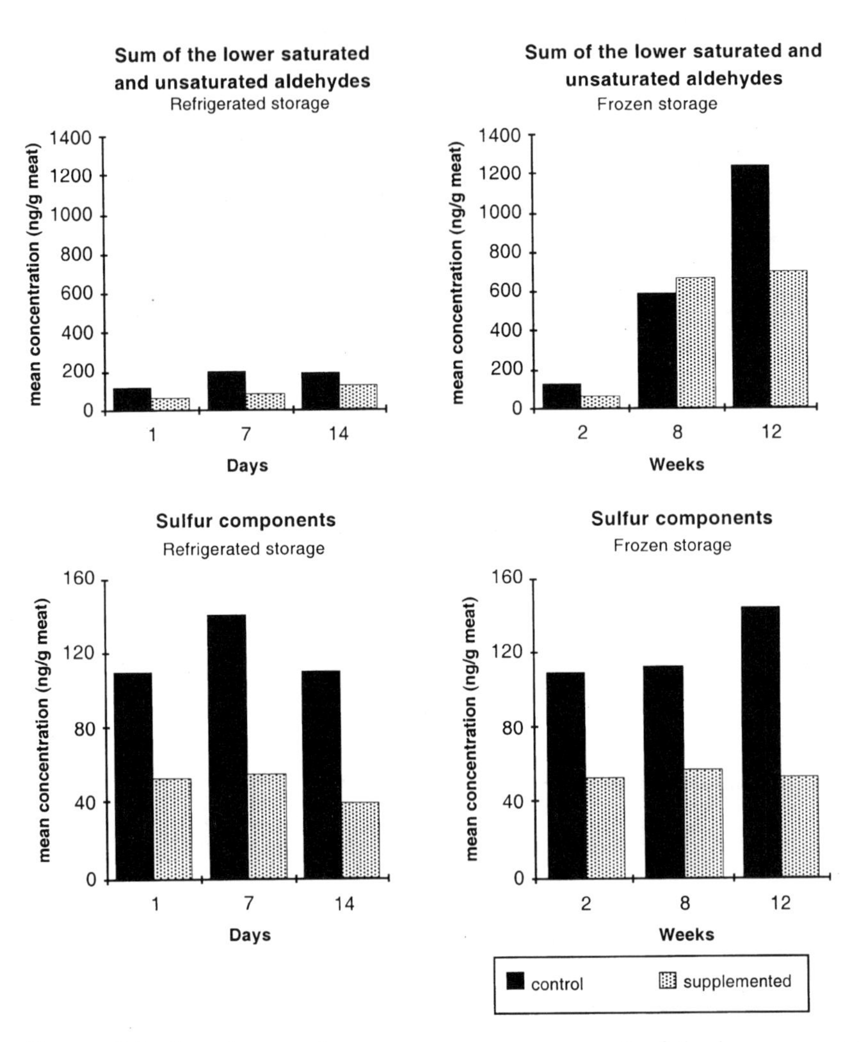


**FIGURE 4.9** Sum (expressed as nanograms per gram meat) of the lower saturated aldehyde, the unsaturated aldehydes, and the sulfur components as a function of storage in the refrigerated unit (6°C) and the freezer (−18°C). (From Ref. 77.)

residual nitrite in the sausage. Harms and colleagues (82) stressed that further research is needed to define limits for the reduction of nitrite concentration in cured sausages in the presence of antioxidants.

Kingston et al (71). examined the individual and combined effects of muscle vitamin E levels, cooking conditions (duration, temperature, and rate), and packaging on lipid oxidation in refrigerated cooked pork. The oxidation stability of cooked pork was higher in samples containing 4.3 μg/g α-T when compared to muscles containing 1 μg/g α-T (control group). The vitamin E effect was observed regardless of the cooking conditions or types of packaging. Oxidative stability was higher in pork cooked at a lower temperature, for a shorter time, at a faster rate and stored in vacuum packs. A combination of approaches is likely to be more effective than a single approach to limit oxidation of cooked chilled pork. Increased muscle α-T levels and improved packaging systems were recommended as practical and easily implemented industrial applications.

### 4.4.3. Effect of Dietary Fat and Vitamin E on Lipid Oxidation

**4.4.3.1. Fat Composition.** Increasing the proportions of unsaturated fatty acids and/or decreasing the levels of saturated fatty acids in pork can be beneficial to the consumer; however, increased levels of the PUFA in pork increase the susceptibility of the meat to lipid oxidation, leading to quality deterioration. Modification of the diet along with supplementation of α-TAC to the diet can neutralize the negative effects of increased PUFA level in the muscle. Monahan and associates (69) investigated the effects of dietary fat on the fatty acid profiles of porcine muscle and adipose tissue lipid levels and on the susceptibility of muscle tissue to lipid oxidation in combination with dietary vitamin E supplementation. Pigs were fed diets containing 3% soybean oil or 3% beef tallow with either a basal (10–15 mg/kg feed) or supplemented (200 mg/kg feed) level of α-TAC. The neutral lipids of muscle had significantly lower proportions of C16:0 and C18:1 and a higher proportion of C18:2 in animals fed the soybean oil diet than in those fed the tallow diet. Polar lipid fractions from pigs fed the soybean oil diet had a significantly lower level of C18:1 and significantly higher levels of C18:2 and C20:5 than those from pigs receiving tallow. In adipose tissue, total lipids from pigs fed the soybean oil diets had significantly lower levels of C14:0, C16:0, C16:1, and C18:1 and significantly higher levels of C18:2 and C20:4 compared to pigs receiving tallow (Table 4.14). Dietary α-TAC supplementation did not influence the deposition of fatty acids in the muscle or adipose tissue of pigs fed either the tallow or the soybean oil diet. α-Tocopherol concentrations in plasma and muscle from pigs fed the soybean oil diet were lower than those from pigs fed the tallow diet with the basal level of α-TAC. Increased linoleic acid in tissues of pigs receiving the soybean oil diet was thought to decrease the absorption of α-T. Muscle homogenates from pigs fed the soybean oil diet with a basal α-TAC level were significantly more susceptible to iron-induced lipid oxidation than those from pigs fed the tallow diet with the same level of α-TAC because of the increased proportions of unsaturated fatty acids and the decrease in the concentration of α-TAC in the muscle. Dietary α-TAC supplementation significantly increased the oxidative

**TABLE 4.14** Fatty Acid Profiles of the Neutral, Polar, and Total Lipid Fraction of Muscle from Pigs Fed Tallow and Soybean Oil Diets

| | Neutral lipid | | Polar lipid | | Total lipid | |
|---|---|---|---|---|---|---|
| Fatty acid[a] | Tallow diet[b] | Soybean oil diet[b] | Tallow diet[b] | Soybean oil diet[b] | Tallow diet[b] | Soybean oil diet[b] |
| C14:0 | 0.6a | 0.9a | 0.4a | 1.0a | 1.0a | 0.8a |
| C16:0 | 27.2a | 24.3b | 19.7a | 18.8a | 26.6a | 22.1b |
| C16:1 | 4.3a | 3.5a | 2.8a | 0.9a | 4.1a | 2.5b |
| C18:0 | 13.6a | 13.3a | 11.8a | 13.6a | 12.1a | 11.3a |
| C18:1 | 45.2a | 40.8b | 23.6a | 15.6b | 40.5a | 33.2b |
| C18:2 | 5.9b | 13.4a | 28.9b | 37.8a | 11.2b | 24.4a |
| C18:3 | 2.3a | 3.0a | 2.2a | 2.1a | 4.0a | 4.9a |
| C20:0 | 0.2a | 0.4a | 6.7a | 8.5a | — | — |
| C20:4 | 0.4a | Trace a | 0.9a | 1.9b | 0.3b | 0.5a |
| C20:5 | 0.3a | Trace a | 0.8a | Trace a | — | — |
| C22:6 | 0.1a | 0.3a | 1.3a | 0.9a | 0.2a | 0.2a |
| Total saturates | 41.6a | 38.9b | 32.7a | 33.4a | 39.6a | 34.2b |
| Total unsaturates | 58.4b | 61.1a | 67.3a | 66.6a | 60.4b | 65.8a |
| Ratio | | | | | | |
| Unsaturates/saturates | 1.4b | 1.6a | 2.1a | 2.0a | 1.5b | 1.9a |
| C18:2/C18:1 | 0.1b | 0.3a | 1.2b | 2.4a | 0.3b | 0.7a |

[a]Means in the same row within the same lipid fraction followed by different letters are significantly different ($p < 0.05$).
[b]Percentage of total peak area of fatty acid listed.
*Source*: Modified from Ref. 69.

stability of muscle in both cases. The same trend was observed for the cooked muscle samples (Figure 4.10).

Investigation of the influence of dietary fat (100 g/kg diet rapeseed or 200 g/kg full-fat soybean) on fatty acid composition indicated that feeding rapeseed increased the percentage of C18:2 and C18:3 and lowered the proportions of saturated fatty acids of the backfat (86). A full-fat soybean diet significantly decreased the percentage of C16:1. This result was confirmed by Jensen et al. (87), who reported that a 6% rapeseed oil diet slightly increased the content of monounsaturated and polyunsaturated fatty acids and slightly reduced the amount of saturated fatty acids in meat patties. Susceptibility of precooked patties to lipid oxidation increased during chill storage as a result of the rapeseed. Supplementation of 200 mg $\alpha$-TAC/kg feed effectively counteracted the effects of the rapeseed oil on lipid oxidation by increasing $\alpha$-T concentration in the

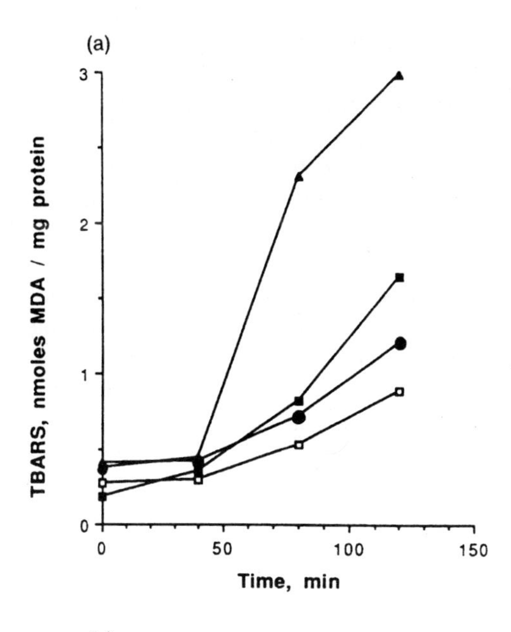


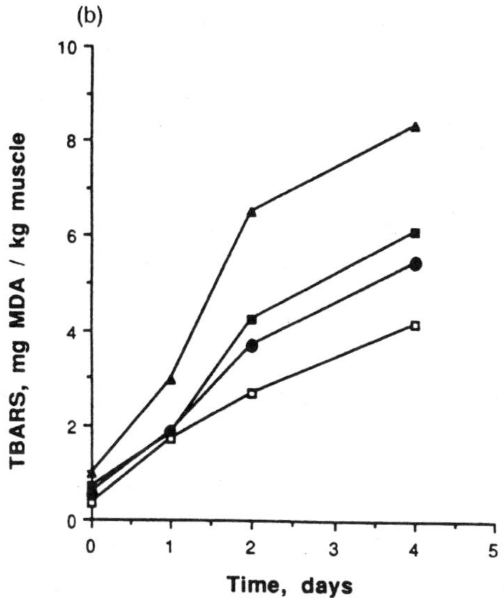


**FIGURE 4.10** Effect of dietary fat and $\alpha$-T supplementation on (a) iron-induced lipid peroxidation in porcine muscle and (b) the TBARS numbers of cooked pork patties stored at 4°C; tallow with basal $\alpha$-TAC (■), tallow with supplemented $\alpha$-TAC (□), soy oil with basal $\alpha$-TAC (▲), soy oil with supplemented $\alpha$-TAC (●). $\alpha$-T, $\alpha$-tocopherol; TBARS, thiobarbituric acid–reactive substance; $\alpha$-TAC, $\alpha$-tocopherol acetate; MDA, malondialdehyde. (From Ref. 69.)

patties from 3.31 to 6.26 mg $\alpha$-T/kg dry matter. Similar results were obtained with dietary linseed oil (88).

The effect of copper intake on the quality of pork in relation to dietary fats and vitamin E has been extensively studied. Copper salt is often added to pig diets as a growth promoter to ensure maximal growth rate. However, increased dietary copper levels may decrease the stability of the pork meat by interacting with reducing agents including cysteine, glutathione, ascorbate, and $\alpha$-T; oxidizing them, and decreasing the antioxidant capacity of the meat (89). Jensen et al (90). studied the effect of addition of rapeseed oil, copper sulfate ($CuSO_4$), and vitamin E on pork meat quality. Pigs were fed either a control diet (no supplementation) or a 6% rapeseed oil diet supplemented with $CuSO_4$ and vitamin E. The diet supplemented with rapeseed oil and vitamin E increased the concentration of $\alpha$-T in muscle, and $CuSO_4$ did not affect the $\alpha$-T level (Table 4.15). Feeding increased levels of $CuSO_4$ and vitamin E did not influence color of chops from pigs fed rapeseed oil diets as measured by the Minolta a value. However, the color of chops from the pigs fed rapeseed oil had significantly higher a values compared to that of chops from pigs fed the control diet (Table 4.15). Dietary levels of $CuSO_4$ did not affect the development of lipid oxidation in the pork chops. The addition of rapeseed oil or $CuSO_4$ did not adversely affect the quality of chilled and stored pork chops. Other research (91,92) supports these findings; however, Lauridsen and associates (93) reported reduced susceptibility to lipid oxidation with increasing level of dietary copper.

**4.4.3.2. Dietary Fat Quality.** Evaluation of the effects of dietary vitamin E and oxidized oil on the oxidative stability of membranal lipids in porcine muscles and pork products during refrigerated and frozen storage showed that microsomal and mitochondrial lipids from pigs fed a supplemental diet (200 mg $\alpha$-TAC/kg) for 10 weeks (long-term $\alpha$-T group) were much more stable to oxidation than those from the control pigs (94). Feeding pigs a 200-mg $\alpha$-TAC/kg diet only for the last 4 weeks of feeding (short-term $\alpha$-T group) did not influence the stability of the lipids. Long-term supplementation (10 weeks) with natural mixed tocopherols (200 mg/kg diet) had no effect on the stability of the microsomal and mitochondrial lipids. Feeding oxidized corn oil (3% for 10 weeks) increased rates of lipid oxidation compared to those of the control group (Figure 4.11). Oxidized oils in the diet became a source of free radicals that could reduce the stability of the lipids of subcellular membranes to oxidation. Similar trends were observed for pork products, pork patties, and pork chops. Monahan and colleagues (95) also studied the effect of oxidized corn oil and $\alpha$-TAC in pig diets on oxidation of lipids in raw and cooked pork. Pigs were fed either 3% fresh corn oil or 3% oxidized corn oil with 10, 100, or 200 mg of $\alpha$-TAC/kg of diet. Plasma and muscle $\alpha$-T levels were significantly influenced by dietary $\alpha$-TAC (Table 4.16). The $\alpha$-T concentrations in plasma and muscle were increased by

**TABLE 4.15** Concentration of $\alpha$-Tocopherol in Feed and Muscle and Color Stability Measured as Minolta a Values During Chill Storage of Chops from Pigs Fed Different Levels of Rapeseed Oil, $CuSO_4$, and Vitamin E

| Feed No. | Rapeseed oil (%) | $CuSO_4$ (mg/kg feed) | $\alpha$-TAC (mg/kg feed) | Analyzed vitamin E | | Red color (a value)[a] | | | |
|---|---|---|---|---|---|---|---|---|---|
| | | | | Feed | Muscle | Day 0 | Day 2 | Day 5 | Day 8 |
| Control | 0 | 0 | 0 | 9 | 1.6a[b] | 4.61 | 5.23 | 4.00 | 3.88 |
| 1 | 6 | 0 | 0 | 18 | 2.7b | 6.64 | 6.71 | 5.47 | 5.17 |
| 2 | 6 | 0 | 100 | 78 | 4.3c | 6.32 | 6.52 | 5.36 | 5.32 |
| 3 | 6 | 0 | 200 | 131 | 5.4d | 5.52 | 5.43 | 4.87 | 4.03 |
| 4 | 6 | 35 | 0 | 23 | 2.9b | 6.02 | 5.77 | 4.66 | 4.67 |
| 5 | 6 | 35 | 100 | 77 | 4.0c | 5.19 | 5.22 | 4.43 | 3.81 |
| 6 | 6 | 35 | 200 | 133 | 5.6d | 5.90 | 6.19 | 4.32 | 4.75 |
| 7 | 6 | 175 | 0 | 19 | 3.0b | 5.33 | 4.88 | 4.37 | 4.29 |
| 8 | 6 | 175 | 100 | 81 | 4.3c | 5.54 | 6.15 | 5.46 | 4.79 |
| 9 | 6 | 175 | 200 | 139 | 5.5d | 5.42 | 5.43 | 4.18 | 4.22 |

[a]Chops from pigs fed control diet (no rapeseed oil addition) had significantly ($p < 0.01$) lower a values during storage than chops from pigs fed feed 1 (6% rapeseed oil). No difference in color stability was observed between pigs fed rapeseed oil diets (feed 1–9). $\alpha$-TAC, $\alpha$-tocopherol acetate.
[b]Numbers with a different letter within a column are significantly different ($p < 0.01$).
*Source*: Modified from Ref. 90.

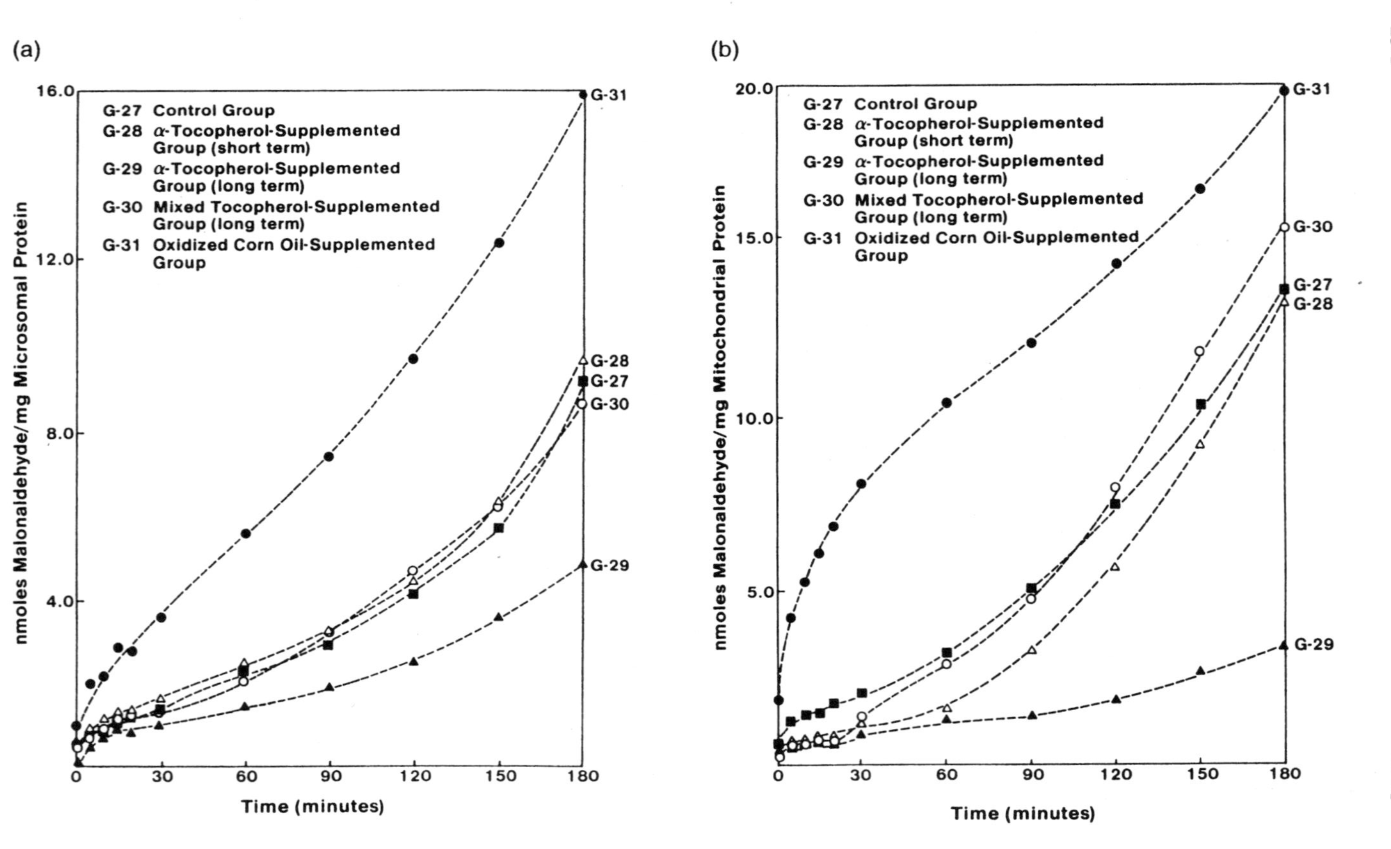


**FIGURE 4.11** Metmyoglobin/hydrogen peroxide–initiated peroxidation in (a) mitochondria and (b) microsomes isolated from the semitendinosus muscles of pigs fed various diets. (From Ref. 94.)

**TABLE 4.16** Mean α-Tocopherol Content of Pig Diets and of Plasma and Muscle from Pigs Fed Diets Containing Oxidized or Fresh Corn Oil with 10, 100, or 200 mg of α-Tocopherol Acetate/kg of Diet[a]

| | | α-T concentration | | |
|---|---|---|---|---|
| Group | Dietary treatment | Diet (mg/kg) | Plasma (μg/mL) | Muscle (μg/g) |
| 1 | Oxidized oil + α-T (10 mg/kg) | 12.7 | 0.20 | 0.45 |
| 2 | Fresh oil + α-T (10 mg/kg) | 23.5 | 0.53 | 0.78 |
| 3 | Oxidized oil + α-T (100 mg/kg) | 135.0 | 2.01 | 2.98 |
| 4 | Fresh oil + α-T (100 mg/kg) | 140.6 | 1.47 | 2.58 |
| 5 | Oxidized oil + α-T (200 mg/kg) | 226.3 | 3.10 | 4.19 |
| 6 | Fresh oil + α-T (200 mg/kg) | 214.7 | 3.54 | 4.07 |

[a]α-T, α-tocopherol.
*Source*: Modified from Ref. 95.

increasing the level of dietary vitamin E, but dietary oil had no effect. The TBARS values were significantly influenced by dietary vitamin E but not by the dietary oil. Supplemental vitamin E significantly increased the stability of raw and cooked pork chops. Lipid oxidation of porcine muscle microsomal fractions and pork chops was significantly influenced by dietary α-TAC but not by the degree of oxidation of dietary corn oil (96,97).

### 4.4.4. Effect of Vitamin E on Other Meat Quality Parameters

**4.4.4.1. Color Stability.** Dietary supplementation with α-TAC increases the color stability of pork meat, exact mechanisms for the increased color stability are not known. L (luminance, whiteness) and b (yellowness) values of pork chops decreased along with storage period regardless of the levels of dietary vitamin E (73). The a values (redness) of pork chops also decreased with length of storage at 4°C; however, changes in a values were relatively slow in pork chops from the pigs fed 100 and 200 IU α-TAC/kg feed compared to those in pork chops from the pigs fed the control diet containing 10 IU α-TAC/kg feed (Table 4.17). Other studies show increased color stability of pork and pork products that is due to vitamin E supplementation (97–100).

Whereas the studies described show a positive effect of vitamin E supplementation on color stability, other research shows little impact. Studies on vacuum-packed ham (101), low-oxygen modified atmosphere packaged ham (101), minced pork (79), and cured pork sausage (81) showed limited ability of vitamin E supplementation to improve color stability of the products.

**TABLE 4.17** Changes in Color (Hunter L, a, b Values) in Pork Chops from Vitamin E–Supplemented Pigs When Stored Under Fluorescent Light at 4°C

| Storage (days) | Hunter parameter | Vitamin E supplementation (mg/kg feed) | | |
|---|---|---|---|---|
| | | 10 | 100 | 200 |
| 0 | L Value | 44.8a | 45.5a | 44.0a |
| 3 | | 38.1b | 39.5a | 37.4b |
| 6 | | 33.6b | 34.7a | 33.1b |
| 10 | | 30.6a | 30.2a | 29.1b |
| 0 | a Value | 10.7a | 11.6ab | 12.6b |
| 3 | | 10.1a | 11.1ab | 12.4b |
| 6 | | 7.0a | 9.3b | 10.0b |
| 10 | | 7.0a | 7.9a | 8.7a |
| 0 | b Value | 12.5a | 12.7a | 12.5a |
| 3 | | 12.3a | 12.2a | 12.3a |
| 6 | | 11.3a | 10.8a | 10.2a |
| 10 | | 9.4a | 9.4a | 9.7a |

*Mean values having the same letter in the same row are not significantly different ($p > 0.05$).
*Source*: Modified from Ref. 73.

**4.4.4.2. Drip Loss.** Dietary supplementation of $\alpha$-TAC affects drip loss of fresh and thawed pork. Frozen pork chops from pigs fed three levels of dietary vitamin E showed significantly different rates of drip loss on thawing during storage at 4°C under fluorescent light for 10 days (Table 4.18) (73). Pork chops from the pigs fed 200 IU $\alpha$-TAC/kg feed had decreased drip loss compared to

**TABLE 4.18** Percentage Drip Loss from Frozen Pork Chops from Pigs Fed Vitamin E–Supplemented Diets When Stored Under Fluorescent Light at 4°C

| Storage (days) | Vitamin E supplementation (mg/kg feed) | | |
|---|---|---|---|
| | 10 | 100 | 200 |
| 3 | 19.0a | 16.2a | 10.2b |
| 6 | 20.1a | 19.5a | 12.2b |
| 9 | 21.3a | 21.2a | 14.1b |

*Mean values having the same letter in the same row are not significantly different ($p>0.05$).
*Source*: Modified from Ref. 73.

those from pigs fed 10 or 100 IU $\alpha$-TAC/kg feed. Protection of the integrity of cell membranes by $\alpha$-T by preventing phospholipid oxidation and destruction of membranes by phospholipase action was suggested. Dietary supplementation of 500 mg $\alpha$-TAC/kg feed for 46 days reduced drip loss by 54% and 46% in unfrozen Longissimus thoracis (LT) (102). Reduced erythrocyte fragility and phospholipase $A_2$ activity was noted, suggesting that dietary vitamin E stabilizes membranes by inhibiting the activity of phospholipase $A_2$, which decreases the stability of membrane integrity of erythrocytes and water-holding capacity. Monahan and coworkers (103) found that lipid oxidation and drip loss are not directly related, although dietary vitamin E supplementation led to a reduction in both lipid oxidation and drip loss. The drip loss and lipid oxidation were reduced by dietary vitamin E supplementation (200 $\alpha$-TAC/kg feed). However, drip loss increased at a more rapid initial rate than TBARS in control pork, and in the supplemented pork, considerable drip loss occurred even though lipid oxidation was negligible (Figure 4.12). They suggested that measurement of primary oxidative changes, such as the formation of peroxides, would give a better estimate of lipid oxidation to evaluate the relationship between lipid oxidation and drip loss. Other research indicated that dietary vitamin E supplementation did not influence drip loss of fresh pork even though supplementation significantly reduced lipid oxidation. (75,104)

**4.4.4.3. Cholesterol Oxidation.** Cholesterol is believed to function as an integral part of the lipid bilayer of cell membranes. Its close association with phospholipids in the membrane where initiation of lipid oxidation occurs has led investigators to postulate that cholesterol oxidation proceeds concomitantly with phospholipid oxidation (95). Research has shown that supplementation of animal diets with vitamin E is effective in inhibiting the formation of cholesterol oxidation products such as 5$\beta$, 6$\beta$-epoxycholestan-3$\beta$-ol, cholest-5-ene-3$\beta$, 7$\beta$-diol, and 7-oxocholest-5-ene-3$\beta$-ol. Studies on ground pork showed that cholesterol oxidation was significantly influenced by dietary $\alpha$-TAC but not by the type of dietary oil (Table 4.19) (95). Lipid oxidation and cholesterol oxidation were linearly related. Increasing the $\alpha$-T content of muscle by diet supplementation appears to be an effective way to reduce cholesterol oxidation in pork (82,85,95,105).

## 4.5. BEEF

Lipid oxidation, overall meat color changes, including metmyoglobin formation, and drip loss are the most important attributes influencing the display life of retail beef. Research suggests that the supplementation of cattle rations with $\alpha$-TAC increases tissue $\alpha$-T levels and appears to be an effective way for improving the color and oxidative stability of beef and its products. Pertinent research that

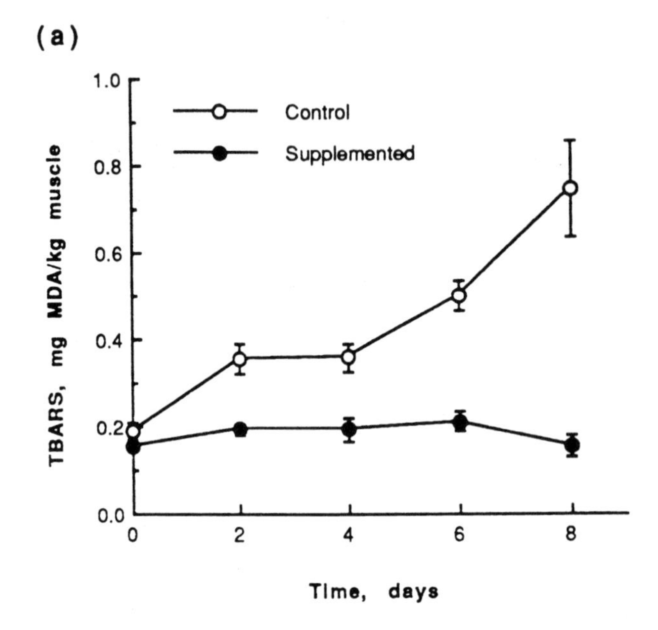


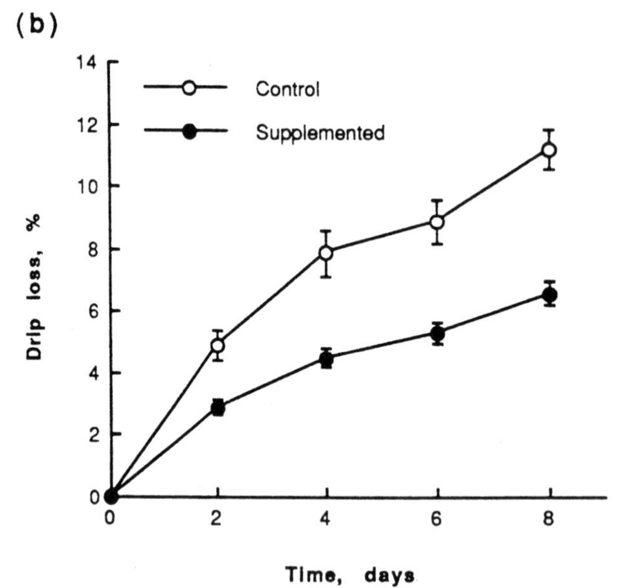


**FIGURE 4.12** Effect of dietary $\alpha$-T supplementation on (a) lipid oxidation and (b) drip loss from pork steaks in refrigerated storage. TBARS, thiobarbituric acid–reactive substance; MDA, malondialdephyde. (From Ref. 103.)

**TABLE 4.19** Effect of Dietary Oil and α-Tocopherol Supplementation on Cholesterol Oxide Content (μg/g) of Cooked Pork During Storage at 4°C

| Dietary oil | Dietary α-TAC (mg/kg feed) | Day 4 | | | |
|---|---|---|---|---|---|
| | | β-Epoxide | 7β-OH | 7-Keto | Total COPs |
| Oxidized | 10 | 7.21b | 5.35b | 10.92b | 23.48b |
| | 100 | 4.93a | 4.41a | 9.31a | 18.64a |
| | 200 | 5.65a | 4.28a | 8.41a | 18.34a |
| Fresh | 10 | 5.67a | 5.07b | 9.79b | 20.53b |
| | 100 | 5.64a | 4.54ab | 7.85a | 18.03a |
| | 200 | 5.15a | 4.05a | 8.79ab | 17.99a |

*For each oil type, means in the same column bearing different letters are significantly different ($p < 0.05$). COPs, cholesterol oxidations products; α-TAC, α-tocopherol acetate.
*Source*: Modified from Ref. 95.

shows the effects of feeding supplemental levels of vitamin E on the oxidative and storage stability and on the other quality parameters of beef is discussed in the following sections and summarized in Table 4.20.

## 4.5.1. Vitamin E Supplementation and Tissue Levels

Faustman et al (112). reported higher α-T levels in ground sirloin from vitamin E–supplemented Holstein steers compared to ground sirloin from the control group after feeding 370 mg α-TAC/animal/day throughout the feeding period. In a later study, Holstein calves were fed whole milk twice a day (control group) while supplemented animals received 500 mg α-TAC powder added directly to the milk for 12 weeks after birth (113). Concentrations of α-T in the plasma, liver, heart, lung, kidney, adipose tissue, muscle, mitochondria, and microsomes from supplemented animals were significantly higher than those in the corresponding parts from the control group. The concentrations of α-T for organs from the supplemented group decreased in the following order: adipose tissue > liver > kidney > lung > heart. Other research reported increased α-T levels in muscles from supplemented animals compared to those from control animals (114–116)

Liu and colleagues (117) investigated the effects of four levels of α-TAC (0, 250, 500, and 2000 mg/head/day) and duration of supplementation (24 and 126 days) on α-T concentrations in fresh and cooked muscle. Tissue α-T levels of supplemented steers were higher than those of nonsupplemented steers for both fresh and cooked muscle *M. gluteus medius* (GM). Both level and duration of dietary α-TAC supplementation significantly affected muscle α-T concentration (Figure 4.13). Cooking did not affect concentration of α-T in the muscle. Garber and coworkers (118) also examined dose–response effects of dietary α-TAC

**TABLE 4.20** Selected Summaries of Research Supplementing Beef Rations with Vitamin E[a]

| Research topic | Vitamin E forms | Amount/ head/day | Cofactor | Observations | Ref. |
|---|---|---|---|---|---|
| Effect of α-TAC supplementation on frozen storage stability | α-TAC | 500 mg | Coconut oil, corn oil | α-TAC supplementation enhanced tissue levels of α-T and retarded lipid oxidation of LL tissues during frozen storage | 1981, 121 |
| Concentration of α-T in plasma and tissues after oral administration of different tocopherols | *all-rac*-α-T, *RRR*-α-T, *all-rac*-α-TAC, *RRR*-α-TAC | 1000 IU | | *RRR*-α-T and its ester increased plasma α-T level faster than racemic products; greatest response occurred with *RRR*-α-T; highest α-T concentrations were noted in adrenal gland and liver, lowest in muscle and thyroid tissues | 1988, 119 |
| Effect of α-TAC supplementation on a and chroma values of fresh sirloin steaks | α-TAC | 370 mg | | Chroma and Hunter a values of steaks from vitamin E–supplemented were significantly higher | 1989, 124 |
| Effect of α-TAC supplementation on pigment changes and oxidative stability | α-TAC | 370 mg | | Meat containing 0.3 mg α-T/100 g tissue displayed least oxidation of both pigments and lipids | 1989, 112 |
| Effect of α-TAC supplementation on color and lipid stability | α-TAC | 1200 mg | Vitamin C | Dietary vitamin E supplementation retarded MetMb formation and suppressed lipid oxidation | 1991, 131 |

| | | | | | |
|---|---|---|---|---|---|
| Effect of dosage strategy, rate, and extent of α-T equilibration in plasma, muscle, and liver of steers on muscle display life after slaughter | α-TAC | Varies with days | Length of dosage | Maximal accretion or depletion of α-T in plasma and liver occurred before 42 d, but accretion required 120 d and depletion required 180 d in LL; vitamin E supplementation elevated concentration of α-T in liver, lung, subcutaneous fat, omental fat, perirenal fat, kidney, diaphragm, spinal cord, LL, and plasma at slaughter; vitamin E inhibited oxidation at surface and center of LL steaks displayed for 19 d | 1993, 120 |
| Effect of dietary vitamin E supplementation and vitamin E addition after grinding on pigment and lipid stability | α-TAC | 1500 mg | White mineral oil, oil + vitamin E | Dietary α-TAC supplementation delayed MetMb increase and suppressed lipid oxidation in ground beef during 9 d of display; postmortem addition of vitamin E (oil + vitamin E) was slightly effective in retarding oxidation of pigment and lipid | 1993, 123 |
| Effect of long-term feeding of α-TAC on meat quality | α-TAC | 0, 360, 1290 mg | Level of α-TAC | Color display life of fresh beef under simulated retail conditions was extended 2 to 5 d by vitamin E, lipid oxidation was markedly reduced | 1993, 132 |
| Effect of α-TAC supplementation on color stability | α-TAC | 2100 mg | Freeze–thaw cycle, storage time, light and film permeability | α-TAC supplementation increased color stability of frozen samples | 1993, 125 |

*(continued)*

**TABLE 4.20** *Continued*

| Research topic | Vitamin E forms | Amount/ head/day | Cofactor | Observations | Ref. |
|---|---|---|---|---|---|
| Effect of α-TAC supplementation on oxidative stability | α-TAC | 500 mg | — | α-TAC increased muscle and membranal α-T concentrations; oxidative stability of mitochondrial and microsomal lipids was enhanced by dietary supplementation; muscle lipid and cholesterol stability also improved | 1993, 113 |
| Effect of α-TAC supplementation on pigment and lipid stability | α-TAC | 2100 mg | Light, film permeability | Dietary supplementation improved pigment and lipid stability of meats stored in darkness and under constant illumination | 1994, 129 |
| Effect of α-TAC supplementation on lipid stability of cooked sirloin | α-TAC | 0, 250, 500, 2000 mg | — | α-T concentration increased in fresh and cooked muscle as a result of level and duration of supplementation; cooking did not affect α-T concentration in muscle; dietary α-TAC delayed accumulation of lipid oxidation products in cooked muscle | 1994, 117 |
| Effect of α-TAC supplementation on drip and cooking losses | α-TAC | 298 mg/ kg Diet | — | α-TAC supplementation produced meat that had smaller increases in drip loss during 14 d of display but higher cooking loss; cooking yield was reduced by supplementation; supplementation reduced muscle cell disruption in beef steak displayed for 14 d | 1995, 136 |

| | | | | | |
|---|---|---|---|---|---|
| Effect of $\alpha$-T levels on storage quality | $\alpha$-TAC | 500 mg | — | Meat from cattle fed supplemental $\alpha$-TAC contained higher levels of $\alpha$-T and exhibited less lipid oxidation, brighter lean color, and lower discoloration; increased levels of $\alpha$-T in beef extended case life and decreased incidence of discounted beef products | 1995, 114 |
| Effect of $\alpha$-TAC supplementation on color stability | $\alpha$-TAC | 0, 500, 2000 mg | Storage temperature | LL muscle from supplemented steers showed less surface MetMb accumulation | 1995, 126 |
| Effect of $\alpha$-TAC supplementation on color stability | $\alpha$-TAC | 1204 mg | | $\alpha$-TAC supplementation delayed oxymyoglobin oxidation in muscle and increased color shelf life of muscles without affecting total microbial load; panelists preferred appearance of vitamin E-treated beef steaks | 1996, 127 |
| Effect of $\alpha$-TAC supplementation on MetMb accumulation | $\alpha$-TAC | 0, 250, 500, 2000 mg | Levels of vitamin E | MetMb formation was delayed with supplementation dosage and duration | 1996, 128 |
| Dose-response effects of $\alpha$-TAC supplementation on growth performance, carcass and meat sensory characteristics, serum and tissue $\alpha$-T levels | $\alpha$-TAC | 0, 500, 1000, 2000 mg | Levels of vitamin E | Serum $\alpha$-T level increased with $\alpha$-TAC intake; growth performance was not affected; there were no effects of vitamin E on sensory attributes of frozen steaks; surface MetMb formation was delayed by supplementation | 1996, 118 |

(continued)

**Table 4.20** *Continued*

| Research topic | Vitamin E forms | Amount/head/day | Cofactor | Observations | Ref. |
|---|---|---|---|---|---|
| Effect of α-TAC supplementation on color stability | α-TAC | 0, 250, 500, 2000 mg | Level and length of dosage | Effects of vitamin E dosage on a, b, and chroma values and hue angle were 2000 > 500 > 250 > 0; effectiveness of dosage duration on color parameters was 126 d > 42 d; dietary supplementation stabilized redness and color saturation, decreased yellowness, and extended color display life of fresh beef | 1996, 130 |
| Effect of α-T supplementation on drip loss | α-T | 2150 IU | | Effect of supplementation on drip loss seemed to depend on muscle studied; drip loss of LL was not significantly influenced, whereas supplemented ST had significantly less drip loss and supplemented PM had significantly more drip loss than did control counterparts | 1997, 138 |
| Effect of α-TAC supplementation on retail display characteristics after vacuum-packaged storage | α-TAC | 0, 1000, 2000 mg | | Supplementation resulted in steaks that exhibited superior lean color, less surface discoloration, more desirable overall appearance, and less lipid oxidation during retail display | 1997, 139 |
| Effect of α-T supplementation on drip loss, color, and oxidative stability | α-T | 5000 mg | | Vitamin E supplementation maintained redness and retarded MetMb formation, delayed lipid oxidation, and reduced drip loss | 1998, 137 |

| | | | | | |
|---|---|---|---|---|---|
| Effect of α-TAC supplementation, packaging, and storage time on α-T content, oxidative properties, color, and shelf life of ground beef held under refrigerated display | α-TAC | 2000 mg | Packaging, storage time | α-T concentrations were significantly higher in minced meat samples from supplemented group; significant reduction in α-T concentrations in supplemented meat samples was observed with increased concentrations of oxygen in different packaging systems; TBARS values were reduced over whole retail display period for all packaging systems with α-TAC-supplemented beef; supplementation in combination with vacuum packaging and MAP improved color stability | 1998, 115 |
| Effect of dietary α-TAC on color, bacteriological characteristics, and case life | α-TAC | 1000 mg | Packaging | Dietary vitamin E increased a values and reduced MetMb accumulation irrespective of packaging atmosphere; vitamin E acted synergistically with $CO_2$ packaging treatment to increase color case life | 1998, 140 |
| Effect of α-TAC supplementation and α-T concentration in different tissues on oxidative stability | α-TAC | 600, 2000 mg | Length and level of vitamin E | Vitamin E supplementation delayed increase of MetMb and reduced fat oxidation and drip loss | 1998, 122 |

(*continued*)

**Table 4.20** *Continued*

| Research topic | Vitamin E forms | Amount/ head/day | Cofactor | Observations | Ref. |
|---|---|---|---|---|---|
| Effect of α-TAC supplementation on susceptibility of fresh, frozen, and vacuum-packaged beef to lipid oxidation and color deterioration | α-TAC | 20 and 2000 mg/kg feed | | α-T level was higher in muscle from supplemented animals; supplemented fresh, frozen, and vacuum-packed beef showed greater color and oxidative stability | 1999, 116 |
| Effect of α-TAC supplementation on color stability and drip loss | α-TAC | 2025 mg | | α-TAC supplementation did not affect color or drip loss; basal diet was high with vitamin E (330 mg/head/day); oxidation was inhibited by α-TAC supplementation | 2000, 133 |
| Effect of α-TAC supplementation on color and oxidative stability | α-TAC | 2500 IU | Pastured and grain-fed | α-TAC supplementation reduced lipid oxidation in grain-fed beef but not in pasture-fed; α-T level in muscle of pasture-fed beef was not changed by supplementation; color stability was not changed | 2002, 134 |
| Effect of α-T supplementation on pasture- and grain-fed beef | | 2500 IU | β-Carotene | α-T level in plasma, muscle, and fat was not modified in pasture-fed cattle but increased in grain-fed animals with supplementation | 2002, 135 |

[a] α-TAC, α-tocopherol acetate; α-T, α-tocopherol; LL, M. longissimus lumborum; MetMb, Metmyoglobin; ST, M. semitendinosus; PM, M. psoas major; TBARS, thiobarbituric acid–reactive substance; MAP, modified atmosphere packaging.

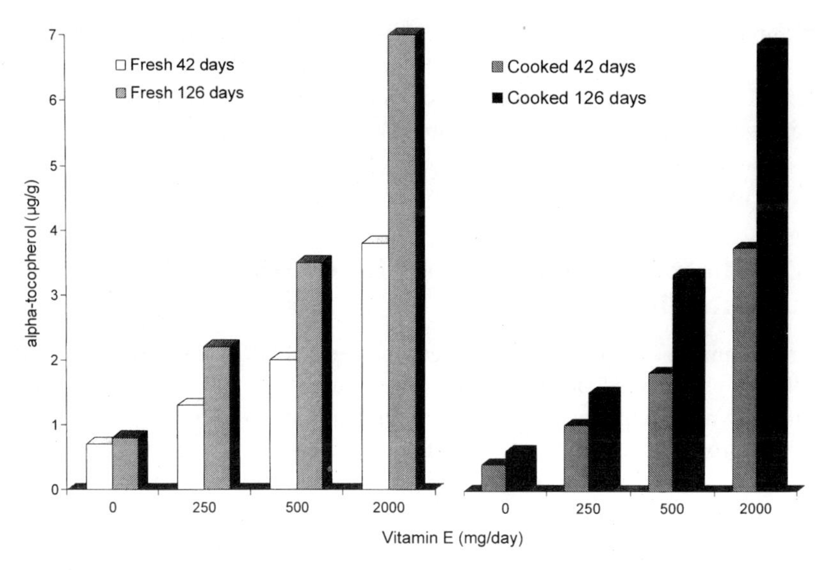


**FIGURE 4.13** α-Tocopherol concentrations in fresh ($n = 24$) and cooked ($n = 24$) GM muscle from Holstein steers fed four dosages of vitamin E for 42 or 126 days. Across both fresh and cooked meat, means with different letters differ ($p < 0.01$). GM, glutens medius. (Modified from Ref. 117.)

supplementation on α-T concentrations. Steers were fed a ration supplemented with 0, 250, 500, 1000, or 2000 mg α-TAC/head/day. The levels of α-T in serum, muscle (*M. gluteus medius*), *M. semimembranosus* muscle, perirenal and subcutaneous fat, and liver increased linearly with increasing levels of dietary vitamin E (Table 4.21).

**TABLE 4.21** The α-Tocopherol Concentration in Serum, GM and SM Muscles, Liver, and Subcutaneous Fat of Finishing Beef Fed Various Supplemental Levels of Dietary Vitamin E

| Dietary vitamin E (IU/head/day) | α-Tocopherol (µg/g tissue) | | | | |
|---|---|---|---|---|---|
| | Serum | GM[a] | SM[a] | Liver | Subcutaneous fat |
| 0 | 1.9 | 2.7 | 2.0 | 8.6 | 5.2 |
| 250 | 3.3 | 4.5 | 2.7 | 17.9 | 9.6 |
| 500 | 4.1 | 5.0 | 3.0 | 15.3 | 10.5 |
| 1000 | 4.9 | 6.1 | 3.8 | 16.2 | 13.0 |
| 2000 | 5.2 | 6.9 | 4.0 | 25.2 | 15.9 |

[a]GM, *Gluteus medius*; SM, *M. Semi Membranosus*.
*Source*: Modified from Ref. 118.

Supplementation of *all-rac-α*-T, *RRR-α*-T, *all-rac-α*-TAC, and *RRR-α*-TAC showed that the *RRR-α*-T and its acetate ester increased plasma α-T concentration faster than the racemic forms of tocopherol (119). The greatest increase was observed with *RRR-α*-T supplementation. The α-T concentration in adrenal gland, kidney, liver, and lung was higher for cattle fed *RRR-α*-T than for those fed the racemic forms of tocopherol (Table 4.22).

## 4.5.2. Effect of Dietary Vitamin E on Oxidative Stability

Dietary vitamin E supplementation of veal showed TBARS values were lowered in both raw and cooked steaks stored at 4°C (Table 4.23) (113). Mitochondrial and microsomal membranes of the control animals oxidized to a greater extent than those from calves fed the vitamin E supplement. These results agree with other findings that supplemental vitamin E retarded lipid oxidation of fresh, frozen and vacuum-packed beef during frozen storage (Figure 4.14).[116,120,121] Formanek and associates (115) examined the effect of dietary vitamin E supplementation, packaging, and storage time on oxidative stability of ground beef stored at refrigerated (4°C) display conditions. Friesian cattle were fed a diet supplemented with 2000 mg α-TAC/kg feed/day for 50 days. After frozen storage (−20°C for 8 weeks), semimembranosus muscles from the basal and supplemented groups were minced and vacuum packaged, aerobically packaged, or packaged under modified atmosphere packaging (MAP, 30% $O_2$:70% $CO_2$; 70% $O_2$:30% $CO_2$; 80% $O_2$:20% $CO_2$). Samples were stored under refrigerated display (fluorescent lighting, 616 lux) for 8 days. The changes

**TABLE 4.22** Tissue α-Tocopherol Concentrations in Cattle Fed Various Vitamin E Preparations[a]

| | Dietary form (μg/g fresh tissue) | | | |
|---|---|---|---|---|
| Tissue | *RRR-α*-TAC | *RRR-α*-T | *all-rac-α*-T | *all-rac-α*-TAC |
| Adrenal gland | 38.4 | 38.1 | 27.9 | 28.8 |
| Heart | 20.4 | 18.7 | 18.4 | 16.1 |
| Kidney | 12.1 | 13.1 | 8.8 | 12.3 |
| Liver | 24.2 | 27.0 | 15.7 | 19.9 |
| Lung | 15.7 | 16.5 | 10.6 | 15.0 |
| Muscle | 5.3 | 5.8 | 5.7 | 5.8 |
| Spleen | 18.0 | 15.8 | 11.8 | 13.9 |
| Thyroid | 3.4 | 4.4 | 5.6 | 4.4 |

[a] α-TAC, α-tocopherol acetate; α-T, α-tocopherol.
*Source*: Modified from Ref. 119.

**TABLE 4.23** Thiobarbituric Acid–Reactive Substance Values (mg Malonaldehyde/kg Meat) for Raw and Cooked Veal Steak from Control and Vitamin E–Supplemented Animals Held at 4°C for 4 Days[a]

| | Raw | | Cooked | |
|---|---|---|---|---|
| Days | Control | Supplemented | Control | Supplemented |
| 0 | 3.8 | 0.3 | 6.2 | 0.4 |
| 2 | 6.3 | 0.4 | 9.7 | 1.9 |
| 4 | 7.6 | 0.4 | 12.4 | 5.0 |

[a]Control different from supplemented ($p < 0.001$).
*Source*: Modified from Ref. 113.

in TBARS values during storage at 4°C are shown in Table 4.24. Increases in TBARS values were significantly lower for vacuum-packed minced beef samples compared with samples packaged aerobically or in MAP. In all cases, the supplemented beef with 2000 mg $\alpha$-TAC/kg feed/day had lower TBARS values than meat from animals fed the basal diet (20 mg $\alpha$-TAC/kg feed/day).

Dietary supplementation with vitamin E at four dosage levels (0, 250, 500, and 2000 mg/head/day) and two durations (42 or 126 days) showed that dietary $\alpha$-TAC delayed TBARS accumulation during refrigerated display (Figure 4.15) (117). The TBARS responded to dietary $\alpha$-TAC supplementation levels linearly, although no difference was observed between the control group and the group supplemented with 250 mg $\alpha$-TAC/head/day. Dosage duration showed no effect. Other research showed that lipid oxidation rates were decreased by dietary vitamin E supplementation in beef, and oxidation rates decreased with increasing levels of vitamin E supplementation (118,122,123). Dietary vitamin E supplementation to cattle greatly improved lipid stability in ground beef compared with that in the control, and postmortem vitamin E treatment was slightly effective in retarding the oxidation of lipid. Postmortem addition of $\alpha$-T to beef in amounts equivalent to those deposited in beef by dietary vitamin E supplementation was ineffective in controlling lipid oxidation and suggested that a much higher postmortem addition of $\alpha$-T would be needed to obtain better oxidative stability (123).

### 4.5.3. Effect of Vitamin E on Other Meat Quality Parameters

**4.5.3.1. Color Stability.** Control of discoloration of fresh beef is most important in maintaining a stable display of retail meat because the consumer's perception of beef quality is strongly influenced by the color. The undesirable brown metmyoglobin results from oxidation of the red oxymyoglobin and purple

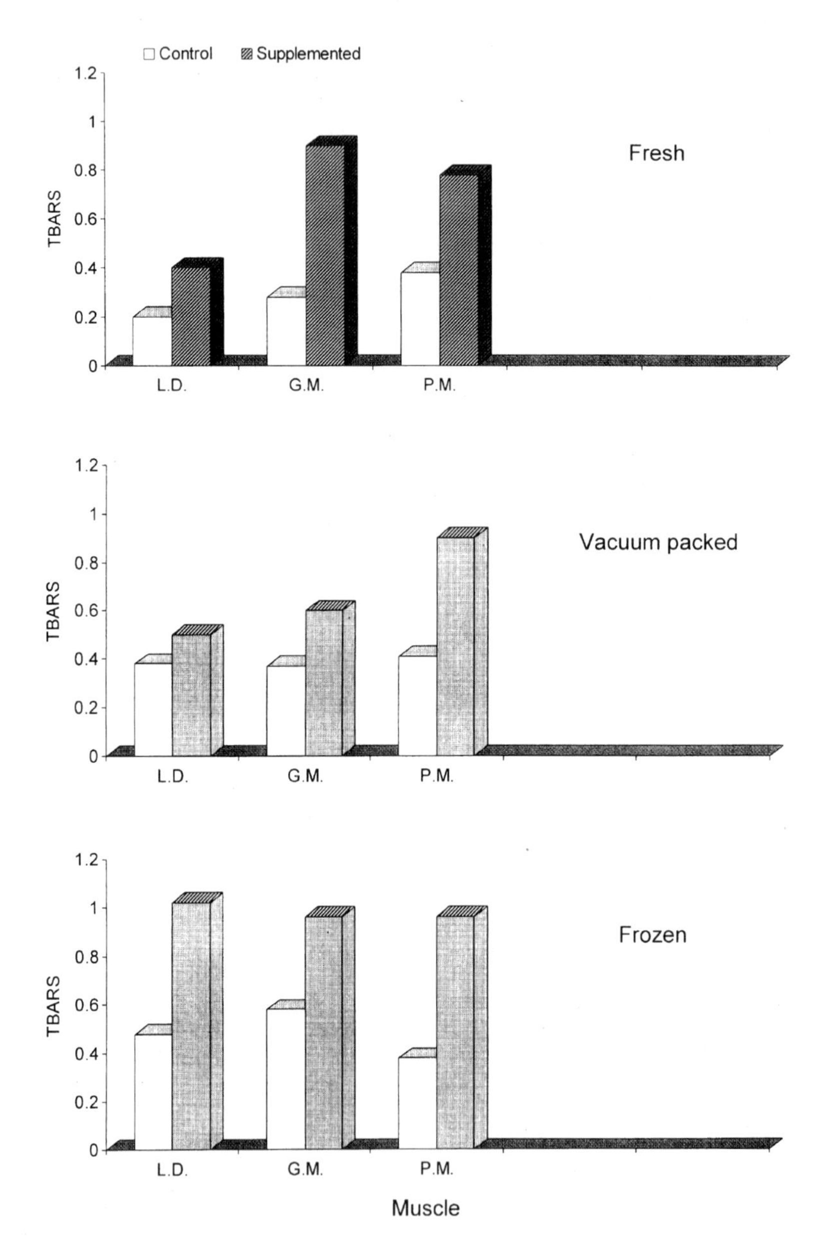


**FIGURE 4.14** Effect of $\alpha$-T supplementation on TBARS formation in (a) fresh, (b) vacuum-packaged, and (c) frozen beef LD, GM, and PM muscles after 7-day storage at 4°C. TBARS, thiobarbituric acid–reactive substance; LD,*M. longissimus dorsi*; GM, *M. gluteus medius*; PM, *M. psoas major*. (Modified from Ref. 116.)

**TABLE 4.24** Effect of Feeding of Beef Cattle Basal (20 mg/head/day) or Supplemented (2000 mg/head/day) Diets Containing α-Tocopherol Acetate and Various Packaging Conditions on the Oxidative Stability (Thiobarbituric Acid–Reactive Substance mg Malonaldehyde/kg Meat) of Raw Mince Held Under Refrigerated (4°C) Display Conditions for 8 Days

| Packaging conditions | Time (days) | | | |
|---|---|---|---|---|
| | 2 | 4 | 6 | 8 |
| Vacuum | | | | |
| Basal | 0.79aw | 0.67aw | 0.67aw | 0.44aw |
| Supplemented | 0.83aw | 0.48ax | 0.37ax | 0.35ax |
| Aerobic | | | | |
| Basal | 2.29bw | 2.71bw | 2.63bw | 3.01bw |
| Supplemented | 1.39bw | 1.55cw | 1.71cw | 1.80cw |
| 30% $O_2$ : 70% $CO_2$ | | | | |
| Basal | 2.12bw | 2.65bw | 3.45dx | 3.00bw |
| Supplemented | 1.70bw | 1.77cw | 3.24dx | 3.82bx |
| 70% $O_2$ : 30% $CO_2$ | | | | |
| Basal | 3.01bw | 3.62bx | 5.48ex | 4.78dx |
| Supplemented | 2.04bw | 2.88bw | 2.48dw | 4.74dx |
| 80% $O_2$ : 20% $CO_2$ | | | | |
| Basal | 2.26bw | 3.48bx | 5.29ex | 5.64dx |
| Supplemented | 1.78bw | 2.33bw | 4.44ex | 4.85dx |

Different letters within the same column (*a–e*) and across the same row (*w–x*) indicate significant ($p < 0.05$) differences.
*Source*: Modified from Ref. 115.

deoxymyoglobin. Various attempts have been made to extend the stability of the desirable pigments by dietary vitamin E supplementation (124–132).

Faustman et al (7). summarized the role of vitamin E in beef color stability as follows:

1. Delivery of α-T through dietary supplementation with α-TAC is effective in stabilization of red meat color.
2. The relative color stability of different muscles is not changed by α-T. Compositional and metabolic differences that are not directly related to oxidative stability of microsomal fractions influence color stability.
3. Several potential mechanisms enable vitamin E to stabilize oxymyoglobin. However, α-T most likely exerts an indirect effect on oxymyoglobin stability by direct inhibition of lipid oxidation. Products of lipid oxidation are more water-soluble than nonoxidized lipids and enter the cytoplasm, where they interact with oxymyoglobin.

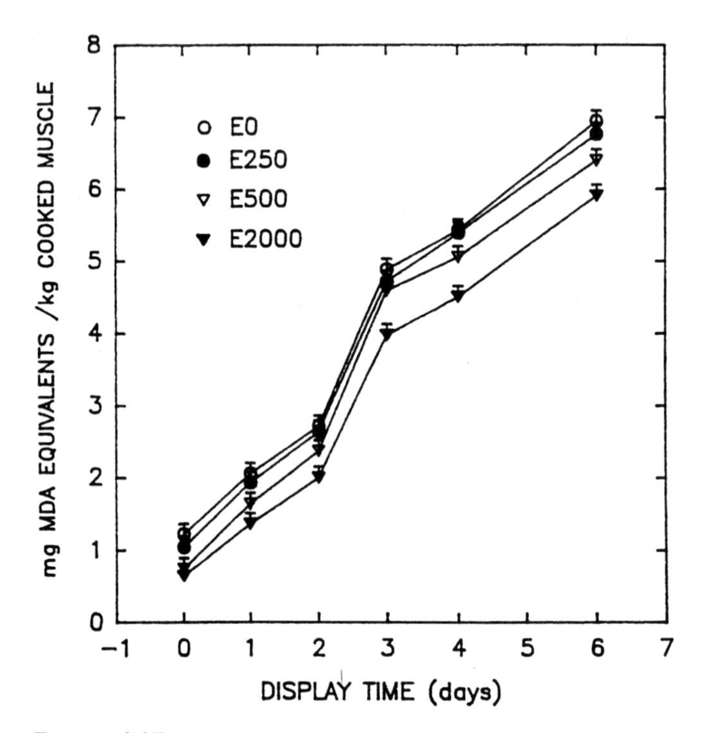


**FIGURE 4.15** Effects of level (0, 250, 500 or 2000 mg/head/day) of *all-rac-α*-tocophenyl acetate E on lipid oxidation in cooked GM muscle during illuminated display at 4°C. MDA, malondialdehyde; GM, *M. gluteus medius*. (From Ref. 117.)

4. Low-oxygen partial pressure (4–10 mm Hg) favors oxidation of oxymyoglobin. Formation of metmyoglobin at low-oxygen partial pressure can be delayed by supplemental vitamin E.

Figure 4.16 (124) shows color changes in sirloin steak from vitamin-supplemented and control animals under refrigerated storage. Figure 4.17 (129) shows changes in oxymyoglobin and metmyoglobin under dark and illuminated storage. Effects of vitamin E dosage on storage duration life under vacuum are given in Table 4.25 (130).

Faustman and colleagues (112) investigated the effect of dietary vitamin E supplementation (370 mg α-TAC/animal/day for 10 months) of Holstein steers on pigment and lipid oxidation of fresh ground sirloin. During 6 days of storage at 4°C, metmyoglobin accumulation and lipid oxidation (TBA) were greater for

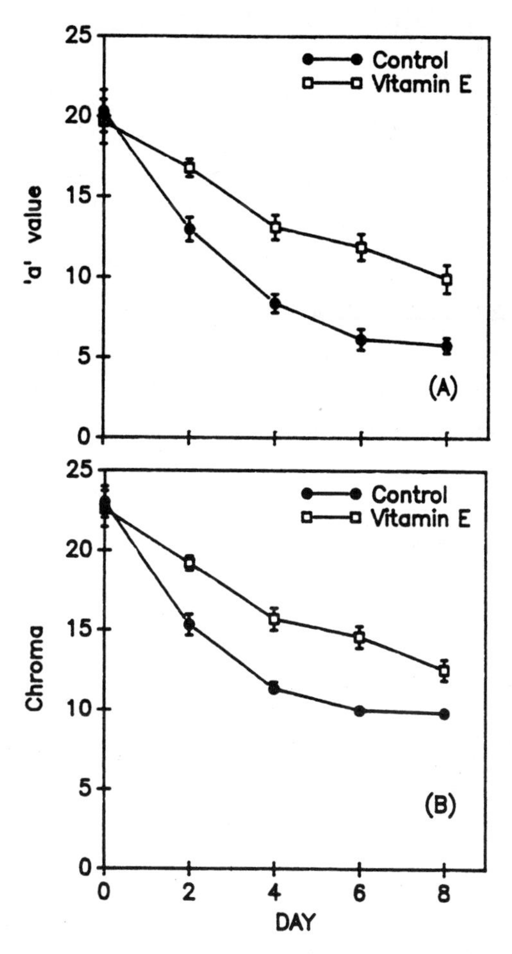


**FIGURE 4.16** Objective color measurements of sirloin steaks, from control and vitamin E–supplemented Holstein steers, during storage at 4°C. (A) a value (redness) and (B) chroma (color intensity); $n = 17$ for each treatment group. (From Ref. 124.)

control animals than for those supplemented with vitamin E. The TBA values and metmyoglobin percentage (% metmyoglobin) were highly correlated in the control ($r = 0.91$) and supplemented ($r = 0.72$) groups. These results correspond with other studies that reported that dietary vitamin E supplementation retarded metmyoglobin formation of LD muscles and highly suppressed lipid oxidation compared to those from nonsupplemented animals (131,132). Faustman et al (112). concluded that dietary vitamin E supplementation should be maintained at

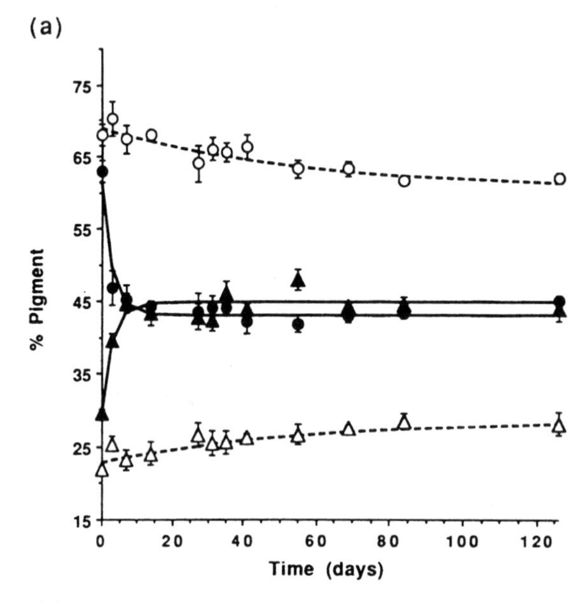


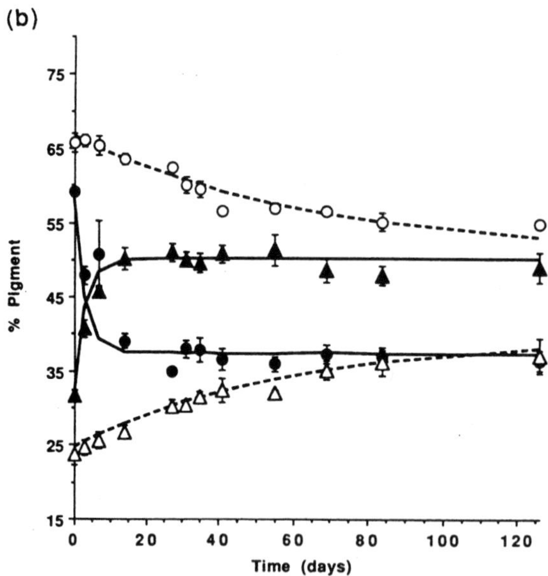


**FIGURE 4.17** Oxymyoglobin (●, ○) and metmyoglobin (▲, △) concentrations during (a) aerobic storage in the dark and (b) aerobic illuminated display at −20°C of control (●, ▲) and supplemented (○, △) LL packaged in polyethylene. Solid and dashed lines represent pigment concentrations predicted by the kinetic model for the respective treatments. LL, *M. longissimus lumborum*. (From Ref. 129.)

**TABLE 4.25** Dosage and Duration Effects of Supplemental Vitamin E on Color Display Life of Bovine Longissimus Muscle Held in Vacuum Storage for Three Periods

| Vitamin E (mg/day) | Aged 14 days | | Aged 28 days | | Aged 56 days | |
|---|---|---|---|---|---|---|
| | 42[a] | 126[a] | 42[a] | 126[a] | 42[a] | 126[a] |
| 0 | 3.3[b] | 4.7 | 3.3 | 3.0 | 2.3 | 3.0 |
| 250 | 5.7 | 6.7 | 5.0 | 6.0 | 3.3 | 4.0 |
| 500 | 6.0 | 7.7 | 5.3 | 6.3 | 2.7 | 4.3 |
| 2000 | 8.7 | 10.0 | 7.3 | 8.3 | 4.3 | 6.0 |

[a]Dose duration.
[b]Color display life.
*Source*: Modified from Ref. 130.

a level that produces 3.5-mg $\alpha$-T/kg meat. Therefore, the accumulation of sufficient levels of $\alpha$-T in muscle seems to be the critical factor to reduce pigment oxidation.

Studies (133,134) in 2000 and 2002 did not show an effect of supplemental vitamin E on color stability, in this research, $\alpha$-T levels in control animals were quite high. Yang and associates (135) reported that cattle grazed on good pasture can maintain $\alpha$-T levels in muscles comparable to levels found in vitamin E–supplemented, grain-fed cattle.

**4.5.3.2. Drip Loss.** Various studies indicated positive effects of dietary vitamin E supplementation on drip loss of beef during refrigerated display (136–140). However, the influence of supplementation on drip loss of muscles is not always consistent and can vary among different muscles. The differences on a percentage weight loss basis comparing meat cuts from supplemented and nonsupplemented animals are usually quite low. Mitsumoto and colleagues (136) concluded that vitamin E supplementation shifted weight loss from drip loss to cooking loss and could be beneficial to meat retailers. Increased concentrations of $\alpha$-T most likely stabilize membrane stability and enhance the ability of cells to retain sarcoplasmic components during refrigerated shore display. Effects of vitamin E supplementation for muscle from steers supplemented with 5000 mg $\alpha$-T/day for 7 days before slaughter are shown in Figure 4.18 (137).

**4.5.3.3. Cholesterol Oxidation in Beef.** Relatively few studies have been published on the effects of dietary supplementation on cholesterol oxidation in beef. Engeseth and coworkers (113) and Engeseth and Gray (141) showed that vitamin E supplementation was effective in controlling the development of

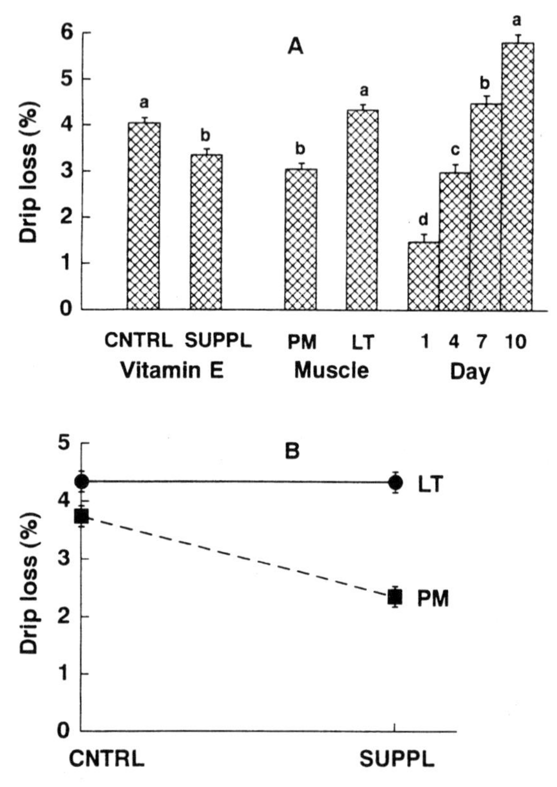


**FIGURE 4.18** (A) Effect of vitamin E supplementation, muscle, and day on drip loss percentage. Least-squares means and standard error bars are shown. Within main effects, means with different letters differ ($p < 0.05$). CNTRL, no vitamin E supplementation; SUPPL, vitamin E supplementation. (B) Dietary vitamin E supplementation multiplied by muscle interaction for drip loss percentage. PM, *M. psoas major*; LT, *M. longissimus thoracis*. (From Ref. 137.)

cholesterol oxides in raw and cooked muscles during storage (Table 4.26). Cholesterol oxidation in vacuum-packaged cooked beef steaks was inhibited during refrigerated and frozen storage; however, the effect varied with muscle type (142).

## 4.6. MILK AND EGGS

### 4.6.1. Milk

Oxidation of milk fat and development of spontaneous oxidized flavor are widespread problems in the milk and dairy industry. They may be caused by an

**TABLE 4.26** Cholesterol Oxide Concentration (μg/g Sample) in Cooked Veal Held at 4°C for 4 days[a]

| | Day 0 | | Day 4 | |
|---|---|---|---|---|
| Oxide | Control | *all-rac-α*-TAC[b] | Control | *all-rac-α*-TAC[b] |
| β-Epoxide | 1.1 | 6.4 | 4.4 | 1.1 |
| α-Epoxide | 0.1 | 0.5 | 0.3 | 0.2 |
| 7-β-OH | 2.7 | 1.5 | 4.0 | 1.8 |
| Triol | ND[c] | ND | ND | ND |
| 7-Keto | 5.5 | 0.2 | 7.2 | 2.7 |
| 25-OH | ND | ND | 0.9 | ND |
| Total | 9.4 | 8.6 | 16.8 | 5.8 |

[a]Mean of four samples.
[b]500 mg α-TAC per day.
[c]ND, not detected (detection limit: 1 ng).
*Source*: Modified from Ref. 113.

imbalance in levels of pro- and antioxidants in milk or by physical or chemical alteration of the structure of the fat globule membrane during processing (143). As early as 1967, Dunkley and associates (144) studied the effect of supplementing cow rations with vitamin E to control oxidized flavor in milk. Cows were fed an alfalfa-hay-concentrate ration supplemented with α-TAC at a rate of 0.0025% of dry matter intake for 4 weeks. Supplementary α-TAC

**TABLE 4.27** Influence of Supplementary Tocopherol on Tocopherol Content of Milk and Oxidative Stability of Milk and Milk Fat for 5-Day Storage

| Item | Control | Tocopherol supplemented |
|---|---|---|
| α-Tocopherol (μg/g lipid) | 21.0 | 23.4 |
| Oxidative stability of milk | | |
| TBA[a] | 25.6 | 19.4 |
| TBA, Cu[b] | 88.1 | 63.7 |
| Score[c] | 1.2 | 1.2 |
| Score, Cu | 2.4 | 1.8 |
| Oxidative stability of fat (induction period, h) | 82.0 | 96.0 |

[a]TBA, increase in absorbance of the thiobarbituric acid test, $A \times 10^3$.
[b]Cu, copper added to milk at 0.1 μg/g.
[c]Flavor score: 0, no oxidized flavor; 4, strong oxidized flavor.
*Source*: Modified from Ref. 144.

increased the concentration of $\alpha$-T in the milk and increased the oxidative stability of the milk and of the milk fat as measured by TBA test and flavor scores (Table 4.27). More recent research has confirmed these results (145–147).

St. Laurent and colleagues (148) determined the effect of $\alpha$-T supplementation to lactating dairy cows on milk and plasma $\alpha$-T concentrations. Holstein cows ($n = 12$) were assigned to one of three dietary $\alpha$-TAC levels, 0, 700, or 3000 mg/cow/day for 5 weeks. The highest levels of milk $\alpha$-T were observed at week 1 for the 700-mg $\alpha$-TAC group and at week 2 for the 3000-mg $\alpha$-TAC group. During weeks 2 to 5, milk $\alpha$-T concentrations were the highest for the 3000-mg $\alpha$-TAC group and peaked at 22.0 μg/g lipid; plasma $\alpha$-T levels increased by 0.7 and 1.3 μg/mL for the 700- and 3000-mg $\alpha$-TAC groups. By the end of posttreatment phase, in the animals that had no supplementation, milk $\alpha$-T concentration had returned to week 0 levels.

### 4.6.2. Eggs

The micronutrient and PUFA contents of egg yolk are easily modified by supplementation of the diet. Various studies have shown the ability of laying hens to respond to supplemented $\alpha$-T and produce eggs with increased $\alpha$-T content with improved oxidative stability of yolk lipids (149–155). Increases in $\alpha$-T and $\beta$-carotene levels were noted after feeding supplemental $\alpha$-TAC up to 400 mg $\alpha$-TAC/kg diet together with $\beta$-carotene (149). $\alpha$-Tocopherol level in the yolks increased from 144 (control) to 477 mg/g (400 mg $\alpha$-TAC). Egg production and weight were not changed (Table 4.28). Pál and colleagues (155) noted that $\beta$-carotene level in egg yolk did not increase with increasing levels of $\beta$-carotene in non-$\alpha$-TAC-supplemented hens fed pumpkin seed oil.

Increased dietary intake of $\alpha$-T decreases PUFA and cholesterol oxidation (149–154). The increase in oxidative stability is particularly significant in eggs produced with increased PUFA or n-3 fatty acid levels. However, a prooxidant effect was noted in yolk when hens were fed quite high levels of $\alpha$-T (152,153). A prooxidant effect occurred with 120 mg $\alpha$-T/kg (150). A vitamin E supplementation rate of 80 IU/kg diet has been recommended to protect eggs produced with increased content of n-3 fatty acids (153).

## 4.7. FISH

### 4.7.1. Vitamin E Supplementation and Tissue Levels

In general, vitamin E is recognized as the primary antioxidant defense mechanism to prevent oxidative stress in fish. Tocher and coworkers (156) reported on the effects of dietary vitamin E on antioxidant defense mechanisms in turbot, halibut, and sea bream. In each species, relationships were observed in tissue vitamin E and the ratio of PUFA to vitamin E levels in response to levels of vitamin E in the diet. Liver catalase, superoxide dismutase, and glutathione

**Table 4.28** Influence of $\alpha$-Tocopherol and $\beta$-Carotene on Deposition, Production, Yield, and Egg Weight of Yolk Throughout 5 Weeks of Feeding

| Treatments | $\alpha$-Tocopherol (μg/g Yolk) | $\beta$-Carotene (μg/g Yolk) | Egg production (% hen-day) | Egg yield (kg Feed/12 eggs) | Egg weight (g/Egg) |
|---|---|---|---|---|---|
| $\alpha$-Tocopherol acetate (mg/kg diet) | | | | | |
| 0 | 134.77 | 0.14 | 78.77 | 1.84 | 66.03 |
| 50 | 164.42 | 0.13 | 78.29 | 1.77 | 67.58 |
| 100 | 235.57 | 0.15 | 73.43 | 2.08 | 67.43 |
| 200 | 245.76 | 0.14 | 75.71 | 1.80 | 66.55 |
| 400 | 390.08 | 0.10 | 66.00 | 2.37 | 64.81 |
| $\beta$-Carotene (mg/kg diet) | | | | | |
| 0 | 134.77 | 0.14 | 78.77 | 1.84 | 66.03 |
| 50 | 133.07 | 1.81 | 68.29 | 2.24 | 64.61 |
| 100 | 134.02 | 2.68 | 71.43 | 2.14 | 67.14 |
| 200 | 121.81 | 5.19 | 65.71 | 2.34 | 64.96 |
| 400 | 126.60 | 4.81 | 66.29 | 2.14 | 66.22 |
| $\alpha$-Tocopherol + $\beta$-carotene (mg/kg diet) | | | | | |
| 0 + 0 | 134.77 | 0.14 | 78.77 | 1.84 | 66.03 |
| 50 + 50 | 126.68 | 1.39 | 69.14 | 2.17 | 64.71 |
| 100 + 100 | 116.74 | 2.71 | 72.00 | 1.90 | 65.45 |
| 200 + 200 | 166.23 | 4.78 | 71.14 | 2.25 | 65.94 |
| 400 + 400 | 225.65 | 3.85 | 69.14 | 2.13 | 65.65 |

*Source*: Modified from Ref. 149.

peroxidase levels were the highest in fish fed the lowest levels of vitamin E. The TBARS and isoprostane levels used as indicators of oxidative stress were lowest in fish fed the highest level. Because of higher dietary and tissue PUFA levels, the minimal requirement for vitamin E for cold water fish is 50 mg $\alpha$-TAC/kg diet (156,157). The dietary requirement for vitamin E increases with increasing PUFA intake (158,159).

Hamre and Lie (160) showed that $\alpha$-T concentration in the whole body of Atlantic salmon could be increased five to seven times with a diet supplemented with 300 mg $\alpha$-TAC/kg. Whole body $\alpha$-T levels were above 7.5 compared to <1.5 mg/100 g for nonsupplemented fish. Several other studies have shown the ability of supplemented vitamin E to increase tissue and organ $\alpha$-T concentrations (154,159,161–163).

## 4.7.2. Effect of Dietary Vitamin E on Oxidative Stability

Various studies show the importance of dietary supplementation of vitamin E to quality maintenance of fresh and processed fish (159,162,163). Supplemental vitamin E becomes more essential for quality maintenance if the species contains normally high n-3 fatty acid levels or the diet has been modified to increase n-3 tissue levels. Waagbo and associates (159) found that in fillets of Atlantic salmon fed a high-n-3 fatty acid diet and low vitamin E levels an oxidized, rancid flavor developed to a greater extent than in those fed a high-PUFA–high-vitamin E (300 mg $\alpha$-TAC/kg diet) diet. Oxidative stability of trout and channel catfish fillets is significantly improved by feeding diets containing up to 200 mg $\alpha$-TAC/kg diet for trout (163) and 400 mg $\alpha$-T/kg diet for channel catfish (164).

## REFERENCES


1. Jensen, C.; Lauridsen, C.; Bertelsen, G. Dietary vitamin E: quality and storage stability of pork and poultry. Trends. Food Sci. Technol. **1998**, *9*, 62–72.
2. Frigg, M.; Buckley, D.J.; Morrissey, P.M. Influence of $\alpha$-tocopheryl acetate supplementation on the susceptibility of chicken or pork tissues to lipid oxidation. Mh. Vet. Med. **1993**, *48*, 79–83.
3. Morrissey, P.A.; Buckley, D.J.; Sheehy, P.J.A. Vitamin E and meat quality. Proc. Nutr. Soc. **1994**, *53*, 289–295.
4. Buckley, D.J.; Morrissey, P.A.; Gray, J.I. Influence of dietary vitamin E on the oxidative stability and quality of pig meat. J. Anim. Sci. **1995**, *73*, 3122–3130.
5. Liu, Q.; Lanari, M.C.; Schaefer, D.M.; A review of dietary vitamin E supplementation for improvement of beef quality. J. Anim. Sci. **1995**, *73*, 3131–3140.
6. Sheehy, P.J.A.; Morrissey, P.A.; Buckley, D.J.; Wen, J. Effects of vitamins in the feed on meat quality in farm animals: vitamin E. In Recent Advances in Animal Nutrition; Garnsworthy, P.C., Wiseman, J., Eds.; Nottingham University Press, England, Nottingham, 1997.
7. Faustman, C.; Chan, W.K.M.; Shaefer, D.M.; Havens, A. Beef color update: the role for vitamin E. J. Anim. Sci. **1998**, *76*, 1019–1026.
8. Morrissey, P.A.; Kerry, J.P.; Galvin, K. Lipid oxidation on muscle foods. In Freshness and Shelf Life of Foods; Cadwallader, K.R., Weenen, H., Eds.; Washington, DC: ACS Symposium Series 836, 2003.
9. Kummerow, F.A.; Vail, G.E.; Conrad, R.M.; Avery, T.B. Fat rancidity in eviscerated poultry. Poult. Sci. **1948**, *27*, 635–640.
10. Mecchi, E.P.; Pool, M.F.; Behman, G.A.; Hamachi, M.; Klose, A.A. The role of tocopherol content in the comparative stability of chicken anf turkey fat. Poult. Sci. **1956**, *35*, 1238–1246.
11. Webb, J.E.; Brunson, C.C.; Yates, J.D. Effects of feeding antioxidants on rancidity development in pre-cooked, frozen broiler parts. Poult. Sci. **1972**, *51*, 1601–1605.
12. Webb, R.W.; Marion, W.W.; Hayse, P.L. Effect of tocopherol supplementation on the quality of precooked and mechanically deboned turkey meat. J. Food Sci. **1972**, *37*, 853–856.

13. Webb, J.E.; Brunson, C.C.; Yates, J.D. Effects of feeding fish meal and tocopherol on flavor of precooked, frozen turkey meat. Poult. Sci. **1973**, *52*, 1027–1034.
14. Webb, J.E.; Brunson, C.C.; Yates, J.D. Effects of dietary fat and *dl*-$\alpha$-tocopheryl acetate on stability characteristics of precooked frozen broiler parts. J. Food Sci. **1974**, *39*, 133–136.
15. Hayse, P.L.; Marion, W.W.; Paulson, R.J. The effectiveness of tocopherol in controlling oxidative rancidity in turkey. Poult. Sci. **1974**, *53*, 1934–1934.
16. Marusich, W.L.; De Ritter, E.; Ogrinz, E.F.; Keating, J.; Mitrovic, M.; Bunnell, R.H. Effect of supplemental vitamin E in control of rancidity in poultry meat. Poult. Sci. **1975**, *54*, 831–844.
17. Bartov, I.; Bornstein, S. Effects of degree of fatness in broilers on other carcass characteristics: relationship between fatness and the stability of meat and adipose tissue. Br. Poult. Sci. **1976**, *17*, 29–38.
18. Bartov, I.; Bornstein, S. Stability of abdominal fat and meat of broilers: the interrelationship between the effects of dietary fat and vitamin E supplements. Br. Poult. Sci. **1977**, *18*, 47–57.
19. Bartov, I.; Bornstein, S. Stability of abdominal fat and meat of broilers: effects of duration and feeding antioxidants. Br. Poult. Sci. **1978**, *19*, 129–135.
20. Sheehy, P.J.A.; Morrissey, P.A.; Flynn, A. Influence of dietary $\alpha$-tocopherol on tocopherol concentrations in chick tissues. Br. Poult. Sci. **1991**, *32*, 391–397.
21. Morrissey, P.A.; Brandon, S.; Buckley, D.J.; Sheehy, P.J.A.; Frigg, M. Tissue content of $\alpha$-tocopherol and oxidative stability of broilers receiving dietary $\alpha$-tocopheryl acetate supplement for various periods pre-slaughter. Br. Poult. Sci. **1997**, *38*, 84–88.
22. Galvin, K.; Morrissey, P.A.; Buckley, D.J. Cholesterol oxides in processed chicken muscle as influenced by dietary $\alpha$-tocopherol supplementation. Meat. Sci. **1998**, *48*, 1–9.
23. Ruiz, J.A.; Pérez-Vendrell, A.M.; Esteve-Grací, E. Effect of $\beta$-carotene and vitamin E on oxidative stability in leg meat of broilers fed different supplemental fats. J. Agric. Food Chem. **1999**, *47*, 448–454.
24. Gray, J.I.; Pearson, A.M. Rancidity and warmed-over flavor. Adv. Meat. Res. **1987**, *3*, 221–269.
25. Webb, J.E.; Brunson, C.C.; Yates, J.D. Effects of feeding antioxidants on rancidity development in pre-cooked, frozen broiler parts. Poult. Sci. **1972**, *51*, 1601–1605.
26. Bartov, I.; Bornstein, S. Stability of abdominal fat and meat of broilers: relative effects of vitamin E, butylated hydroxytoluene and ethoxyquin. Br. Poult. Sci. **1977**, *18*, 59–68.
27. Winne, A.D.; Dirinck, P. Studies on vitamin E and meat quality. 2. Effect of feeding high vitamin E levels on chicken meat quality. J. Agric. Food Chem. **1996**, *44*, 1691–1696.
28. Harel, S.; Kanner, J. Muscle membranal lipid peroxidation initiated by hydrogen peroxide–activated metmyoglobin. J. Agric. Food Chem. **1985**, *33*, 1188–1192.
29. Asghar, A.; Lin, C.F.; Gray, J.I.; Buckley, D.J.; Booren, A.M.; Crackel, R.L.; Flegal, C.J. Influence of oxidised dietary oil and antioxidant supplementation on membrane-bound lipid stability in broiler meat. Br. Poult. Sci. **1989**, *30*, 815–823.

30. Lauridsen, C.; Buckley, D.J.; Morrissey, P.A. Influence of dietary fat and vitamin E supplementation on $\alpha$-tocopherol levels and fatty acid profiles in chicken muscle membranal fractions and on susceptibility to lipid peroxidation. Meat. Sci. **1997**, *46*, 9–22.
31. Bartov, I.; Frigg, M. Effect of high concentrations of dietary vitamin E during various age periods on performance, plasma vitamin E and meat stability of broiler chicks at 7 weeks of age. Br. Poult. Sci. **1992**, *33*, 393–402.
32. Jakobsen, K.; Engberg, R.M.; Andersen, J.O.; Jensen, S.K.; Lauridsen, C.; Søren, P.; Henkel, P.; Bertelsen, G.; Skibsted, L.H.; Jensen, C. Supplementation of boiler diets with *all-rac-*$\alpha$- or a mixture of natural source *RRR-*$\alpha$-, $\gamma$-, $\delta$-tocopheryl acetate. 1. Effect on vitamin E status of boilers *in vivo* and at slaughter. Poult. Sci. **1995**, *74*, 1984–1994.
33. Jensen, C.; Skibsted, L.H.; Jakobsen, K.; Bertelsen, G. Supplementation of broiler diets with *all-rac-*$\alpha$- or a mixture of natural source *RRR-*$\alpha$-, $\gamma$-, $\delta$-tocopheryl acetate. 2. Effect on the oxidative stability of raw and precooked broiler meat products. Poult. Sci. **1995**, *74*, 2048–2056.
34. Olivo, R.; Soares, A.L.; Ida, E.I.; Shimokomaki, M. Dietary vitamin E inhibits poultry PSE and improves meat functional properties. J. Food Biochem. **2001**, *25*, 271–283.
35. O'Neill, L.M.; Gavlvin, K.; Morrissey, P.A.; Buckley, D.J. Effect of carnosine, salt and dietary vitamin E on the oxidative stability of chicken meat. Meat. Sci. **1999**, *52*, 89–94.
36. Grau, A.; Guardiola, F.; Grimpa, S.; Barroeta, A.C.; Codony, R. Oxidative stablility of dark chicken meat through frozen storage: influence of dietary fat and $\alpha$-tocopherol and ascorbid acid supplementation. Poult. Sci. **2001**, *80*, 1630–1642.
37. Grau, A.; Codony, R.; Grpimpa, S.; Baucells, M.D.; Guardiola, F. Cholesterol oxidation in frozen dark chicken meat: influence of dietary fat source, and $\alpha$-tocopherol and ascorbic acid supplementation. Meat. Sci. **2001**, *57*, 197–208.
38. Lin, C.F.; Gray, J.I.; Asghar, A.; Buckley, D.J.; Booren, A.M.; Flegal, C.J. Effects of dietary oils and $\alpha$-tocopherol supplementation on lipid composition and stability of broiler meat. J. Food Sci. **1989**, *54*, 1457–1460, 1484.
39. Asghar, A.; Lin, C.F.; Gray, J.I.; Buckley, D.J.; Booren, A.M.; Flegal, C.J. Effects of dietary oils and $\alpha$-tocopherol supplementation on membranal lipid oxidation in broiler meat. J. Food Sci. **1990**, *55*, 46–50.
40. Nam, K.T.; Lee, H.A.; Min, B.S.; Kang, C.W. Influence of dietary supplementation with linseed and vitamin E on fatty acids, $\alpha$-tocopherol and lipid peroxidation in muscles of broiler chicks. Anim. Feed. Sci. Technol. **1997**, *66*, 149–158.
41. O'Neill, L.M.; Galvin, K.; Morrissey, P.A.; Buckley, D.J. Comparison of effects of dietary olive oil, tallow and vitamin E on the quality of broiler meat and meat products. Br. Poult. Sci. **1998**, *39*, 365–371.
42. Sheehy, P.J.A.; Morrissey, P.A.; Flynn, A. Influence of heated vegetable oils and $\alpha$-tocopheryl acetate supplementation on $\alpha$-tocopherol, fatty acids and lipid peroxidation in chicken muscle. Br. Poult. Sci. **1993**, *34*, 367–381.
43. Lin, C.F.; Asghar, A.; Gray, J.I.; Buckley, D.J.; Booren, A.M.; Crackel, R.L.; Flegal, C.J. Effects of oxidised dietary oil and antioxidant supplementation on broiler growth and meat stability. Br. Poult. Sci. **1989**, *30*, 855–864.

44. Sheehy, P.J.A.; Morrissey, P.A.; Flynn, A. Consumption of thermally-oxidized sunflower oil by chicks reduces $\alpha$-tocopherol status and increases susceptibility of tissues to lipid oxidation. Br. J. Nutr. **1994**, *71*, 53–65.
45. Galvin, K.; Morrissey, P.A.; Buckley, D.J. Influence of dietary vitamin E and oxidised sunflower oil on the storage stability of cooked chicken muscle. Br. Poult. Sci. **1997**, *38*, 499–504.
46. Bartov, I.; Bornstein, S. Stability of abdominal fat and meat of broilers: combined effect of dietary vitamin E and synthetic antioxidants. Poult. Sci. **1981**, *60*, 1840–1845.
47. Bartov, I.; Sklan, D.; Friedman, A. Effect of vitamin A on the oxidative stability of broiler meat during storage: lack of interactions with vitamin E. Br. Poult. Sci. **1997**, *38*, 255–257.
48. Galvin, K.; Morrissey, P.A.; Buckley, D.J. Effect of dietary $\alpha$-tocopherol supplementation and gamma-irradiation on $\alpha$-tocopherol retention and lipid oxidation in cooked minced chicken. Food Chem. **1998**, *62*, 185–190.
49. Calabotta, D.F.; Shermer, W.D. Controlling feed oxidation can be rewarding. Feedstuffs. **1985**, *57*, 24–33.
50. Criddle, J.E.; Morgan, A.F. The effect of tocopherol feeding on the tocopherol and peroxide content of turkey tissues. Fed. Proc. **1947**, *6*, 247–252.
51. Sheldon, B.W. Effect of dietary tocopherol on the oxidative stability of turkey meat. Poult. Sci. **1984**, *63*, 673–681.
52. Wen, J.; Morrissey, P.A.; Buckley, D.J.; Sheehy, P.J.A. Oxidative stability and $\alpha$-tocopherol retention in turkey burgers during refrigerated and frozen storage as influenced by dietary $\alpha$-tocopheryl acetate. Br. Poult. Sci. **1996**, *37*, 787–795.
53. Walsh, M.M.; Kerry, J.F.; Buckley, D.J.; Arendt, E.K.; Morrissey, P.A. Effect of dietary supplementation with $\alpha$-tocopheryl acetate on the stability of reformed and restructured low nitrite cured turkey products. Meat. Sci. **1998**, *50*, 191–201.
54. Mercier, Y.; Gatellier, P.; Viau, M.; Remignon, H.; Renerre, M. Effect of dietary fat and vitamin E on colour stability and on lipid and protein oxidation in turkey meat during storage. Meat. Sci. **1998**, *48*, 301–318.
55. Renerre, M.; Poncet, K.; Mercier, Y.; Gatellier, P.; Metro, B. Influence of dietary fat and vitamin E on antioxidant status of muscles of turkey. J. Agric. Food Chem. **1999**, *47*, 237–244.
56. Marusich, W.L.; Ritter, E.D.; Ogrinz, E.F.; Keating, J.; Mitrovic, M.; Bunnell, R.H. Effect of supplemental vitamin E in control of rancidity in poultry meat. Poult. Sci. **1975**, *54*, 831–844.
57. Webb, R.W.; Marion, W.W.; Hayse, P.L. Effect of tocopherol supplementation on the quality of precooked and mechanically deboned turkey meat. J. Food Sci. **1972**, *37*, 853–856.
58. Webb, R.W.; Marion, W.W.; Hayse, P.L. Tocopherol supplementation and lipid stability in the turkey. J. Food. Sci. **1972**, *37*, 496.
59. Webb, J.E.; Brunson, C.C.; Yates, J.D. Effects of feeding fish meal and tocopherol on flavor of precooked, frozen turkey meat. Poult. Sci. **1973**, *52*, 1029–1034.
60. Bartov, I.; Basker, D.; Angel, S. Effect of dietary vitamin E on the stability and sensory quality of turkey meat. Poult. Sci. **1983**, *62*, 1224–1230.

61. Sheldon, B.W.; Curtis, P.A.; Dawson, P.L.; Ferket, P.R. Effect of dietary vitamin E on the oxidative stability, flavor, color, and volatile profiles of refrigerated and frozen turkey breast meat. Poult. Sci. **1997**, *76*, 634–641.
62. Ahn, D.U.; Sell, J.L.; Jo, C.; Chen, X.; Wu, C.; Lee, J.I. Effects of dietary vitamin E supplementation on lipid oxidation and volatiles content of irradiated, cooked turkey meat patties with different packaging. Poult. Sci. **1998**, *77*, 912–920.
63. Ahn, D.U.; Sell, J.L.; Jeffery, M.; Jo, C.; Chen, X.; Wu, C.; Lee, J.I. Dietary vitamin E affects lipid oxidation and total volatiles of irradiated raw turkey meat. J. Food Sci. **1997**, *62*, 954–958.
64. Sklan, D.; Tenne, Z.; Budowski, P. The effect of dietary fat and tocopherol on lipolysis and oxidation in turkey meat stored at different temperatures. Poult. Sci. **1983**, *62*, 2017–2021.
65. Bartov, I.; Kanner, J. Effect of high levels of dietary iron, iron injection, and dietary vitamin E on the oxidative stability of turkey meat during storage. Poult. Sci. **1996**, *75*, 1039–1046.
66. Soto-Salanova, M.F.; Sell, J.L. Efficacy of dietary and injected vitamin E for poults. Poult. Sci. **1996**, *75*, 1393–1403.
67. Monahan, F.J.; Buckley, D.J.; Gray, J.I.; Morrissey, P.A.; Asghar, A.; Hanrahan, T.J.; Lynch, P.B. Effect of dietary vitamin E on the stability of raw and cooked pork. Meat. Sci. **1990**, *27*, 99–108.
68. Monahan, F.J.; Buckley, D.J.; Morrissey, P.A.; Lynch, P.B.; Gray, J.I. Effect of dietary $\alpha$-tocopherol supplementation on $\alpha$-tocopherol levels in porcine tissues and on susceptibility to lipid peroxidation. Food Sci. Nutr. **1990**, *42F*, 203–212.
69. Monahan, F.J.; Buckley, D.J.; Morrissey, P.A.; Lynch, P.B.; Gray, J.I. Influence of dietary fat and $\alpha$-tocopherol supplementation on lipid oxidation in pork. Meat. Sci. **1992**, *31*, 229–241.
70. Pfalzgraf, A.; Frigg, M.; Steinhart, H.; $\alpha$-Tocopherol contents and lipid oxidation in pork muscle and adipose tissue during storage. J. Agric. Food Chem. **1995**, *43*, 1339–1342.
71. Kingston, E.R.; Monahan, F.J.; Buckley, D.J.; Lynch, P.B. Lipid oxidation in cooked pork as affected by vitamin E, cooking and storage conditions. J. Food Sci. **1998**, *63*, 386–389.
72. Isabel, B.; Lopez-Bote, C.J.; de la Hoz, L.; Timón, M.; Garcia, C.; Ruiz, J. Effects of feeding elevated concentrations of monounsaturated fatty acids and vitamin E to swine on characteristics of dry cured hams. Meat. Sci. **2003**, *64*, 475–482.
73. Asghar, A.; Gray, J.I.; Booren, A.M.; Gomaa, E.A.; Abouzied, M.M.; Miller, E.R. Effects of supranutritional dietary vitamin E levels on subcellular deposition of $\alpha$-tocopherol in the muscle and on pork quality. J. Sci. Food Agric. **1991**, *57*, 31–41.
74. Wen, J.; Morrissey, P.A.; Buckley, D.J.; Sheehy, P.J.A. Supranutritional vitamin E supplementation in pigs: influence on subcellular deposition of $\alpha$-tocopherol and on oxidative stability by conventional and derivative spectrophotometry. Meat. Sci. **1997**, *47*, 301–310.
75. Jensen, C.; Guidera, J.; Skovgaard, I.M.; Staun, H.; Skibsted, L.H.; Jensen, S.K.; Møller, A.J.; Buckley, J.; Bertelsen, G. Effects of dietary $\alpha$-tocopheryl acetate supplementation on $\alpha$-tocopherol deposition in porcine *m. psoas major* and *m.*

*longissimus dorsi* and on drip loss, colour stability and oxidative stability of pork meat. Meat. Sci. **1997**, *45*, 491–500.

76. Rosenvold, K.; Lærke, H.N.; Jensen, S.K.; Karlsson, A.H.; Lundström, K.; Andersen, H.J. Manipulation of critical quality indicators and attributes in pork through vitamin E supplementation, muscle glycogen reducing finishing feeding and pre-slaughter stress. Meat. Sci. **2002**, *62*, 485–496.
77. Winne, A.D.; Dirinck, P. Studies on vitamin E and meat quality. 3. Effect of feeding high vitamin E levels to pigs on the sensory and keeping quality of cooked ham. J. Agric. Food Chem. **1997**, *45*, 4309–4317.
78. Isabel, B.; Lopez-Bote, C.J.; Rey, A.I.; Arias, R.S. Influence of dietary $\alpha$-tocopheryl acetate supplementation of pigs on oxidative deterioration and weight loss in sliced dry-cured ham. Meat. Sci. **1999**, *51*, 227–232.
79. Houben, J.H.; Eikelenboom, G.; Hoving-Bolink, A.H. Effect of the dietary supplementation with vitamin E on colour stability and lipid oxidation in packaged, minced pork. Meat. Sci. **1998**, *48*, 265–273.
80. Walsh, M.M.; Kerry, J.F.; Buckley, D.J.; Morrissey, P.A.; Lynch, P.B.; Arendt, E. The effect of dietary supplementation with $\alpha$-tocopheryl acetate on the stability of low nitrite cured pork products. Food Res. Int. **1998**, *31*, 59–63.
81. Zanardi, E.; Novelli, E.; Ghiretti, G.P.; Chizzolini, R. Oxidative stability of lipids and cholesterol in salame Milano, coppa and Parma ham: dietary supplementation with vitamin E and oleic acid. Meat. Sci. **2000**, *55*, 169–175.
82. Harms, C.; Fuhrmann, H.; Nowak, B.; Wenzel, S.; Sallmann, H-P. Effect of dietary vitamin E supplementation on the shelf life of cured pork sausage. Meat. Sci. **2003**, *63*, 101–105.
83. Miles, R.S.; McKeith, F.K.; Bechtel, P.J.; Novakofski, J. Effect of processing, packaging and various antioxidants on lipid oxidation of restructured pork. J. Food Prot. **1986**, *49*, 222–225.
84. Coronado, S.A.; Trout, G.R.; Dushea, F.R.; Shah, N.P. Effect of dietary vitamin E, fishmeal and wood and liquid smoke on the oxidative stability of bacon during 16 weeks' frozen storage. Meat. Sci. **2002**, *62*, 51–60.
85. Rey, A.I.; Kerry, J.P.; Lynch, P.B.; Lopez-Bote, C.J.; Buckley, D.J.; Morrissey, P.A. Effect of dietary oils and $\alpha$-tocopheryl acetate supplementation on lipid (TBARS) and cholesterol oxidation in cooked pork. J. Anim. Sci. **2001**, *79*, 1201–1208.
86. Flachowsky, G.; Schöne, F.; Schaarmann, G.; Lübbe, F.; Böhme, H. Influence of oilseeds in combination with vitamin E supplementation in the diet on backfat quality of pigs. Anim. Feed Sci. Technol. **1997**, *64*, 91–100.
87. Jensen, C.; Flensted-Jensen, M.; Skibsted, L.H.; Bertelsen, G. Warmed-over flavour in chill-stored pork patties in relation to dietary rapeseed oil and vitamin E supplementation. Z. Lebensm Unters Forsch A **1998**, *207*, 154–159.
88. D'Arrigo, M.; Hoz, L.; Lopez-Bote, C.J.; Cambero, I.; Pin, C.; Rey, A.I.; Ordonez, J.A. Effect of dietary linseed oil and $\alpha$-tocopherol on selected properties of pig fat. Can. J. Anim. Sci. **2002**, *82*, 339–346.
89. Kanner, J.; Hazan, B.; Doll, L.; Catalytic "free" iron in muscle foods. J. Agric. Food Chem. **1988**, *36*, 412–415.

90. Jensen, C.; Flensted-Jensen, M.; Skibsted, L.H.; Bertelsen, G. Effects of dietary rape seed oil, copper(II) sulfate and vitamin E on drip loss, colour and lipid oxidation of chilled pork chops packed in atmospheric air or in a high oxygen atmosphere. Meat. Sci. **1998**, *50*, 211–221.
91. Zanardi, E.; Novelli, E.; Nanni, N.; Ghiretti, G.P.; Delbono, G.; Campanini, G.; Dazzi, G.; Madarena, G.; Chizzolini, R. Oxidative stability and dietary treatment with vitamin E, oleic acid and copper of fresh and cooked pork chops. Meat. Sci. **1998**, *49*, 309–320.
92. Jensen, C.; Skibsted, L.H.; Bertelsen, G. Oxidative stability of frozen-stored raw pork chops, chill-stored pre-frozen raw pork chops, and frozen-stored pre-cooked sausages in relation to dietary $CuSO_4$, rapeseed oil and vitamin E. Z. Lebensm. Unters. Forsch. A **1998**, *207*, 363–368.
93. Lauridsen, C.; Nielsen, J.H.; Henckel, P.; Sørensen, M.T. Antioxidative and oxidative status in muscles of pigs fed rapeseed oil, vitamin E, and copper. J. Anim. Sci. **1999**, *77*, 105–115.
94. Buckley, D.J.; Gray, J.I.; Asghar, A.; Price, J.F.; Crackel, R.L.; Booren, A.M.; Pearson, A.M.; Miller, E.R. Effects of dietary antioxidants and pork product quality. J. Food Sci. **1989**, *54*, 1193–1197.
95. Monahan, F.J.; Gray, J.I.; Booren, A.M.; Miller, E.R.; Buckley, D.J.; Morrissey, P.A.; Gomaa, E.A. Influence of dietary treatment on lipid and cholesterol oxidation in pork. J. Agric. Food Chem. **1992**, *40*, 1310–1315.
96. Monahan, F.J.; Gray, J.I.; Asghar, A.; Haug, A.; Shi, B.; Buckley, D.J. Effect of dietary lipid and vitamin E supplementation on free radical production and lipid oxidation in porcine muscle microsomal fractions. Food Chem. **1993**, *46*, 1–6.
97. Monahan, F.J.; Asghar, A.; Gray, J.I.; Buckley, D.J. Effect of oxidized dietary lipid and vitamin E on the colour stability of pork chops. Meat. Sci. **1994**, *37*, 205–215.
98. Lanari, M.C.; Schaefer, D.M.; Scheller, K.K. Dietary vitamin E supplementation and discoloration of pork bone and muscle following modified atmosphere packaging. Meat Sci. **1995**, *41*, 237–250.
99. Dirinck, P.; Winne, A.D.; Casteels, M.; Frigg, M. Studies on vitamin E and meat quality. 1. Effect of feeding high vitamin E levels on time-related pork quality. J. Agric. Food Chem. **1996**, *44*, 65–68.
100. Hoving-Bolink, A.H.; Eikelenboom, G.; van Diepen, J.T.M.; Jongbloed, A.W.; Houben, J.H. Effect of dietary vitamin E supplementation on pork quality. Meat Sci. **1998**, *49*, 205–212.
101. Houben, J.H.; Gerris, C.V.M. Effect of dietary supplementation with vitamin E on colour stability of packaged, sliced pasteurized ham. Meat Sci. **1998**, *50*, 421–428.
102. Cheah, K.S.; Cheah, A.M.; Krausgrill, D.I. Effect of dietary supplementation of vitamin E on pig meat quality. Meat Sci. **1995**, *39*, 255–264.
103. Monahan, F.J.; Gray, J.I.; Asghar, A.; Haug, A.; Strasburg, G.M.; Buckley, D.J.; Morrissey, P.A. Influence of diet on lipid oxidation and membrane structure in porcine muscle microsomes. J. Agric. Food Chem. **1994**, *42*, 59–63.
104. Cannon, J.E.; Morgan, J.B.; Schmidt, G.R.; Tatum, J.D.; Sofos, J.N.; Smith, G.C.; Delmore, R.J.; Williams, S.N. Growth and fresh meat quality characteristics of pigs supplemented with vitamin E. J. Anim. Sci. **1996**, *74*, 98–105.

105. Amer, M.A.; Elliot, J.I. Influence of supplemental dietary copper and vitamin E on the oxidative stability of porcine depot fat. J. Anim. Sci. **1973**, *37*, 87–90.
106. Thode Jensen, P.; Nielsen, H.E.; Danielsen, V.; Leth, T. Effect of dietary fat quality and vitamin E on the antioxidant potential of pigs. Acta Vet. Scand. **1983**, *24*, 135–147.
107. Cannon, J.E.; Morgan, J.B.; Schmidt, G.R.; Delmore, R.J.; Sofos, J.N.; Smith, G.C.; Williams, S.N. Vacuum-packaged precooked pork from hogs fed supplemental vitamin E: chemical, shelf-life and sensory properties. J. Food Sci. **1995**, *60*, 1179–1182.
108. Leonhardt, M.; Gebert, S.; Wenk, C. Stability of $\alpha$-tocopherol, thiamin, riboflavin and retinol in pork muscle and liver during heating as affected by dietary supplementation. J. Food Sci. **1996**, *61*, 1048–1051.
109. Onibi, G.E.; Scaife, J.R.; Murray, I.; Fowler, V.R. Use of $\alpha$-tocopherol acetate to improve pig meat quality of full-fat rapeseed-fed pigs. JAOCS **1998**, *75*, 189–198.
110. Zanardi, E.; Novelli, E.; Ghiretti, G.P.; Dorigoni, V.; Chizzolini, R. Colour stability and vitamin E content of fresh and processed pork. Food Chem. **1999**, *67*, 163–171.
111. van Heugten, E.; Hasty, J.L.; See, M.T.; Larick, D.K. Storage stability of pork from Berkshire and Hampshire sired pigs following dietary supplementation with vitamin E. J. Muscle Foods **2003**, *14*, 67–80.
112. Faustman, C.; Cassens, R.G.; Schaefer, D.M.; Buege, D.R.; Williams, S.N.; Sheller, K.K. Improvement of pigment and lipid stability in Holstein steer beef by dietary supplementation with vitamin E. J. Food Sci. **1989**, *54*, 858–962.
113. Engeseth, N.J.; Gray, J.I.; Booren, A.M.; Asghar, A. Improved oxidative stability of veal lipids and cholesterol through dietary vitamin E supplementation. Meat Sci. **1993**, *35*, 1–15.
114. Sherbeck, J.A.; Wulf, D.M.; Morgan, J.B.; Tatum, J.D.; Smith, G.C.; Williams, S.N. Dietary supplementation of vitamin E to feedlot cattle affects beef retail display properties. J. Food Sci. **1995**, *60*, 250–252.
115. Formanek, Z.; Kerry, J.P.; Buckley, D.J.; Morrissey, P.A.; Farkas, J. Effects of dietary vitamin E supplementation and packaging on the quality of minced beef. Meat Sci. **1998**, *50*, 203–210.
116. Lynch, M.P.; Kerry, J.P.; Buckley, D.J.; Faustman, C.; Morrissey, P.A. Effect of dietary vitamin E supplementation on the color and lipid stability of fresh, frozen and vacuum-packaged beef. Meat Sci. **1999**, *52*, 95–99.
117. Liu, Q.; Scheller, K.K.; Schaefer, D.M.; Arp, S.C.; Williams, S.N. Dietary $\alpha$-tocopheryl acetate contributes to lipid stability in cooked beef. J. Food Sci. **1994**, *59*, 288–290.
118. Garber, M.J.; Roeder, R.A.; Davidson, P.M.; Pumfrey, W.M.; Schelling, G.T. Dose–response effects of vitamin E supplementation on growth performance and meat characteristics in beef and dairy steers. Can. J. Anim. Sci. **1996**, *76*, 63–72.
119. Hidiroglou, N.; Laflamme, L.F.; McDowell, L.R. Blood plasma and tissue concentrations of vitamin E in beef cattle as influenced by supplementation of various tocopherol compounds. J. Anim. Sci. **1988**, *66*, 3227–3234.

120. Arnold, R.N.; Arp, S.C.; Scheller, K.K.; Williams, S.N.; Schaefer, D.M. Tissue equilibration and subcellular distribution of vitamin E relative to myoglobin and lipid oxidation in displayed beef. J. Anim. Sci. **1993**, *71*, 105–118.
121. Shorland, F.B.; Igene, J.O.; Pearson, A.M.; Thomas, J.W.; McGuffey, R.K.; Aldridge, A.E. Effects of dietary fat and vitamin E on the lipid composition and stability of veal during frozen storage. J. Agric. Food Chem. **1981**, *29*, 863–871.
122. Schwarz, F.J.; Augustini, C.; Timm, M.; Kirchgeßner, M.; Steinhart, H. Effect of vitamin E on $\alpha$-tocopherol concentration in different tissues and oxidative stability of bull beef. Livestock Prod. Sci. **1998**, *56*, 165–171.
123. Mitsumoto, M.; Arnold, R.N.; Schaefer, D.M.; Cassens, R.G. Dietary versus postmortem supplementation of vitamin E on pigment and lipid stability in ground beef. J. Anim. Sci. **1993**, *71*, 1812–1816.
124. Faustman, C.; Cassens, R.G.; Schaefer, D.M.; Buege, D.R.; Scheller, K.K. Vitamin E supplementation of Holstein steer diets improves sirloin steak color. J. Food Sci. **1989**, *54*, 485–486.
125. Lanari, M.C.; Cassens, R.G.; Schaefer, D.M.; Scheller, K.K. Dietary vitamin E enhances color and display life of frozen beef from Holstein steers. J. Food Sci. **1993**, *58*, 701–704.
126. Chan, W.K.M.; Hakkarainen, K.; Faustman, C.; Schaefer, D.M.; Scheller, K.K.; Liu, Q. Color stability and microbial growth relationships in beef as affected by endogenous $\alpha$-tocopherol. J Food Sci **1995**, *60*, 966–971.
127. Chan, W.K.M.; Hakkarainen, K.; Faustman, C.; Schaefer, D.M.; Scheller, K.K.; Liu, Q. Dietary vitamin E effect on color stability and sensory assessment of spoilage in three beef muscles. Meat Sci. **1996**, *42*, 387–399.
128. Lanari, M.C.; Schaefer, D.M.; Liu, Q.; Cassens, R.G. Kinetics of pigment oxidation in beef from steers supplemented with vitamin E. J. Food Sci. **1996**, *61*, 884–889.
129. Lanari, M.C.; Cassens, R.G.; Schaefer, D.M.; Scheller, K.K. Effect of dietary vitamin E on pigment and lipid stability of frozen beef: a kinetic analysis. Meat Sci. **1994**, *38*, 3–15.
130. Liu, Q.; Scheller, K.K.; Arp, S.C.; Schafer, D.M.; Frigg, M. Color coordinates for assessment of dietary vitamin E effects on beef color stability. J. Anim. Sci. **1996**, *74*, 106–116.
131. Mitsumoto, M.; Cassens, R.G.; Schaefer, D.M.; Arnold, R.N.; Scheller, K.K. Improvement of color and lipid stability in beef longissimus with dietary vitamin E and vitamin C dip treatment. J. Food Sci. **1991**, *56*, 1498–1492.
132. Arnold, R.N.; Scheller, K.K.; Arp, S.C.; Williams, S.N.; Schaefer, D.M. Dietary $\alpha$-tocopheryl acetate enhances beef quality in Holstein and beef breed steers. J. Food Sci. **1993**, *58*, 28–33.
133. Eikelenboom, G.; Hoving-Bolink, A.H.; Kluitman, I.; Houben, J.H.; Klont, R.E. Effect of dietary vitamin E supplementation on beef colour stability. Meat Sci. **2000**, *54*, 17–22.
134. Yang, A.; Lanari, M.C.; Brewster, M.; Tume, R.K. Lipid stability and meat colour of beef from pasture- and grain-fed cattle with or without vitamin E supplement. Meat Sci. **2002**, *60*, 41–50.

135. Yang, A.; Brewster, M.J.; Lanari, M.C.; Tume, R.K. Effect of vitamin E supplementation on $\alpha$-tocopherols and $\beta$-carotene concentration in tissues from pasture- and grain-fed cattle. Meat Sci. **2002**, *60*, 35–40.
136. Mitsumoto, M.; Arnold, R.N.; Schaefer, D.M.; Cassens, R.G. Dietary vitamin E supplementation shifted weight loss from drip to cooking loss in fresh beef longissimus during display. J. Anim. Sci. **1995**, *73*, 2289–2294.
137. Mitsumoto, M.; Ozawa, S.; Mitsuhashi, T.; Koide, K. Effect of dietary vitamin E supplementation for one week before slaughter on drip, colour and lipid stability during display in Japanese black steer beef. Meat Sci. **1998**, *49*, 165–174.
138. den Hertog-Meischke, M.J.A.; Smulders, F.J.M.; Houben, J.H.; Eikelenboom, G. The effect of dietary vitamin E supplementation on drip loss of bovine *longissimus lumborum*, *psoas major* and *semitendinosus* muscles. Meat Sci. **1997**, *45*, 153–160.
139. Sanders, S.K.; Morgan, J.B.; Wulf, D.M.; Tatum, J.D.; Williams, S.N.; Smith, G.C. Vitamin E supplementation of cattle and shelf-life of beef for the Japanese market. J. Anim. Sci. **1997**, *75*, 2634–2640.
140. Greer, G.G.; Jones, S.D.M.; Dilts, B.D.; Robertson, W.M. The effect of dietary vitamin E and controlled atmosphere packaging on the storage life of beef. Can. J. Anim. Sci. **1998**, *78*, 57–67.
141. Engeseth, N.J.; Gray, J.I. Cholesterol oxidation in muscle tissue. Meat Sci. **1994**, *36*, 309–320.
142. Galvin, K.; A-Lynch, M.; Kerry, J.P.; Morrissey, P.A.; Buckley, D.J. Effect of dietary vitamin E supplementation on cholesterol oxidation in vacuum packaged cooked beef steaks. Meat Sci. **2000**, *55*, 7–11.
143. Charmley, E.; Nicholson, J.W.G.; Zee, J.A. Effect of supplemental vitamin E and selenium in the diet on vitamin E and selenium levels and control of oxidized flavor in milk from Holstein cows. Can. J. Anim. Sci. **1993**, *73*, 453–457.
144. Dunkley, W.L.; Ronning, M.; Franke, A.A.; Robb, J. Supplementing rations with tocopherol and ethoxyquin to increase oxidative stability of milk. J. Dairy Sci. **1967**, *50*, 492–499.
145. Focant, M.; Mignolet, E.; Marique, M.; Clabots, F.; Breyne, T.; Dalemans, D.; Larondelle, Y. The effect of vitamin E supplementation of cow diets containing rapeseed and linseed on the prevention of milk fat oxidation. J Dairy Sci **1998**, *81*, 1095–1101.
146. Nicholson, J.W.G.; StLaurent, A.M. Effect of forage type and supplemental dietary vitamin E on milk oxidative stability. Can. J. Anim. Sci. **1991**, *71*, 1181–1186.
147. Atwal, A.S.; Hidiroglou, M.; Kramer, J.K.G. Effects of feeding Protec and $\alpha$-tocopherol on fatty acid composition and oxidative stability of cow's milk. J. Dairy Sci. **1991**, *74*, 140–145.
148. St Laurent, A.M.; Hidiroglou, M.; Snoddon, M.; Nicholson, J.W.G. Effect of $\alpha$-tocopherol supplementation to dairy cows on milk and plasma $\alpha$-tocopherol concentrations and on spontaneous oxidized flavor in milk. Can. J. Anim. Sci. **1990**, *70*, 561–570.
149. Jiang, Y.H.; McGeachin, R.B.; Bailey, C.A. $\alpha$-Tocopherol, $\beta$-carotene, and retinol enrichment of chicken eggs. Poult. Sci. **1994**, *73*, 1137–1143.

150. Chen, J.Y.; Latshaw, J.D.; Lee, H.O.; Min, D.B. $\alpha$-Tocopherol content and oxidative stability of egg yolk as related to dietary $\alpha$-tocopherol. J. Food Sci. **1998**, *63*, 919–922.
151. Li, S.X.; Cherian, G.; Sim, J.S. Cholesterol oxidation in egg yolk powder during storage and heating as affected by dietary oils and tocopherol. J. Food Sci. **1996**, *61*, 721–725.
152. Cheriam, G.; Wolfe, F.W.; Sim, J.S. Dietary oils with added tocopherols. Effect on egg or tissue tocopherols, fatty acids and oxidative stability. Poult. Sci. **1996**, *75*, 423–431.
153. Grune, T.; Kramer, K.; Hoppe, P.P.; Siems, W. Enrichment of eggs with n-3 polyunsaturated fatty acids: effects of vitamin E supplementation. Lipids **2001**, *36*, 833–838.
154. Flachowsky, G.; Engelman, D.; Sunder, A.; Halle, I.; Sallmann, H.P. Eggs and poultry meat as tocopherol sources in dependence on tocopherol supplementation of poultry diets. Food Res. Int. **2002**, *35*, 239–243.
155. Pál, L.; Dublecz, K.; Husvéth, F.; Wágner, L.; Bortos, Á.; Kovács, G. Effects of dietary fats and vitamin E on fatty acid composition, vitamin A and E content and oxidative stability of egg yolk. Arch. Geflügelk **2002**, *66*, 251–257.
156. Tocher, D.R.; Mourente, G.; Vander Eecken, A.; Evjemo, J.O.; Diaz, E.; Bell, J.G.; Geurden, I.; Lavens, P.; Olsen, Y. Effects of dietary vitamin E on antioxidant defense mechanisms of juvenile turbot (*Scophthalmus maximus L.*), halibut (*Hippoglossus hippoglossus L.*) and sea breams (*Sparus aurata L.*). Aquacult. Nutr. **2002**, *8*, 195–207.
157. National Research Council. Nutrient requirement of fish. In *Nutrient Requirement of Domestic Animals*; National Academic Press: Washington, D.C., 1999; 26, 63 pp.
158. Waagbo, R.; Sanders, K.; Sandvin, A.; Lie, O. Feeding three levels of n-3 polyunsaturated fatty acids at two levels of vitamin E to Atlantic salmon (*Salmo salar*): growth and chemical composition. Fisk. Dir. Skr. Ser. Ernaering **1991**, *4*, 51–63.
159. Waagbo, R.; Sandnes, K.; Torrissen, O.J.; Sandvin, A.; Lie, O. Chemical and sensory evaluation of fillets from Atlantic salmon (*Salmo salar*) fed three levels of n-3 polyunsaturated fatty acids at two levels of vitamin E. Food Chem. **1993**, *46*, 361–366.
160. Hamre, K.; Lie, O. $\alpha$-Tocopherol levels in different organs of Atlantic salmon (*Salmo salar L.*)—effect of smoltification, dietary levels of n-3 polyunsaturated fatty acids and vitamin E. Comp. Biochem. Physiol. **1995**, *111*, 547–554.
161. Cowey, C.B.; Degener, E.; Tacon, A.G.J.; Youngson, A.; Bell, J.G. The effect of vitamin E and oxidized fish oil on the nutrition of rainbow trout (*Salmo gairdneri*) grown at natural, varying water temperatures. Br. J. Nutr. **1984**, *51*, 443–451.
162. Boggio, S.M.; Hardy, R.W.; Babbitt, J.K.; Brannon, E.L. The influence of dietary lipid source and $\alpha$-tocopheryl acetate level on product quality of rainbow trout (*Salmo gairdneri*). Aquaculture **1985**, *51*, 13–24.
163. Frigg, M.; Prabucki, A.L.; Ruhdel, E.U. Effect of dietary vitamin E levels on oxidative stability of trout fillets. Aquaculture **1990**, *84*, 145–158.
164. O'Keefe, T.M.; Noble, R.L. Storage stability of channel catfish (*Ictalurus punctatus*) in relation to dietary level of $\alpha$-tocopherol. J. Fish Res. Board Can. **1978**, *35*, 457–460.

# 5

# Stability of Vitamin E During Food Processing

## 5.1. INTRODUCTION

Because of the interaction of tocopherols and tocotrienols with oxidative events in foods through their function as antioxidants, physical handling associated with harvesting and storage of raw commodities and, then, further processing and marketing can produce significant changes in vitamin E levels. Depending on environmental factors and the oxidative stress placed on the commodity by the required chain of events necessary to deliver the fresh or processed food to the consumer, these changes can be quite severe with the potential for complete loss. Such events leading to loss of vitamin E can be initiated at any point during the harvesting, storage, processing, and marketing chain. Likewise, storage of the product and food preparation by the consumer can have dramatic effects on the retention of vitamin E in the food at the point of consumption. Because of vitamin E's relative instability, a large degree of variability exists in reported vitamin E contents for similar products. Many researchers have documented the stability of tocopherols and tocotrienols under various agronomic, storage, processing, and food preparation conditions for many commodities and their processed foods.

One of the first reviews that summarized effects of varietal differences, harvesting, processing, and storage on vitamin E levels was published in 1973 by

Kivimäe and Carpena (1). This review included 45 references covering 1942–1969. These authors provided the following observations regarding the stability of vitamin E in foods and animal feeds:

1. The level of vitamin E is variable, depending on stage of growth, time of harvesting, genetic variety, processing, and storage.
2. The level in green fodder falls as growth proceeds.
3. Different cultivars have different natural levels of tocopherols.
4. Losses during harvesting depend on the weather and drying conditions.
5. High temperature, prolonged storage, and high moisture content increase losses.
6. All processing steps produce some loss of vitamin E.
7. Milling, flaking, and shredding produce large losses.
8. Oil refining leads to small losses.
9. Losses during storage depend on time and temperature conditions.

Later reviews (2,3) covering the period through the mid-1970s to 1980, included drying, organic acid treatment, milling, expanding, puffing, rolling and shredding, irradiation, fumigation, refining of edible oils, food preparation methods, and conventional processes of dehydration, canning, and freezing. More recent reviews provide updates on processing effects, including milling, refining steps, irradiation, and heating (4,5). This chapter provides information on the stability of vitamin E under various processing and handling conditions significant to the current food processing industry. However, it is evident that observations and conclusions drawn from earlier research (2,3) were accurate, providing a sound basis for understanding factors that influence the stability of vitamin E in edible oils and processed foods.

## 5.2. EDIBLE OILS

### 5.2.1. Edible Oil Refining

It is generally recognized that oxidative events in raw commodities during harvesting and storage lead to considerable variation in vitamin E levels in crude oil before refining. Bauernfeind's reviews (2,3) showed that some tocopherol loss inevitably occurs during refining and that deodorization and bleaching processes were points at which substantial losses can occur. However, research reports on refining losses are difficult to compare because studies are completed on different oils under different conditions. Eitenmiller (6) stated that up through 1997 studies on the effects of refining were difficult to interpret, ranging from highly significant losses to minimal (7,8). Again, the highly variable nature of the oil, the initial oil quality, and processing parameters studied in the available literature make generalizations difficult.

Table 5.1 provides summaries of pertinent literature showing the effects of refining on the vitamin E content of edible oils. Excellent studies on soybean oil (8–10) show that vitamin E content decreases throughout the refining process and that largest losses can be expected at the deodorization stage. A well-presented study by Jung et al. (9) followed the refining process from the crude oil through the deodorization stage and reported tocopherol content at each stage. Total losses (percentage) at each stage were degumming, 5%; alkaline refining, 7%; bleaching, 12%; and deodorization, 32%. Similar orders but varying magnitudes of losses were reported for soybean oil by Ferrari et al. (8) and Gutfinger and Letan (10). Relative ratios of $\alpha$-, $\beta$-, $\gamma$-, and $\delta$-tocopherol (T) remained almost constant throughout the refining process (9). Each of the three studies cited showed minor changes in tocopherol content of soybean oil due to degumming and alkali refining.

Studies on the refining of other oils also indicate that all stages produce some loss of tocopherols (8,11–28). Prior et al. (13) reported relatively large losses of vitamin E through degumming and bleaching of canola press oils. $\alpha$-Tocopherol was lost to a greater extent than other tocopherols, representing 8%, 30%, and 33% of the total tocopherols on a weight basis in bleached, degummed, and crude oils, respectively. Large losses of $\alpha$-T can dramatically decrease the nutritional worth of the oil to meet $\alpha$-T requirements of the human. Prior et al. (13) noted that the higher loss of $\alpha$-T compared to that of the other tocopherols could be due to a selective adsorption of $\alpha$-T on the bleaching clay and/or greater sensitivity to the processes leading to preferential destruction. The observed loss of $\alpha$-T, whether induced chemically or physically, during refining of canola oil agrees with earlier work (12) that indicated greater loss of $\alpha$-T compared to $\gamma$-T in rapeseed oil processed to the refined, bleached, deodorized (RBD) stage. Gogolewski et al. (14) reported on the effects of refining of low–erucic acid rapeseed oil. Changes in tocopherols due to the refining process are listed in Table 5.2. In this study, $\delta$-T was lost to a greater extent on a percentage basis when compared to $\alpha$- and $\gamma$-T. However, losses of $\alpha$- and $\gamma$-T, although not as great on a percentage basis, represent almost all of the total tocopherols lost on a weight basis. Losses due to the deodorization step account for approximately two-thirds of the processing loss. Overall, the refining process led to a 30% decrease in total tocopherol content. Losses noted for $\alpha$- and $\gamma$-T were similar (Table 5.2).

In oils containing primarily $\alpha$-T at low levels such as coconut and marine oils, refining can have quite significant effects on residual tocopherols. Effects of various processing conditions on $\alpha$-T stability in coconut oil showed that a combined degumming and bleaching process led to reduced losses of total tocopherol (7.4%) (15). Sequential degumming and bleaching produced losses of 46% for citric acid degummed and bleached oil and 58% for phosphoric acid degummed and bleached oil. Alkali refining used with degumming and

**TABLE 5.1** The Effects of Refining on the Vitamin E Content of Edible Oils

| Oil | Process | Percentage Loss of Vitamin E[a] | References |
|---|---|---|---|
| Soybean | Degumming, alkali refining, bleaching, deodorization | Degumming: <1<br>Alkali refining: 12<br>Bleaching: 24 (RB)<br>Deodorization: 36 (RBD)<br>Total losses range from 31–47 through refining of three batches of soybean oil | 1974, 10 |
| Rapeseed | Degumming, alkali refining, bleaching, deodorization | Degumming: 3<br>Alkali refining: 42<br>Bleaching: 54<br>Deodorization: 75<br>Oil stored for 9 mo before analysis<br>$\alpha$-T percentage loss > $\gamma$-T percentage loss | 1975, 12 |
| Rice bran | Steam refining, alkali refining | Higher vitamin E levels of steam refined oil than of alkali refined oil | 1985, 21 |
| Olive | Alkali refining, bleaching, deodorization | 50 Loss in $\alpha$-T to RBD stage<br>Progressive loss in $\alpha$-T as hydrogenation proceeded | 1987, 19 |
| Soybean | Degumming, alkali refining, bleaching, deodorization | Degummed: 5<br>Alkali refined: 7<br>Bleached: 12 (RB)<br>Deodorized: 32 (RBD)<br>Relative compositions constant | 1989, 9 |
| Menhaden | Bleaching, alkali refining, deodorization | Total process: 46<br>Deodorization: 25 | 1991, 16 |
| Canola press | Degumming, bleaching | $\alpha$-T loss > $\gamma$-T loss<br>Degumming: 20<br>Bleaching: 60 loss | 1991, 13 |

| | | | |
|---|---|---|---|
| Coconut | Degumming, alkali refining, bleaching, deodorization | Degumming: Citric acid: <10<br>Phosphoric acid: <4<br>Bleaching: After citric acid degumming: 45<br>After phosphoric acid degumming: 58<br>Deodorization: After citric acid degumming and bleaching: 57<br>After phosphoric acid degumming and bleaching: 54<br>Alkali refining: 39<br>RBD: 92 | 1991, 15 |
| Soybean | Deodorization | Process optimization at 475°F–492°F: 12–18 loss | 1992, 29 |
| Soybean, rapeseed, corn | Alkali refining, bleaching, deodorization | Deodorized: Corn, 56; SBO, 14; rapeseed, 36<br>No significant changes noted at other processing stages | 1996, 8 |
| Tomato seed | Degumming, alkali refining, bleaching | Total process: 18<br>Loss of $\alpha$-T > $\delta$-T | 1998, 24 |
| Marine | $H_3PO_4$ degumming, alkali refining, bleaching, deodorization | RBD: Seal, 14; cod, 32<br>$\alpha$-T lost during deodorization | 1998, 1999 17, 18 |
| Rapeseed | Refining | Total process: 30<br>Neutralization and bleaching: 10<br>Deodorization: 23 | 2000, 14 |
| Palm | Bleaching, physical refining (acid clay, synthetic silica, steam) | Total process: 20 | 2001, 26 |

*(continued)*

**TABLE 5.1** *Continued*

| Oil | Process | Percentage Loss of Vitamin E[a] | References |
|---|---|---|---|
| Wheat germ | Refining | Deodorization: 28 total T ($\alpha$-T: 25, $\beta$-T: 32) at 290°C for 9 min 63 total T ($\alpha$-T: 60, $\beta$-T: 68) at 290°C for 30 min<br>Neutralization: 14 $\beta$-T | 2001, 27 |
| Vegetable | Deodorization | Little change at 175°C for 4.5 h<br>$\alpha$-T loss (30) > $\gamma$-T loss (17) > $\delta$-T loss (15) at 205°C for 82 h | 2001, 28 |
| Soybean | Deodorization $N_2$ vs. $CO_2$ vs. steam vs. conventional | No effect of laboratory scale deodorization processes on total tocopherols levels, free fatty acid levels, or color | 2002, 32 |

[a]RB, redefined, bleached; RBD, refined, bleached, deodorized; SBO, soybean oil; $\alpha$-T, $\alpha$-tocopherol.

**TABLE 5.2** Changes of Tocopherols in Rapeseed Oil During Refining

| | | | Bleaching | | Refined oil | |
|---|---|---|---|---|---|---|
| | | Crude oil (mg/100 g) | Bleached oil (mg/100 g) | Percentage retention | Refined oil (mg/100 g) | Percentage retention |
| Tocopherols (mg/100 g) | α-Tocopherol | 22.1 | 20.1 | 91.0 | 15.4 | 69.7 |
| | γ-Tocopherol | 32.3 | 26.0 | 80.5 | 22.4 | 69.3 |
| | δ-Tocopherol | 1.1 | 0.9 | 81.8 | 0.7 | 63.4 |
| | Total tocopherol | 55.4 | 47.0 | 84.8 | 38.5 | 69.5 |

*Source*: Modified from Ref. 14.

deodorization to produce a RBD oil resulted in almost complete loss of vitamin E (92%). Unlike in results noted for most oils, deodorization of the coconut oil produced small tocopherol losses.

Commonly used alkali refining, bleaching, and deodorization steps decreased $\alpha$-T levels in marine oils. A 46% loss of $\alpha$-T was noted for the processing of menhaden oil to the RBD stage (16). Slightly over one-half of the loss occurred during deodorization. Primary losses of $\alpha$-T occurred at the deodorization stage for seal blubber and cod liver oil (17,18). However, total losses were quite low for both oils (14% for seal and 32% for cod). Refining of olive oil decreased $\alpha$-T level by up to 50% (19).

Rice bran oil, because of its high initial levels of free fatty acids (2–20%), waxes, and color, requires modified refining processes to decrease processing losses and production of large amounts of soap stock (20). Steam or physical refining is used as either a partial or a complete replacement for alkali refining to remove free fatty acids. Since steam refining is similar to a conventional deodorization step although at higher temperature, losses of vitamin E would be expected. If alkali refining is eliminated completely from the process, then increased vitamin E retention might occur. Early work on steam refining of rice bran oil showed quite higher levels of vitamin E in steam-refined compared to alkali-refined oil (21). De and Bhattacharyya(20) reported that more than 70% of total vitamin E was lost through application of physical or steam refining using steam purging at 235°C to 265°C under 5-mm Hg pressure. Conventional refining with deodorization at 185°C, 5-mm Hg pressure, and alkali refining caused a somewhat higher loss of vitamin E (82%).

Rice bran is processed by extrusion (expansion) with steam injection to inactivate lipoxygenase to improve oxidative stability of the oil. Lloyd et al. (22) followed changes in tocopherol and tocotrienol contents during commercial milling and steam expansion of rice bran (Figure 5.1). Rice bran collected from the various milling breaks had varying levels of tocopherols and tocotrienols. Of significance, steam expansion did not decrease tocopherol and tocotrienol levels in the rice bran. Concentration of oryzanol, another natural antioxidant in rice bran oil, decreased by 26% during steam expansion of the rice bran. Wide variations have been noted in the vitamin E content of commercially available rice bran oil as a result of problems with handling of the bran and variations in processing.(6,22)

Because of the low molecular weight of tocopherols and tocotrienols, the temperature and vacuum used during deodorization of edible oils lead to slight volatilization and steam stripping. Vitamin E is, therefore, concentrated in the distillate. Such distillates are now the source of value-added vitamin E and sterol concentrates used for pharmaceuticals and food fortification. Because of the impact of deodorization and combined steam refining on the quality of RBD oils, Maza et al. (29) optimized deodorization processes for free fatty acid removal

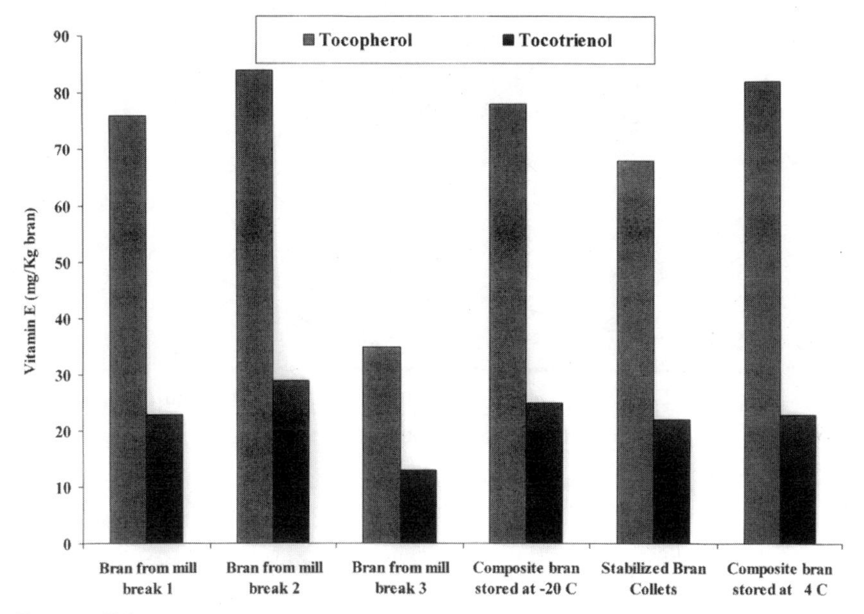


**FIGURE 5.1** Tocopherol and tocotrienol content of rice bran at various processing stages. (Modified from Ref. 22.)

and tocopherol retention for several commercial oils. For soybean oil, optimization of the process at 246–256°C for flow rates of 40,000–50,000 lb/h produced tocopherol retention rates of 82% to 88% (Figure 5.2). With the rapidly increasing natural vitamin E market, the process can be optimized to produce greater vitamin E concentration in the distillate, while maintaining adequate vitamin E levels in the oil to fulfill antioxidant requirements. The authors emphasized that oil quality is the result of multiple characteristics imparted to the oil by the refining process. Parameters used to judge oil quality were free fatty acid content, $\leq 0.02\%$; tocopherol retention, $>50\%$; initial flavor strength ($F_0$) = 2.0 maximum (AOCS Intensity Scale); flavor strength after 4-wk storage with light exposure ($F_1$) = 4.0 and after 8-wk storage in the dark ($F_2$) = 3.6 maximum.

Nitrogen gas stripping can be used in place of conventional steam stripping at higher temperatures to produce a deodorizer distillate of higher quality.(30–32) $N_2$ gas stripping at 150°C for 1 h produced soybean oil with similar total tocopherol levels, free fatty acid levels, and colors to those of a conventionally deodorized oil (32). Under the laboratory scale treatments, none of the deordorization processes, including conventional deordorization, decreased total tocopherol levels as might be expected. The authors attributed the lack of effect

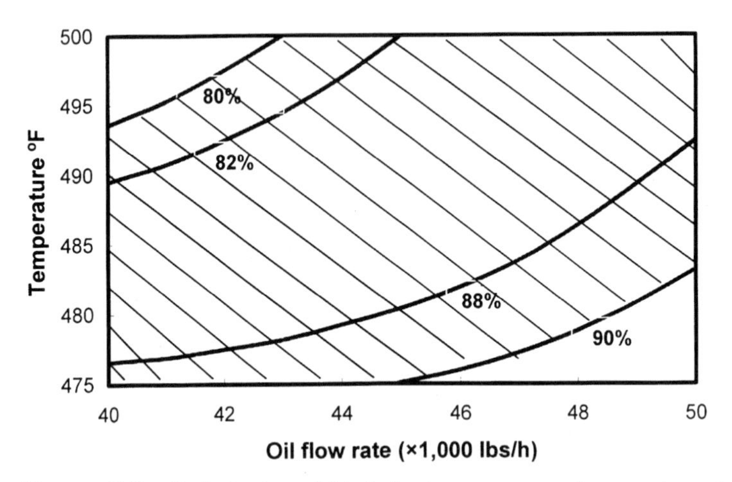


**FIGURE 5.2** Optimization of deodorization parameters for retention of tocopherols in soybean oil. Percentages are retention of vitamin E. (Modified from Ref. 29.)

on residual tocopherols on the short residence time of the laboratory scale deordorizer (9 min at 265°C). Prior work with $N_2$ stripping of olive oil showed that $\alpha$-T level was decreased significantly by both $N_2$ and steam stripping (31).

## 5.2.2. Interesterification and Enzyme Modification

Interesterification is commonly used in the edible oil industry to modify physical properties by rearranging the distribution of fatty acids on the glycerol. This process might become an alternative to hydrogenation to produce plasticized fats with low or zero trans isomers (33). Chemical interesterification is catalyzed most commonly by sodium methoxide. Since the temperature (>70°C) and chemical environment of the reaction are quite severe, effects on vitamin E content could be appreciable. However, few data clearly show the effects of chemical interesterification on vitamin E levels. Park et al. (34) interesterified soybean oil with sodium methoxide and reported that randomization of the glyceride composition had no significant effect on oxidative stability of the oil. Vitamin E levels were, however, decreased substantially by purification procedures after the interestification process to the point that the oil was less stable to autoxidation. The primary loss of tocophoerols occurred at the purification step after interesterification, when soaps and colored materials formed by the process were removed. Overall tocopherol loss was almost complete after purification.

Few reports describe the effects of various enzyme modifications used by the fat and oil industry to produce structured lipids on vitamin E. Production of structured lipids high in eicosapentaenoic acid and docosahexaenoic acid by incorporation of capric acid into fish oil by immobilized lipase from *Rhizomucor miehei* decreased vitamin E to low levels (35). Tocopherols and other antioxidants should be added back to enzymatically modified oils to protect the unsaturated fatty acid from oxidation.

### 5.2.3. Hydrogenation

Few studies have been completed to define adequately the effects of hydrogenation on vitamin E content of edible oils. Available literature up to 1979 indicated that little or no destruction occurred under ordinary hydrogenation conditions (36). However, a more recent study by Rabascall and Riera(19) showed that degradation of vitamin E proceeds in a first-order reaction with time of hydrogenation. With olive oil, approximately, 60% of $\alpha$-T was lost after 5 h of hydrogenation at 2 atm of hydrogen at 180°C with nickel catalyst. Tocotrienols exist as R, trans, trans isomers in nature and would theoretically be subject to isomerization during hydrogenation to cis isomers. However, cis isomers of $\gamma$-tocotrienol ($\gamma$-T3) were not detected in hydrogenated palm oil (37). Drotleff and Ternes(37) incorporated liquid chromatography (LC) methodology using two columns (ET 200/4 NUCLEODEX $\beta$-PM) in series to resolve the four potential cis–trans side chain isomers of $\gamma$-T3. $\alpha$-Tocodienol and $\alpha$-tocomoneol, reduced forms of $\alpha$-T3, were identified in the hardened palm oil. These compounds were previously identified.(38,39) The study indicated that hydrogenation may cause loss of $\gamma$-T3 but does not significantly influence the geometric structure of the double bonds in the T3 side chain. Clearly, not enough work has been completed to define the effects of hydrogenation on the vitamin E content and forms of vitamin E present in hardened edible oils adequately.

### 5.2.4. Effects of Frying on the Vitamin E Content of Oils and Fats

Bunnell et al. (40) in one of the first literature references to loss of vitamin E in edible oil during deep-fat frying indicated that little loss occurs. Later studies clearly showed that this is not the case. McLaughlin and Weihrauch (36) in their 1979 review of the vitamin E content of food cited only five references showing the effects of heating on vitamin E loss in vegetable oils. This work was primarily conducted on oils under carefully controlled heating conditions without the introduction of foods for frying. The results of the research showed that different oils lost varying amounts of vitamin E, ranging from 9% in safflower oil to 100% in coconut oil, under similar heat treatments for 10 h. Rate of loss was rapid when oxygen was available during early stages of heating and decreased with prolonged heating. Other factors influencing vitamin E loss included the oil-surface-to-air ratio and physical mixing of oxygen into the oil during heating. Some volatilization of vitamin E can occur during prolonged frying operations, further decreasing the antioxidant capacity of the oil. Table 5.3 summarizes some pertinent literature on the effects of frying on vitamin E stability.

Since vitamin E loss in frying oils indicates its capacity as an antioxidant is being overcome, the loss is critical to oxidative stability of the oil and to the shelf life of the fried product. Hence, rate and extent of loss of tocopherols and tocotrienols have been extensively studied during frying processes, and a highly complex picture influenced by many parameters has been revealed. Lehmann and Slover (41). applied gas chromatography to the quantitation of vitamin E in model oxidative systems and edible oils and provided early, definitive information on the oxidative stability of the individual tocopherols and tocotrienols. During autoxidation of methyl myristate, stabilities were $\alpha$-T = $\alpha$-T3 < $\beta$-T3 < $\gamma$-T3 < $\beta$-T3 < $\delta$-T3 < $\gamma$-T < $\delta$-T. $\alpha$-Tocopherol was the least stable in both systems. The relative stabilities were similar to those reported earlier for antioxidant activities for lard and methyl linoleate ($\gamma$-T > $\delta$-T > $\beta$-T > $\alpha$-T) (42) $\alpha$-Tocopherol protected $\gamma$- and $\delta$-T in mixtures, but $\gamma$- and $\delta$-T had no appreciable protective effect for $\alpha$-T. From these observations, Lehmann and Slover (41) theorized that stabilities and antioxidant activities during protection of fats and oils vary in the same direction, the most stable, $\delta$-T, is the best antioxidant. However, when considering interactions among the tocopherols, $\alpha$-T is the better antioxidant, protecting $\gamma$- and $\delta$-T. It was assumed that $\alpha$-T level would decrease first during cooking and storage of vegetable oil because of its protective role for other forms of vitamin E. Various studies indicated more rapid loss of $\alpha$-T than of other tocopherols in model systems and frying oils.(43–47) Barrera-Arellano et al. (47), in a 2002 study of several vegetable oils and oils stripped of natural antioxidants that were supplemented with known levels of tocopherols, found that $\alpha$-T was the least stable at 180°C for 2h. Formation of polymeric and polar compounds was more dependent on the natural content and type of tocopherol than on the degree of unsaturation of the oil. For natural oils, tocopherols were less stable in the oils with lower degrees of unsaturation.

$\alpha$-Tocopherol is not the least stable form of vitamin E under all frying conditions. Frying of potato chips in cottonseed and peanut oil on an industrial scale over 5 days showed that rates of loss of $\alpha$- and $\gamma$-T vary with time of heating and with the oil (48). In peanut oil, $\gamma$-T loss was greater than that of $\alpha$-T at 26h but less at the end of the frying time (103h). In cottonseed oil, $\gamma$-T loss was greater than $\alpha$-T loss over the entire time of heating. Over time of use, losses of $\alpha$- and $\gamma$-T in cottonseed oil decreased and stabilized (Figure 5.3) with apparent stabilization of the oil. Then, vitamin E levels increased, apparently from oil added as replacement oil. Carlson and Tabacch(49) studied the relationship between $\alpha$- and $\gamma$-T losses in partially hydrogenated soybean oil containing tertiary butylhydroquinone (TBHQ), citric acid, and dimethyl siloxane. Oil was

**TABLE 5.3** The Effects of Frying on the Vitamin E Content of Fats and Oils[a]

| Food | Frying oils | Conditions | Other parameters | Observations | References |
|---|---|---|---|---|---|
| Potato chips, french fries | Cottonseed oil | Deep frying: 200–210°C | $\alpha$-T acetate addition (100 mg/100 g oil), storage (fried foods): −12°C, room temperature | 11% Loss of total tocopherols in one frying | 1965, 40 |
| Potato slices | Mixture of soybean and rapeseed oils | Deep frying: 180°C, 0–9 h = 17 min, 32 times | Tempura coating ingredients: wheat flour, egg, water | Decomposition rates: $\gamma$-T $\geq$ $\delta$-T $\geq$ $\alpha$-T | 1991, 50 |
| Potatoes | Rapeseed oil | Deep frying: 162°C | Rosemary extract (0.1%), ascorbyl palmitate (0.02%) | $\alpha$-T loss greater than $\beta$, $\gamma$-, and $\delta$-T loss; 50% $\alpha$-T loss after 4–5 fryings; vitamin E loss reduced by rosemary extract and ascorbyl palmitate | 1995, 46 |
| Chicken nuggets, breaded shrimp | Soybean oil, corn oil, palm olein | Deep frying: 185°C, 0–30 h | None | Relative stabilities: soybean oil $\alpha$-T > $\delta$-T > $\beta$-T > $\gamma$-T corn oil $\alpha$-T > $\gamma$-T > $\delta$-T > $\gamma$-T3 palm olein $\alpha$-T > $\delta$-T3 > $\alpha$-T3 > $\gamma$-T3 | 1998, 51 |

(continued)

**TABLE 5.3** *Continued*

| Food | Frying oils | Conditions | Other parameters | Observations | References |
|---|---|---|---|---|---|
| Potatoes | High-oleic sunflower oil, regular sunflower oil | Discontinuous, Continuous frying: 175°C, 0–5.7h | Storage (fried potatoes): 60°C, 0–30 days | $\alpha$-T loss greater in more saturated oils | 1999, 55 |
| French fries | Canola oils: regular, high-oleic, low-linoleic, high-oleic and low-linoleic | Deep frying: 72h | None | See Table 5.5 | 2001, 57 |
| Marinated and nonmarinated chicken | Peanut oil | Pressure frying: 168°C | None | After 1 day frying, $\alpha$-, $\beta$, $\gamma$-, and $\delta$-T degraded by 20%, 40%, 33%, and 22% | 2001, 58 |
| Fish and peanut snack extrudates | Soybean oil | Deep frying: 200°C, 1.5 min | None | Total tocopherol of soybean oil reduced by 6% and 3% during frying of fish and peanut snacks, respectively | 2001, 59 |
| Common vegetable oils | Common vegetable oils | 180°C, 2h, Rancimat | Natural oils and stripped oils supplemented with tocopherols | $\alpha$-T less stable; tocopherol loss greater in less unsaturated oils | 2002, 47 |
| Potatoes | Olive oil | Deep frying vs. pan frying | None | $\alpha$-T more stable during deep frying | 2002, 56, 158 |

[a] $\alpha$-T, $\alpha$-tocopherol; $\gamma$-T3, $\gamma$-tocotrienol.

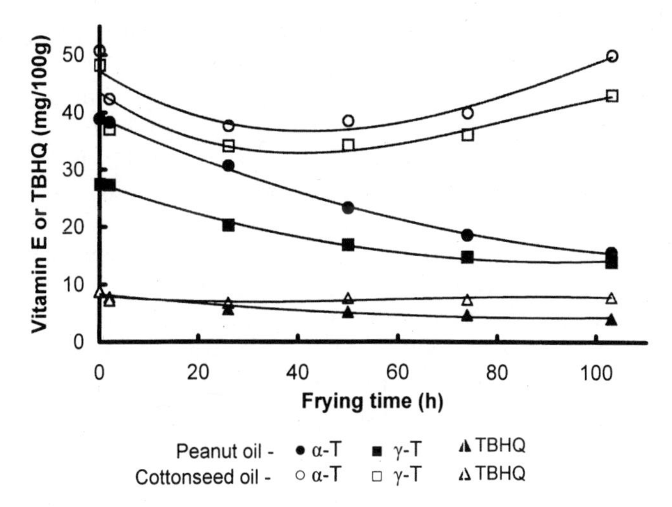


**FIGURE 5.3** Changes in $\alpha$- and $\gamma$-T and TBHQ in peanut and cottonseed oils during frying (160°C). $\alpha$-T, $\alpha$-tocopherol; TBHQ, tertiary butylhydroquinone. (Modified from Ref. 48.)

sampled under commercial frying of french fries at 177°C over a 4-day period. During the frying, oil was added to replenish oil lost during use. Tocopherols were monitored on each day over 4 days of continuous use, which represented frying of more than 310 kg of frozen french fries in the larger of two replicate studies. At the end of the study, $\gamma$-T retention was slightly higher than $\alpha$-T retention. The authors concluded that the type of food being fried, the duration of the use of the oil, and the addition of fresh oil during food service operations affect the rate of vitamin E loss. $\alpha$-Tocopherol loss in various heated oils held at 177°C without introduction of food was decreased by use of partially hydrogenated oil and addition of antioxidants. In later work, Miyagawa et al. (50) studied tocopherol stability in a mixture of soybean and rapeseed oils used for deep-fat frying of tempura-coated and -noncoated potato slices. Decomposition rates were $\gamma$-T $>$ $\delta$-T $\geq$ $\alpha$-T for both procedures over repeated fryings (32 times, 17 min per frying, 180°C $\pm$ 10°C) for a total of 9 h, 4 min. Introduction of the tempura coating changed the rate of loss of the different tocopherols but not the order. Changes in vitamin E levels and increasing amounts of fluorescent substances in the oil correlated with other quality characteristics of the used oil.

In another large study of the stability of tocopherols and tocotrienols in frying oils, vitamin E changes in soybean oil, corn oil, and palm olein were followed during simulated frying over 30 h using wet cotton balls (185°C) and frying of various breaded products (176°C) (51). In the simulated frying study, the relative stabilities of the vitamin E homologues in the oils were $\alpha$-T > $\delta$-T > $\beta$-T > $\gamma$-T (soybean oil), $\alpha$-T > $\gamma$-T > $\delta$-T > $\gamma$-T3 (corn oil), and $\alpha$-T > $\delta$-T3 > $\alpha$-T3 > $\gamma$-T3 (palm olein) (Table 5.4). $\alpha$-Tocopherol equivalent ($\alpha$-TE) levels decreased significantly in each oil; vitamin E was completely absent in palm olein after 30h of frying. Corn oil retained 63.3% of the $\alpha$-TE after 30h, whereas soybean oil retained only 11.8% of the $\alpha$-TE activity. The stabilities of the specific vitamin E homologues under simulated frying conditions vary according to the oils under study and the experimental parameters. The relative stabilities of the vitamin E homologues after 6h of simulated deep-fat frying were $\alpha$-T > $\delta$-T > $\beta$-T > $\gamma$-T (soybean oil), $\alpha$-T > $\beta$-T > $\delta$-T > $\gamma$-T3 (corn oil), and $\alpha$-T > $\delta$-T3 > $\alpha$-T3 > $\gamma$-T3 (palm olein).

It appears that the tocotrienols are less stable under thermal oxidation than the tocopherols. Thus, it can be assumed that they are interacting as more effective antioxidants in the simulated frying environment. The complexity of the simulated frying curves (time versus concentration) prohibited calculation of accurate half-lives for the total vitamin E activity or for the individual vitamin E homologues. Reaction rates did not follow first-order kinetics. Under the conditions of the study, the stabilities of vitamin E homologues were not directly related to the degree of unsaturation of the oils. The rapid loss of vitamin E in palm olein was not unexpected because Frankel et al. (52) showed tocopherol loss to be less in highly unsaturated oils than in more saturated oils during autoxidation at 60°C and 100°C. These authors suggested that polyunsaturated fat hydroperoxides decomposed quickly during initial autoxidation and that the decomposition products did not appear to react with tocopherols. Yuki and Ishikawa (53) also reported greater tocopherol stability in more highly unsaturated oils during simulated deep-fat frying. They postulated that decreasing stabilities of more saturated oils as temperatures approach frying temperature led to rapid tocopherol loss during thermal oxidation. Studies on the formation of degradation compounds in model systems (triolein, trilinolein, and a 1 : 1 mixture of both) during heating at 180°C indicated that the antipolymerization effect of tocopherols at high temperature depends on the degree of unsaturation, which affects the less unsaturated substrate, triolein, to a greater extent (54). In this study, $\alpha$-T losses were very rapid and dependent on the unsaturation of the triacylglycerol system, although degradation of substrate was higher as the degree of unsaturation increased. Yoshida et al. (45) also found that after 8–10min of microwave heating, the amount of tocopherol decreased substantially in linseed, olive, and palm oils, whereas 90% of tocopherols remained in corn and soybean oils. They concluded that the reduction in level of tocopherols in oils is not necessarily in agreement with chemical properties of the oils.

Evaluation of the oxidative stability of fried potatoes in oils with varying levels of unsaturation and degree of degradation due to use showed that the length

**TABLE 5.4** Total Vitamin E (mg/100 g), Vitamin E Homologues (mg/100 g), and α-Tocopherol Equivalents (mg) of Soybean Oil, Corn Oil, and Palm Olein During Simulated Frying

| Vegetable oil | Time (h) | mg/100g | | | | | | | | | mg |
|---|---|---|---|---|---|---|---|---|---|---|---|
| | | α-T | β-T | γ-T | δ-T | α-T3 | β-T3 | γ-T3 | δ-T3 | Total[a] | α-TE[b] |
| Soybean oil | 0 | 7.9 | 1.1 | 47.4 | 12.0 | | | | | 68.3 | 12.7 |
| | 1 | 7.4 | 1.0 | 42.0 | 11.5 | | | | | 61.5 | 12.3 |
| | 3 | 7.2 | 0.8 | 41.6 | 11.3 | | | | | 61.2 | 11.9 |
| | 6 | 6.9 | 0.8 | 38.9 | 10.8 | | | | | 57.2 | 11.4 |
| | 10 | 6.0 | 0.7 | 27.5 | 9.8 | | | | | 43.9 | 9.4 |
| | 14 | 5.9 | 0.7 | 26.8 | 8.6 | | | | | 42.2 | 9.2 |
| | 20 | 5.3 | 0.7 | 26.0 | 6.7 | | | | | 38.6 | 8.5 |
| | 25 | 2.8 | 0.5 | 8.9 | 6.2 | | | | | 19.4 | 4.2 |
| | 30 | 0.7 | 0.4 | 0.9 | 3.9 | | | | | 5.9 | 1.5 |
| Corn oil | 0 | 12.3 | 0.5 | 58.5 | 2.6 | 1.2 | | 1.1 | | 76.7 | 18.8 |
| | 1 | 12.0 | 0.3 | 53.5 | 2.3 | 1.1 | | 0.9 | | 71.3 | 18.1 |
| | 3 | 11.8 | 0.3 | 53.5 | 2.2 | 1.0 | | 0.9 | | 66.1 | 16.8 |
| | 6 | 11.8 | 0.3 | 52.6 | 2.2 | 0.9 | | 0.8 | | 66.1 | 16.3 |
| | 10 | 11.7 | 0.2 | 51.7 | 2.1 | 0.9 | | 0.8 | | 65.6 | 16.0 |
| | 14 | 11.5 | 0.2 | 49.7 | 2.1 | 0.8 | | 0.7 | | 61.8 | 15.9 |
| | 20 | 11.1 | 0.2 | 46.1 | 1.9 | 0.8 | | 0.6 | | 60.4 | 15.2 |
| | 25 | 10.4 | 0.2 | 36.9 | 1.7 | 0.7 | | 0.5 | | 48.0 | 13.6 |
| | 30 | 9.3 | 0.2 | 20.6 | 1.5 | 0.7 | | 0.2 | | 33.1 | 11.9 |
| Palm olein | 0 | 15.5 | | | 1.5 | 16.5 | 1.4 | 20.7 | 4.2 | 59.6 | 19.4 |
| | 1 | 12.5 | | | 0.8 | 12.8 | 0.9 | 15.6 | 3.1 | 45.7 | 16.3 |
| | 3 | 10.2 | | | 0.5 | 10.0 | 0.8 | 9.7 | 2.6 | 34.2 | 13.0 |

*(continued)*

**TABLE 5.4** *Continued*

| Vegetable oil | Time (h) | mg/100 g | | | | | | | | | mg |
|---|---|---|---|---|---|---|---|---|---|---|---|
| | | α-T | β-T | γ-T | δ-T | α-T3 | β-T3 | γ-T3 | δ-T3 | Total[a] | α-TE[b] |
| | 6 | 7.7 | | | 0.1 | 6.8 | 0.6 | 4.8 | 2.0 | 22.1 | 8.9 |
| | 10 | 6.4 | | | | 5.2 | 0.5 | 3.3 | 1.9 | 17.5 | 3.4 |
| | 14 | 5.2 | | | | 4.1 | 0.3 | 2.2 | 1.3 | 13.3 | 0.8 |
| | 20 | 4.4 | | | | 3.1 | 0.2 | 0.8 | 0.9 | 9.5 | 0.7 |
| | | | | | | 1.3 | | 0.2 | 0.3 | 4.7 | 0.3 |
| | | | | | | | | | | 0.5 | |

[a]Rounded means of four observations.
[b]One milligram α-TE is equal to 1 mg of α-T; activities of other homologues are β-T, 0.5; γ-T, 0.1; δ-T, 0.03; α-T3, 0.3; β-T3, 0.05. Activities of γ- and δ-T3 are unknown.
α-T, α-tocopherol; α-TE, α-tocopherol equivalent; α-T3, α-tocotrienol.
*Source*: Modified from Ref. 51.

of the induction period for oxidation in the fried product could not be explained by the levels of unsaturation of the oil or polar compounds in the oil (55). However, low levels of $\alpha$-T in the oils led to rapid oxidation in the fried product. $\alpha$-Tocopherol was lost more rapidly in more saturated oils during frying. In the products, $\alpha$-T level decreased more rapidly in those fried in more highly unsaturated oils. Pan frying is known to be more destructive to frying oil quality because of large surface area exposure compared to that for deep-fat frying. $\alpha$-Tocopherol in olive oil exposed to pan-fry operations using potatoes decreased from 29 to 3.1 mg/100 g during 10 fryings compared to 8.7 mg/100 g after the same exposure to deep-fat frying.(56,158)

Studies on canola oil, high-oleic canola oil, high-oleic low-linolenic canola oil, and low-linolenic canola oil showed that intermittent frying of french fries at 175°C produced varying rates of vitamin E degradation among the oils (57). Regular canola with the lowest level of tocopherols had the slowest degradation rate (Table 5.5). An inverse relationship was found between total polar compounds and tocopherol loss. Oils with higher rates of tocopherol degradation showed higher rates of total polar compound formation. It was emphasized by the authors that plant breeders should not ignore changes in tocopherol content of modified oils resulting from modification of fatty acid profiles.

Edible films on raw products reduced $\gamma$-T losses in peanut oil used to fry marinated and nonmarinated chicken strips (58). Hydroxypropylmethyl cellulose was an effective protector of $\gamma$-T when applied as a coating or as an ingredient in the breading. The authors believed that the edible film acted as a hydrophilic barrier to migration of acetic acid (prooxidant) from the product to the oil. Changes in the vitamin E content of frying oils occur rapidly in fresh, high-quality oils on use. Suknark et al. (59) reported measurable losses in vitamin E content in soybean oil after frying one batch of extruded fish or peanut half-products at 200°C for 1.5 min, including a 30-min heating time to reach the frying temperature.

**TABLE 5.5** Degradation Rates of Tocopherols in Canola Oils

| | Tocopherols | | |
|---|---|---|---|
| Canola oils | Total[a,b] | $\alpha$-T | $\gamma$-T |
| Regular | >72 (3.3) | >72 (1.4) | 60–72 (2.6) |
| High-oleic | 3–6 (50.1) | 3–6 (15) | 3–6 (35.1) |
| High-oleic, low-linoleic | 48–60 (7.4) | >72 (8) | 36–48 (6.3) |
| Low-linoleic | 3–6 (33) | 3–6 (12.5) | 3–6 (26.5) |

[a]Time (h) required to reduce original levels by 50%.
[b]Rate of degradation, ppm/h.
*Source*: Modified from Ref. 57.

## 5.3. VITAMIN E STABILITY DURING PROCESSING

### 5.3.1. Dehydration

Kivimäe and Carpena(1) summarized the effects of dehydration of fresh green animal fodder as reported by early studies completed before 1966. Losses reported ranged from 30% to 68% in common animal feeds when artificially dried at temperatures of 60°C or higher.(60–62) Sun drying was shown to produce higher vitamin E losses when compared to artificial drying.(63,64) Thalvelin and Oksanen(64) provided an in-depth study of the production of hay from red clover, timothy, and tufted hair grass, showing that vitamin E levels depended on the method of drying and the length of the drying period. Tocopherol and linolenic acid contents were shown to be closely related, highest levels were found in short-term artificially dried (not sun-dried) hays.

Because of the significance of alfalfa hay to animal agriculture, older studies (Table 5.6) report the effects of drying on the vitamin E content of alfalfa (65,66). Again, as noted in other early work, artificial drying produced a product with higher vitamin E levels when compared to sun-drying. Mean tocopherol levels were 11.5 and 20.1 mg/100 g for sun-cured and dehydrated alfalfa meal, respectively. $\alpha$-Tocopherol losses ranged from 5% to 33% for dehydration of fresh alfalfa into meal (66). Largest loss occurred in production of low-moisture meals ($<3\%$). Dehydration of fresh, green animal feeds can lead to oxidative losses of vitamin E, and use of ethoxyquin can reduce vitamin E loss (66).

One of the first reports on the effects of freeze drying on the vitamin E content of human foods was completed in conjunction with studies on military rations completed at the Nutrition Branch of the Armed Forces Quartermaster Food and Container Institute (67). Results of this study are given in Figure 5.4. For beef and chicken, $\alpha$-T level decreased significantly as a result of freeze drying. Little decrease in $\alpha$-T content was noted for pork. Freeze-dried foods must be carefully packaged to prevent oxidation during storage since the porous structure allows easy penetration of oxygen and rapid rates of oxidation.

Dehydration of Capsicum annuum L. to produce paprika leads to quite significant losses of vitamin E. Daood et al. (68) reported vitamin E losses attributable to dehydration ranging from 12.4% to 41.2%. Vitamin C losses approximated 70%. Highest retention of $\alpha$-T was obtained by drying overripe fruit with high dry matter content, and lowest retention was found with forced-air drying of fresh high-moisture fruits. Carvajal et al. (69) reported that drying of red pepper fruit to produce paprika by forced-air drying at 50°C for 2 days led to a 25–30% decrease in $\alpha$-T level. Retention of the red paprika color was directly related to the total antioxidant capacity of the dehydrated product.

**TABLE 5.6** The Effects of Processing on Vitamin E

| Food | Process | Observations | References |
|---|---|---|---|
| **Dehydration** | | | |
| Alfalfa | Commercial dehydration, sun curing | α-T levels 2 times higher in dehydrated meal than in sun-cured hay | 1961, 65 |
| Alfalfa | Drying: forced draft oven, 110°C, 24h; freezing | α-T loss range from 5–33%; higher losses when meal <3% moisture produced | 1968, 66 |
| Red pepper (paprika) | Natural drying: fruit; forced-air drying | Higher retention of vitamin E in forced-air drying than in natural drying | 1996, 68 |
| Red pepper (paprika) | Drying: forced air, 50°C, 2 days | Decreases of ascorbic acid level (75%), red color (14–58%), and α-T level (25–30%) due to drying and grinding | 1998, 69 |
| **Canning and freezing** | | | |
| Spinach | Washing, blanching, filling, sterilization (121°C, 30 min), freezing (−18°C), storage | 87% Loss of α-T | 1992, 70 |
| Salad tomatoes, processing cultivars | Washing, chopping, hot break extraction (90°C, 5–10 min), sieving, vacuum evaporation (60°C–70°C, 4h), filling, sterilization (100°C, 30 min), storage | α- and γ-T levels decreased by 20% and 33%, respectively | 2000, 71 |
| **Microwave processing** | | | |
| Soybean | 2450 MHz, 0.5 kW, 0–12 min | 6-min Processing, soybeans suitable for preparation of full-fat four with 10% loss of tocopherols; 12-min, ≥40% loss; progressive lipid deterioration during microwave treatment | 1989, 73 |

*(continued)*

**TABLE 5.6** *Continued*

| Food | Process | Observations | References |
|---|---|---|---|
| Linseed, soybean, corn, olive, palm | 2450 MHz, 0.5 kW, 0–20 min | Substantial tocopherol level decrease in linseed, olive, and palm oil, but not in corn and soybean oils, after 8–10 min heating; reduction of tocopherol levels not directly related to chemical properties of oils, such as degree of unsaturation | 1990, 74 |
| Tocopherol stripped coconut, palm oil, safflower oil | 2450 MHz, 0.5 kW, 0–20 min | Tocopherol stability in presence of saturated fatty acid ethyl esters, $\delta$-T > $\beta$-T > $\gamma$-T $\gg$ $\alpha$-T; in oils, tocopherols in more unsaturated oils more stable than in saturated oils during microwave heating, greater loss of tocopherols with shorter chain length and higher level of fatty acids in oil | 1991, 1991, 1992, 75–77 |
| Beef tallow, lard | 2450 MHz, 0.5 kW, 0–20 min | Stability of tocopherols, $\delta$-T > $\beta$-T > $\gamma$-T > $\alpha$-T; order of stability not depend on type of fat | 1992, 78 |
| Ethyl linoleate rapeseed, palm oil, soybean oil | 2450 MHz, 0.5 kW, 0–20 min | Optimal concentrations of tocopherols to increase oxidative stability 100 ppm for $\alpha$-T, 150–200 ppm for $\beta$- and $\gamma$-T, 500 ppm for $\delta$-T; antioxidant effect of tocopherols, $\alpha$-T > $\beta$-T = $\gamma$-T > $\delta$-T in all substrates; no tocopherol antioxidant effect increase above 500 ppm | 1993, 79 |
| Milk | 2450 MHz, 0.7 kW, 2 min, dark | Heating to 56.2°C: no effect on $\alpha$-T in whole milk; in low-fat milk, 14% loss at 80.2°C no more $\alpha$-T decrease than at 56.2°C | 1994 83 |
| Olive oil | 2450 MHz, 8 min, pan frying | $\alpha$-T loss greater with microwave heating (51%) than with pan frying (38%) | 1995 84 |

| | | | |
|---|---|---|---|
| Sesame oil | 2450 MHz, 15 min, roasting: 200°C, steaming: 100°C | With microwave treatment γ-T 40% decreased after storage at 35 days at 60°C | 1997 85 |
| Grapeseed oil | 60 MHz, 0.95 kW, 24 min, air dry, fluid bed, 2 h, 50°C | With microwave conditioning of grapeseed before oil extraction: chlorophyll level decrease and α-T, α-T3, and γ-T3 level increase of oil when compared to air-drying | 1998 86 |
| Rapeseed oil, soybean oil, safflower oil | 2450 MHz, 0.5 kW, 0–25 min | With addition of sesamol or tocopherols and their mixtures significant retardation of oxidation during microwave processing; sesamol combined with γ-T more efficient antioxidant than sesamol alone or other tocopherols; 400 ppm tocopherols or 40–400 ppm sesamol effective concentration | 1999 80 |
| Soybean | 2450 MHz, 0.5 kW, 0–20 min | 80% Retention after 20 min at 2450 MHz | 1999 81 |
| Soybean | 2450 MHz, 0.5 kW, 0–20 min | Retention percentage (total tocopherols)<br>60%, seed coat<br>80%, cotyledons and axis | 1999 82 |
| Eggs | 1.5 kW microwave boiling, 3 and 10 min, omelette preparation | Retention percentage (α-TE)<br>Boiling (3 min): 79<br>Boiling (10 min): 78<br>Omelette: 49<br>Microwave: 57 | 1999 87 |
| Sunflower seed | 2450 MHz, 0.5 kW, 0–30 min | 92% Retention of total vitamin E after 30 min | 2002 154 |
| **Ultraviolet and visible irradiation** | | | |
| Cucumber, pea | 400 W Incandescent, 100% RH | Irradiance decline of α-T | 1987 88, 89 |

*(continued)*

**TABLE 5.6** *Continued*

| Food | Process | Observations | References |
|---|---|---|---|
| Spinach | UV-B, 9h/days, 12 days | With UV-B radiation no change in lipid oxidation measured by TBARS of thylakoid membrane lipid; $\alpha$-T level increase compared to photosynthetically active form | 1997 92 |
| **Gamma irradiation** | | | |
| Milk, evaporated milk, cream, cheese, mutter, margarine | Vitamin A, ascorbic acid, cobalt-60, $-2.2^\circ C$ | In whole milk, >60% loss of tocopherols after 12h irradiation (80,000 roentgens/h; tocopherol loss < vitamin A and ascorbic acid loss | 1953 106 |
| Whole wheat | Cobalt-60 $10^5$–$10^7$ rad | Occurence of induction of autooxidation tocopherol decrease from 38–79% depending on wheat cultivar | 1965 105 |
| Chicken breast muscle | 137Cs, 1–10kGy, 4°C, aerobic | At 3kGy, 15% and 30% reduction for $\gamma$- and $\alpha$-T, respectively | 1992 99 |
| Pork | Freeze-dried, rehydrated, $^{137}C_s$, 0.114kGy/min, 0–6kGy | With increasing water content of rehydrated ground pork, decreased loss of $\alpha$- and $\gamma$-T; with NaCl, decreased loss of $\alpha$- and $\gamma$-T due to competition of $Cl^-$ for hydroxyl radicals | 1994 101 |

| | | | |
|---|---|---|---|
| Black bream, redfish | 1, 2, and 6 kGy, 0°C | $\alpha$-T loss 0–42% | 1994 103 |
| Red meats, turkey | $^{137}Cs$, 0–9.4 kGy, 5°C | With irradiation significant decrease in $\alpha$-T level in all species; rate of loss greater in turkey breast | 1995 101 |
| Tilapia, spanish mackerel | Cobalt-60, 1.5–10 kGy | In tocopherols decrease with increased dose; effect of postirradiation storage minimal | 1996 104 |
| Exotic meats | $^{137}Cs$, 0–10 kGy, 5°C | With irradiation significant decrease in $\alpha$-T level in all species | 1998 102 |
| Pork sausage | 2.5 and 4.5 kGy, aerobic and vacuum packaging | With irradiation accelerated lipid oxidation and increased volatile level in aerobic-packaged sausage during storage; influence of tocopherol content in sausage on production of volatiles at different levels of unsaturated fatty acids | 2000 98 |
| Turkey breast | 2.4 to 2.9 kGy, cooking, storage, aerobic, nitrogen flush | With irradiation reduced $\alpha$- and $\gamma$-T levels by 33% and 21%, respectively; slightly higher levels of both $\alpha$- and $\gamma$-T in nitrogen-packed samples than in air-packed samples during storage | 2001 107 |

$\alpha$-T, $\alpha$-tocopherol; UV-B, ultraviolet B; RH, relative humidity; $\alpha$-TE, $\alpha$-tocopherol equivalent; TBARS, thiobarbituric acid–reactive substance.

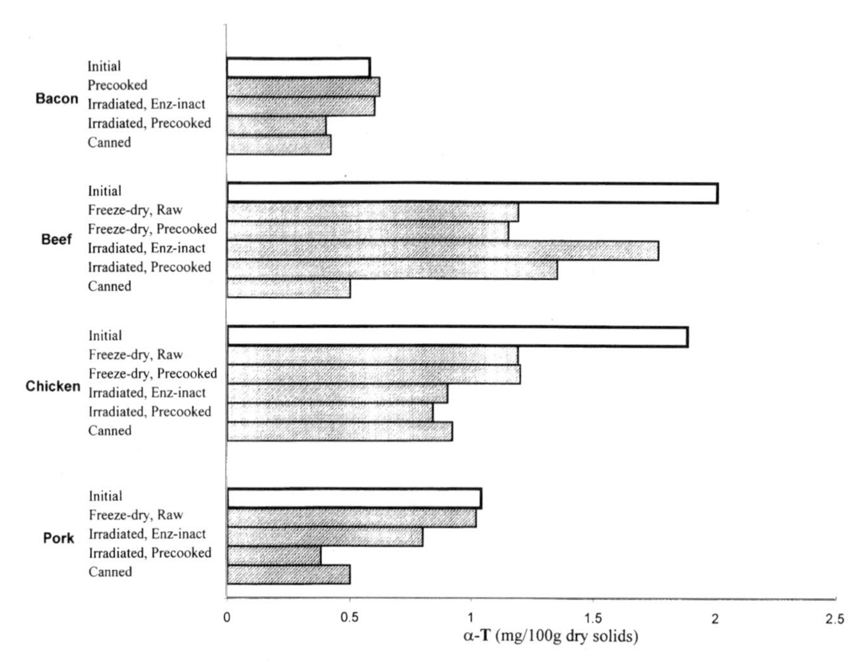


**FIGURE 5.4** $\alpha$-Tocopherol ($\alpha$-T) in processed animal products. Enz-inact, enzyme inactivated before irradiation. (Modified from Ref. 67.)

## 5.3.2. Canning and Freezing

Whereas extensive data exist on the effects of commercial canning and freezing on water-soluble vitamins, few definitive data exist for vitamin E. Bauernfeind's reviews of early studies (2, 3) cited two studies that showed greater than 50% loss of vitamin E in canned beans, corn, and peas. Thomas and Calloway (67) showed that canning of meats reduced vitamin E level to a greater extent than dehydration or irradiation (Figure 5.4). Canning of spinach at 121°C for 30 min decreased $\alpha$-T level by approximately 90% (70). However, no significant losses were noted between fresh spinach and frozen spinach (70). It can be concluded that freezing as a process does not change vitamin E content of foods. However, frozen storage can produce large losses due to oxidation, which progresses with prolonged freezer storage.

Processing of tomatoes into paste yields a product that contains approximately 80% of the $\alpha$-T originally present in the raw material (71). $\alpha$-Tocopherol contribution to the loss was greater than that of $\alpha$-tocopheryl quinone and $\gamma$-T. Thirty percent of the $\alpha$-T in the paste was quantified as $\alpha$-tocopheryl quinone, suggesting that $\alpha$-tocopheryl quinone can be important to the antioxidant capacity of processed foods.

### 5.3.3. Irradiation

*Food irradiation* is defined as the process of exposing food to radiant energy in order to reduce or eliminate bacteria, making it safer and more resistant to spoilage (72). Radiant energy includes microwave, infrared, visible, and ultraviolet (UV) light and ionizing radiation. Of these, ionizing radiation was cleared for use on various meats and has received much attention in the press because of its usefulness associated with Escherichia coli O157 : H7 and other pathogenic bacteria. Chemical changes produced in food by various irradiation processes have been well characterized over the past decades, and considerable information about their effects on vitamin E content has been published. Pertinent literature is summarized in Table 5.6.

**5.3.3.1. Microwave Radiation.** Microwave heating varies from conventional heating in that heat is generated by molecular excitation resulting from friction from the interaction of an electromagnetic field with chemical components of the food. Because of advantages of time, energy savings, excellent control, and convenience when compared to conventional heat processing procedures, microwave heating has been adapted to commercial processing, particularly drying applications. Additionally, laboratory use is rapidly increasing to speed extractions and organic synthesis processes. Because of the speed and frictional heat generation, research has been conducted in many areas of food chemistry to characterize chemical changes induced by microwave heating compared to conventional processes. In this line, extensive work has been conducted to define the effects of microwave energy on oxidation, oxidative stability, and vitamin E components of microwave processed foods.

Some of the most comprehensive work showing the effects of microwave heating on vitamin E has been conducted by Yoshida and colleagues (73–82,154). This work covers a broad field, including heating of soybeans before production of full-fat flour, quality of seed oils during microwave treatment, and antioxidative efficiences of tocopherols in oils during microwave heating. Conclusions drawn from Yoshida's collective research include the following:

1. Microwave processing can be used to condition soybeans for preparation of full-fat flour with little loss of vitamin E level (73).
2. During microwave heating, reduction of vitamin E level does not closely relate to the chemical properties of the oils, including level of unsaturation (74).
3. In tocopherol stripped oils containing added-back tocopherol, the order of stability was $\delta$-T $>$ $\beta$-T $>$ $\gamma$-T $\gg$ $\alpha$-T (75).

4. Greater reduction of tocopherol level occurred in the presence of shorter-chain-length ethyl esters of fatty acids and more saturated fatty acids.(76,77)
5. Reduction of vitamin E levels during microwave processing increased with increasing levels of free fatty acids (76,77).
6. In more saturated animal fats, the order of stability of tocopherols was $\delta$-T > $\beta$-T > $\gamma$-T > $\alpha$-T. After 12 min of microwave heating, peroxide values, carbonyl values, and anisidine values increased, showing that antioxidant capacity can be overcome quite easily during microwave heating (Figure 5.5) (78).
7. Optimal concentrations of tocopherols in stripped oils to increase oxidative stability were 100 ppm for $\alpha$-T, 150–200 ppm for $\beta$- or $\gamma$-T, and 500 ppm for $\delta$-T. Antioxidant effects of the tocopherols did not increase at concentrations above 500 ppm (79).
8. A mixture of sesamol and $\gamma$-T was more effective as an antioxidant than sesamol and other tocopherols at concentrations of 400 ppm and 50–400 ppm for the tocopherols and sesamol, respectively (80).
9. The exposure of soybeans to microwaves for 6–8 min caused no significant loss in the content of tocopherols in the hypocotyl oils. Tocopherol retention was greater than 80% after 20 min of roasting (81).
10. Microwave energy affected the composition of tocopherols and the fatty acid distribution of soybeans (82).
11. Roasting of sunflower seeds by microwave heating had very little impact on quality of the seeds or vitamin E content (154).

Other research on the effects of microwave processing on vitamin E include studies on milk (83), olive oil (84), sesame oil (85), grapeseed (86), and eggs (87). These studies, collectively, show both beneficial and negative aspects of microwave processing of foods on vitamin E content and oil quality. Whereas extensive heating by microwave energy can induce oxidation with rapid loss of vitamin E components, careful control of the process can be beneficial, depending on the food product. For example, the study by Oomah et al. (86) showed that microwave heating of grapeseed before oil extraction improved oil yield with decreased chlorophyll levels and with increased levels of $\alpha$-T, $\alpha$-T3, and $\gamma$-T3.

**5.3.3.2. Visible and Ultraviolet Radiation.** Little work has been completed on the effects of visible and UV radiation on vitamin E content of food. Ultraviolet radiation is considered to be only a surface treatment for killing microorganisms. Because of the low penetrating power of visible and UV radiations, significant impact on nutrient quality would not be expected except on green leafy vegetables with high surface-to-volume ratios. Extensive studies with

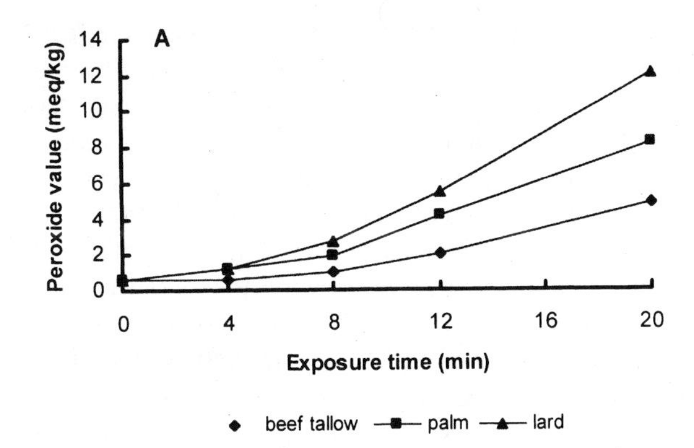


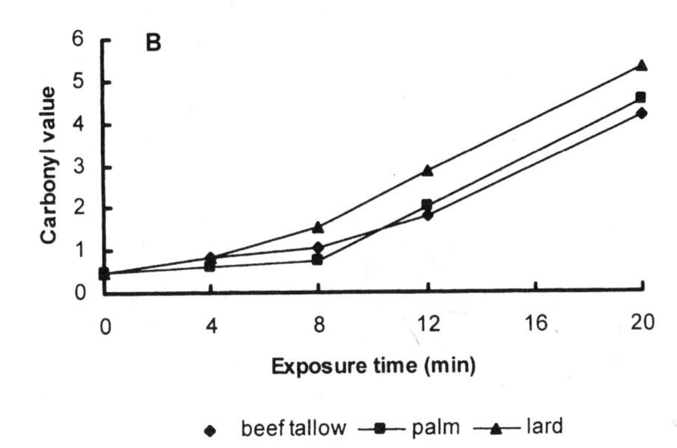


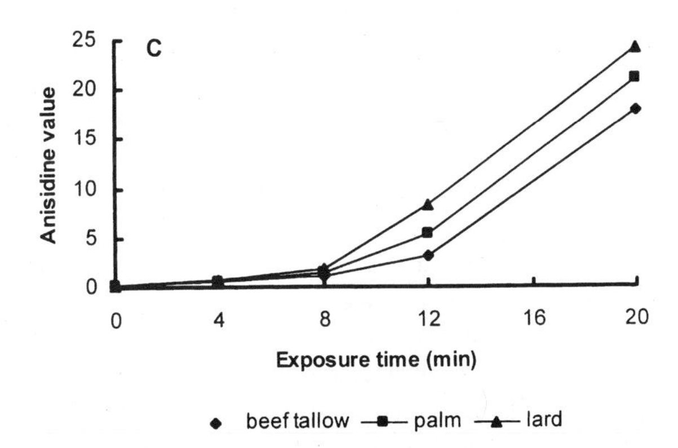


**FIGURE 5.5** Changes in peroxide value (A), carbonyl value (B), and anisidine value (C) of purified fats by microwave heating. (Modified from Ref. 78.)

a plant metabolism aspect have been completed to show photooxidative effects when leaf tissue is irradiated under high-intensity light in relation to the role of vitamin E in membrane stability. Wise and Naylor (88,89) reported that chlorophylls *a* and *b*, $\beta$-carotene, and xanthophylls were degraded at a similar rate by high-irradiance light. Lipid oxidation was dependent on the presence of oxygen and ascorbic acid, and glutathione and $\alpha$-T levels declined with the extent of light exposure. Antioxidant studies indicated that singlet oxygen and superoxide radicals participated in the decomposition of the pigments and endogenous antioxidants. $\alpha$-Tocopherol level decreased in chill-injury-sensitive cucumber leaves but not in chill-injury-resistant peas on irradiation, indicating increased oxidative stress in the chill-injury-sensitive cucumber (88).

Although $\alpha$-T level decreases in specific membranes as a first sign of lipid oxidation, the role of $\alpha$-T as a protective agent against oxidative stress is difficult to differentiate from that of other plant antioxidants (90). Ultraviolet B (UV-B) irradiation–induced damage in plants occurs within the photosynthetic apparatus of plants (91,92). DeLong and Steffen(92) however, were not able to show UV-B damage to the lipid matrix of thylakoid membranes. $\alpha$-Tocopherol level increased in the thylakoid membranes during the first 8 days of irradiation and then decreased as overall antioxidant capacity of the chloroplasts was overcome. Therefore, enhanced UV-B radiation may represent an environmental signal that up-regulates the antioxidant capacity of the chloroplasts (92).

Several excellent reviews consider the antioxidant function of vitamin E in plants (90,93–95). Hess(93) states, "Although the source of dietary vitamin E is from plants, limited experimental data directly establish the antioxidant function of vitamin E in plants." Hess (93) divided the function of vitamin E in plant structure and metabolism into the categories of membrane stabilization and antioxidant activity, highly interrelated roles. Vitamin E is one component of a dynamic system that responds to environmental factors including development and life-cycle effects, chilling stress and cold acclimation, storage, nutrient effects, drought and other climatic conditions, and herbicide treatment (93). Shewfelt and colleagues (90,94,95) published several interpretative reviews on the role of lipid peroxidation in storage disorders of fruits and vegetables. In their discussions, a model for lipid oxidation of specific membranes was proposed to indicate that peroxidative processes in plant tissues could function to cause tissue disorders (Figure 5.6). Lipid deterioration would produce changes in membrane integrity, physical structure, and membrane fluidity—effects that would modify the function of protein. Loss of a critical enzyme within a specific membrane could induce metabolic imbalances, eventually leading to the visible symptoms of a disorder (e.g., chill injury) (90). The total plant antioxidant system, including $\alpha$-T, $\beta$-carotene, lycopene, reducing agents (ascorbic acid and glutathione), and enzymes that respond to oxidative stress (catalase, peroxidase, superoxide dismutase), participates actively to provide protective agents against lipid

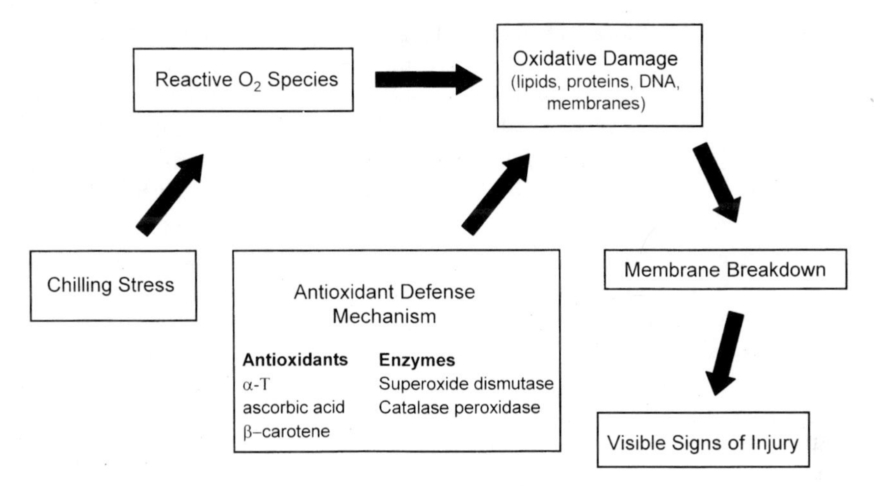


**FIGURE 5.6** Proposed model for lipid oxidation in chilling injury and other membrane disorders of plant tissue. DNA, deoxyribonucleic acid; $\alpha$-T, $\alpha$-tocopherol. (Modified from Ref. 90.)

oxidation (90). Shewfelt and coworkers' discussions stress that antioxidant degradation in localized areas can be a useful marker for the onset of quality loss; however, measurements of more than one antioxidant are needed to determine whether changes in concentrations precede evidence of oxidative damage.

**5.3.3.3. Gamma Radiation.** Application of gamma irradiation to foods can effectively reduce or eliminate pathogens and spoilage microorganisms without decreasing wholesomeness and sensory qualities.(72,96) Low doses of irradiation kill bacteria and delay spoilage. Because of the need for increased control in fresh and processed meat demonstrated by hazards increasingly apparent from outbreaks of food-borne illness due to E. coli O157 : H7, Salmonella spp., and other food pathogens, the United States Department of Agriculture (USDA) through the Food Safety and Inspection Service (FSIS) proposed regulations in 1999 covering the use of ionizing radiation for processing of refrigerated or frozen uncooked meat, meat by-products, and other meat food products, including poultry, to reduce levels of food-borne pathogens and to extend shelf life (97). The rule, which became effective on February 22, 2000, expands the use of irradiation to red meats. Irradiation had previously been approved for use in fresh, frozen, uncooked, and packaged poultry products. Maximal safe adsorbed doses approved by the Food and Drug Administration (FDA) and included in USDA's final rule are 4.5 and 7.0 kGy for refrigerated and frozen meat, respectively, and 3 kGy for poultry.

At these low doses, chemical changes induced by gamma radiation are minimal; however, it is well recognized that lipid components of the food are most susceptible to ionization and formation of free radicals. At the approved doses, small numbers of free radicals initially produced can catalyze oxidation in the food. A recent study by Jo and Ahn (98) reported that the formation of oxidation products in pork sausage by irradiation was influenced by dosage of irradiation, fat sources, tocopherol content, and packaging methods. They stated that sausage prepared with flaxseed oil produced lower lipid oxidation than sausage prepared with other treatments probably because of the high tocopherol content present in flaxseed oil. Results indicated that an oxygen-free environment minimizes off-odors from lipid oxidation, but vacuum packaging would not completely control production of volatiles by irradiation. Such compounds can be produced through radiolysis as well as through lipid oxidation. Catalysis of lipid oxidation as influenced by gamma radiation has been a fertile area of food chemistry research. Further, because of the effect of irradiation on antioxidant levels in foods, including vitamin E, considerable information on the overall effects of irradiation on nutritional quality is available. Information in Table 5.6 summarizes research showing specific effects of gamma irradiation on vitamin E levels in various foods.

Because of recent regulatory activities and food safety problems associated with meats, research that shows the effects of gamma radiation on $\alpha$-T in meats at the levels approved for industry use has been completed. The most pertinent studies were completed at the Food Safety Research Unit of the Eastern Regional Research Center, USDA (99–102). This work provided the following conclusions regarding the stability of $\alpha$- and $\gamma$-T in irradiated meat products:

1. At 3 kGy, $\alpha$- and $\gamma$-T levels were reduced by 30% and 15%, respectively, in poultry breast muscle at 4–6°C. The decrease was linear with increasing dose levels.
2. Losses of $\alpha$- and $\gamma$-T levels in rehydrated, freeze-dried pork muscle were dependent upon the level of rehydration. Smallest losses occurred at higher rehydration levels, indicating the competition of water molecules for hydroxyl radicals, thereby providing some protection for the tocopherols from the ionizing radiation.
3. NaCl addition decreased vitamin E loss due to competition for hydroxyl radicals by chloride ions.
4. The rate of tocopherol loss in turkey breast muscle was greater than that found in turkey leg, beef, pork, and lamb, possibly as a result of the lower lipid content of turkey breast meat. Irradiation significantly decreased $\alpha$-T level in all meats at similar rates except in the turkey breast muscle.

5. $\alpha$-Tocopherol loss due to irradiation of exotic meats (alligator, bison, caiman, and ostrich) was similar to that noted for domestic species.

From this work, Lakritz and coworkers (99–102) concluded that meat pasteurization by irradiation can be used without regard for species. Studies on fish (103,104), wheat (105), milk (106), and turkey (107) show that vitamin E level decreases with increasing radiation doses. Al-Kahtani et al. (104) reported increasing losses of $\alpha$- and $\gamma$-T levels in tilapia and of $\alpha$-, $\beta$-, $\gamma$-, and $\delta$-T levels in Spanish mackerel with increasing doses of radiation. Little further loss occurred during 20 days of postirradiation storage in ice.

Most current work on irradiation of foods has centered on lethality to pathogenic microorganisms; loss of sensory and nutritional quality must also be prevented to ensure consumer acceptance. Approaches available to the industry to minimize overall quality loss, of which loss of vitamin E is crucial to the stability of other quality measures, include proper temperature control during irradiation; use of proper packaging; atmosphere control, which varies with the product and packaging material; exclusion of catalysts and initiators of autoxidation; use of minimal doses; use of various protective agents (104) such as hydroxyl radical scavengers and other antioxidants(100) and control of water concentration and/or water activity (100,104).

## 5.3.4. Cereal Processing

Cereal grains are important sources of vitamin E. Hamburger rolls, alone, made from wheat flour provide 1% of the vitamin E available in the U.S. market (108). A Finnish study (109) indicated that as much as 30% of the recommended dietary allowance in Finland originates from cereal products. Vitamin E in cereal is largely located in the bran and germ fractions. Since the oil content is largely contained in the germ fraction, most vitamin E is in this fraction. The vitamin E content in cereal is influenced by plant genetics, environmental conditions during growing and harvest, maturity at harvest, and significant loss of vitamin E that occurs during processing after harvesting (1–3,110,111). Herting and Drury's comprehensive study on corn, wheat, oats, and rice (110) found that cereal processing could reduce vitamin E content by as much as 90%. The lipid content of the grain that is usually reduced by processing correlates with the vitamin E content. Herting and Drury (110) suggested that vitamin E be restored to compensate for processing losses.

Changes in tocopherols and tocotrienols in cereals vary widely, depending on the type and severity of the process (110,112). Vitamin E loss in wheat products ranged from 20% for shredded corn cereal to 92% for refined wheat flour. Puffing of rice reduced $\alpha$-T level by 40%. Rice products showed more than 70% loss of $\alpha$-T level. The more highly processed cereal products showed relatively greater loss (110). Bauernfeind (2,3) stated that virtually any type of cereal processing, including milling, expanding, puffing, rolling, and shredding, resulted in a lower level of vitamin E in the final products. He also showed that the degree of vitamin E loss increased as the severity of the process increased. Different types of processing lead to different degrees of fractionation of the grain; therefore, the levels of vitamin E in the various fractions of kernel differ, as does the proportion of $\alpha$-T to total tocopherol (113–116). It is often difficult to distinguish clearly between loss of vitamin E caused by physical removal and loss caused by chemical reactivity. Summaries of pertinent literature dealing with the effects of cereal processing on vitamin E content are provided in Table 5.7.

**5.3.4.1. Drying.** Harvested grains usually require drying before storage. Artificial drying of corn, when well controlled, can be carried out effectively without the destruction of vitamin E or unsaturated fatty acids. No differences were observed in total vitamin E content or in the proportions of the tocopherol isomers in corn after drying in a forced air or a fluidized bed drier at temperatures ranging from ambient to 290°F (117). Pond et al. (118) showed that air and oven drying of corn had very little effect on vitamin E content. They also indicated that the $\alpha$- and $\gamma$-T concentrations were slightly higher for air-dried (20°C for 2 wk) compared to oven-dried (90°C for 24 h) corn.

On the other hand, drum drying (roller drying) of wheat flour reduces the vitamin E activity by 90%. Hàkansson et al. (119,120) showed that drum drying destroyed 90% of the $\alpha$-T in white wheat flour. Among thermal processes studied by Hàkansson et al. (119) (steam flaking, autoclaving, popping, extrusion, and drum drying), extrusion and drum drying caused the most loss of vitamin E. Another similar study by Hàkansson et al. (120) showed that less than 10% of the vitamin E in whole meal and white wheat flour was retained after drum drying. Wennermark et al. (121) indicated that 28% and 42% of $\alpha$-T was retained, respectively, after mild (0.4 MPa, 40 min, 12 rpm/min) and severe (0.4 MPa, 40 min, 4 rpm/min) drum drying after scalding and fermentation of freshly milled whole meal wheat flour. These observations (119,121) clearly show that drum drying causes severe loss of vitamin E in cereal. A 2002 study by Bryngelsson et al. (122) reported the effects of steaming, autoclaving, and drum drying on antioxidants in oats. Drum drying of steamed rolled oats reduced tocopherols and tocotrienols to practically nondetectable levels.

The main causes of loss of vitamin E during the processing of cereals undoubtedly are fractionation of the kernel coupled with lipid oxidation. Lipids in whole grain wheat and corn are 70–80% mono- and polyunsaturated fatty acids (123). To what extent the vitamin E losses can be ascribed to enzymatic (lipoxygenase) or nonenzymatic oxidation is not known. Various studies (119,120,124) support the hypothesis that the retention of vitamin E during processing of cereals is related to lipid oxidation. Chow and Draper (117) stated that oxidation of unsaturated fatty acids would not be anticipated in the absence

**Table 5.7** The Effects of Processing on Vitamin E Content of Cereals

| Cereal | Process | Observations | References |
|---|---|---|---|
| **Dehydration** | | | |
| Corn | Artificial drying (forced-air, model fluidized bed drier): 36–60%, 90°F, 140°F, 190°F, 240°F, 290°F for 48, 7, 2.5, 1.2, 0.8, 0.5 h, respectively | No differences observed in total vitamin E content or proportions of tocopherol isomers in dried corns at temperature ranging from ambient to 290°F; no significant effect of drying on vitamin E content of the corn | 1969, 117 |
| High-, low-selenium corns | Oven-drying: 90°C, 24 h Air-drying: 20°C, 2 wk | Very little effect of oven and air drying of corn on tocopherol content; $\alpha$- and $\gamma$-T concentrations slightly higher for air-dried corn compared to oven-dried corn; tocopherol in high-selenium corn than low-selenium corn at both drying temperatures | 1971, 118 |
| Wheat flour | Drum drying: mild (60 min, 0.69 MPa, 13 rpm), severe (55 min, 0.98 MPa, 5 rpm) | In white wheat flour 10% of $\alpha$-TE retained by drum drying among vitamin E isomers, $\alpha$-TE least stable | 1987, 119 |
| Freshly milled wholemeal, white wheat flour | Drum drying (0.7 MPa, 160–170°C, 13 rpm); steam flaking | Vitamin E in wholemeal and white wheat flours destroyed after drum drying without steam flaking; vitamin E loss begun immediately on mixing of flour with water and increased with increased temperature of flour–water slurry | 1990, 120 |

*(continued)*

**Table 5.7** *Continued*

| Cereal | Process | Observations | References |
|---|---|---|---|
| Freshly milled and stored whole wheat flour | Drum drying: mild (40 min, 0.4 MPa, 12 rpm), severe (40 min, 0.4 MPa, 4 rpm); scalding; fermentation | Retention of α-T 28% and 42% during mild and severe drum drying | 1994, 121 |
| Oats | Steaming and flaking, autoclaving, drum drying | Tocopherols and tocotrienols almost completely destroyed by drum drying; increased by autoclaving whole grains | 2002, 122 |
| **Milling** | | | |
| Wheat | Milling | Vitamin E contents of whole wheat, germ, bran, shorts, patent flour 0.91, 15.84, 0.3, 3.18, and 0.03 mg/100 g, respectively | 1941, 125 |
| Corn | Wet and dry milling | Recoveries of α- and total tocopherols (68% and 73%) after dry milling much better than those (18% and 27%) after wet milling | 1971, 127 |
| Triticale | Milling | Triticale grain α-T content range 7.0–14.5 μg/g; α-T content of whole grain, flour, bran, and shorts of spring triticales 13.5–14.5, 1.1–3.3, 18.7–19.8, and 10.1–11.5 μg/g, respectively | 1974, 113 |
| Rice bran | Milling (very low, low, medium degrees) | About 50% oil of total oil of whole grain removed by medium milling; varying vitamin E content of bran with degree of milling; increased percentage of tocopherols removed from brown rice with degree of milling | 1984, 132 |

| | | | |
|---|---|---|---|
| Waxy hullless barley | Pearling, milling | Pearling more effective than milling as means of concentrating total vitamin E and oil in barley flour; in pearling flour (20% of kernel weight) higher concentrations of $\alpha$-T3, $\alpha$-T, total vitamin E, and oil than those of the whole grain | 1993, 114 |
| Amaranth seed (whole seed, bran fraction, collets, oils) | Milling (gaps: 0.71 to 0.89 mm), extrusion (twin-screw) | Percentage weight of bran fraction enriched in oil decrease with increasing milling gap; with milling, extrusion, and extraction increased FFA content and peroxide value and changed in vitamin E content of oil | 1995, 133 |
| Corn | Steeping: time (18, 24, 48 h), solutions (0.1%, 0.2%, 0.3% $SO_2$, 1% vitamin C), Saponification: 5,15, 40 times, at 26°C, 50°C, 70°C, 90°C | Little effect of steeping conditions on $\alpha$-T and $\alpha$-T3 contents; in corn steeped in vitamin C solution much higher tocopherol content than in corn steeped in $SO_2$ solution | 1998, 129 |
| Long- and medium-grain rice | Multibreak milling, steam-extrusion (120°C), storage | Varied vitamin E levels in rice bran according to degree of milling of rice kernel; highest vitamin E content in bran from milling break 2, in long-grain rice bran collected from milling break 1 average 30% more tocopherol than in medium-grain rice bran | 2000, 22 |
| **Extrusion, flaking, puffing, rolling, shredding** | | | |
| Corn, rice, oats, wheat | Flaking, shredding, puffing, expanding, rolling | Cereal processing cause of extensive loss of vitamin E: expanded rice (97%), shredded rice (94%), puffed wheat (22%), shredded wheat (99%), rolled oat (14–39%) | 1969, 110 |

(continued)

**TABLE 5.7** *Continued*

| Cereal | Process | Observations | References |
|---|---|---|---|
| Wheat flour, whole grain wheat | Drum drying, steam flaking, popping, autoclaving, extrusion cooking | Vitamin E loss ($\alpha$-T) percentage<br>Extrusion, 85<br>Drum drying, 63<br>Steam flaking, 40–45<br>Popping, 40–45 | 1987, 119 |
| Soybeans, corn | Extrusion: exit temperature −127°C, 138°C, 149°C, 160°C | Soybean trypsin inhibitor activity destroyed 49% to 99% as exit temperature increased; no major extrusion temperature effect on tocopherol isomers; lipoxygenase completely inactivated by extrusion | 1989, 142 |
| Rice bran | Extrusion: 110°C, 120°C, 130°C, 140°C, postholding time: 0, 3, 6 min | With increased extrusion temperatures reduced retention of vitamin E; with increased holding time significantly reduced total vitamin E content; no holding time effect on free fatty acid levels in extruded rice bran | 1997, 138 |
| Oat flour | Heat treatment: 100°C, 30 min<br>Extrusion: control of moisture, starch levels, dietary fiber | With extrusion about 50% degradation of phenolic compounds; with heat treatment no significant tocopherol content reduction in oat flour | 1999, 137 |

| | | | |
|---|---|---|---|
| Grass pea seeds | Grinding: hammer mill Extrusion: moistures 140, 180, 220, 260, 300 g water/kg sample Temperatures: 90/100/120/100°C, 120°C/140°C/170°C/160°C, 140°C/180°C/220°C/200°C | Extrusion decrease of α- and γ-T; significant γ-T decrease with increasing moisture content; most distinctive decrease of α-T content with increasing cooking temperature | 1999, 139 |
| Tapioca starch, minced fish, peanut flour | Extrusion, drying, deep-frying (soybean oil) | Total tocopherol losses in fish and peanut extrudates 39% and 27%, respectively, during extrusion; α-, β-, γ-, and δ-T losses in peanut extrudate were 18%, 11%, 28%, and 30%, respectively; with exception of β-T, tocopherol loss during drying after extrusion 1% to 5%; in final products more tocopherol than in intermediates because of high tocopherol content in frying oil and its uptake | 2001, 59 |
| **Bleaching** | | | |
| Manitoba flour, mixed grist flour | Bleaching: chlorine dioxide, persulfate, agene, bromate (10 times at 30 ppm) | Tocopherol content of untreated flour reduced by about 70% compared with that of untreated flour | 1953, 146 |
| Flours | Bleaching: chlorine dioxide (30 ppm) | As much as 95% of total reducing value of unsaponifiable fraction destroyed after treatment with chlorine dioxide at ordinary commercial level (30 ppm) | 1954, 147 |

*(continued)*

**TABLE 5.7** *Continued*

| Cereal | Process | Observations | References |
|---|---|---|---|
| Wheat flour | Bleaching: chlorine dioxide (1, 10 times at normal level) | Changes in vitamin E content that occur with chlorine dioxide treatment not significant in terms of human nutrition | 1956, 151 |
| Wheat flour | Bleaching: chlorine dioxide | Chlorine dioxide cause of almost complete destruction of tocopherols; in biological tests, various signs of vitamin E deficiency in rats given treated flour; in untreated flour enough tocopherol to satisfy requirement | 1957, 148 |
| Wheat flour | Bleaching: azodicarbonamide, benzoyl peroxide, chlorine dioxide, chlorine, acetone peroxide | RRR-α-tocopheryl acetate resistant to destruction by bleaching; natural vitamin E significantly destroyed | 1981, 153 |

α-T, α-tocopherol; α-TE, α-tocopherol equivalent; α-T3, α-tocotrienol; FFA, free fatty acid.

of tocopherol destruction. Processing studies indicated that lipid oxidation and vitamin E degradation begin as soon as water is added to the flour, the first stage in drum drying (120). Further losses may occur when the slurry is transferred and heated on the drum. Nonenzymatically induced lipid oxidation may continue also when the process temperature has passed the point at which the enzymes are heat-inactivated. Autooxidation is likely to occur since the concentrations of copper and iron increase noticeably during the drum drying. Whole grain wheat, when steam-flaked to inactivate lipoxygenases, retains most of the vitamin E (120). However, subsequent drum drying of the steam-flaked wheat destroys 50% of original vitamin E activity. It is a well-known fact that rice bran oil is subject to wide variations in vitamin E levels due to variations in handling of the unprocessed bran and methods of oil refining. Oxidative changes can largely be prevented through inactivation of lipoxygenase activity by extrusion of the raw bran before extraction of the oil. The stabilized bran can be stored without loss of antioxidant activity before oil extraction (22) (Figure 5.1). Such research shows the practical significance of lipoxygenase inactivation to vitamin E stability.

**5.3.4.2. Milling.** Preparation of cereal-based foods usually requires some degree of processing of whole grains. It is generally recognized that the losses of the tocopherols and tocotrienols present in the whole grains occur during milling and that these losses increase when the processing is extensive (1). Early work (2,3) showed that some vitamin E loss occurs during the milling process, and the extent of loss varies with factors including the degree of milling, the extent of fractionation of the kernel, and the distribution of vitamin E in the kernel. Since the oil content is high in the germ fraction, the most significant portion of vitamin E is in this fraction. During milling, the vitamin E in the whole grain is fractionated into the bran and germ fractions so that flours have lower levels of vitamin E than are present in the whole grain. Removal of the hull and most of the germ from corn produced losses of 35% to 70% of the tocopherol initially present in the whole grain (110). In milling of rice, most of the $\alpha$-T originally present in the rough rice was lost with removal of the bran fraction during milling of brown rice (110). Vitamin E is not equally distributed in cereal grains and in the milling fractions (111,114,125). Moreover, since the loss of vitamin E by physical removal occurs along with the oxidative destruction of tocopherols and tocotrienols (115) it is difficult to distinguish routes of loss.

Mechanical fractionation of cereal grain leads to products with varying vitamin E content. The distribution of tocopherols and tocotrienols in wheat (115), corn (116), and barley (126) fractions by hand dissection has been studied. For wheat, the endosperm fraction of the wheat grain had more than 90% of the tocotrienols and more than 50% of the tocopherols isolated from the whole grain (115). For corn, the endosperm vitamin E content varied from 27% in normal corn to 11% in high-lysine corn, and the germ fraction contained 94–96% of the $\alpha$-T extracted from the whole grain (116).

The effects of dry and wet milling on vitamin E content in corn were studied by Grams et al. (127). Respective recoveries of $\alpha$-T and total vitamin E (68% and 73%) after dry milling were much better than those (18% and 27%) after wet milling. Recoveries of tocopherols (23%) and tocotrienols (38%) varied during wet milling. Commercial wet milling had little effect on the content of $\alpha$-and $\gamma$-T in corn germ oil (128). Steeping conditions during wet milling only slightly changed the vitamin E content. Wang et al. (129) reported that corn kernels steeped in a vitamin C solution had a much higher concentration of tocopherols than those steeped in $SO_2$ solution. However, a higher concentration of $SO_2$ and a shorter steeping time yielded slightly higher $\gamma$-T3 and lower $\gamma$-T contents.

Because most of the vitamin E in cereals is located either in the germ or in the bran, the vitamin E content of milled products is dependent on the extraction rate. In 1942, the effects of the milling rate on the level of tocopherol was studied by Engel (130). In wheat, the level of vitamin E in the first fraction (0–70% extraction) was 71% higher than in the last fraction (82–100% extraction). In rye, the level in the first fraction (0–60% milling) was 44% higher than in the last fraction (74–100% extraction). Therefore, the lower the flour extraction rate in the first fraction, the higher the vitamin E content (131). Milling of triticale resulted in flour fractions of increasingly lower tocopherol content (113). For rice, the vitamin E content of the bran varied with the degree of milling, but the percentage of tocopherols removed from brown rice increased with the degree of milling (132). About 50% of the total oil of the whole grain was removed when the rice was milled to a medium degree. Also, the comprehensive survey by Piironen et al. (109) demonstrated that the rate of extraction in wheat milling had a great effect on the content of $\alpha$-T and other vitamin E components.

The oil content of the milled kernel is affected by processing. Milling gap significantly affects the distribution of oil between the bran and perisperm fraction in amaranth milled fractions (133). When the milling gap was increased from 0.710 to 0.755 mm, the percentage weight of the bran decreased significantly, but the percentage of oil remaining in the bran fraction did not decrease significantly. However, the decrease in the percentage weight of bran from gaps of 0.755 to 0.890 mm was not significant (133). Becker et al. (134) had previously shown that the percentage weight of the bran fraction in amaranth seed decreased with increasing milling gap.

Parboiling is often used for cereal products before or after milling. During production of milled rice from rough rice both before and after parboiling, a significant loss was noted for $\alpha$-T (110). Then, the remaining $\alpha$-T in the parboiled rice decreased by more than 50% during milling. Sondi et al. (135) reported that the oil content of the residual milled kernel was lower and the content of bran higher in parboiled as compared to raw rice at all degrees of milling. They also indicated that the oil in rice migrated outward on parboiling whereas the total oil content of the grain was unchanged after parboiling. In addition, further destruction of vitamin E during the processing of wheat, rye, or barley into flour occurs at the bleaching or improving stage, as discussed in Sec. 5.3.4.5.

**5.3.4.3. Extrusion Cooking.** Extrusion cooking utilizes pressure, high temperature (150–160°C) and short processing times (60–120 s) at moisture of 15–25%. As the cereal product is moved through the extruder, the temperature of the cooking cereal dough in the extruder barrel increases, primarily as a result of the internal shear forces and external heat sources. The severe conditions of temperature, pressure, and intense mechanical shear active during extrusion affect physical and chemical properties. Changes in chemical composition are generated by thermal degradation, depolymerization, and recombination of fragments (136). With these changes, vitamin E loss through oxidation can be quite pronounced. The extent of loss is affected by extrusion conditions and food matrix composition.

Wheat flour lost 70% and 83% of total vitamin E during mild (148°C) and severe (197°C) extrusion, respectively (119). Another study reported that extrusion resulted in about 50% degradation of phenolic compounds, whereas heat treatment (100°C for 30 min) did not significantly reduce the vitamin E in oat flour (137). Increased extrusion temperatures reduced the retention of vitamin E and increased postextrusion holding time significantly in rice bran (138). Therefore, stabilization of rice bran by extrusion should be done at the lowest possible temperature, preferably below 120°C, and no postextrusion holding at elevated temperatures should be allowed. The order of stability of the vitamin E forms in extruded rice bran for all extrusion temperatures was $\gamma$-T3 < $\alpha$-T < $\alpha$-T3 < $\gamma$-T < $\delta$-T3 < $\beta$-T < $\delta$-T (138). Moisture conditioning and extrusion significantly decreased the content of $\alpha$- and $\gamma$-T in grass pea (139). In particular, $\gamma$-T content significantly decreased with increasing moisture content, and $\alpha$-T was most sensitive to increasing extrusion temperature.

Destruction of natural antioxidants during extrusion is a major factor responsible for the susceptibility of extruded materials to lipid oxidation (140). Low-cost extruder (LCE) cookers, which are being used in developing countries to produce nutritious, precooked foods based on legumes and cereals(141) can improve retention of vitamin E. A study by Guzman et al. (142) of properties of soybean–corn mixtures processed by low-cost extrusion indicated that extrusion temperature (127–160°C) had no major effect on the tocopherol isomers whereas lipoxygenase was completely inactivated (up to 98.8%). Cowpea–corn blends processed at 170°C with LCE resulted in 84% trypsin inhibitor activity destruction (143) Lorenz and Jansen (144) recommended an extrusion temperature of 143°C for production of full-fat soy flour by LCE.

#### 5.3.4.4. Expanding, Flaking, Puffing, Rolling, and Shredding.

Processing of grain by flaking, shredding, and puffing usually causes extensive loss of vitamin E (110). Hàkansson et al. (119) investigated the effects of steam flaking, autoclaving, popping, extrusion cooking, and drum drying on vitamin E content in wheat. Processing under mild conditions did not reduce the amounts of any of the tocopherols and tocotrienols in whole grain wheat. However, steam flaking and popping performed under severe conditions resulted in 40–45% losses of $\alpha$- and $\beta$-T. Although steam flaking is a relatively mild heating process, the substantial losses may have been due to considerable mechanical disruption during processing, providing a greater opportunity for lipoxygenase activity with acceleration of the oxidation. The low-temperature processes, such as steam flaking and drum drying, or the high-temperature–short-time-process extrusion cooking, generally, with the exception of vitamin E, led to higher nutrient quality when compared to popping and autoclaving. Mild steaming and flaking of dehulled oats caused only moderate losses of tocotrienols (122).

#### 5.3.4.5. Bleaching.

Bleaching is known to destroy much of the vitamin E in flour (1,145). The destructive effect of bleaching on the natural vitamin E in flour has been reported by many researchers. The loss of vitamin E differs slightly with the degrees of extraction of flour and treatment and bleaching. In 1942, partial destruction of vitamin E in wheat flour during bleaching or improvement was first reported by Engel (130). Later, Moran et al. (146) investigated the destruction of vitamin E in flour by chlorine dioxide. After the application of the improver at the rate of 30 ppm, 70% loss of the vitamin E content in flour was observed. These same researchers (147) showed that as much as 95% of the total reducing value of the unsaponifiable fraction was destroyed after treatment with chlorine dioxide at the ordinary commercial level (30 ppm), whereas Moore et al. (148), working with 80% extraction wheat flour, found that total tocopherol decreased from 15.7 to 1.9 $\mu$g/g after treatment of the flour (80% extraction wheat flour) with chlorine dioxide at a level of approximately 30 ppm. Vitamin E in 72% extraction flour decreased from 15.5 to 7.2 $\mu$g/g with 16.5 ppm of chlorine dioxide (149). The data obtained by Mason and Jones's work (149) indicate that $\delta$-T is considerably more stable to chlorine dioxide than $\alpha$-T.

Wheat flour (78% extraction) contained 1.5 mg $\alpha$-T/100 g, reduced to 0.2 mg/100 g after treatment with chlorine dioxide (150). These authors stated in another study (151) that the chlorine dioxide treatment of flour does not have any significant deleterious effect on its nutritional value. Also, they concluded that the changes in vitamin E content during chlorine dioxide treatment are not considered to be significant in terms of human intake. On the other hand, Moore et al. (152) found in biological tests that in rats given treated flour various signs of vitamin E deficiency developed, whereas untreated flour provided enough vitamin E to satisfy the requirement. After the destruction of the vitamin E by chlorine dioxide was confirmed, interest in the fortification of vitamins into flour increased. Ranum et al. (153) investigated the effect of typical flour treatments on vitamin E and reported that among bleaching agents–azodicarbonamide, benzoyl peroxide, chlorine dioxide, and acetone peroxide—chlorine destroyed natural vitamin E by the largest extent (91%) and azodicarbonamide decreased it by the smallest extent (58%).

### 5.3.5. Dairy Processing

Whole cow's milk contains 0.05 to 0.10 mg of total tocopherols, primarily composed of $\alpha$-T (84–92%) (see Chapter 8, Table 8.3) (155,156). As with any food that is fractionated to remove fat, the vitamin E in fluid milk decreases with the production of reduced-fat or skim fluid dairy products. This effect was documented in 2001 by Kaushik et al. (156). Data obtained in the study (Table 5.8) clearly show the fractionation effect on the vitamin E content of fluid dairy products. With fat removal, vitamin E content decreased from approximately 0.07 to 0.006 mg/100 g in nonfat milk. Likewise, addition of milk fat to produce half and half increased the total vitamin E to 0.2 mg/100 g. Conclusions from the study indicate that substitution of reduced-fat milk for whole milk could impact $\alpha$-T intake for consumers who consume large amounts of milk. The authors suggested that the decreasing consumption trends evident for whole milk in the United States make reduced-fat products logical vehicles for vitamin E fortification.

Pasteurization of fluid milk has little effect on vitamin E content. Since deaeration is universally employed, the process most likely has a stabilization effect on vitamin E during subsequent heat processing. Ultrahigh-temperature (UHT) processing at 138°C for 2 s or 145°C for 3–4 s followed by evaporative or

**TABLE 5.8** Vitamin E Contents of Dairy Products

| Product | Fat content (g/100 g) | (mg/100 g) $\alpha$-T | $\gamma$-T | $\alpha$-T3 | $\alpha$-T/Cholesterol (μg/mg) |
|---|---|---|---|---|---|
| Raw | 3.5 | 0.045 | 0.019 | 0.002 | 2.8 |
| Whole | 3.4 | 0.044 | 0.002 | 0.002 | 3.1 |
| Reduced-fat | 2.1 | 0.026 | 0.001 | 0.001 | 3.7 |
| Low-fat | 1.1 | 0.014 | 0.001 | 0.001 | 4.0 |
| Nonfat | 0.3 | 0.005 | 0.001 | — | 2.6 |
| Half and half | 12.0 | 0.193 | 0.012 | 0.007 | 4.0 |

$\alpha$-T, $\alpha$-tocopherol; $\alpha$-T3, $\alpha$-tocotrienol.
*Source*: Modified from Ref. 156.

indirect cooling did not change $\alpha$-T levels in the milk (157). Likewise, commercial pasteurization of milk used in the Kaushik et al. study (156) did not decrease $\alpha$-T levels. Little information is available on the effect of concentration processes applied to fluid milk such as multiple-effect evaporation and spray drying. Dried whole milk powder contains 0.5–0.8 mg/100 g, content that is approximately 10 times greater than that of fluid whole milk (Chapter 8, Table 8.3). Therefore, one can postulate that the effect of concentration processes on vitamin E is minimal for production of concentrated and dried products.

## REFERENCES


1. Kivimäe, A.; Carpena, C. The level of vitamin E content in some conventional feeding stuffs and the effects of genetic variety, harvesting, processing and storage. Acta Agric. Scand. Suppl. **1973**, *19*, 161–168.
2. Bauernfeind, J.C. The tocopherol content of food and influencing factors. Crit. Rev. Food Sci. Nutr. **1977**, *8*, 337–382.
3. Bauernfeind, J.C. Tocopherols in foods. In *Vitamin E: A Comprehensive Treatise*; Machlin, L.J., Ed.; Marcel Dekker: New York, 1980.
4. Bramley, P.M.; Elmadfa, I.; Kafatos, A.; Kelly, F.J.; Manios, Y.; Roxborough, H.E.; Schuch, W.; Sheehy, P.J.A.; Wagner, K.-H. Review: Vitamin E. J. Sci. Food Agric. **2000**, *80*, 913–938.
5. Čmolík, J.; Pokorný, J. Physical refining of edible oils. Eur. J. Lipid Sci. Technol. **2000**, *102*, 472–486.
6. Eitenmiller, R.R. Vitamin E content of fats and oils—nutritional implications. Food Technol. **1997**, *51*, 78–81.
7. Dick, W. Vitamin E content of foods and feeds for human and animal consumption. Agric Bull 435; Laramie: University of Wyoming, 1965.
8. Ferrari, R.; Schulte, E.; Esteves, W.; Brühl, L.; Mukherjee, K.D. Minor constituents of vegetable oils during industrial processing. JAOCS **1996**, *73*, 587–592.
9. Jung, M.Y.; Yoon, S.H.; Min, D.B. Effects of processing steps on the contents of minor compounds and oxidation of soybean oil. JAOCS **1989**, *66*, 118–120.
10. Gutfinger, T.; Letan, A. Quantitative changes in some unsaponifiable components of soy bean oil due to refining. J. Sci. Food Agric. **1974**, *25*, 1143–1147.
11. Rutkowski, A. The influence of expelling, extraction, de-acidification and bleaching on the stability of rapeseed oil. Fette Seifen. Anstrichm. **1959**, *61*, 1216–1218.
12. Walker, B.L.; Slinger, S.J. Effect of processing on the tocopherol content of rapeseed oils. J. Inst. Can. Sci. Technol. Alminet. **1975**, *8*, 179–180.
13. Prior, E.M.; Vadke, V.S.; Sosulski, F.W. Effect of heat treatments on canola press oils: Non-triglyceride components. JAOCS **1991**, *68*, 401–406.
14. Gogolewski, M.; Nogala-Kalucka, M.; Szeliga, M. Changes of the tocopherol and fatty acid contents in rapeseed oil during refining. Eur. J. Lipid Sci. Technol. **2000**, *102*, 618–623.

15. Gordon, M.H.; Rahman, I.A. Effect of processing on the composition and oxidative stability of coconut oil. JAOCS **1991**, *68*, 574–596.
16. Scott, K.C.; Latshaw, J.D. Effects of commercial processing on the fat-soluble vitamin content of manhadden fish oil. JAOCS **1991**, *68*, 234–236.
17. Wanasundara, U.N.; Shahidi, F.; Amarowicz, R. Effect of processing on constituents and oxidative stability of marine oils. J. Food Lipids **1998**, *5*, 29–41.
18. Shahidi, F.; Wanasundra, U.N. Effects of processing and squalene on composition and oxidative stability of seal blubber oil. J. Food Lipids **1999**, *6*, 159–172.
19. Rabascall, N.J.; Riera, J.B. Variaciones del contenido en tocoferoles y tocotrienoles durante los procesos de obtención, refinacion e hidrogenacion de aceites comestibles. Fasc. **1987**, *3*, 145–148.
20. De, B.K.; Bhattacharyya, D.K. Physical refining of rice bran oil in relation to degumming and dewaxing. JAOCS **1998**, *75*, 1683–1686.
21. Kim, S.; Kim, C.; Cheigh, H.; Yoon, S. Effect of caustic refining, solvent refining and steam refining on the deacidification and color of rice bran oil. JAOCS **1985**, *62*, 1492–1495.
22. Lloyd, B.J.; Siebenmorgen, T.J.; Beers, K.W. Effect of commercial processing on antioxidants in rice bran. Cereal Chem. **2000**, *77*, 551–555.
23. Hassapidou, M.N.; Balatsouras, G.D.; Manoukas, A.G. Effect of processing upon the tocopherol and tocotrienol composition of tale olives. Food Chem. **1994**, *50*, 111–114.
24. Lazos, E.S.; Tsaknis, J.; Lalas, S. Characteristics and composition of tomato seed oil. Grasas Aceites **1998**, *49*, 440–445.
25. Ranalli, A.; Cabras, P.; Iannucci, E.; Contento, S. Lipochromes, vitamins, aromas and other components of virgin olive oil are affected by processing technology. Food Chem. **2001**, *73*, 445–451.
26. Rossi, M.; Gianazza, M.; Alamprese, C.; Stanga, F. The effect of bleaching and physical refining on color and minor components of palm oil. JAOCS **2001**, *78*, 1051–1055.
27. Wang, T.; Johnson, L.A. Refining high-free fatty acid wheat germ oil. JAOCS **2001**, *78*, 71–76.
28. Kemény, Z.; Recseg, K.; Hénon, G.; Kővri, K.; Zwobada, F. Deodorization of vegetable oils: Prediction of trans polyunsaturated fatty acid content. JAOCS **2001**, *78*, 973–979.
29. Maza, A.; Ormsbee, R.A.; Strecker, L.R. Effects of deodorization and steam-refining parameters on finished oil quality. JAOCS **1992**, *69*, 1003–1008.
30. Ruiz-Méndez, M.V.; Garrido-Fernandez, A.; Rodriguez-Berbel, F.C.; Graciani-Constante, E. Relationships among the variables involved in the physical refining of olive oil using nitrogen as stripping gas. Fett/Lipid **1996**, *98*, 121–125.
31. Ruiz-Méndez, M.V.; Márqquez-Ruiz, G.; Dobarganes, M.C. Comparative performance of steam and nitrogen as stripping gas in physical refining of edible oils. JAOCS **1996**, *73*, 1641–1645.
32. Wang, X.; Wang, T.; Johnson, L.A. Composition and sensory qualities of minimum-refined soybean oils. JAOCS **2002**, *79*, 1207–1214.

33. Liu, L.; Lampert, D. Monitoring chemical interesterification. JAOCS **1999**, *76*, 783–787.
34. Park, D.K.; Terao, J.; Matsushita, S. Influence of interestification on the autoxidative stability of vegetable oils. Agric. Biol. Chem. **1983**, *47*, 121–123.
35. Jennings, B.H.; Akoh, C.C. Enzymatic modification of triacylglycerols of high eicosapentaenoic and docosahexaenoic acids content to produce structured lipids. JAOCS **1999**, *76*, 1133–1137.
36. McLaughlin, P.J.; Weihrauch, J.L. Vitamin E content of foods. J. Am. Diet Assoc. **1979**, *79*, 647–665.
37. Drotleff, A.M.; Ternes, W. Cis/trans isomers of tocotrienols—occurrence and bioavailability. Eur. Food Res. Technol. **1999**, *210*, 1–8.
38. Konings, E.J.M.; Roomans, H.H.S.; Beljaars, P.R. Liquid chromatographic determination of tocopherols and tocotrienols in margarine, infant foods and vegetables. JAOAC Int. **1996**, *79*, 902–906.
39. Rammell, C.G.; Hoogenboom, J.L. Separation of tocols by HPLC on an amino-cyano polar phase column. J. Liq. Chromatogr. **1985**, *8*, 707–717.
40. Bunnell, R.H.; Keating, J.; Quarasimo, A.; Parman, G.K. Alpha-tocopherol content of foods. Am. J. Clin. Nutr. **1965**, *17*, 1–10.
41. Lehmann, J.; Slover, H.T. Relative autoxidative and photolytic stabilities of tocols and tocotrienols. Lipids **1976**, *11*, 853–856.
42. Lea, C.H.; Ward, R.J. Relative antioxidant activities of the seven tocopherols. J. Sci. Food Agric. **1959**, *10*, 537–548.
43. Niki, E.; Tsuchiya, J.; Yoshikawa, Y.; Yamamoto, Y.; Kamiya, Y. Antioxidant activities of $\alpha$-, $\beta$-, $\gamma$- and $\delta$- tocopherols. Bull. Chem. Soc. Jpn **1986**, *59*, 497–501.
44. Yoshida, H.; Hirooka, N.; Kajimoto, G. Microwave energy effects on quality of some seed oils. J. Food Sci. **1990**, *55*, 1412–1416.
45. Yoshida, H.; Tatsumi, M.; Kajimoto, G. Relationship between oxidative stability of vitamin E and production of fatty acids in oils during microwave heating. JAOCS **1991**, *68*, 566–570.
46. Gordan, M.H.; Kourimska, L. Effect of antioxidants on losses of tocopherols during deep-fat frying. Food Chem. **1995**, *52*, 175–177.
47. Barrera-Arellano, D.; Ruiz-Méndez, V.; Velasco, J.; Márqquez-Ruiz, G.; Dobarganes, C. Loss of tocopherols and formation of degradation compounds at frying temperatures in oils differing in degree of unsaturation and natural antioxidant content. J. Sci. Food Agric. **2002**, *82*, 1696–1702.
48. DuPlessis, L.M.; Van Twisk, P.; van Niekerk, P.J.; Steyn, M. Evaluation of peanut and cottonseed oils for deep frying. JAOCS **1981**, *58*, 575–578.
49. Carlson, B.L.; Tabacch, M.H. Frying oil deterioration and vitamin loss during food service operation. J. Food Sci. **1986**, *51*, 218–221, 230.
50. Miyagawa, K.; Hirai, K.; Takezoe, R. Tocopherol and fluorescence levels in deep-frying oil and their measurement for oil assessment. JAOCS **1991**, *68*, 163–167.
51. Simonne, A.H.; Eitenmiller, R.R. Retention of vitamin E and added retinyl palmitate in selected vegetable oils during deep-fat frying and in fried breaded products. J. Agric. Food Chem. **1998**, *46*, 5273–5277.

52. Frankel, E.; Evans, C.; Cooney, P. Tocopherol oxidation in natural fats. J. Agric. Food Chem. **1959**, *7*, 438–440.
53. Yuki, E.; Ishikawa, Y. Tocopherol contents of nine vegetable frying oils and their changes under simulated deep-fat frying conditions. JAOCS **1976**, *53*, 673–676.
54. Barrera-Arellano, D.; Ruiz-Méndez, V.; Ruiz, G.M.; Dobarganes, C. Loss of tocopherols and formation of degradation compounds in triacylglycerol model systems heated at high temperature. J. Sci. Food Agric. **1999**, *79*, 1923–1928.
55. Ruiz, G.M.; Polvillo, M.M.; Jorge, N.; Mendez, M.V.R.; Dobarganes, M.C. Influence of used frying oil quality and natural tocopherol content on oxidative stability of fried potatoes. JAOCS **1999**, *76*, 421–425.
56. Andrikopoulos, N.K.; Kalogeropoulos, N.; Falirea, A.; Barbagianni, M.N. Performance of virgin olive oil and vegetable shortening during domestic deep-frying and pan-frying of potatoes. Int. J. Food Sci. Technol. **2002**, *37*, 177–190.
57. Normand, L.; Eskin, N.A.M.; Przybylski, R. Effect of tocopherols on the frying stability of regular and modified canola oils. JAOCS **2001**, *78*, 369–373.
58. Holownia, K.I.; Erickson, M.C.; Chinnan, M.S.; Eitenmiller, R.R. Tocopherols losses in peanut oil during pressure frying of marinated chicken strips coated with edible films. Food Res. Int. **2001**, *34*, 7–80.
59. Suknark, K.; Lee, J.; Eitenmiller, R.R.; Phillips, R.D. Stability of tocopherols and retinyl palmitate in snack extrudates. J. Food Sci. **2001**, *66*, 897–902.
60. Cabell, C.A.; Ellis, N.R. The vitamin E content of certain varieties of corn, wheat, grasses and legumes as determined by rat assay. J. Nutr. **1942**, *23*, 633–644.
61. Brown, F. The tocopherol content of farm feeding-stuffs. J. Food Sci. Agric. **1953**, *4*, 161–165.
62. Akopyan, G.O. Variations in the tocopherol content of plants as affected by process and duration of drying and storage. Izv. Nauk. Armyan SSR Ser. Biol. **1962**, *15*, 29–35.
63. Akopyan, O. The content of vitamin E in Vetches of the Stepanavan region. Izv. Akad. Nauk. Armyan SSR Ser. Biol. **1958**, *11*, 95–97.
64. Thalvelin, B.; Okamen, H. Vitamin E and linolenic acid content of hay as related to different drying conditions. J. Dairy Sci. **1966**, *49*, 282–286.
65. Charkey, L.W.; Pyke, W.E.; Kano, A.; Carlson, R.E. Carotene and tocopherol content of dehydrated and sun-cured alfalfa meals. J. Agric. Food Chem. **1961**, *9*, 70–77.
66. Livingston, A.L.; Nelson, J.W.; Kohler, G.O. Stability of $\alpha$-tocophoerol during alfalfa dehydration and storage. J. Agric. Food Chem. **1968**, *16*, 492–495.
67. Thomas, M.H.; Calloway, D.H. Nutritional value of dehydrated foods. J. Am. Diet Assoc. **1961**, *39*, 105–116.
68. Daood, H.G.; Vinkler, M.; Markus, F.; Hebshi, E.A.; Biacs, P.A. Antioxidant vitamin content of spice red pepper (paprika) as affected by technological and varietal factors. Food Chem. **1996**, *55*, 365–372.
69. Carvajal, M.; Gimenez, J.L.; Riquelme, F.; Alcaraz, C.F. Antioxidant content and color level in different varieties of red pepper (Capsicum annuum L.) affected by plant-leaf $Ti^4$ spray and processing. Acta Aliment. **1998**, *27*, 365–375.
70. Murcia, M.A.; Vera, A.; Garcia-Carmona, F. Determination by HPLC of changes in tocopherol levels in spinach after industrial processing. J. Sci. Food Agric. **1992**, *60*, 81–84.

71. Abushita, A.A.; Daood, H.G.; Biacs, P.A. Change in carotenoids and antioxidant vitamins in tomato as a function of varietal and technological factors. J. Agric. Food Chem. **2000**, *48*, 2075–2081.
72. Food Safety and Inspection. Backgrounder, USDA Issues Final Rule on Meat and Poultry Irradiation. December, 1999.
73. Yoshida, H.; Kajimoto, G. Effects of microwave energy on the tocopherols of soybean seeds. J. Food Sci. **1989**, *54*, 1596–1600.
74. Yoshida, H.; Hirooka, N.; Kajimoto, G. Microwave energy effects on quality of some seed oils. J. Food Sci. **1990**, *55*, 1412–1416.
75. Yoshida, H.; Tatsumi, M.; Kajimoto, G. Relationship between oxidative stability of vitamin E and production of fatty acids during microwave heating. JAOCS **1991**, *68*, 566–570.
76. Yoshida, H.; Hirooka, N.; Kajimoto, G. Microwave heating effects on relative stabilities of tocopherols in oils. J. Food Sci. **1991**, *56*, 1042–1046.
77. Yoshida, H.; Tatsumi, M.; Kajimoto, G. Influence of fatty acids on the tocopherol stability in vegetable oils during microwave heating. JAOCS **1992**, *69*, 119–125.
78. Yoshida, H.; Kondo, I.; Kajimoto, G. Effects of microwave energy on the relative stability of vitamin E in animal fats. J. Sci. Food Agric. **1992**, *58*, 531–534.
79. Yoshida, H.; Kajimoto, G.; Emura, S. Antioxidant effects of $\alpha$-tocopherols at different concentrations in oils during microwave heating. JAOCS **1993**, *70*, 989–995.
80. Yoshida, H.; Takagi, S. Antioxidative effects of sesamol and tocopherols at various concentrations in oils during microwave heating. J. Sci. Food Agric. **1999**, *79*, 220–226.
81. Yoshida, H.; Takagi, S.; Mitsuhashi, S. Tocopherol distribution and oxidative stability of oils prepared from the hypocotyl of soybeans roasted in a microwave oven. JAOCS **1999**, *76*, 915–920.
82. Takagi, S.; Ienaga, H.; Tsuchiya, C.; Yoshida, H. Microwave roasting effects on the composition of tocopherols and acyl lipids with each structural part and section of a soya bean. J. Sci. Food Agric. **1999**, *79*, 1155–1162.
83. Medrano, A.; Hernandez, A.; Prodanov, M.; Vidal-Valverde, C. Riboflavin, $\alpha$-tocopherol and retinol retention in milk after microwave heating. Lait. **1994**, *74*, 153–159.
84. Ruiz-Lopez, M.O.; Artacho, R.; Pineda, M.A.; Garcia de la Serrana, H.; Martinez, M.C. Stability of $\alpha$-tocopherol in virgin olive oil during microwave heating. Lebensm. Wiss. u. Technol. **1995**, *28*, 644–646.
85. Shahidi, F.; Amarowicz, R.; Abou-Gharbia, H.A.; Adel-Shehata, A. Endogenous antioxidants and stability of sesame oil as affected by processing and storage. JOACS **1997**, *74*, 143–148.
86. Oomah, B.D.; Liang, J.; Godfrey, D.; Mazza, G. Microwave heating of grapeseed: Effect on oil quality. J. Agric. Food Chem. **1998**, *46*, 4017–4021.
87. Murcia, M.A.; Martínez-Tomé, M.; Cerro, I.; Sotillo, F.; Ramírez, A. Proximate composition and vitamin E levels in egg yolk: Losses by cooking in a microwave oven. J. Sci. Food Agric. **1999**, *79*, 1550–1556.
88. Wise, R.R.; Naylor, A.W. Chilling-enhanced photooxidation. The peroxidative destruction of lipids during chilling injury to photosynthesis and ultrastructure, a comparision of cucumber and pea. Plant Physiol. **1987**, *83*, 272–277.

89. Wise, R.R.; Naylor, A.W. Chilling-enhanced photooxidation: Evidence for the role of singlet oxygen and superoxide and endogenous antioxidants. Plant Physiol. **1987**, *83*, 278–282.
90. Shewfelt, R.L.; del Rosario, B.A. The role of lipid peroxidation in storage disorders of fresh fruits and vegetables. Hortic. Sci. **2000**, *35*, 575–579.
91. Teramura, A.H.; Sullivan, J.H. Effects of UV-B radiation on photosynthesis and growth of terrestrial plants. Photosynth. Res. **1994**, *39*, 463–473.
92. DeLong, J.M.; Steffen, K.L. Photosynthetic function, lipid peroxidation, and $\alpha$-tocopherol content in spinach leaves during exposure to UV-B radiation. Can. J. Plant Sci. **1997**, *77*, 453–459.
93. Hess, J.L. Vitamin E, $\alpha$-tocopherol. In *Antioxidants in Higher Plants*; Alscher, R.G., Hess, J.L., Eds.; CRC Press: Boca Raton, FL, 1993.
94. Shewfelt, R.L.; Purvis, A.C. Toward a comprehensive model for lipid peroxidation in plant tissue disorders. Hortic. Sci. **1995**, *30*, 213–217.
95. Erickson, M.C.; Shewfelt, R.L.; del Rosario, B.A.; Wang, G.D.; Purvis, A.C. Localized antioxidant degradation in relation to promotion of lipid oxidation. In *Chemical Markers for Processed and Stored Foods*; Lee, T.C., Kim, H.J., Eds.; ACS Symposium Series 631, American Chemical Society: Washington DC, 1996.
96. Expert Panel on Food Safety and Nutrition. Irradiation of Food. Institute of Food Technologists, Scientific Status Summary, January, 1998.
97. Federal Register. 9CFR, Parts 381 and 424, December 23, 1999.
98. Jo, C.; Ahn, D.U. Volatiles and oxidative changes in irradiated pork sausage with different fatty acid composition and tocopherol content. J. Food Sci. **2000**, *65*, 270–275.
99. Lakritz, L.; Thayer, D.W. Effect of ionizing radiation on unesterified tocopherols in fresh chicken breast muscle. Meat Sci. **1992**, *32*, 257–265.
100. Fox, J.B., Jr.; Lakritz, L.; Kohout, K.H.; Thayer, D.W. Water concentration/activity and loss of vitamins B-1 and E in pork due to gamma radiation. J. Food Sci. **1994**, *59*, 1291–1295.
101. Lakritz, L.; Fox, J.B., Jr.; Hampson, J.; Richardson, R.; Kohout, K.; Thayer, D.W. Effect of gamma radiation on levels of $\alpha$-tocopherol in red meats and turkey. Meat Sci. **1995**, *41*, 261–271.
102. Lakritz, L.; Fox, J.B., Jr.; Thayer, D.W. Thiamin, riboflavin and $\alpha$-tocopherol content of exotic meats and loss due to gamma radiation. J. Food Protect. **1998**, *61*, 1681–1683.
103. Armstrong, S.G.; Wyllie, S.G.; Leach, D.N. Effects of preservation by gamma-irradiation on the nutritional quality of Australian fish. Food Chem. **1994**, *50*, 351–357.
104. Al-Katani, H.; Abu-Tarboush, H.; Bajaber, A.; Atia, M.; Abou-Arab, A.; El-Mojaddidi, M. Chemical changes after irradiation and post-irradiation storage in Tilapia and Spanish mackerel. J. Food Sci. **1996**, *61*, 729–733.
105. Tipples, K.H.; Norris, F.W. Some effects of high levels of gamma irradiation on the lipids of wheat. Cereal Chem. **1965**, *42*, 437–451.
106. Kung, H.C.; Gaden, E.L.; King, C.G. Effect of gamma irradiation on activity—vitamins and enzymes in milk. J. Agric. Food Chem. **1953**, *1*, 142–144.

107. Bagorogoza, K.; Bowers, J.; Okot-Kotber, M. The effect of irradiation and modified atmosphere packaging on the quality of intact chill-stored turkey breast. J. Food Sci. **2001**, *66*, 367–372.
108. Haytowitz, D. Personal communication. United States Department of Agriculture, 2000.
109. Piironen, V.; Syväoja, E.L.; Varo, P.; Salminen, K.; Koivistoinen, P. Tocopherols and tocotrienols in cereal products from Finland. Cereal Chem. **1986**, *63*, 78–81.
110. Herting, D.C.; Drury, E.J. Alpha-tocopherol content of cereal grains and processed cereals. J. Agric. Food Chem. **1969**, *17*, 785–790.
111. Slover, H.T.; Lehmann, J. Effects of fumigation on wheat in storage. IV. Tocopherols. Cereal Chem. **1972**, *49*, 412–415.
112. Peterson, D.M.; Qureshi, A.A. Genotype and environment effects on tocols of barley and oats. Cereal Chem. **1993**, *70*, 157–162.
113. Lorenz, K.; Limjaroenrat, P. The alpha-tocopherol content of triticales and triticale milling fractions. Lebensm. Wiss. Technol. **1974**, *7*, 86–88.
114. Wang, L.; Xue, Q.; Newman, R.K.; Newman, C.W. Enrichment of tocopherols, tocotrienols, and oil in barley fractions by milling and pearling. Cereal Chem. **1993**, *70*, 499–501.
115. Hall, G.S.; Laidman, D.L. The determination of tocopherols and isoprenoid quinones in the grain and seedlings of wheat (Triticum vulgare). Biochem. J. **1968**, *108*, 465–473.
116. Grams, G.W.; Blessin, C.W.; Inglett, G.E. Distribution of tocopherols within the corn kernel. Cereal Chem. **1970**, *47*, 337–339.
117. Chow, C.K.; Draper, H.H. Effect of artificial drying on tocopherols and fatty acids of corn. J. Agric. Food Chem. **1969**, *17*, 1316–1317.
118. Pond, W.G.; Allaway, W.H.; Walker, E.F., Jr.; Krook, L. Effects of corn selenium content and drying temperature and of supplemental vitamin E on growth liver selenium and blood vitamin E content of chicks. J. Anim. Sci. **1971**, *33*, 996–1000.
119. Hàkansson, B.; Jägerstad, M.; Öste, R.; Akesson, B.; Jonsson, L. The effects of various thermal processes on protein quality, vitamins and selenium content in whole-grain wheat and white flour. J. Cereal Sci. **1987**, *6*, 269–282.
120. Hàkansson, B.; Jägerstad, M. The effect of thermal inactivation of lipoxygenase on the stability of vitamin E in wheat. J. Cereal Sci. **1990**, *12*, 177–185.
121. Wennermark, B.; Ahlmén, H.; Jägerstad, M. Improved vitamin E retention by using freshly milled whole-meal wheat flour during drum-drying. J. Agric. Food Chem. **1994**, *42*, 1348–1351.
122. Bryngelsson, S.; Dimberg, L.H.; Kamal-Eldin, A. Effects of commercial processing on levels of antioxidants in oats (Avena sativa L.). J. Agric. Food Chem. **2002**, *50*, 1890–1896.
123. Mattern, P.J. Wheat. In *Handbook of Cereal Science and Technology*; Lorenz, K.J., Kulp, K., Ed.; Marcel Dekker: New York, 1991; 1–53.
124. Wennermark, B.; Jägerstad, M. Breadmaking and storage of various wheat fractions affect vitamin E. J. Food Sci. **1992**, *57*, 1205–1209.
125. Binnington, D.S.; Andrews, J.S. The distribution of vitamin E in products of cereal milling. Cereal Chem. **1941**, *18*, 618–686.

126. Peterson, D.M. Barley tocols: Effects of milling, malting, and mashing. Cereal Chem. **1994**, *71*, 42–44.
127. Grams, G.W.; Blessin, C.W.; Inglett, G.E. Distribution of tocopherols in wet- and dry-milled corn products. Cereal Chem. **1971**, *48*, 356–359.
128. Howland, D.W.; Pienkowski, J.J.; Reiners, R.A. The effect of wet-milling on the tocopherols in corn germ oil. Cereal Chem. **1973**, *50*, 661–665.
129. Wang, C.; Ning, J.; Krishnan, P.G.; Matthees, D.P. Effects of steeping conditions during wet-milling on the retentions of tocopherols and tocotrienols in corn. JAOCS **1998**, *75*, 609–613.
130. Engel, C. The tocopherol (vitamin E) content of milling products from wheat, rye and barley and the influence of beaching. Z. Vitaminforsch. **1942**, *12*, 220–224.
131. Slover, H.T.; Lehmann, J.; Valis, R.J. Nutrient composition of selected wheats and wheat products. III. Tocopherols. JAOCS **1969**, *46*, 635–641.
132. Krishna, A.G.G.; Prabhakar, J.V.; Sen, D.P. Effect of degree of milling on tocopherol content of rice bran. J. Food Sci. Technol. **1984**, *21*, 222–224.
133. Sun, H.; Wiesenborn, D.; Rayas-Duarte, P.; Mohamed, A.; Hagen, K. Bench-scale processing of Amaranth seed for oil. JAOCS **1995**, *72*, 1551–1555.
134. Becker, R.; Irving, D.W.; Saunders, R.M. Production of Debranned Amaranth Flour by Stone Mill. London: Academic Press, 1986; 372–375.
135. Sondi, A.B.; Reddy, I.M.; Bhattacharya, K.R. Effect of processing conditions on the oil content of parboiled-rice bran. Food Chem. **1980**, *5*, 277–282.
136. Camire, M.E. Chemical changes during extrusion cooking: recent advances. In *Process-Induced Chemical Changes in Food*; Shahidi, F., Ho, C.T., Chuyen, N.V., Eds.; New York and London: Plenum Press, 1998.
137. Zadernowski, R.; Nowak-Polakowska, H.; Rashed, A.A. The influence of heat treatment on the activity of lipo-and hydrophlic components of oat grain. J. Food Proc. Pres. **1999**, *23*, 177–191.
138. Shin, T.S.; Godber, J.S.; Martin, D.E.; Wells, J.H. Hydrolytic stability and changes in E vitamers and oryzanol of extruded rice bran during storage. J. Food Sci. **1997**, *62*, 704–708.
139. Grela, E.R.; Jensen, S.K.; Jakobsen, K. Fatty acid composition and content of tocopherols and carotenoids in raw and extruded grass pea. J. Sci. Food Agric. **1999**, *79*, 2075–2078.
140. Mustakas, G.C.; Albretch, W.J.; Bookwalter, G.N.; McGhee, J.E.; Kwolek, W.F.; Griffin, E.L., Jr. Extruder processing to improve nutritional quality, flavor and keeping quality of full-fat soy flour. Food Technol. **1970**, *24*, 102–108.
141. Harper, J.M.; Jansen, G.R. Production of nutritious precooked foods in developing countries by low-cost extrusion technology. Food Rev. Int. **1985**, *1*, 27–97.
142. Guzman, G.J.; Murphy, P.A.; Johnson, L.A. Properties of soybean-corn mixtures processed by low-cost extrusion. J. Food Sci. **1989**, *54*, 1590–1593.
143. Ringe, M.L.; Love, M.H. Kinetics of protein quality change in an extruded cowpea-corn flour blend under varied steady-state storage. J. Food Sci. **1988**, *53*, 584–588.
144. Lorenz, K.; Jansen, G.R. Nutrient stability of full-fat soy flour and corn-soy blends produced by low-cost extrusion. Cereal Foods World **1980**, *25*, 161–162, 171–172.

145. Frazier, A.C.; Lines, J.G. Studies on changes in flour tocopherols following aging and treatment of the flour with chlorin dioxide. J. Sci. Food Agric. **1967**, *18*, 203–207.
146. Moran, T.; Pace, J.; McDermott, E.E. Interaction of chlorine dioxide with flour: Certain chemical aspects. Nature **1953**, *171*, 103–106.
147. Moran, T.; Pace, J.; McDermott, E.E. The lipids in flour: Oxidative changes induced by storage and improver treatment. Nature **1954**, *174*, 449–452.
148. Moore, T.; Sharman, I.M.; Ward, R.J. The destruction of vitamin E in flour by chlorine dioxide. J. Sci. Food Agric. **1957**, *8*, 97–104.
149. Mason, E.L.; Jones, W.L. The tocopherol contents of some Australian cereals and flour milling products. J. Sci. Food Agric. **1958**, *9*, 524–529.
150. Frazer, A.C.; Hickman, J.R.; Sammons, H.G.; Sharratt, M. Studies on the effects of treatment with chlorine dioxide on the properties of wheat flour. III. Lipid changes and vitamin content of treated flours. J. Sci. Food Agric. **1956**, *7*, 375–380.
151. Frazer, A.C.; Hickman, J.R.; Sammons, H.G.; Sharratt, M. Studies on the effects of treatment with chlorine dioxide on the properties of wheat flour. IV. The biological properties of untreated, normally treated and overtreated flours. J. Sci. Food Agric. **1956**, *7*, 464–470.
152. Moore, T.; Sharman, I.M.; Ward, R.J. Flour and bread, prepared with or without treatment with chlorine dioxide, as long-term sources of vitamin E for rats. Br. J. Nutr. **1958**, *12*, 215–226.
153. Ranum, P.M.; Loewe, R.J.; Gordon, H.T. Effect of bleaching, malting, and oxidizing agents on vitamins added to wheat flour. Cereal Chem. **1981**, *58*, 32–35.
154. Yoshida, H.; Hirakawa, Y.; Abe, S.; Mizushina, Y. The content of tocopherols and oxidative quality of oils prepared from sunflower (*Helianthus annuus* L.) seeds roasted in a microwave oven. Eur. J. Lipid Sci. Technol. **2002**, *104*, 116–122.
155. Dial, S.; Eitenmiller, R.R. Tocopherols and tocotrienols in key foods in the U.S. Diet. In *Nutrition, Lipids, Health and Disease*; Ong, As H, Nike, E., Packer, L., Eds.; AOCS Press: Champaign, IL, 1995.
156. Kaushik, S.; Wander, R.; Leonard, S.; German, B.; Traber, M.G. Removal of fat from cow's milk decreases the vitamin E contents of the resulting dairy products. Lipids **2001**, *36*, 73–78.
157. Ford, J.E.; Porter, J.W.G.; Thompson, S.Y.; Toothill, J.; Edwards-Webb, J. Effects of ultra high-temperature (UHT) processing and of subsequent storage on the vitamin content of milk. J. Dairy Res. **1969**, *36*, 447–454.
158. Andrikopoulos, N.K.; Dedoussis, G.V.Z.; Falirea, A.; Kalogeropoulos, N.; Hatzinikola, H.S. Deterioration of natural antioxidant species of vegetable edible oils during the domestic deep-frying and pan-frying of potatoes. Int. J. Food Sci. Nutr. **2002**, *53*, 351–363.

# 6

# Effects of Food Preparation and Storage on the Vitamin E Content of Food

## 6.1. INTRODUCTION

Food preparation either in a commercial setting or in a household can significantly impact levels of vitamin E in the food at the ready-to-consume stage. Changes during cooking can be beneficial or detrimental and depend on many variables. Increased vitamin E concentrations can be expected if ingredients such as vegetable oils with relatively high vitamin E content compared to that of the primary components are added to a mixed dish. Likewise, the method of preparation influences vitamin E content at the point of consumption. Deep-fat frying of raw foods low in vitamin E, e.g., vegetables, produces a consumable product with potentially high vitamin E content. The tocopherol and tocotrienol profiles become similar to that of the frying oil because of fat uptake from the oil into the fried food. Other preparation methods such as broiling, roasting, and baking can be quite destructive to vitamin E, depending on time and temperature effects and the degree of lipid oxidation taking place in the food during cooking and during storage of the cooked product.

Storage of raw and processed foods can produce significant decreases in vitamin E level. Packaging methods and materials, length and temperature of storage, characteristics of the food and its susceptibility to lipid oxidation, availability of other natural or synthetic antioxidants in the food, and many other factors affect the stability of vitamin E during storage. Ames(1) in his early review on the occurrence of vitamin E in food stated that foods are normally exposed to deleterious factors during processing and storage that can lead to large losses in vitamin E level. Normally, storage losses are related to lipid oxidation occurring in the food and the interaction of vitamin E as an antioxidant. This chapter is presented in two sections to examine the effects of food preparation and storage on vitamin E level.

## 6.2. EFFECTS OF FOOD PREPARATION ON THE VITAMIN E CONTENT OF FOODS

Bauernfeind (2,3) reported that most forms of heating used in common cooking methods adversely affect the vitamin E content of the prepared food. As discussed in Chapter 5, thermal processes, including dehydration and extrusion, can be quite destructive with regard to vitamin E level during commercial food processing operations. In the following sections, effects of home preparation of foods are discussed. Summaries of pertinent literature are provided in Table 6.1.

### 6.2.1. Effect of Deep-Fat Frying on the Vitamin E Content of Food

Deep-fat frying is simply defined as cooking of food by immersion in hot oil (4). Because of the high ratio of oil to food, oil absorption readily occurs; therefore, the quality of the cooking oil becomes a primary consideration in the quality and shelf stability of the fried product. The vitamin E content of the fried food is variable, depending on the oil type, oil quality, degree of oil uptake, and many other factors that control oil absorption during the frying process. Because of the significance of the effects of oil absorption on product quality and cost, the phenomenon has been the subject of extensive research. Mechanisms involve fluid flow into the porous food structure produced by the volatilzation of water; the level of surfactants produced in the oil through use and oil degradation; the food matrix; the properties of the breading material, if used; and factors that control oil absorption during postfrying or cooling phases of the process. Continuing research shows the physical and chemical complexity of deep-fat frying. Blumenthal (5) summarized the significance of surfactants to oil absorption and final quality of the fried product with the following observations:

1. Low levels of surfactants in the oil lead to introduction of low levels of oxygen into the oil.

**TABLE 6.1** The Effect of Cooking on the Vitamin E Content of Foods

| Food | Cooking methods | Observations | References |
|---|---|---|---|
| **Meat and fish** | | | |
| Beef | Broiling, roasting, braising | Losses on dry weight basis 33–44%; greatest loss of vitamin E from broiling least from roasting | 1982, 16 |
| Channel catfish | Cooking: 177°C, 7 min, conventional household oven | No loss of vitamin E | 1991, 21 |
| Refrigerated minced channel catfish | Refrigeration: 0–7 days<br>Cooking: 177°C, 5 min | Loss of γ-T on cooking fairly constant (15%); losses of α-T greater in 2-day and 5-day refrigerated samples (40%) than in 7-day refrigerated samples (14%) | 1992, 24 |
| Boneless pork chops | Grilling: 93°C, 121°C, 148°C, 176°C, 204°C | In chops grilled at 204°C significantly lower vitamin E retention values when compared to 121°C, 148°C, and 176°C | 1998, 20 |
| Bison patties | Broiling, grilling: 71°C | α-T retention 76–83% | 1999, 21 |
| **Vegetables** | | | |
| Cereal, grain, tortilla, nut, legume, oil | Cooking by package instructions | Cooking loss for most grains 22% to 55%, loss for legumes 9% for garbanzo bean to 59% for bayo bean; almost all vitamin E destroyed by processing into tortillas | 1998, 27 |
| Bean, chick pea, lentils | Soaking (12 h, room-temperature, water), cooking | α-T losses<br>Soaking: 4%<br>Cooking: 10%<br>γ-T losses<br>Soaking: 2–5%<br>Cooking: 5–10%<br>3–10% Vitamin E transferred to cooking broth | 1998, 28 |

(*continued*)

**TABLE 6.1** *Continued*

| Food | Cooking methods | Observations | References |
|---|---|---|---|
| *Dhals* (peas, India) | Steam pressure cooking (10–20 min), drying, flaking, freezing–thawing, storage | α-T losses<br>Flaking and drying process: 23–32%<br>Cooking, drying, freeze–thaw drying: 11–16% | 2000, 29 |
| Cereals | | | |
| French bread (wheat/rye) | Scalding, fermentation, dough making, baking | No reduction of vitamin E content by scalding or fermentation; for sourdough preparation and dough making 20–60% reduction in vitamin E content | 1992, 36 |
| Milled barley | Heating: 75°C, 90°C, 105°C, 120°C, 48 h | 92% Loss of vitamin E in barley during heating at 120°C for 24 h; at 105°C and 120°C relative content of α-T3 increase at expense of other isomers | 1985, 38 |
| Sesame seed | Roasting (200°C, 20 min), steaming (100°C, 20 min), roasting (200°C, 15 min) + steaming (100°C, 7 min) | γ-T losses<br>Roasting: 20–33%<br>Steaming: 14–26%<br>Roasting plus steaming: 4–10% | 1997, 52 |
| Sunflower oil, high-oleic sunflower oil, olive oil, lard, virgin olive oil | Conventional heating: 180°C, 120 min, electric oven<br>Microwave heating: 170°C, 120 min | α-T losses by conventional heating<br>Sunflower oil: 39%<br>High-oleic sunflower oil: 46%<br>Virgin olive oil: 46%<br>Olive oil: 72%<br>α-T loss by microwave heating > by conventional heating | 1997, 53 |
| Egg yolk | Boiling: 3, 10 min, microwave heating, grilling: frying pan (omelette) | α-T losses<br>Boiling: 20%<br>Grilling: 46%<br>Microwave heating: 52%<br>No difference in α-T loss by boiling time | 1999, 32 |

γ-T, γ-tocopherol; α-T3, α-tocotrienol.

2. Moderate levels of surfactants lead to oxygenation and subsequent thermal oxidation. Oxidative degradation produces good heat-transfer properties in the oil and desirable volatiles.
3. The rate of oil degradation increases as surfactant levels increase. High surfactant concentrations, high oxygenation, and thermal oxidation of the oil produce short-chain fatty acids and a complex mixture of secondary oxidation products and polymeric materials that dramatically modify surfactant properties.
4. Low surfactant concentrations produce low absorption of the oil into the food and little cooking of the exterior and interior of the product. Residence time of the food in the oil moderates oil absorption.
5. Moderate surfactant levels produce a desired rate of oil absorption and proper cooking of the food. Surfactant concentrations at moderate to high levels produce longer contact times between the hot oil and the aqueous food surfaces. Better heat transfer increases the rate of dehydration at the surface, leading to increased water migration from the center to the exterior of the frying food.
6. High surfactant levels produce oil-soaked food that can be overcooked on the exterior and undercooked in the interior.
7. Higher surfactant concentrations produce greater deposition of polymeric material.

A better understanding of the surfactant theory of frying can lead to enhanced production efficiencies and higher-quality fried foods(5) Because of the degree of oil uptake, the lipid profile of the fried food often takes on the characteristics of the frying oil. If the oil is high-quality and contains residual antioxidant capacity, autoxidation during subsequent storage would be expected to be delayed. Likewise, the vitamin E profile of the fried food closely resembles the vitamin E profile of the frying oil. Content of vitamin E in the fried food, therefore, depends on oil absorption and the content of vitamin E in the frying oil, the native vitamin E content of the food being fried, and loss of vitamin E from the food matrix through transfer of the lipid in the food undergoing frying with the frying oil. With the inherent variability of the vitamin E levels in frying oils and the many factors affecting oil absorption and the final level of fat in the finished product, it is difficult to predict the vitamin E content of the fried food.

Surprisingly, few analytical values exist in the literature that accurately provide the vitamin E content of deep-fat fried foods (see Chapter 8). Dial and Eitenmiller (6) reported that corn and potato chips contained from 5.1 to 11.4 $\alpha$-tocopherol equivalent ($\alpha$-TE) units/100 g and that the $\alpha$-TE level depended upon the oil used for frying. Carlson and Tabacch (7) followed vitamin E levels in french fries with prolonged frying oil use in a commercial food service frying operation and found little correlation between vitamin E levels in the product and deterioration of the frying oil. The data (Table 6.2) showed that although tocopherol concentrations in the oil decreased with increasing usage, there was no significant change in the vitamin E in the french fries over the period of frying oil use. The effect of decreasing vitamin E levels in the oil was countered by a significant increase in fat uptake as the oil deteriorated, a finding that supports Blumenthal's (5) thoughts on factors impacting oil absorption. The rapid decrease in $\alpha$-tocopherol ($\alpha$-T) level in sunflower oil used for successive fryings of potatoes is shown in Figure 6.1 (8). Oil uptake by the french fries ranged from 10.9–12.8% for deep-frying and from 5.7–6.5% for pan frying. Some oil uptake variation was noted for different frying oils. The $\alpha$-T content of the oil and, thus, the $\alpha$-T content of the fried food depend on the type of frying oil, duration of use of the oil, and whether fresh oil was added to the used oil to compensate for oil absorbed by the food.

Levels of vitamin E in chicken nuggets and breaded shrimp before and after frying in palm olein are given in Table 6.3.(9) Because the chicken nuggets were flash-fried before deep-fat frying, the increase in total vitamin E level was not substantial (from 4.6 mg/100 g before frying to 4.9 mg/100 g after frying). However, in breaded shrimp, total vitamin E level increased from 0.6 to 5.8 mg/100 g. Similar trends were noted for products fried in corn oil and soybean oil, and the vitamin E profiles of the fried foods closely resembled those of the specific frying oils. Stability of vitamin E in the frying oils is discussed in Chapter 5. Ruiz et al. (10) followed changes in $\alpha$-T level in potatoes fried in oils of varying quality for 30 days at 60°C to evaluate oxidative stability. The decrease of $\alpha$-T level during storage was more rapid during storage in potatoes fried in more unsaturated oils. $\alpha$-Tocopherol in oil extracted from potatoes fried

**TABLE 6.2** $\alpha$- and $\gamma$-Tocopherol Content of French Fries Prepared in Used Frying Oils

| | | Vitamin E (mg/100 g) | | |
|---|---|---|---|---|
| Stage of use[a] | Percentage of french fries | $\alpha$-T | $\gamma$-T | Free fatty acids[b] ($\times 10^{-2}$M) |
| Before cooking | 5.3 | 0.06 | 0.36 | 0.28 |
| Day 1 initial | 7.7 | 0.15 | 1.27 | 0.38 |
| Day 1 final | 11.0 | 0.14 | 0.89 | 0.46 |
| Day 2 | 12.4 | 0.14 | 1.31 | 0.54 |
| Day 3 | 14.4 | 0.14 | 1.03 | 1.25 |
| Day 4 | 15.8 | 0.12 | 1.28 | 1.47 |

$\alpha$-T, $\alpha$-tocopherol.
[a]Total product load was approximately 300 kg over the usage period.
[b]Fatty acid content of the frying oil, partially hydrogenated soybean oil with tertiary butylhydroquinone (TBHQ) and citric acid.
*Source*: Modified from Ref. 7.

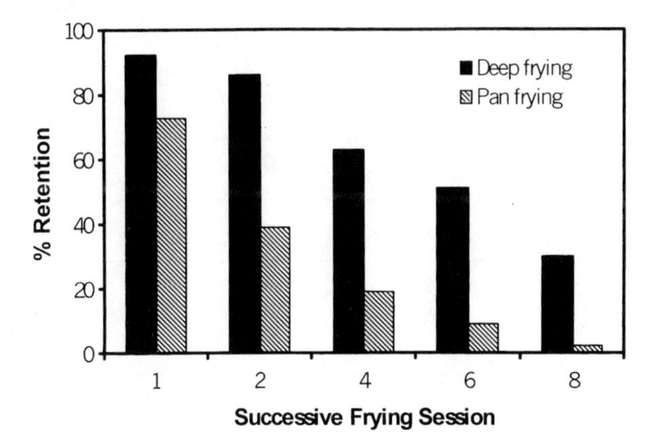


**FIGURE 6.1** Retention of α-tocopherol level during successive deep-fat frying (10 min each frying) and pan frying of french fries in sunflower oil. (Modified from Ref. 8.)

in sunflower oil reached nondetectable levels after 14 days of storage, whereas α-T in oil from potatoes fried in high-oleic sunflower oil was still at detectable levels at 21 days of storage (Table 6.4). Likewise, peroxide values and oil stability index values indicated more rapid oxidative deterioration in the potatoes fried in oils containing lower α-T levels. Overall, the length of the induction period could not be correlated to the degree of unsaturation or polar compound levels in the fried potatoes before storage. The work showed the significance of residual antioxidants in the frying oil to oxidative stability of the fried product during storage. Further, the authors concluded that antioxidant protection is

**TABLE 6.3** Vitamin E Content of Products Before and After Deep-Fat Frying in Palm Olein

| | Vitamin E (mg/100 g) | | | | | | | |
|---|---|---|---|---|---|---|---|---|
| | α-T | β-T | γ-T | δ-T | α-T3 | γ-T3 | δ-T3 | Total |
| Chicken nuggets | | | | | | | | |
| Initial | 0.8 | 0.1 | 3.1 | 0.7 | ND | ND | ND | 4.6 |
| After frying | 1.1 | 0.6 | ND[a] | 0.9 | 1.0 | 1.4 | 0.3 | 4.9 |
| Breaded shrimp | | | | | | | | |
| Initial | 0.5 | ND | 0.1 | ND | ND | ND | ND | 0.6 |
| After frying | 1.7 | 0.2 | ND | 0.1 | 1.4 | 1.8 | 0.4 | 5.8 |

α-T, α-tocopherol; α-T3, α-tocotrienol. ND, not detected.
*Source*: Modified from Ref. 9.

TABLE 6.4 α-Tocopherol Content (mg/100 g) of Oils Extracted From Fried Potatoes Stored at 60°C

| | Days | | | | | |
|---|---|---|---|---|---|---|
| | 0 | 3 | 5 | 7 | 9 | 21 |
| Oils | mg/100g | | | | | |
| Sunflower | 55 | 55 | 40 | 25 | 7 | — |
| High-oleic sunflower | 39 | NA | NA | 38 | NA | 21 |

NA, Not assayed.
*Source*: Modified from Ref. 10.

essential for preparation of fried foods that require storage before consumption to prevent rapid oxidative deterioration. Added ascorbyl palmitate (500 mg/kg) to potatoes fried in sunflower oil and stored at 100°C significantly increased the induction time of oxidation and decreased loss of the tocopherols (Table 6.5) (11).

Application of edible coating on the surface of meats before frying influences oil absorption during frying and, thus, influences vitamin E content in the food and stability in the frying oil. Such effects have been noted in battered and tempura-coated foods (12,13) and in foods coated with hydroxypropylmethylcellulose (14).

### 6.2.2. Effect of Various Preparation Methods

As noted in the previous section for deep-fat fried foods, surprisingly few detailed studies define the effects of other cooking methods on the vitamin E content of foods. The USDA Nutrient Database for Standard Reference, Release 16 (15) provides cooking retention factors for 18 nutrients, but not for vitamin E. The following sections summarize the available studies that give specific information on cooking effects on vitamin E. Tabular summaries are given in Table 6.1.

**6.2.2.1. Meat and Fish.** The vitamin E content of meat and fish is composed almost exclusively of α-T usually at levels less than 0.5 mg/100 g (Chapter 8). Bennik and Ono (16) completed a comprehensive study of the vitamin E content of raw and cooked beef that included differentiation by carcass grade and by cooking methods. Vitamin E levels were assessed by several different methods (Emmerie-Engle, fluorescence, and liquid chromatography [LC]), and the data are of generally excellent quality. Data for the study are given

**TABLE 6.5** Induction Times at 100°C and Tocopherols (mg/kg) in Lipids Extracted from Potato Chips Fried in Sunflower Oil After Storage at 60°C

| Sample | Storage days (60°C) | IT (h) | α-T | β-T | γ-T | Total-T |
|---|---|---|---|---|---|---|
| Without ascorbyl palmitate | 0 | 12.7 | 672 | 22 | 8 | 701 |
| | 2 | 13.4 | 639 | 22 | 8 | 669 |
| | 4 | 4.6 | 562 | 22 | 8 | 592 |
| | 6 | 3.3 | 249 | 19 | 7 | 275 |
| | 8 | 0 | 115 | 5 | 0 | 120 |
| | 10 | 0 | 0 | 0 | 0 | 0 |
| | 12 | — | — | — | — | — |
| | 16 | 0 | 0 | 0 | 0 | 0 |
| With ascorbyl palmitate | 0 | 20.3 | 662 | 22 | 8 | 692 |
| | 2 | — | — | — | — | |
| | 4 | 16.9 | 541 | 21 | 7 | 570 |
| | 6 | 11.4 | 513 | 19 | 8 | |
| | 8 | 7.4 | 497 | 15 | 2 | 514 |
| | 10 | 1.7 | 175 | 15 | 5 | 195 |
| | 12 | — | — | — | — | — |
| | 16 | 1.0 | 20 | 4 | 0 | 24 |

IT, induction time; α-T, α-tocopherol.
*Source*: Modified from Ref. 11.

in Table 6.6. The overall study included vitamin E assay of 464 samples. Conclusions included the following:

1. On an edible weight basis, no differences in vitamin E content were apparent in raw, broiled, braised, and roasted beef.
2. On a dry weight basis, cooking losses were 35% to 44%, depending on the method. Vitamin E content of cooked meat is dependent upon moisture and fat losses in the drip. Therefore, on an edible weight basis, the extent of moisture and fat loss masks the true loss of vitamin E from the raw product.
3. On a dry weight basis, broiling produced the greatest loss of vitamin E when compared to roasting and braising.
4. No differences in vitamin E content were found among primal cuts or carcass grades.

In a later study, Ono et al. (17) reported the percentage retention values for vitamin E for veal cooked by methods best for each retail cut. This information

**TABLE 6.6** Tocopherol Content of Raw and Cooked Separable Lean Beef[a]

| Carcass grade[b] | Tocopherols (mg/100 g of edible weight) | | | | |
|---|---|---|---|---|---|
| | Raw | Broiled | Roasted | Braised | Mean value |
| Prime | 0.15 ± 0.02[c] (56)[c] | 0.13 ± 0.03 (20) | 0.13 ± 0.04 (16) | 0.12 ± 0.02 (20) | 0.13 ± 0.03 (112) |
| Choice | 0.22 ± 0.04 (27) | 0.18 ± 0.04 (9) | 0.24 ± 0.07 (8) | 0.20 ± 0.05 (10) | 0.21 ± 0.05 (54) |
| Good | 0.09 ± 0.01 (53) | 0.07 ± 0.01 (18) | 0.08 ± 0.01 (16) | 0.14 ± 0.03 (20) | 0.10 ± 0.01 (107) |
| Standard | 0.31 ± 0.04 (13) | 0.10 ± 0.04 (5) | 0.22 ± 0.02 (4) | 0.21 ± 0.03 (4) | 0.21 ± 0.04 (26) |
| Mean value | 0.16 ± 0.02 (149) | 0.12 ± 0.03 (52) | 0.14 ± 0.03 (44) | 0.15 ± 0.03 (54) | 0.15 ± 0.02 (299) |
| | mg/100g of dry meat | | | | |
| All grades | 540 | 300 | 350 | 320 | |
| | mg/100g of nitrogen | | | | |
| All grades | 4610 | 2570 | 3070 | 2980 | |

[a]Vitamin E content was determined colorimetrically.
[b]Samples were obtained from 14 retail cuts from 4 carcasses for the prime and good grades, 2 carcasses from the choice grade and 1 carcass from the choice grade, and 1 carcass from the standard grade.
[c]Mean ± SE. Numbers in brackets are the numbers of samples analyzed.
*Source*: Modified from Ref. 16.

(Table 6.7) shows that for each method true retention(15,18) was greater than 100%.

True retention (*% TR*) is calculated by the following formula:

$$\% \, TR = (Nc \times Gc)/Nr \times Gr \times 100$$

where

$Nc$ = nutrient content per gram of cooked food
$Gc$ = gram of cooked of food
$Nr$ = nutrient content per gram of raw food
$Gr$ = gram of food before cooking

This is the acceptable method to calculate nutrient retention values to account for loss of weight and solids from the raw product during preparation and cooking.

True retention values for cooking of pork were 44% for roasting (mean of several treatments) and approximately 80% retention for grilling pork chops to an

**TABLE 6.7** Retention of Vitamin E in Cooked Retail Cuts of Special Fed Veal

| Retail cut | Cooking method | Percentage retention |
|---|---|---|
| Arm steak | Braise, 164°C, 30 min | 103 |
| Blade steak | Braise, 164°C, 30 min | 101 |
| Loin chop | Braise, 164°C, 30 min | 103 |
| Sirloin chop | Braise, 164°C, 30 min | 101 |
| Rib roast | Roast, 164°C to internal temperature of 76°C | 133 |
| Cutlets | Pan fry, 192°C with vegetable oil, 6–12 min | 110 |

*Source*: Modified from Ref. 17.

internal temperature of 71°C at grill temperatures ranging from 93°C to 176°C (Figure 6.2) (19,20). At 204°C, the vitamin E content decreased significantly compared to that at the lower grill temperatures. Studies in 1999 on bison patties (21) and in 2001 on rabbit meat (22) indicated retention values of 76% for bison and 79–88% for rabbit, depending on the cooking method used. $\alpha$- and $\gamma$-Tocopherol in channel catfish muscle baked at 177°C for 5 min showed little loss (23,24). However, when refrigerated samples were stored minced and then cooked up to 40% of the $\alpha$-T was destroyed, indicating that disruption of the

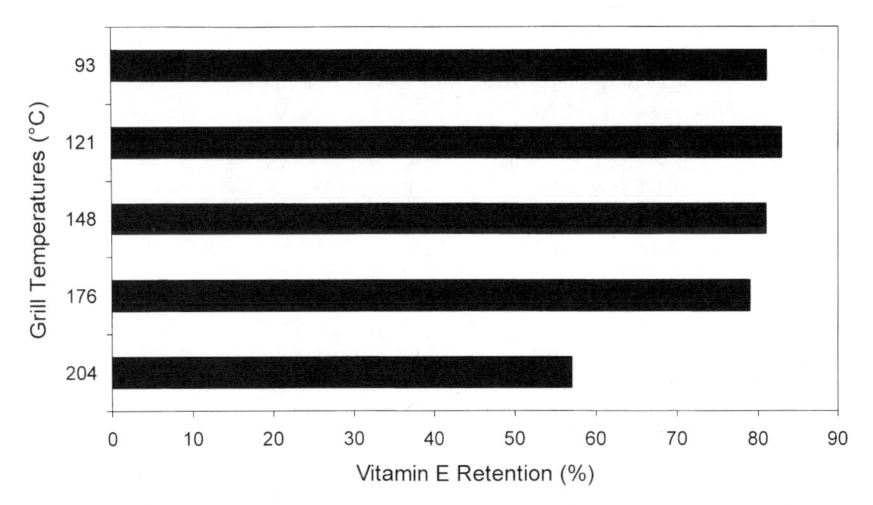


**FIGURE 6.2** True retention (percentage) of vitamin E level in grilled pork chops. (Modified from Ref. 20.)

integrity of the muscle and increased oxidative events can influence cooking stability (24).

**6.2.2.2. Vegetables.** Few definitive studies show the effect of home preparation procedures on vitamin E content of vegetables. Tocopherols and tocotrienols are not severely affected by home cooking procedures because of their fat-solubility (25). The fat-soluble vitamins, in general, are not subject to water leaching losses, which can significantly decrease concentrations of water-soluble vitamins and minerals in cooked vegetables. The few literature sources that provide cooking loss information for vitamin E tend to support the finding that normal cooking of vegetables does not dramatically decrease vitamin E levels on an edible weight basis. Only a 10–20% decrease in vitamin E resulted from boiling carrots, cabbage, brussels sprouts, and leeks (26) Data presented in Chapter 8, Table 8.3, from a variety of sources show that boiling and freezing have little effect on vitamin E content on an edible weight basis. From the authors' own experience, vitamin E content of blanched vegetables, when reported on a dry weight basis, is higher than in the fresh product because of leaching losses of water-soluble solids during the blanching process.

Several studies are available on cooking of legumes (27–30). Wide ranges of loss were reported for total vitamin E and α-tocopherol equivalents (α-TEs) in several legumes common in the Mexican diet (Table 6.8) (27). Losses ranged from 9% for garbanzo beans to 59% for bayo beans. The wide discrepancies in percentage loss for the various beans were not explained. Atienza et al. (28) reported minimal losses of less than 10% by cooking in different beans, chick

**TABLE 6.8** Changes in α- and γ-Tocopherol Levels Due to Cooking in Legumes in the Mexican Diet

| | α-T (mg/100 g) | | γ-T (mg/100 g) | | % Cooking loss (dry weight) | |
|---|---|---|---|---|---|---|
| Legume | Raw | Cooked | Raw | Cooked | α-T + γ-T | α-TE |
| Bayo bean | — | — | 2.6 | 1.1 | 59 | 60 |
| Black bean | — | — | 0.9 | 0.8 | 12 | 10 |
| Pinto bean | 0.2 | 0.1 | 2.1 | 1.7 | 17 | 21 |
| Garbanzo | 2.8 | 2.2 | 7.3 | 6.8 | 9 | 17 |
| Faba bean | 1.0 | 0.6 | 5.2 | 3.0 | 38 | 27 |
| Lentils | 1.0 | 0.3 | 4.7 | 2.9 | 44 | 58 |
| Split peas | 0.1 | 0.2 | 4.7 | 2.5 | 48 | 54 |

α-T, α-tocopherol; α-TE, α-tocopherol equivalents.
*Source*: Modified from Ref. 27.

peas, and lentils (Table 6.9). Soaking and cooking losses were similar for the different legumes. Only small amounts of $\alpha$- and $\gamma$-T were found in the cooking broth. Other studies have noted small cooking losses for various legumes common in the Indian diet (29,30). Dial and Eitenmiller (6) reported vitamin E and $\alpha$-tocopherol equivalent ($\alpha$-TE) levels in several legumes that were cooked by boiling and found little change attributable to cooking when the data were reported on a dry weight basis. In some cases, the vitamin E levels were higher in the cooked product as a result of loss of solids during the cooking process.

**6.2.2.3. Cereals.** Some cooking processes can have quite significant effects on the vitamin E content of cereals. Rice, oats, wheat, and corn lost appreciable vitamin E when the whole grains were ground and cooked in water (27). Losses ranged from 22% to 55%. Cereal flours consumed in baked products are staples in most areas of the world and constitute significant nutrient sources. Milling- and other processing-induced changes (Chapter 5) can significantly alter nutrient profiles. For vitamin E, various studies have documented losses incurred by bread-making procedures (31–37). The most definitive of these (36) (Table 6.10) showed 20–60% reductions in vitamin E levels with the most significant reductions occurring at the dough-making stage. Other published studies indicate similar effects on the tocopherol and tocotrienol contents of baked cereal products.(25) Thermal stability of vitamin E level in milled barley

**TABLE 6.9** Changes in $\alpha$- and $\gamma$-Tocopherol in Beans, Chick Peas, and Lentils Due to Cooking

| | Dry gain | | Soaked grain | | Cooked broth | | Cooked grain | |
|---|---|---|---|---|---|---|---|---|
| | $\alpha$-T | $\gamma$-T | $\alpha$-T | $\gamma$-T | $\alpha$-T | $\gamma$-T | $\alpha$-T | $\gamma$-T |
| Legume | mg/100g (Dry weight basis) | | | | | | | |
| Beans (*Phaseolus vulgaris*) | | | | | | | | |
| Riñón de León | ND | 3.4 | ND | 3.8 | ND | 0.5 | ND | 3.6 |
| Morada larga | ND | 2.6 | ND | 2.5 | ND | 2.5 | ND | 2.3 |
| Chick peas (*Cicer arietinum*) | | | | | | | | |
| Fuentesaúco | 2.6 | 11.2 | 2.5 | 10.9 | 0.1 | 0.6 | 2.3 | 10.6 |
| Turkish | 1.8 | 7.9 | 1.7 | 7.7 | 0.1 | 0.2 | 1.7 | 7.6 |
| Lentils (*Lens culinaris*) | | | | | | | | |
| Armuña | 0.1 | 4.5 | 0.1 | 4.3 | n.d. | 0.2 | 0.1 | 4.2 |
| Verdina | 0.4 | 4.3 | 0.3 | 4.2 | n.d. | 0.2 | 0.3 | 4.1 |

ND, Not determined; $\alpha$-T, $\alpha$-tocopherol. n.d., Not detected.
*Source*: Modified from Ref. 28.

**TABLE 6.10** Effects of Baking on Vitamin E in Wheat/Rye Bread

| | Tocopherol | | | Tocotrienol | |
|---|---|---|---|---|---|
| | α | β (mg/100 Dry matter) | γ | α | β |
| | | | Batch I | | |
| Scalding | | | | | |
| Scalding, freshly mixed | 3.1 | 1.0 | — | 1.1 | 1.2 |
| Scalding, after fermentation | 3.2 | 1.1 | — | 1.0 | 1.1 |
| Sourdough | | | | | |
| Whole rye flour, raw | 1.3 | 0.4 | — | 1.5 | 1.4 |
| Sourdough, freshly mixed | 0.4 | 0.2 | — | 0.6 | 0.8 |
| Sourdough, after fermentation | 0.4 | 0.2 | — | 0.6 | 0.6 |
| Wheat/rye bread | | | | | |
| Ingredients | 1.3 | 0.4 | 0.4 | 0.3 | 1.2 |
| Dough, freshly mixed | 0.8 | 0.4 | 0.4 | 0.3 | 1.1 |
| Dough, after fermentation | 0.9 | 0.4 | 0.4 | 0.3 | 1.1 |
| Bread, freshly baked | 0.8 | 0.3 | 0.3 | 0.2 | 0.9 |
| | | | Batch II | | |
| Scaling | | | | | |
| Scaling, freshly mixed | 3.9 | 1.3 | — | 1.1 | 1.3 |
| Scalding, after fermentation | 3.9 | 1.3 | — | 1.0 | 1.1 |
| Sourdough | | | | | |
| Whole rye flour, raw | 1.5 | 0.4 | — | 2.0 | 1.5 |
| Sour dough, freshly mixed | 0.5 | 0.2 | — | 0.6 | 0.6 |
| Sourdough, after fermentation | 0.6 | 0.2 | — | 0.9 | 0.8 |
| Wheat/rye bread | | | | | |
| Ingredients | 1.3 | 0.4 | 0.4 | 0.3 | 1.1 |
| Dough, freshly mixed | 1.0 | 0.4 | 0.3 | 0.3 | 1.2 |
| Dough, after fermentation | 1.0 | 0.4 | 0.3 | 0.3 | 1.1 |
| Bread, freshly baked | 0.9 | 0.3 | 0.3 | 0.2 | 1.0 |

*Source*: Modified from Ref. 36.

was temperature-dependent; $\alpha$-tocotrienol ($\alpha$-T3) showed greater stability than other vitamin E constituents in the barley flour(38) At ambient temperature, the flour lost about 5% of total vitamin E level per week (Figure 6.3). This rate of loss is quite rapid and is directly related to the experimental design of the study. Barley flour was stored on open shelves in 2-cm-thick layers exposed to the atmosphere. Under these conditions, one would expect rapid lipid oxidation with concomitant, extensive loss of vitamin E.

## 6.3. STORAGE AND ITS EFFECTS ON THE STABILITY OF VITAMIN E

Previous reviews(1,2,25,39) reported highly variable data on the stability of vitamin E in various raw and processed foods under widely varying storage conditions. Such studies have shown that vitamin E stability is quite good if the food is adequately protected from conditions conducive to lipid oxidation. Even under thermal abuse, if lipid oxidation is not proceeding, vitamin E can be expected to remain stable. If, however, oxidation is not controlled, rapid and extensive loss of vitamin E occurs. The following sections discuss factors affecting storage stability of vitamin E in various commodities. Pertinent literature is summarized in Table 6.11.

### 6.3.1. Model Food Systems

Widicus et al.(40) and Widicus and Kirk(41) provided extensive information on the storage stability of $\alpha$-T under variable storage conditions designed to show

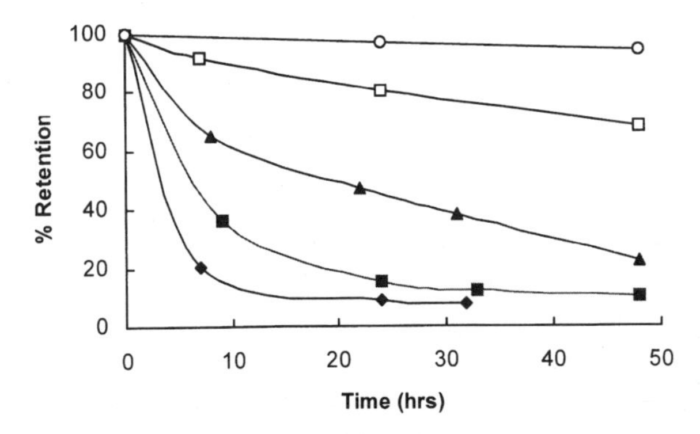


**FIGURE 6.3** Effect of storage temperature on vitamin E stability in milled barley. 0, ambient; □, 75°C; ▲, 90°C; ■, 105°C, ◆, 120°C. (Modified from Ref. 38.)

**Table 6.11** Effects of Storage on the Vitamin E Content of Foods

| Food | Storage conditions | Other factors | Observations | References |
|---|---|---|---|---|
| **Model system** | | | | |
| α-T | 20°C, 30°C, 37°C | Oxygen content α-T molar ratio: 15 : 1 to 1450 : 1 Water activity: 0.1, 0.24, 0.4, 0.65 | α-T loss increase with water activity, storage temperature, and molar ratio of oxygen: α-T increase; first-order rate kinetics noted | 1980, 40 |
| Methyl linoleate | 20°C, 30°C, 37°C | Water activity: 0.11, 0.23, 0.42, 0.67; oxygen content: 4.8, 0.05 mmol | Degradation rate of α-T best described by zero-order kinetics; effects of storage parameters of water activity, storage container oxygen content, and storage temperature on rate of α-T loss | 1981, 41 |
| **Oils** | | | | |
| Soybean | 30°C | — | For α-, β-, and γ-T in intreated soybean oil gradual decrease with storage time; α-T constant for 3 mo | 1991, 42 |
| Sunflower | Ambient | Container: plastics, tin, stainless steel, glass, polythene polypacks | Vitamin E decrease with storage; no effect of type of container | 1995, 50 |
| Virgin olive oils | Ambient, 18 mo, diffused light or dark | — | Significant loss of α-T during 3 mo under diffused light | 1998, 45 |
| Rapeseed | 40°C, dark, 16 days | Different levels of α-, γ-T and mixtures of α- and γ-T | At low levels (<50 μg/g), α-T more stable and more effective antioxidant than γ-T; γ-T more effective antioxidant than α-T at levels above 100 μg/g; in mixture of α- and γ-T, α-T protection of γ-T from oxidization at addition levels of 5 + 5 and 10 + 10 μg/g | 1999, 49 |

| | | | | |
|---|---|---|---|---|
| Rapeseed | 5°C, 20°C, 40°C, open and closed flasks, 6 mo | — | Vitamin E stable in oil at 5°C and 20°C for 24 wk; 90% decrease after 16 wk at 40°C; in intact seeds slight loss only in seeds incubated at 40°C and in open flasks | 2000, 48 |
| Virgin olive oils | 6°C (winter), 12°C (summer); 18 mo; in green bottles; in the dark | Cultivars, harvest time | α-T content change significant after 6 mo storage but no significant variations due to varieties and harvest times | 2001, 46 |
| **Dairy products and eggs** | | | | |
| Milk | 15–19°C, 90 days | Indirect and direct heating (UHT) | Vitamin E stable during processing and during storage for 90 days | 1969, 54 |
| Milk | 4°C | Pasteurization, $CO_2$ treatment | With $CO_2$ addition inhibition of growth of microorganisms and extenssion of cold-storage period of raw milk with no effect on vitamin E stability | 1998, 57 |
| Milk | −20°C, 30°C–50°C | UHT treatment: Indirect heating: 139°C (3 s), 141.5°C (22 s) Direct heating: 150°C (4.6 s), 144°C (5 s) | α-T loss in UHT milk after 1 mo storage at 30°C; for short periods (up to 60 days) of frozen storage of UHT milk no effect on α-T | 1993, 55 |
| Whole milk powder | −40°C, −18°C, 4°C, 25°C, 30°C, 37°C | — | No change in α-T content of whole milk powder during storage at −18°C and 4°C; after storage at 42°C for 2 wk degradation of α-T | 1993, 58 |
| Eggs | 4°C; 40 days | Feeding to laying hens: menhaden, flax, palm, sunflower oils | With dietary tocopherols increase of tocopherol content of eggs; with storage decrease of δ-T in flax and sunflower oil eggs | 1996, 62 |

(*continued*)

**Table 6.11** *Continued*

| Food | Storage conditions | Other factors | Observations | References |
|---|---|---|---|---|
| Liquid infant milks (follow-on and junior milks) | 20°C, 30°C, 37°C; 12 mo | — | No significant changes in vitamin E content during storage at all temperatures for 1 yr | 2000, 59 |
| Powdered and liquid infant milks | 20°C, 30°C, 37°C; 12 mo | — | No difference in vitamin E stability between powdered and liquid infant milks; no significant changes in vitamin E content during storage at all temperatures for 1 yr | 2000, 60 |
| Commercial enteral feeding formulas | 4°C, 20°C, 30°C; 0–9 mo, dark | Different protein content | At 4°C, after 3, 6, and 9 mo, vitamin E decrease 2–5%, 23–25%, and 37–42%, respectively; vitamin E decrease greater with storage temperature increase; after 9-mo storage at 30°C, vitamin E loss 51%–55% | 2001, 61 |
| **Margarine** | | | | |
| Margarine | 4°C, 20°C, 136 days | — | During 136-day storage, α- and γ-T 12% and 8% losses at 4°C; 50% and 47% losses at 20°C, respectively | 2000, 63 |
| **Meat and fish** | | | | |
| Herring fillet | −22°C, 0–6 mo | — | α-T frozen herring fillets stable for 2 mo, then slow decrease; after 6 mo, more than 70% of α-T remaining | 1985, 74 |
| Blue tilapia, red tilapia | −18°C to −6°C, 6–9 mo | — | No significant losses of α- and γ-T observed in first 3 mo; 82% and 88% α-T of initial values in red tilapia and blue tilapia, respectively, after 6 mo | 1994, 77 |

| | | | | |
|---|---|---|---|---|
| Pork | 4°C, 2–14 days, 20% $CO_2$, 80% $O_2$ | Basal diets (40 mg/kg) or α-tocopheryl acetate (200 mg/kg) | α-T lower in muscle (4.1 mg/kg) and adipose tissue (20.3 mg/kg) from supplemented group; no change of α-T in muscle tissue; decrease in adipose tissue during storage | 1995, 67 |
| Turkey burgers | −20°C and 4°C | Feeding of supplemented diet containing 300 (E300) or 600 (E600)mg α-tocopheryl acetate/kg for 21 wk | No change in α-T levels in raw and cooked burgers during storage at 4°C; for α-T values of raw turkey burgers from E600 and E300 decrease from 5.7 to 3.5 and from 3.6 to 2.3 μg/g after 4 mo at −20°C, respectively; for α-T values decrease from 5.6 to 2.9 and from 3.3 to 1.9 μg/g in cooked burgers from turkeys from E600 and E300, respectively, after 5 mo at −20°C | 1996, 72 |
| Tilapia, Spanish mackerel | 2°C ± 2°C | Irradiation: $CO_{60}$ source (Nutronic), 1.5–10 kGy, 96–640 min | For tocopherols in tilapia and Spanish mackerel decrease with increased irradiation dose; dose of 3.0 kGy best for tocopherol retention; rate of α-T loss slightly higher in tilapia than in Spanish mackerel | 1996, 75 |
| Restructured beef roasts | 4°C, 0–8 days, polyethylene bags | Rice bran oil addition | α-T and γ-T3 decrease during storage; α-T3 and γ-T stable until 4 days of storage, decreased at 8 days of storage | 2000, 65 |
| **Cereals** | | | | |
| Wheat | Ambient temperature, 32°F; 3 yr | Fumigation: methyl bromide, ethylene dichloride/carbon tetrachloride, phosphine | No effect of fumigation on tocopherol content of wheat; minor losses of tocopherols caused by storage | 1972, 78 |

(continued)

**TABLE 6.11** *Continued*

| Food | Storage conditions | Other factors | Observations | References |
|---|---|---|---|---|
| Barley, oat | Propionic acid, sealed silo, conventional with/without hot air drying | — | Vitamin E levels of propionic acid–treated barley considerably lower than those from hot air–dried conventionally stored barley; in conventionally stored grain persisting high vitamin E levels | 1974, 79 |
| Barley | Moisture: 20%, 28%; 1 yr | Air control air: $CO_2$, $NH_3$, expansion sack volume (10%, 25%) | In 20% moisture barley, vitamin E content increased until mid-April, after 10 mo final levels similar to those at harvest except in the bin treated with ammonia; for 28% moisture barley tocopherol isomer fraction increased at cost of tocotrienols; with treatment of barley with 1% ammonia gas vitamin E loss; for barley at 28% moisture, apparent preservative effect on vitamin E of external supply of $CO_2$ | 1983, 81 |
| Barley | 12°C–15°C;; moisture: 18%, 25%, 35%; aerobic, anaerobic | Propionic acid, sodium hydroxide | With propionic acid and sodium hydroxide treatment of moist barley vitamin E loss, though no detrimental effect of moisture or anaerobic storage; vitamin E loss most severe and rapid with alkali treatment; order of susceptibility to decay $\alpha$-T > $\gamma$-T > $\alpha$-T3 > $\gamma$-T3 | 1985, 84 |
| Wheat fractions | 20°C, 1 yr | — | % Vitamin E loss: wholemeal, 60; white flour, 62; bran, 72; germ, 60 | 1992, 36 |

| | | | | |
|---|---|---|---|---|
| Oat products | −24°C, room temperature, 7 mo | Container: jars, envelope | Tocopherol degradation faster in envelopes than in jars at room temperature; α-T decrease faster than that of other homologues during room temperature storage in envelopes; tocopherols stable for 7 mo in oat products in jars at −24°C; at room temperature all tocopherols degraded in all processed oat products except undried goat | 1995, 87 |
| Extruded rice bran | Ambient temperature, 1 yr | Extrusion: 100°C–140°C, Postextrusion holding times: 0–6 min | Raw rice bran loss of 44% and 73% of total vitamin E after 35-day and 1-yr storage, respectively; total vitamin E content decreased by 21% and 46% after 7- and 105-day storage of rice bran extruded at 110°C with 0-min holding time; reduced vitamin E retention during storage caused by increased temperature | 1997, 88 |
| **Nuts** | | | | |
| Almond, pecan, macadamia | 30°C, 16 mo, 55% RH | — | Total tocopherol content decrease in all nuts during storage; no significant differences in rancidity detected by taste panel in almonds after 16 mo of storage; significant differences detected in pecan and macadamia after 4 and 2 mo of storage, respectively | 1989, 91 |
| Walnut | 4°C, 12 mo | Geographic origin (U.S., France), variety (Franquette, Hartley) | Vitamin E losses during 3 mo; δ-T (30%) > α-T (29%) > γ-T (28%)<br>Effect of geographic origin > effect of variety | 1997, 95 |

(continued)

**TABLE 6.11** *Continued*

| Food | Storage conditions | Other factors | Observations | References |
|---|---|---|---|---|
| Roasted and salted cashew nut | 30°C, 360 days, 80% RH, −18°C (control) | Packaging: polypropylene/polyethylene, metallized polyethylene terethalate/polyethylene, polyethylene terethalate/aluminum foil/low-density polyethylene | No vitamin E loss in shelled, roasted, and salted cashew nuts during storage in flexible packaging materials with lower water vapor permeability rate at 30°C for 1 yr | 1998, 96 |
| **Miscellaneous** | | | | |
| Potato tubers | 3°C, 9°C | — | α-T in tuber lowest at zero time storage; α-T level fourfold increase during storage; no significant differences between two storage temperatures | 1990, 101 |
| Broccoli | MAP 75% $CO_2$ | 5°C | With MAP no improvement in vitamin E retention, decrease after 6 days in all treatments | 1996, 102 |
| Redgram *Dhals* | −10°C Polypropylene pouches | Cooking and drying<br>Flaking and drying<br>Freeze–thaw drying | Rate of α-T loss highest in freeze–thaw dehydrated redgram *dhal*, followed by flaked and dried *dhal*; 16–25% and 34–78% of α-T losses during 8-mo in storage at −10°C and 37°C, respectively | 2000, 30 |
| Potato chips | 60°C | Addition of ascorbyl palmitate | With addition of ascorbyl palmitate increase in induction period of oxidation and decrease in rate of tocopherol degradation | 2002, 11 |

α-T, α-tocopherol; UHT, ultrahigh temperature; γ-T3, γ-tocotrienol; RH, relative humidity; MAP, modified atmosphere packaging.

effects of water activity, temperature, and oxygen content, and availability. Observations included the following in a fat-free system:

1. The degradation rate of $\alpha$-T increased as the water activity increased in the range 0.10–0.65$A_w$ (Figure 6.4).
2. The degradation rate of $\alpha$-T increased as the storage temperature increased from 20°C to 37°C (Table 6.12).
3. The degradation rate of $\alpha$-T increased as the molar ratio of oxygen: $\alpha$-T increased from 15 : 1 to 1450 : 1.
4. Activation energies ranged from 8.85 to 13.05 kcal/mol.
5. Degradation products included $\alpha$-tocopherol oxide and $\alpha$-tocopheryl quinone.

When methyl linoleate was included in the system (41) the degradation rate was zero-order and dependent on the initial concentration of $\alpha$-T, water activity, storage container oxygen content, and temperature. Comparison of the fat-free dehydrated food to that containing methyl linoleate showed that the rate of $\alpha$-T loss was greater in the presence of the unsaturated lipid.

## 6.3.2. Oils and Oilseeds

Vitamin E stability in edible oils depends on the initial oil quality. In refined, bleached, deodorized (RBD) oils protected by proper packaging under normal storage conditions, little progressive loss in vitamin E would be expected. Most

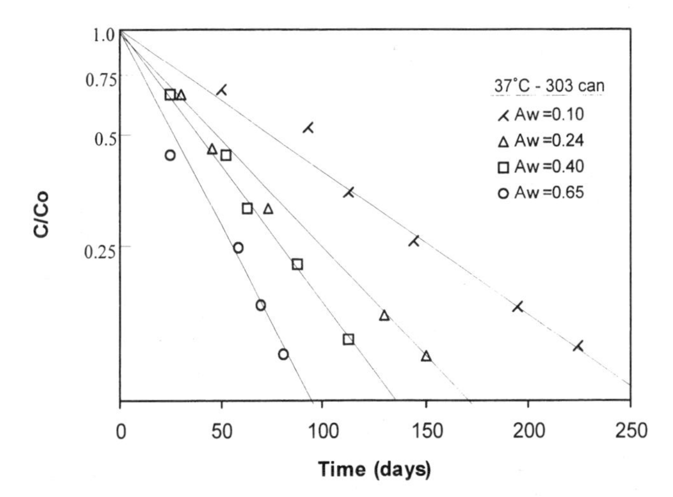


**FIGURE 6.4** Effect of water activity on $\alpha$-tocopherol in a fat-free model system stored at 37°C. (Modified from Ref. 40.)

**Table 6.12** Rate Constants and Half-Lives for α-Tocopherol as a Function of Water Activity, Storage Container, and Storage Temperature

| | | 303 Can[a] | | 208 × 006 Can (TDT)[b] | |
|---|---|---|---|---|---|
| Temperature (°C) | $A_w$ | $k$[c] | $t_{1/2}$[d] | $k$[c] | $t_{1/2}$[d] |
| 37 | 0.65 | 15.94 | 43.5 | 13.4 | 51.7 |
| | 0.4 | 14.85 | 46.7 | 13.15 | 52.7 |
| | 0.24 | 12.84 | 53.9 | 11.38 | 60.9 |
| | 0.1 | 8.02 | 86.4 | 8.63 | 80.3 |
| 30 | 0.65 | 7.11 | 97.5 | 6.49 | 106.8 |
| | 0.4 | 6.28 | 110.4 | 6.03 | 114.9 |
| | 0.24 | 6.22 | 111.4 | 5.91 | 117.3 |
| | 0.1 | 4.97 | 139.4 | 4.7 | 147.5 |
| 20 | 0.65 | 5.18 | 133.8 | 5.54 | 125.1 |
| | 0.4 | 5.23 | 132.5 | 4.53 | 152.9 |
| | 0.24 | 4.47 | 155 | 3.26 | 212.6 |
| | 0.1 | 3.24 | 213.9 | 3.23 | 214.6 |

[a]1450 : 1 Calculated molar ratio of oxygen: α-tocopherol.
[b]15 : 1 Calculated molar ratio of oxygen : α-tocopherol. TDT, thermal death time.
[c]First-order rate constant, $\times 10^{-3}$/day.
[d]Half-life, days.
*Source*: Modified from Ref. 40.

changes are attributable to abuse leading to oxidative changes. Storage studies exist for soybean oil.(42,43) olive oil (44–47) canola and rapeseed oil (48,49), sunflower oil (50), sesame oil (51) and various other edible oils (52,53). This work, summarized in Table 6.11, covers a wide variety of storage conditions that can promote degradation of vitamin E in the edible oil. Generalizations that can be made from the studies center on quality factors of the RBD oil and interactions of the vitamin E with natural prooxidants in the product as well as the storage environment.

Factors to be considered include the following:

1. Absence of prooxidants
2. Maintenance of the absence of oxygen and metals
3. Proper packaging that prevents oxygen transfer into the oil
4. Proper temperature control
5. Absence of high-intensity light and other types of irradiation

Under proper storage of high-quality RBD oil, little loss of vitamin E occurs even after prolonged storage. Studies in our laboratory of RBD soybean oil used as an in-house quality assurance sample for analytical work show that under ambient temperature and absence of light little change occurs in the tocopherols over 6-month storage (Figure 6.5).

Although vitamin E is stable in RBD oil under proper storage, considerable losses have been reported in the literature. For example, Jaimand and Rezaee (50) reported extensive losses in sunflower oil over 6 months at ambient temperature. However, all conditions considered in the study led to extensive oxidative changes in the oil, so extensive loss of vitamin E followed.

Little has been reported on the stability of vitamin E in intact oilseeds during storage. Chu and Lin (43) investigated factors affecting the vitamin E content in soybean oils as related to the storage conditions of the soybeans. They prepared soybeans in several forms, including soybean flour, cracked beans, and three different thicknesses of flakes, and then adjusted moisture content in the range of 12%–18% before 4 weeks of storage. The state of soybeans before extraction, moisture content, and storage time were important factors affecting the total oil yield and the tocopherol content of crude soybean oils. The following observations regarding the stability of vitamin E in soybeans were obtained from the work:

1. Soybean flakes with a thickness of 0.16–0.33 mm had a higher extracted oil yield but a slightly lower tocopherol content of the oils than did cracked beans and thicker bean flakes.
2. High moisture content and long storage of soybeans resulted in lower tocopherol content in oils.
3. Soybean oil from stored beans with 15% moisture content had a more significant decrease (31%) in tocopherol content than did oil from stored beans with low (12%) or high (18%) moisture contents.
4. As the bean moisture content increased to 18%, the length of bean storage time had no effect on the reduction of tocopherol content of the extracted oils.
5. Soybean flakes with high and medium thickness had no significant difference in the tocopherol content of the oils, whereas oils from thin flakes had a significantly lower tocopherol content, indicating enzymatic vitamin E destruction.
6. Levels of cracked beans included with the intact beans affected tocopherol losses only for long storage (>1 wk).

Goffman et al. (48) investigated the effects of storage temperature on the tocopherol content in intact rapeseed during storage. No total tocopherol loss was observed in intact rapeseeds during storage at 5°C and 25°C. However, the analysis of the tocopherol composition showed a decrease in the $\alpha$-T content and an increase in the $\gamma$-T content, resulting in a decreasing $\alpha$-T/$\gamma$-T ratio. This trend was most apparent at high storage temperature (40°C).

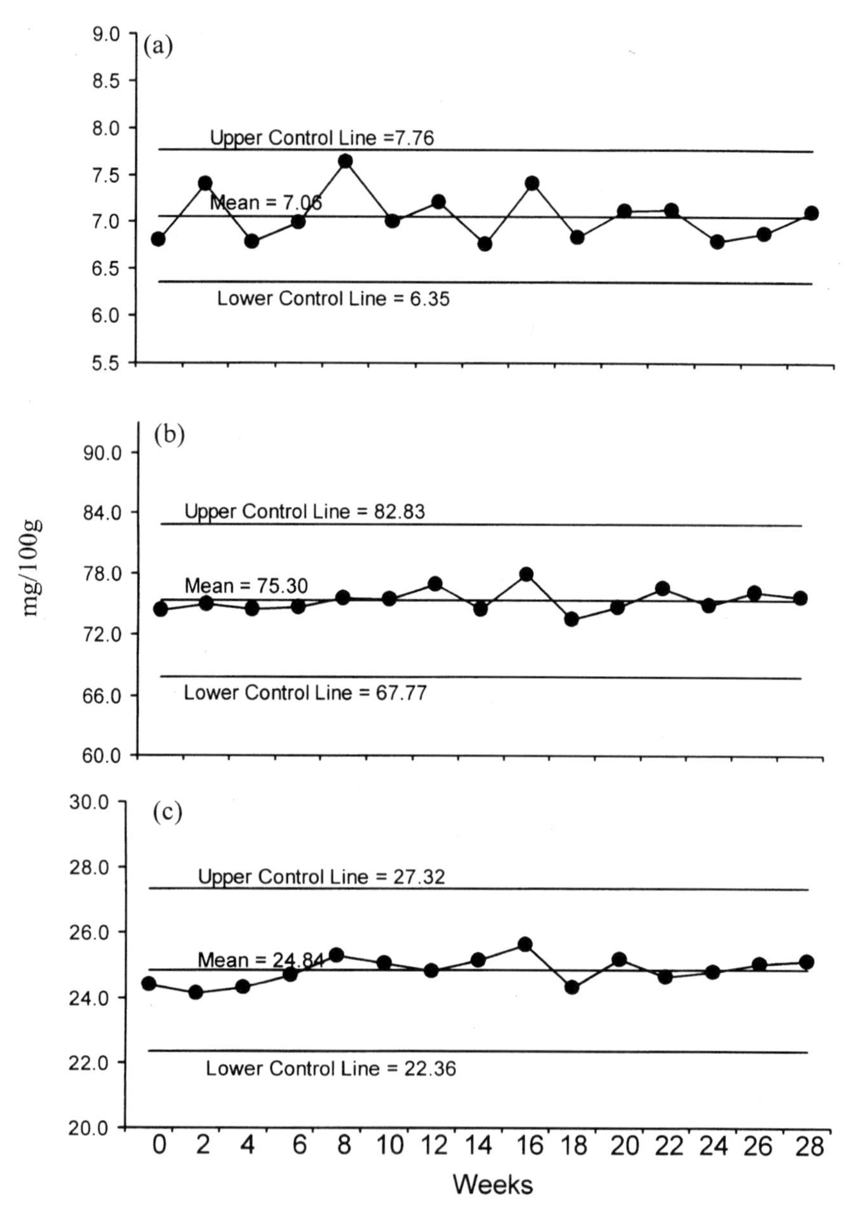


**FIGURE 6.5** Effect of storage at ambient temperature in the dark on tocopherols in refined, bleached, deodorized (RBD) soybean oil. (a), $\alpha$-Tocopherol; (b), $\gamma$-T; (c), $\delta$-T.

### 6.3.3. Dairy Products, Infant and Enteral Formulas, and Eggs

**6.3.3.1. Whole Milk and Whole Milk Powder.** Bovine milk, unless partially defatted or skimmed, contains between 0.05 and 0.1 mg of $\alpha$-T/100 g along with trace amounts of $\gamma$-T (Chapter 8, Table 8.3). Processing and storage of whole milk have little effect on vitamin E content. Deaeration of fluid milk most likely has a stabilization effect. Ford et al.(54) showed that ultrahigh-temperature (UHT) processing at 138°C for 2 s or at 145°C for 3–4 s followed by evaporative or indirect cooling did not change $\alpha$-T levels in the milk. The vitamin E was stable over a 90-day storage period when packaged in 0.5 L or 1 pt cartons (Tetra Pak) at 15–19°C. Abusive storage of UHT milk at temperatures above ambient and long-term freezing can decrease $\alpha$-T levels (55). Also, acidification with $CO_2$ to extend the storage life of raw milk does not decrease $\alpha$-T level over 7-day storage at 4–7°C (56,57).

Production of whole milk powder causes little loss of $\alpha$-T, as indicated by the literature values of 0.5–0.8 mg/100 g reported in Table 8.3. These levels are about what would be expected at high retention; however, definitive data are not available to provide a retention factor for the spray drying process. $\alpha$-Tocopherol level is stable in whole milk powder when stored properly. Storage studies on a whole milk powder food reference material (CRM 380) indicated that $\alpha$-T level was stable at storage temperature of −18°C and 4°C for 24 mo (58). Losses were noted after 6 wk at 24°C and 30°C.

**6.3.3.2. Infant and Enteral Feeding Formulas.** $\alpha$-Tocopheryl acetate ($\alpha$-TAC) is used as the vitamin E source in infant formulas. The $\alpha$-TAC level is stable in both liquid and powdered formulas for 6 mo at abusive storage at 37°C (59,60). Storage of enteral feeding formulas led to large losses of $\alpha$-T level when stored at 4°C, 20°C, and 30°C for 9 mo.(61)

**6.3.3.3. Eggs.** Storage of shell eggs under normal conditions of temperature and relative humidity has no effect on vitamin E content (62). Effects of processing on vitamin E stability are not available.

### 6.3.4. Margarine

Nogala-Kalucka and Gogolewski (63) found that vitamin E level in full-fat margarine is stable during extended refrigerated storage at 4°C over 136 days. However, at 20°C extensive losses occurred with all tocopherols (Table 6.13). As the peroxide value of the margarine increased, vitamin E degradation accelerated. Greater loss of $\alpha$-T level was noted compared to $\gamma$- and $\delta$-T levels.

**TABLE 6.13** Changes in Peroxide Values and Vitamin E Levels in Margarine During Storage

| | | Days | | | |
|---|---|---|---|---|---|
| | | 4°C | | 20°C | |
| | Initial | 57 | 136 | 57 | 136 |
| Peroxide value (mmol $O_2$/kg) | 0.08 | 0.1 | 0.14 | 2.19 | 4.04 |
| % Loss | | | | | |
| α-Tocopherol | — | 1.7 | 12.1 | 10.3 | 50.6 |
| γ-Tocopherol | — | 0.5 | 8.2 | 6.4 | 47.4 |
| δ-Tocopherol | — | 3.3 | 8.3 | 10 | 36.7 |

*Source*: Modified from Ref. 63.

## 6.3.5. Meat and Fish

Lipid oxidation leads to quality loss in meat and processed meats during refrigerated and freezer storage. As discussed in Chapter 4, the progression of lipid oxidation in muscle foods is somewhat controlled by the α-T concentration in the muscle, which can be increased by supplementation of vitamin E into the diets of meat animals, poultry, and fish. Increased storage life can be achieved for both raw and processed meats quite effectively and economically (64–77). Selected papers that show effects of storage on the vitamin E content in meat and fish are summarized in Table 6.11. Representative of such research, Kim et al.(65) followed changes in vitamin E level in restructured beef formulated with rice bran oil. The α-T and α-T3 levels decreased significantly (>30%) during storage at 4°C for 8 days. The thiobarbituric acid–reactive substance (TBAR) values increased from 0.08 to 0.11 mg/kg over the same period. At this point, the roasts were still organoleptically acceptable. Oxidation in this product could be expected to proceed rapidly because of the high unsaturation of the rice bran oil.

Short-term storage of raw and cooked meats generally does not lead to extensive losses in α-T level. However, long-term freezer storage can reduce α-T levels as oxidation slowly proceeds (72) (Figure 6.6).

## 6.3.6. Plant Products

**6.3.6.1. Cereals.** To ensure optimal quality maintenance during storage, whole cereal grains require careful moisture control initiated by artificial hot air drying before storage. Optimal moisture maintenance then ensures absence of microbial and biochemical degradation that can produce functional, organoleptic,

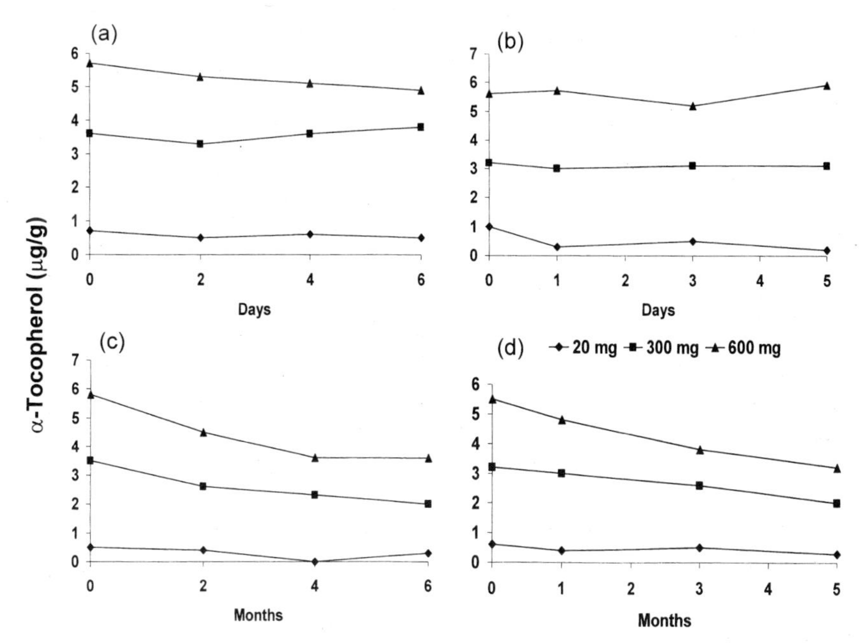


**FIGURE 6.6** Degradation of $\alpha$-tocopherol in turkey burgers. Diets were supplemented with $\alpha$-tocopheryl acetate (mg/kg diet); ◆, 20; ■, 300; ▲, 600. (a) Raw muscle stored at 4°C; (b) cooked muscle stored at 4°C; (c) raw muscle stored at −20°C; (d) cooked muscle stored at −20°C. (Modified from Ref. 72.)

and safety problems with utilization of the grain for animal or human consumption. Stability of vitamin E level is quite good in whole grain cereal if proper storage conditions are maintained (78–81). Slover and Lehmann (78) confirmed vitamin E level stability in wheat over a 3-yr storage study. Likewise, research on corn (80) and barley (81,82) documents that vitamin E level is stable if the moisture levels are such as to maintain overall grain quality. High-moisture, ensiled, and/or propionic/acetate acid–acidified grains are subject to rapid and extensive loss of vitamin E level (79–84). The effect of moisture content and acidification on $\alpha$-T level in corn during long-term storage is shown in Figure 6.7.

Fractionation of cereal grain by milling disrupts natural barriers to oxygen, disrupts cellular structure, exposes membrane-localized unsaturated fatty acids to oxidation, and, thus, promotes degradation of vitamin E. Oxidative stress can easily overcome regenerative capacity of the antioxidant system and rapid loss of vitamin E can occur. Oxidation is recognized to proceed rapidly in whole wheat flour through lipase and lipoxygenase activity. Such degradation affects the functional and organoleptic quality of the flour and undoubtedly the vitamin E

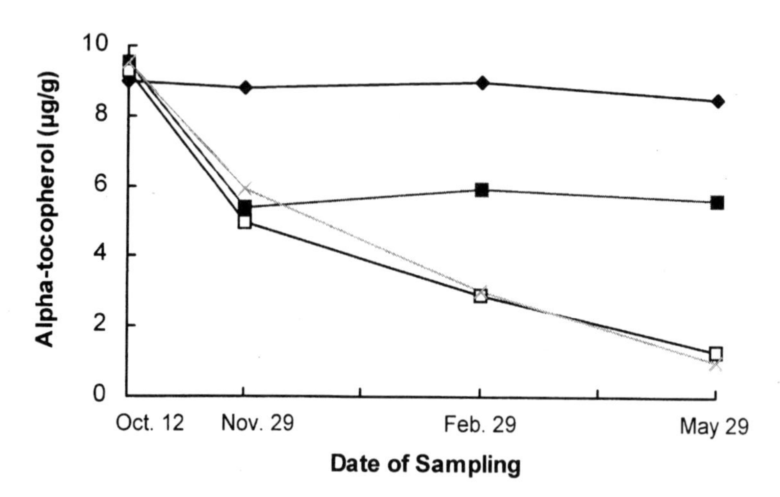


**FIGURE 6.7** $\alpha$-Tocopherol content in shelled corn preserved by various methods. ◆, artificial drying; ■, natural sun drying; □, acid treated; X, high-moisture, ensiled. (Modified from Ref. 80.)

content (85). Wennermark et al. (86) and Wennermark and Jägerstad (36) followed vitamin E retention during processing and storage of several wheat products. Storage effects on wholemeal, white flour, bran, and germ are shown in Figure 6.8. Storage at 20°C for 12 mo decreased vitamin E level in the various fractions by 28–40%. Highest losses occurred with $\alpha$-T level. Studies on oat products also demonstrated decrease in total vitamin E level when stored at ambient temperature (87).

Rice bran, because of its inherent instability to oxidation and hydrolytic rancidity, presents a unique problem in preservation of quality of the bran and oil. Extrusion is commonly used to denature lipiase and lipoxygenase activity in the bran for stabilization (see Chapter 5). Extrusion improves retention of tocopherols, tocotrienols, and oryzanol during long-term storage at ambient temperature (88).

**6.3.6.2. Peanuts and Tree Nuts.** Interest in compositional properties in peanuts and treenuts has greatly increased because of unique nutritional and functional properties that are being clearly delineated by clinical studies. Commodities including peanuts, pecans, almonds, and walnuts, are recognized for their ability to lower serum low-density lipoprotein (LDL) cholesterol level without impacting high-density lipoprotein (HDL) cholesterol level in the human when routinely included in the diet. Although it is not possible to explain completely the beneficial effects of nut consumption on blood lipid profiles, explanations of the effect include the prevalence of unsaturated fatty acids in nut

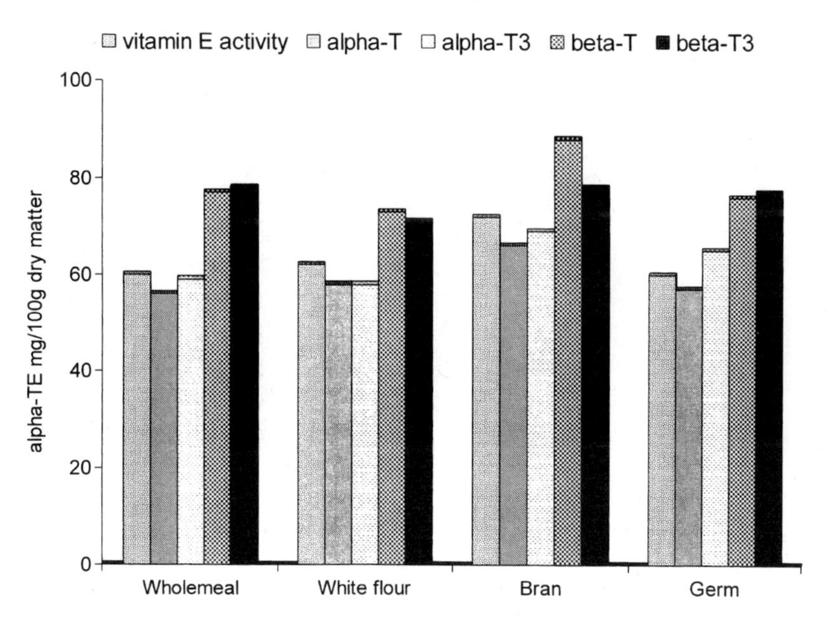


**FIGURE 6.8** Degradation of tocopherols and tocotrienols during storage of wheat fractions at 20°C for 1 year. $\alpha$-T, $\alpha$-tocopherol; $\alpha$-T3, $\alpha$-tocotrienol. (Modified from Ref. 36.)

lipids, the replacement of more hypercholesterolemic fats by nut lipids, and the presence of significant amounts of vitamin E, folate, and sterols that are not as concentrated in animal fats (89).

Because of the highly unsaturated nature of nut lipids, vitamin E plays as integral role in controlling oxidation and maintaining quality of raw and processed products. Storage studies on raw and processed (primarily roasted) nuts usually indicate that roasted whole nuts are less stable to oxidation than raw nuts because of disruption of fat bodies and exposure of membrane phospholipids to oxidation. One would surmise that vitamin E level is, therefore, less stable in roasted nuts than in raw nuts during storage, although little literature documents this postulation. Storage studies have been completed on several tree nuts to document changes in vitamin E level during storage (90–96). In most research, vitamin E content decreases as storage time increases. Rate of loss is temperature-dependent and highly affected by the packaging material and availability of oxygen. Details of several studies are summarized in Table 6.11. Representative of commercial packaging and storage of unroasted pecans, tocopherol levels were stable when stored in commercial cellophane packages in air at 0.6°C for 48 wk. At 23°C, progressive losses were noted for $\gamma$-tocopherol (Figure 6.9).

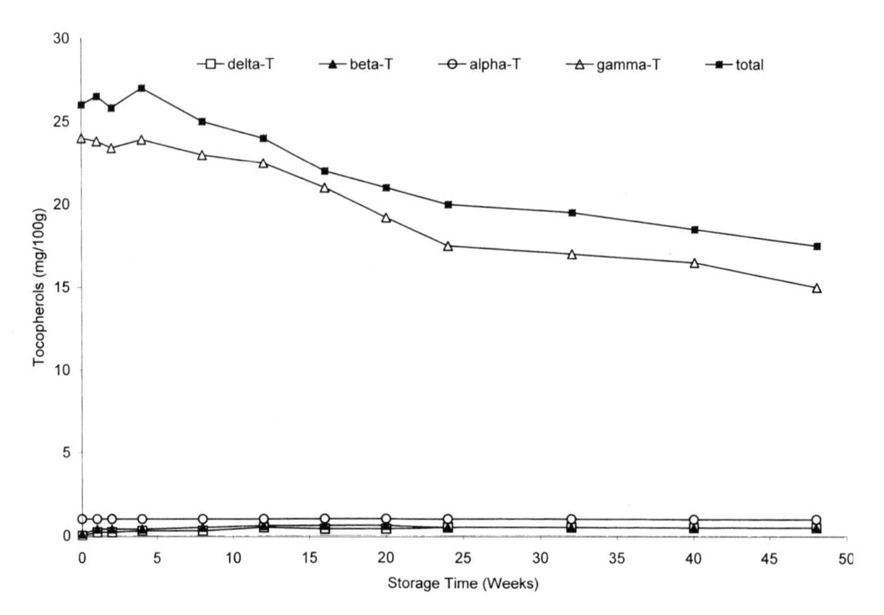


**FIGURE 6.9** Tocopherols in Schley pecans stored at 23.9°C and 60–70% relative humidity (RH). (Modified from Ref. 92.)

**6.3.6.3. Miscellaneous Commodities.** Research covering changes in vitamin E content during storage of paprika (97,98), *dhals* (29,30), potatoes (99), and broccoli florets (100) is summarized in Table 6.11.

## REFERENCES


1. Ames, SR. Tocopherols. V. Occurrence in foods. In *The Vitamins*, Vol. 5; Sebrell, W.H., Jr; Harris, R.S., Ed.; Academic Press: New York, 1972.
2. Bauernfeind, J.C. The tocopherol content of food and influencing factors. Crit. Rev. Food Sci. Nutr. **1977**, *8*, 337–382.
3. Bauernfeind, J.C. Tocopherols in foods. In *Vitamin E: A Comprehensive Treatise*; Machlin, L.J., Ed.; Marcel Dekker: New York, 1980.
4. Moreira, R.G.; Castell-Perez, M.E.; Barrufet, M.A. Deep-Fat Frying: Fundamentals and Applications. Aspen: Gaithersburg, MD, 1999.
5. Blumenthal, M.M. A new look at the chemistry and physics of deep-fat frying. Food. Technol. **1991**, *45*, 68–71.
6. Dial, S.; Eitenmiller, R.R. Tocopherols and tocotrienols in key foods in the U.S. diet. In *Nutrition, Lipids, Health and Disease*; Ong, A.S.H., Nike, E., Packer, L., Eds.; AOCS Press: Champaign, IL: 1995.
7. Carlson, B.L.; Tabacch, M.H. Frying oil deterioration and vitamin loss during foodservice operation. J. Food Sci. **1986**, *51*, 218–230.

8. Andrikopoulos, N.K.; Dedoussis, G.V.Z.; Falirea, A.; Kalogeropoulos, N.; Hatzinikola, H.S. Deterioration of natural antioxidant species of vegetable edible oils during the domestic deep-frying and pan-frying of potatoes. Int. J. Food Sci. Nutr. **2002**, *53*, 351–363.
9. Simonne, A.H.; Eitenmiller, R.R. Retention of vitamin E and added retinyl palmitate in selected vegetable oils during deep-fat frying and in fried breaded products. J. Agric. Food Chem. **1998**, *46*, 5273–5277.
10. Ruiz, G.M.; Polvillo, M.M.; Jorge, N.; Mendez, M.V.R.; Dobarganes, M.C. Influence of used frying oil quality and natural tocopherol content on oxidative stability of fried potatoes. JAOCS **1999**, *76*, 421–425.
11. Masson, L.; Robert, P.; Dobarganes, M.C.; Urra, C.; Romero, N.; Oritiz, J.; Goicoechea, E.; Pérez, P.; Salamé, M.; Torres, R. Stability of potato chips fried in vegetable oils with different degree of unsaturation. Effect of ascorbyl palmitate during storage. Grasas Aceites **2002**, *53*, 191–198.
12. Miyagawa, K.; Hirai, K.; Takezoe, R. Tocopherol and fluorescence levels in deep-frying oil and their measurement for oil assessment. JAOCS **1991**, *65*, 163–166.
13. Balasubramanium, V.M.; Chinnan, M.S.; Mallikarjunan, P.; Phillps, R.D. The effect of edible film on oil uptake and moisture retention of a deep-fat fried poultry product. J. Food Proc. Engin. **1997**, *20*, 17–29.
14. Holownia, K.I.; Erickson, M.C.; Chinnan, M.S.; Eitenmiller, R.R. Tocopherol losses in peanut oil during pressure frying of marinated chicken strips coated with edible films. Food Res. Int. **2001**, *34*, 77–80.
15. United States Department of Agriculture, Agricultural Research Service, USDA Nutrient Database for Standard Reference, Release 16, Nutrient Data Laboratory Home Page, http://www.nal.usda.gov/fnic/foodcomp. Beltsville, MD: Nutrient Data Laboratory, USDA, 2003.
16. Bennik, M.R.; Ono, K. Vitamin $B_{12}$, E and D content of raw and cooked beef. J. Food Sci. **1982**, *47*, 1786–1792.
17. Ono, K.; Berry, B.M.; Douglass, L.W. Nutrient composition of some fresh and cooked retail cuts of veal. J. Food Sci. **1986**, *51*, 1352–1357.
18. Murphy, W.E.; Criner, P.E.; Gray, B.C. Comparisons of methods for calculating retentions of nutrients in cooked foods. J. Agric. Food Chem. **1975**, *23*, 1153–1157.
19. Driskell, J.A.; Sun, J.; Giraud, D.W.; Hamouz, F.L.; Batenhorst, J.H. Selenium and tocopherol content of cooked pork roasts. J. Food. Qual. **1995**, *18*, 455–462.
20. Driskell, J.A.; Giraud, D.W.; Sun, J.; Joo, S.; Hamouz, F.L.; Davis, S.L. Retention of vitamin B-6, thiamin, vitamin E, and selenium in grilled boneless pork chops prepared at five grill temperatures. J. Food. Qual. **1998**, *21*, 201–210.
21. Yuan, X.; Marchello, M.J.; Driskell, J.A. Selected vitamin contents and retentions in bison patties as related to cooking method. J. Food Sci. **1999**, *64*, 462–464.
22. Bosco, A.D.; Castellini, C.; Bernardini, M. Nutritional quality of rabbit meat as affected by cooking procedure and dietary vitamin E. J. Food Sci. **2001**, *66*, 1047–1051.
23. Erickson, M.C. Extraction and quantitation of tocopherol in raw and cooked channel catfish. J. Food Sci. **1991**, *56*, 1113–1114.
24. Erickson, M.C. Changes in lipid oxidation during cooking of refrigerated minced channel catfish muscle. ACS Symp. Ser. **1992**, *500*, 344–351.

25. Bramley, P.M.; Elmadfa, I.; Kafatos, A.; Kelly, F.J.; Manios, Y.; Roxborough, H.E.; Schuch, W.; Sheehy, P.J.A.; Wagner, K.H. Vitamin E. J. Sci. Food Agric. **2000**, *80*, 913–938.
26. Elmadfa, I.; Bosse, W. *Vitamin E*; Wiss Verlagagesellschaft: Stuttgart, 1985; 44–45 pp.
27. Wyatt, C.J.; Carballido, S.P.; Méndez, R.O. $\alpha$- and $\gamma$-Tocopherol content of selected foods in the Mexican diet: Effect of cooking losses. J. Agric. Food Chem. **1998**, *46*, 4657–4661.
28. Atienza, J.; Sanz, M.; Herguedas, A.; Alejos, J.A.; Jiménez, J.J. Note: $\beta$-Carotene, $\alpha$-tocopherol and $\gamma$-tocopherol contents in dry legumes: Influence of cooking. Food Sci. Technol. Int. **1998**, *4*, 437–441.
29. Arya, S.R. Changes in tocopherols during processing and storage of quick cooking *Dhals*. J. Food Sci. Technol. **2000**, *37*, 51–53.
30. Sharma, G.K.; Semwal, A.D.; Mahesh, C.; Arya, S.; Arya, S.S. Studies on changes in carotenoids, tocopherols, and lipids during processing and storage of instant redgram *Dhal* (*Cajanas cajan*). J. Food Sci. Technol. **2000**, *37*, 256–260.
31. Menger, A. Untersuchung uber die Beständigkeit von Vitamin E in Getreidemahlerzeugnissem und Backwaren. Brot. Gebck. **1957**, *8*, 167–173.
32. Moore, T.; Sharman, I.M.; Ward, R.J. The destruction of vitamin E in flour by chlorine dioxane. J. Sci. Food Agric. **1957**, *8*, 97–104.
33. Slover, H.T.; Lehmann, J. Effects of fumigation on wheat in storage. IV. Tocopherols. Cereal Chem. **1972**, *49*, 412–415.
34. Håkansson, B.; Jägerstad, M.; Öste, R.; Åkesson, B.; Jonsson, L. The effects of various thermal processes on protein quality, vitamins and selenium content in whole-grain wheat and white flour. J. Cereal Sci. **1987**, *6*, 269–282.
35. Piironen, V.; Varo, P.; Koivistoinen, P. Stability of tocopherols and tocotrienols in food preparation procedures. J. Food Comp. Anal. **1987**, *1*, 53–58.
36. Wennermark, B.H.; Jägerstad, M. Breadmaking and storage of various wheat fractions affect vitamin E. J. Food Sci. **1992**, *55*, 1195–1209.
37. Håkansson, B.H.; Jägerstad, M. The effect of thermal inactivation of lipoxygenase on the stability of vitamin E in wheat. J. Cereal Sci. **1990**, *12*, 177–185.
38. Työppönen, J.T.; Hakkarainen, R.V.J. Thermal stability of vitamin E in barley. Acta Agric. Scand. **1985**, *35*, 136–138.
39. Kivimäe, A.; Carpena, C. The level of vitamin E content on storage of conventional feeding stuff and the effects of genetic variety, harvesting, processing and storage. Acta Agric. Scand., Suppl **1973**, *19*, 161–168.
40. Widicus, W.A.; Kirk, J.R.; Gregory, J.F. Storage stability of $\alpha$-tocopherol in a dehydrated model food system containing no fat. J. Food Sci. **1980**, *45*, 1015–1018.
41. Widicus, W.A.; Kirk, J.R. Storage stability of $\alpha$-tocopherol in a dehydrated model food system containing methyl linoleate. J. Food Sci. **1981**, *46*, 813–816.
42. Boki, K.; Wada, T.; Ohno, S. Effects of filtration through activated carbon on peroxide, thiobarbituric acid and carbonyl values of autoxidized soybean oil. JAOCS **1991**, *68*, 561–565.
43. Chu, Y.H.; Lin, J. Factors affecting the content of tocopherol in soybean oil. JAOCS **1993**, *70*, 1263–1268.

44. Psomiadou, E.; Tsimidou, M. Simultaneous HPLC determination of tocopherols, carotenoids, and chlorophylls for monitoring their effect on virgin olive oil oxidation. J. Agric. Food Chem. **1998**, *46*, 5132–5138.
45. Manzi, P.; Panfili, G.; Esti, M.; Pizzaferrato, L. Natural antioxidants in the unsaponifiable fraction of virgin olive oils from different cultivars. J. Sci. Food Agric. **1998**, *77*, 115–120.
46. Cinquanta, L.; Esti, M.; Matteo, M.D. Oxidative stability of virgin olive oils. JAOCS **2001**, *78*, 1197–1202.
47. Okogeri, O.; Tasioula-Margari, M. Changes occurring in phenolic compounds and $\alpha$-tocopherol of virgin olive oil during storage. J. Agric. Food Chem. **2002**, *50*, 1077–1080.
48. Goffman, F.D.; Möllers, C. Changes in tocopherol and plastochromanol-8 contents in seeds and oil of oilseed rape (*Brassica napus* L.). During storage as influenced by temperature and air oxygen. J. Agric. Food Chem. **2000**, *48*, 1605–1609.
49. Lampi, A.M.; Kataja, A.; Kamal-Eldin, A.; Vieno, P. Antioxidant activities of $\alpha$- and $\gamma$-tocopherols on the oxidation of rapesed oil triacylglycerols. JAOCS **1999**, *76*, 749–755.
50. Jaimand, K.; Rezaee, M.B. Studies on the storage quality of sunflower oil. Agrochimica **1995**, *XXXIX*, 177–183.
51. Shahidi, F.; Amarowicz, R.; Abou-Gharbia, H.A.; Shehata, A.A.Y. Endogenous antioxidants and stability of sesame oil as affected by processing and storage. JAOCS **1997**, *74*, 143–148.
52. Albi, T.; Lanzón, A.; Guinda, A.; León, M.; Pérez-Camino, M.C. Microwave and conventional heating effects on thermoxidative degradation of edible fats. J. Agric. Food Chem. **1997**, *45*, 3795–3798.
53. Khan, M.A.; Shahidi, F. Tocopherols and phospholipids enhance the oxidative stability of borage and evening primrose triacylglycerols. J. Food Lipids **2000**, *7*, 143–150.
54. Ford, J.E.; Porter, J.W.G.; Thompson, S.Y.; Toothill, J.; Edwards-Webb, J. Effects of ultra-high-temperature (UHT) processing and of subsequent storage on the vitamin content of milk. J. Dairy Res. **1969**, *36*, 447–454.
55. Vidal-Valverde, C.; Ruiz, R. Effects of frozen and other storage conditions on $\alpha$-tocopherol content of cow milk. J. Dairy Sci. **1993**, *76*, 1520–1525.
56. Sierra, I.; Prodanov, M.; Calvo, M.; Olano, A.; Vidal-Valverde, C. Vitamin stability and growth of phychrotrophic bacteria in refrigerated raw milk acidified with carbon dioxide. J. Food Protect **1996**, *59*, 1305–1310.
57. Ruas-Madiedo, P.; Bascarán, V.; Braña, A.F.; Bada-Gancedo, J.C.; Reyes-Gavilán, C.G. Influence of carbon dioxide addition to raw milk on microbial levels and some fat-soluble vitamin contents of raw and pasteurized milk. J. Agric. Food Chem. **1998**, *46*, 1552–1555.
58. Hollmann, P.C.H.; Slangen, J.H.; Finglas, P.M.; Wagstaffe, P.J.; Faure, U. Stability studies of vitamins in three food reference materials. Fresenius J. Anal. Chem. **1993**, *345*, 236–237.
59. Albalá-Hurtado, S.; Veciana-Nogués, M.T.; Riera-Valla, E.; Mariné-Font, A.; Vidal-Carou, M.C. Stability of vitamins during the storage of liquid infant milks. J. Dairy Res. **2000**, *67*, 225–231.

60. Albalá-Hurtado, S.; Veciana-Nogués, M.T.; Vidal-Carou, M.C.; Mariné-Font, A. Stability of vitamins A, E, and B complex in infant milks claimed to have equal final composition in liquid and powdered form. J. Food Sci. **2000**, *65*, 1052–1055.
61. Frian, J.; Vidal-Valverde, C. Stability of thiamine and vitamins E and A during storage of enteral feeding formula. J. Agric. Food Chem. **2001**, *49*, 2313–2317.
62. Cherian, G.; Wolfe, F.H.; Sim, J.S. Feeding dietary oils with tocopherols: effects on internal qualities of eggs during storage. J. Food Sci. **1996**, *61*, 15–18.
63. Nogala-Kalucka, M.; Gogolewski, M. Alteration of fatty acid composition, tocopherol content and peroxide value in margarine during storage at various temperature. Nahrung **2000**, *44*, 431–433.
64. Arnold, R.N.; Scheller, K.K.; Arp, S.C.; Williams, S.N.; Schaefer, D.M. Dietary $\alpha$-tocopheryl acetate enhances beef quality in Holstein and beef breed steers. J. Food Sci. **1993**, *58*, 28–33.
65. Kim, J.S.; Godber, J.S.; Prinaywiwatkul, W. Restructured beef roasts containing rice bran oil and fiber influences cholesterol oxidation and nutritional profile. J. Muscle Foods **2000**, *11*, 111–127.
66. Monahan, F.J.; Bukley, D.J.; Gray, J.I.; Morrissey, P.A.; Asghar, A.; Hanrahan, T.J.; Lynch, P.B. Effect of dietary vitamin E on the stability of raw and cooked pork. Meat Sci. **1990**, *27*, 99–108.
67. Pfalzgraf, A.; Frigg, M.; Steinhart, H. $\alpha$-Tocopherol contents and lipid oxidation in pork muscle and adipose tissue during storage. J. Agric. Food Chem. **1995**, *43*, 1339–1342.
68. Fox, J.B., Jr.; Lakritz, L.; Thayer, D.W. Thiamine, riboflavin and $\alpha$-tocopherol retention in processed and stored irradiated pork. J. Food Sci. **1997**, *62*, 1022–1025.
69. Marusich, W.L.; Ritter, E.D.; Ogrinz, E.F.; Keating, J.; Mitrovic, M.; Bunnell, R.H. Effect of supplemental vitamin E in control of rancidity in poultry meat. Poult. Sci. **1975**, *54*, 831–844.
70. Sheldon, B.W. Effect of dietary tocopherol on the oxidative stability of turkey meat. Poult. Sci. **1984**, *63*, 673–681.
71. Sheehy, P.J.A.; Morrissey, P.A.; Flynn, A. Increased storage stability of chicken muscle by dietary $\alpha$-tocopherol supplementation. Ir. J. Agric. Food Res. **1993**, *32*, 67–73.
72. Wen, J.; Morrissey, P.A.; Buckley, D.J.; Sheehy, P.J.A. Oxidative stability and $\alpha$-tocopherol retention in turkey burgers during refrigerated and frozen storage as influenced by dietary $\alpha$-tocopheryl acetate. Br. Poult. Sci. **1996**, *37*, 787–795.
73. King, A.J.; Uijttenboogaart, T.G.; Vries, A.W. $\alpha$-Tocopherol, $\beta$-carotene and ascorbic acid as antioxidants in stored poultry muscle. J. Food Sci. **1995**, *60*, 1009–1012.
74. Syväoja, E.L.; Salminen, K.; Piironen, V.; Varo, P.; Kerojoki, O.; Koivistoinen, P. Tocopherols and tocotrienols in Finnish foods: Fish and fish products. JAOCS **1985**, *62*, 1245–1248.
75. Al-Kahtani, H.A.; Abu-Tarboush, H.M.; Bajaber, A.A.; Atia, M.; Abou-Arab, A.A.; El-Mojaddidi, M.A. Chemical changes after irradiation and post-irradiation storage in tilapia and Spanish mackerel. J. Food Sci. **1996**, *61*, 729–733.
76. Erickson, M.C. Ability of chemical measurements to differenciate oxidative stabilities of frozen minced muscle tissue from farm-raised striped bass and hybrid striped bass. Food Chem. **1993**, *48*, 381–385.

77. Erickson, M.C.; Thed, S.T. Comparision of chemical measurements to differentiate oxidative stability of frozen minced tilapia fish muscle. Int. J. Food Sci. Technol. **1994**, *29*, 585–591.
78. Slover, H.T.; Lehmann, J. Effects of fumigation on wheat in storage. IV. Tocopherols. Cereal Chem. **1972**, *49*, 412–415.
79. Allen, W.M.; Parr, W.H.; Bradley, R.; Swannack, K.; Barton, C.R.Q.; Tyler, R. Loss of vitamin E in stored cereals in relation to a myopathy of yearling cattle. Vet. Rec. **1974**, April 20, pp 373–375.
80. Young, L.G.; Lun, A.; Pos, J.; Forshaw, R.P.; Edmeades, D. Vitamin E stability in corn and mixed feed. J. Anim. Sci., 1975, *40*, 495–499.
81. Hakkarainen, R.V.J.; Työppönen, J.T.; Bengtsson, S.G. Changes in the content and composition of vitamin E in damp barley stored in airtight bins. J. Sci. Food Agric. **1983**, *34*, 1029–1038.
82. McMurray, C.H.; Blanchflower, W.J.; Rice, D.A. The effect of pre-treatment on the stability of alpha tocopherol in moist barley. Proc. Nutr. Soc. **1980**, *39*, A61–A61.
83. Hakkarainen, R.V.J.; Työppönen, J.T.; Bengtsson, S.G. Relative and quantitative changes in total vitamin E and isomer content of barley during conventional and airtight storage with special reference to annual variations. Acta Agric. Scand. **1983**, *33*, 395–400.
84. Rice, D.A.; Blanchflower, W.J.; McMurray, C.H. The effects of moisture, propionic acid, sodium hydroxide and anaerobiosis on the stability of vitamin E in stored barley. J. Agric. Sci. Camb. **1985**, *105*, 15–19.
85. Galliard, T. Hydrolytic and oxidative degradation of lipids during storage of wholemeal flour: Effect of bran and germ components. J. Cereal Sci. **1986**, *4*, 179–192.
86. Wennermark, B.; Ahlmen, H.; Jägerstad, M. Improved vitamin E retention by using freshly-milled whole-meal wheat flour during drum-drying. J. Agric. Food Chem. **1994**, *42*, 1348–1351.
87. Peterson, D.M. Oat tocols: concentration and stability in oat products and distribution within the kernel. Cereal Chem. **1995**, *72*, 21–24.
88. Shin, T.S.; Godber, J.S.; Martin, D.E.; Wells, J.H. Hydrolytic stability and change in E vitamers and oryzanol of extruded rice bran during storage. J. Food Sci. **1997**, *62*, 704–708, 728.
89. Sabaté, J.; Hook, D.G. Almonds, walnuts, and serum lipids. In *Handbook of Lipids in Human Nutrition*; Soiller, G.A., Ed.; CRC Press: Boca Raton, FL, 1996.
90. Adnan, M.; Argoudelis, C.J.; Rodda, E.; Tobias, J. Lipid oxidative stability of reconstituted partially defatted peanuts. Peanut Sci. **1981**, *8*, 13–15.
91. Fourie, P.C.; Basson, D.S. Changes in the tocopherol content of almond, pecan and macadamia kernels during storage. JAOCS **1989**, *66*, 1113–1115.
92. Yao, F.; Dull, G.; Eitenmiller, R.R. Tocopherol quantification by HPLC in pecans and relationship to kernel quality during storage. J. Food Sci. **1992**, *57*, 1194–1197.
93. Erickson, M.C.; Santerre, C.R.; Malingre, M.E. Oxidative stability in raw and roasted pecans: chemical, physical and sensory measurements. J. Food Sci. **1994**, *59*, 1234–1243.

94. Senesi, E.; Rizzolo, A.; Colombo, C.; Testoni, A. Influence of pre-processing storage conditions on peeled almond quality. Ital. J. Food Sci. **1996**, *2*, 115–125.
95. Lavedrine, F.; Ravel, A.; Poupard, A.; Alary, J. Effect of geographic origin, variety and storage on tocopherol contentrations in walnuts by HPLC. Food Chem. **1997**, *58*, 135–140.
96. Lima, J.R.; Gonçalves, L.A.G.; Silva, M.A.A.P.; Campos, S.D.S.; Garcia, E.E.C. Effect of different packaging conditions on storage of roasted and salted cashew nut. Acta Alimen. **1998**, *27*, 329–339.
97. Daood, H.G.; Vinkler, M.; Márkus, F.; Hebshi, E.A.; Biacs, P.A. Antioxidant vitamin content of spice red pepper (paprika) as affected by technological and varietal factors. Food Chem. **1996**, *55*, 365–372.
98. Márkus, F.; Daood, H.G.; Kapitány, J.; Biacs, P.A. Changes in the carotenoid and antioxidant content of spice red pepper (paprika) as a function of ripening and some technological factors. J. Agric. Food Chem. **1999**, *47*, 100–107.
99. Spychalla, J.P.; Desborough, S.L. Superoxide dismutase, catalase, and $\alpha$-tocopherol content of stored potato tubers. Plant Physiol. **1990**, *94*, 1214–1218.
100. Barth, M.M.; Zhuang, H. Packaging design affects antioxidant vitamin retention and quality of broccoli florets during postharvest storage. Post Biol. Technol. **1996**, *9*, 141–150.

# 7

# Analysis of Tocopherols and Tocotrienols in Foods

## 7.1. HISTORICAL ASPECTS

Bunnell (1) in a 1971 review of procedures for analysis of vitamin E stated, "New or modified tocopherol assay procedures still appear at a frequent rate, even though vitamin E has been with us for over 40 years. The development of reliable assay methodology has been an evolutionary process which has achieved its greatest rate of development in the last 10 years." Now, 70 years after the first characterization of vitamin E, methodology is still in an evolutionary stage and the number of method papers continues to grow rapidly. At the time of Bunnell's review, gas chromatographic (GC) methods for vitamin E analysis were rapidly gaining acknowledgment as the best approach for quantification of the tocopherols and tocotrienols. High-performance liquid chromatographic (HPLC) procedures were not yet in common use. Bunnell (1) reviewed only chromatographic methods, which included paper, thin-layer, column, and GC procedures. For final quantitation, after resolution by paper, thin-layer, or column techniques, Emmerie-Engel or bathophenthroline reagents were usually employed for chromophore development. For GC procedures, detection was by flame ionization.

Parrish (2) in 1980 published a comprehensive review of vitamin E methods that included initial reports on HPLC. He presented HPLC as a method with advantages over other methods. At that time, Parrish cited only 19 publications that applied HPLC to vitamin E analysis. However, Parrish foresaw the power of HPLC techniques for vitamin E assay of biologicals and discussed advantages of the technique over GC. Since 1980, a large number of publications have used HPLC for vitamin E assay of foods, feeds, tissues, and other highly varied biologicals. We doubt that even Dr. Parrish foresaw the rapidity with which HPLC would dominate the field of tocopherol and tocotrienol analysis.

Parrish classified methods for vitamin E analysis into the following categories:

Biological assays: Fertility tests including resorption–gestation, development of encephalomalacia in newly hatched chicks, development of muscular dystrophy and creatinuria in rabbits, vitamin E content of blood or liver in various species, and hemolysis of red blood cells in vitamin E–deficient rats

Physicochemical methods: Ultraviolet (UV), fluorometric, and colorimetric methods

Chromatographic methods: Paper, thin-layer, column, GC, and HPLC

Our intention in this chapter is to discuss GC and HPLC methodology in detail. Older, classical reviews on methods for vitamin E assay are given in Table 7.1 for the convenience of readers who want to read material on the early methods written by some of the pioneers in vitamin E research. Historically significant publications showing the timeline for development of vitamin E methods are summarized in Table 7.2. More recent reviews on vitamin E methods include Nelis et al. (126) Ball (127–129), Desai and Machlin (130), Lang et al. (131) Thompson and Hatina (132), Bourgeous (133), Lumley (134), Eitenmiller and Landen,(135,136) Abidi (137), Piironen (138), and Ruperez et al. (139).

## 7.2. GAS CHROMATOGRAPHY

Early gas chromatographic procedures for vitamin E analysis used packed columns; stationary phases including Apiezon L, SE-30, and OV-17; and flame ionization detection (FID). In most methods, tocopherols and tocotrienols were derivatized to their trimethylsilyl ethers to improve thermal stability and volatility. By the mid-1960s, GC was firmly established as the most precise

**TABLE 7.1** Reviews on Vitamin E Assay Methods to 1980

| |
|---|
| Bunnell, R.H. Modern procedures for the analysis of tocopherols. Lipid 1971, *6*, 245–253 (1). |
| Lehman, R.W. Determination of vitamin E. In *Methods of Biochemical Analysis*, Vol. 2; Glick, D., Ed.; Interscience: New York, 1955 (3). |
| Kofler, M.; Sommer, P.F.; Bollinger, H.R.; Schmidli, B.; Vecchi, M. Physiochemical properties and assay of the tocopherols. In *Vitamins and Hormones*, Vol. 20; Harris, R.S., Wool, I.G., Eds.; Academic Press: New York, 1962 (4). |
| Bunnell, R.H. Vitamin E assay by chemical methods. In *The Vitamins*, Vol. 6; György, P., Pearson, W.N.; Eds.; Academic Press: New York, 1967 (5). |
| Bliss, C.I.; György, P. Bioassays of vitamin E. In *The Vitamins*, Vol. 6; György, P., Pearson, W.N., Eds.; Academic Press: New York, 1967 (6). |
| Brubacher, G. The determination of vitamins and carotenoids in fats. In *Analysis and Characterization of Oils, Fats and Fat Products*, Vol. 2; Boekenoogen, H.A., Ed.; Interscience: New York, 1968 (7). |
| Vogel, P.; Wieske, T. Paper and thin-layer chromatography in fat chemistry. XIV. Tocopherols. In *Analysis and Characterization of Oils, Fats and Fat Products*, Vol. 2; Boekenoogen, H.A., Ed.; Interscience: New York, 1968 (8). |
| Bieri, J.G. Chromatography of tocopherols. In *Lipid Chromatographic Analysis*; Marinetti, G.V., Ed.; Marcel Dekker: New York, 1969 (9). |
| Sheppard, A.J.; Prosser, A.R.; Hubbard, W.D. Gas chromatography of vitamin E. In *Methods in Enzymology, Vitamins and Coenzymes*, Part C; McCormick, D.B., Wright, L.D., Eds.; Academic Press: New York, 1971 (10). |
| Ames, S.R. Tocopherols. IV. Estimation in foods and food supplements. In *The Vitamins*, Vol. 5; Sebrell, W.H., Jr., Harris, R.S., Eds.; Academic Press: New York, 1972.(11) |
| Sheppard, A.J.; Prosser, A.R.; Hubbard, W.D. Gas chromatography of the fat-soluble vitamins: A review. JAOCS 1972, *11*, 619–633 (12). |
| Green, J. Distribution of fat-soluble vitamins and their standardization and assay by biological methods. In *Fat-Soluble Vitamins*; Morton, R.A., Ed.; Pergamon Press: Oxford, 1970 (13). |
| Draper, H.H. Chemical assays of vitamin E. In *Fat-Soluble Vitamins*; Morton, R.A., Ed.; 1970 (14). |
| Laidman, D.L.; Hall, G.S. Adsorption column chromatography of tocopherols. In *Methods in Enzymology, Vitamins and Coenzymes*, Part C; McCormick, D.B., Wright, L.D., Eds.; Academic Press: New York, 1971 (15). |
| Desai, I.D. Assay methods. In *Vitamin E: A Comprehensive Treatise*; Macklin, L.J., Ed.; Marcel Dekker: New York, 1980 (16). |
| Parrish, D.B. Determination of vitamin E in foods—a review. CRC Crit. Rev. Food Sci. Nutr. 1980, 161–187 (2). |

[a]Reference number in parentheses.

**Table 7.2** Historically Significant Methodology Publications for the Analysis of Vitamin E

| Method | Approach | References |
|---|---|---|
| **Biological assays** | | |
| Resorption–gestation | Feed basal diet deficient in vitamin E to young female rats until 34–40 days of age; breed; pregnant females are fed graded doses of test material or vitamin E standards; rats are killed after 16 days gestation; dead and live fetuses are counted. | Joffe and Harris, 1943 (17)<br>Mason and Harris, 1947 (18)<br>Harris and Ludwig, 1949 (19)<br>Bunyan et al., 1961 (20)<br>Ames et al., 1963 (21) |
| Encephalomalacia in chicks | Newly hatched chicks are fed a vitamin E–free diet; feeds and standards are fed from the 4th day after hatching; record deaths occurring in 7 to 10 days. | Dam and Sondergaard, 1964 (22)<br>Hakkarainen et al., 1984 (23) |
| Muscular dystrophy in rabbits | Muscular dystrophy symptoms occur after 1 month with vitamin E–deficient diets; standard and test diets lead to improvements; rabbits die if vitamin E not added to diet. | Hove and Harris, 1947 (24)<br>Fitch and Diehl, 1965 (25) |
| Hemolysis of red blood cells in rats | Young rats (100 g) are fed a vitamin-deficient diet for 3–4 weeks until red blood cells show >90% hemolysis; hemolysis is in vitro with dialuric acid or hydrogen peroxide; vitamin E test doses are administered by stomach tube; biopotency is measured from the reduction in the red blood cell hemolysis of test group compared to that of deficient group. | Rose and György, 1952 (26)<br>Horwitt et al., 1956 (27)<br>Friedman et al., 1958 (28) |

(*continued*)

**Table 7.2** *Continued*

| Method | Approach | References |
|---|---|---|
| Liver storage | Assumes that liver concentrations in rats and chicks respond linearly to dietary levels; 1-day-old chicks are depleted and then given supplements or standard doses for 3 days or 13 days. | Mason, 1942 (29)<br>Bunnell, 1957 (30)<br>Pudelkiwicz et al., 1960 (31)<br>Dicks and Matterson, 1961 (32) |
| **Physicochemical** | | |
| UV spectroscopy | Direct spectrophotometric determination; limited to pure solutions or high concentration pharmaceuticals. | Lambertsen and Braekkan, 1959 (33) |
| Colorimetry | Emmerie-Engel reaction; based on the reduction of ferric ions to ferrous ions, which forms a red complex with $\alpha$,2′-dipyridine; measure at 520 nm; modification uses bathophenanthroline. | Emmerie and Engel, 1938, 1939, 1940 (34,35,36)<br>Emmerie, 1940, 1941 (37,38)<br>Smith et al., 1952 (39)<br>Tsen, 1961 (40) |
| Fluorescence | Free tocopherols fluoresce strongly; esters fluoresce weakly; primary detection mode for HPLC assays. | Duggan, 1959 (41)<br>Thompson et al., 1972 (42) |
| Chromatographic paper | One- and two-dimensional chromatography on paper imprenated with petroleum (Vaseline), paraffin, or zinc carbonate; solvent systems are benzene, benzene-cyclohexane, diethyl ether–petroleum ether and many others; preference given to thin-layer techniques around 1960. | Brown, 1952 (43,44)<br>Eggitt and Ward, 1953 (45,46)<br>Green et al., 1955 (47)<br>Green, 1958 (48)<br>Booth, 1961 (49) |

(*continued*)

**TABLE 7.2** *Continued*

| Method | Approach | References |
|---|---|---|
| Thin-layer | One- and two-dimensional chromatography on alumina magnesium sulfate, silica gel G, calcium phosphate, and diatomaceous earth; mobile phases similar to those used in paper chromatography; detection by spray with Emmerie-Engel reagent, antimony pentachloride, UV, or fluorescence. | Seher, 1961 (50)<br>Dilley and Crane, 1963 (51)<br>Stowe, 1963 (52)<br>Rao et al., 1965 (53)<br>Sturm et al., 1966 (54)<br>Whittle and Pennock, 1967 (55)<br>Chow et al., 1969 (56)<br>Ames, 1971 (57)<br>Lovelady, 1973 (58) |
| Open-column | Primarily used as a cleanup step before other determinative steps such as GC; commonly used solid-phase materials include magnesium phosphate, celite, Florisil, silica gel, alumina, Fuller's earth, hydroxyalkoxypropyl sephadex. | Drummond et al., 1935 (59)<br>Emmerie and Engel, 1939 (35)<br>Kjolhede, 1942 (60)<br>Devlin and Mattill, 1942 (61)<br>Meunier and Vinet, 1942 (62)<br>Tosic and Moore, 1945 (63)<br>Kofler, 1947 (64)<br>Emmerie, 1949 (65)<br>Eggitt and Norris, 1955 (66)<br>Bro-Rasmussen and Hjarde, 1957 (67)<br>Pudelkiewicz and Matterson, 1960 (68)<br>Bieri et al., 1961 (69)<br>Herting and Drury, 1963 (70)<br>Dicks-Bushnell, 1967 (71)<br>Thompson et al., 1972 (42)<br>Strong, 1976 (72) |

(*continued*)

**TABLE 7.2** *Continued*

| Method | Approach | References |
|---|---|---|
| Gas-liquid | Volatile derivatives are usually formed; capillary GC has many advantages over packed column chromatography, detection is with FID; methodology is still useful but most routine assays are completed by HPLC. | Nicolaides, 1960 (73)<br>Wilson et al., 1962 (74)<br>Nair and Turner, 1963 (75)<br>Sweeley et al., 1963 (76)<br>Carrol and Herting, 1964 (77)<br>Libby and Sheppard, 1964 (78)<br>Bieri and Prival, 1965 (79)<br>Nair et al., 1966 (80)<br>Ishikawa and Katsui, 1966 (81)<br>Eisner et al., 1966 (82)<br>Slover et al., 1967, 1968, 1969, 1983, 1985, (83–88)<br>Nair and Machiz, 1967 (89)<br>Nair and Luna, 1968 (90)<br>Mann et al., 1968 (91)<br>Nelson and Milun, 1968 (92)<br>Sheppard et al., 1969 (93)<br>Nelson et al., 1970 (94)<br>Bieri et al., 1970 (95)<br>Lehmann and Slover, 1971 (96)<br>Slover, 1971 (97)<br>Dasilva and Jensen, 1971 (98)<br>Sheppard et al., 1972 (12)<br>Rudy et al., 1972 (99)<br>Lovelady, 1973 (100)<br>Feeter, 1974 (101)<br>Hartman, 1977 (102)<br>Slover and Lanza, 1979 (103)<br>Sheppard and Hubbard, 1979 (104)<br>Slover and Thompson, 1981 (105) |

(*continued*)

**TABLE 7.2** *Continued*

| Method | Approach | References |
|---|---|---|
| HPLC | Normal-phase and reversed-phase chromatography; detection by UV of fluorescence; normal-phase chromatography can resolve the eight vitamin E forms; reversed-phase cannot resolve the positional isomers, β-T and α-T; most widely applicable, easily controlled assay approach for analysis of vitamin E. | Schmit et al., 1971 (106)<br>Van Niekerk, 1973 (107)<br>Cavins and Inglett, 1974 (108)<br>Carr, 1974 (109)<br>Abe et al., 1975 (110)<br>Matsuo and Tahara, 1977 (111)<br>Eriksson and Sörensen, 1977 (112)<br>Vatassery et al., 1978 (113)<br>Nilsson et al., 1978 (114)<br>Söderhjelm and Andersson, 1978 (115)<br>De Leenheer et al., 1978 (116)<br>Cohen and Lapointe, 1978 (117)<br>Barnett and Frick, 1979 (118)<br>Ikenoya et al., 1979 (119)<br>Tagney et al., 1979 (120)<br>Bieri et al., 1979 (121)<br>Carpenter, 1979 (122)<br>McMurray and Blanchflower, 1979 (123)<br>Barnes and Taylor, 1980 (124)<br>Ruggeri et al., 1979 (125) |

Reference numbers in parentheses. UV, ultraviolet; HPLC, high-performance liquid chromatography; GC, gas chromatography; FID, flame ionization detection.

method to assay vitamin E. Parrish (2) summarized advantages and problems of GC methods compared to previously used procedures:

| Advantages |
|---|
| 1. Free and esterified α-tocopherol (α-T) could be quantitified in the same product. |
| 2. Sterols and other fat-soluble vitamins could be quanitified simultaneously. |

3. Assay values were higher, indicating less destruction and/or better extraction.
4. Reproducibility was better.
5. GC was faster.

---

| Problems |
|---|
| 1. GC analysis required higher extract purity when working with low vitamin E levels. |
| 2. Instrument and column parameters had to be carefully controlled. |
| 3. Calibrations of the apparatus and standards had to be constantly checked. |
| 4. Column overloading had to be prevented. |

In order to extract and further purify sample extracts efficiently, analysts relied on saponification, freeze concentration, digitonin precipitation, sublimation, and column and thin-layer chromatography techniques (2). Parrish(2) warned that the preanalysis steps must be carefully controlled to prevent destruction of vitamin E. Even with the problems associated with GC analysis, excellent data, reproducible by today's HPLC methods, were obtained by the investigators who refined the methodology.

Early methods were hampered by the inability of packed column chromatography to resolve $\beta$- and $\gamma$-tocopherols and $\beta$- and $\gamma$-tocotrienols. Additionally, packed column chromatography was labor-intensive and affected by interferences to both the tocopherols and the internal standard peaks, requiring saponification to reduce the interferences and the use of correction factors to correct for unremoved interferences (140). Lang et al. (131) in a review of GC methodology, stated that through 1988, no packed column GC method had been developed to resolve $\beta$- and $\gamma$-T or $\beta$- and $\gamma$-tocotrienol ($\gamma$-T3) adequately. Also, $\alpha$-T3 and $\alpha$-T were not well resolved.

Development of capillary GC solved many of the problems associated with packed column chromatography of tocopherols and tocotrienols. Marks(140) published a capillary GC method for vitamin E in deodorizer sludge and compared the method to packed column chromatography. Comparisons of the parameters of the two procedures are given in Table 7.3. Of significance, saponification was not required for the capillary method, reducing sample preparation time to 5–10 min compared to 2–3 h for the packed column method. Figure 7.1 shows the comparison of the chromatography obtained with the capillary and packed column systems. The method developed by Marks (140) is the basis of AOCS Recommended Practice Ce 7-87 (141) adopted in 1988 (142), "Total Tocopherols in Deodorizer Sludge." Details of the procedure follow:

**TABLE 7.3** Vitamin E Analysis in Deodorizer Distillate by Capillary and Packed Column Gas Chromatography

| Item | Capillary | Packed |
|---|---|---|
| Sample preparation | 5–10 min | 2–3 h |
| Chromatography | Temperature programmed | 40 min Isothermal |
| Resolution | 98% Resolution of β- and γ-T | No resolution between β- and γ-T |
| Interference | None | Possible interference with tocopherols and internal standard |
| Accuracy | 99%+ | Unknown |
| Precision | ±1.1% RSD[a] | ±3.2% RSD[a] |
| Time | 40 min | 4 h |

β-T, β-tocopherol; RSD, relative standard deviation.
*Source*: Modified from Ref. 140.

Apparatus
- Gas chromatograph equipped with FID
- 30-m DB-5 capillary column, 0.25-μm film thickness, 0.25-mm inner diameter (id)

Chromatography
- Helium carrier gas, 2 $cm^3$/min
- Program
- 140°C to 300°C at 10°C/min
- Hold 6 min
- 300°C to 320°C at 5°C/min
- Hold 10 min
- Split flow rate 150 $cm^3$/min
- Injector temperature 240°C
- Detector temperature 345°C

Calculation
- Internal standard heptadecanyl stearate

Full details of procedures are in AOCS Method Ce 7-87 (141). The collaborative study indicated that the four laboratories of the nine that submitted results obtained good agreement of results between analyses completed on different days; however, results between laboratories and between duplicate vials were poor, producing high $RSD_R$ values. The study suffered because samples degraded during cold storage and because one participating laboratory could not meet time frame requirements (142). The method has never been fully collaborated by AOCS.

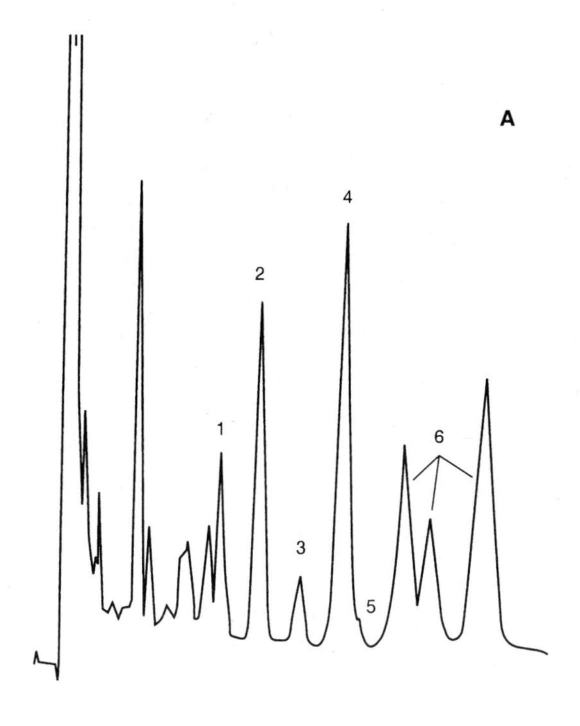


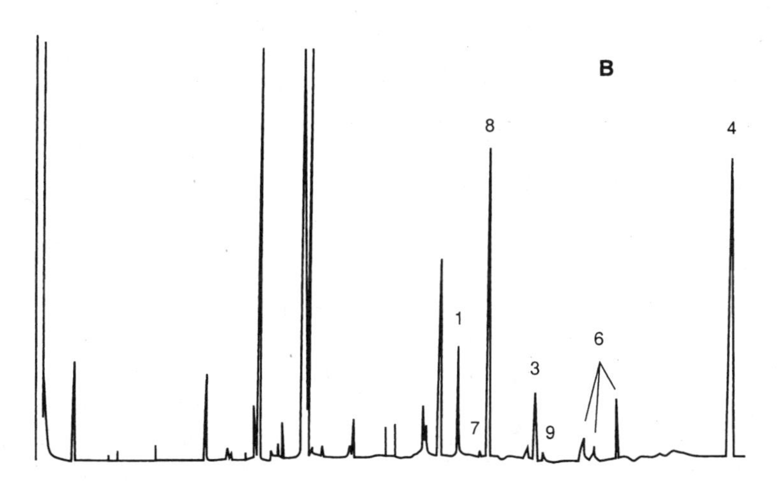


**FIGURE 7.1** Comparison of packed column (A) and capillary column (B) GC of a deodorizer distillate. 1 = $\delta$-T, 2 = $\beta$-T + $\gamma$-T, 3 = $\alpha$-T, 4 = IS, 5 = Brassicasterol, 6 = sterols, 7 = $\beta$-T, 8 = $\gamma$-T, 9 = cholesterol. $\alpha$-T, $\alpha$-tocopherol; IS, internal standard; GS, gas chromatogram. (Modified from Ref. 140.)

Although HPLC is the primary method used for routine vitamin E quantification, GC methods frequently see use in studies requiring identification of analytes from complex matrices that include tocopherols and/or tocotrienols. Such procedures usually rely on the linking of GC and mass spectrometry(143–145). As an example, in 1998 Frega et al. (143) identified and confirmed the presence of several components of annatto, including $\alpha$- and $\beta$-T3. Analysis of the total lipid fraction included saponification, treatment of the extract with diazomethane to methylate free fatty acids, and silanization. Gas chromatography/mass spectrometry (GC/MS) was on a 30-m capillary column containing SPB-5 as the stationary phase. The GC/MS techniques are further discussed in Sec. 7.6.3.

Gas chromatography is still routinely used to assay vitamin E in foods (146–153). Maraschiello and Regueiro (146) used a 30-m column coated with 5% phenylmethylsilicone to assay low levels of $\alpha$-T in poultry tissue. The procedure used saponification and silica SPE to remove cholesterol from the digest before silylating with 33% hexadimethylsilazane and 11% trimethylchlorosilane in pyridine. $\alpha$-Tocopheryl acetate was used as an internal standard. Peaks were confirmed by GC-MS on a GC (Fisons Instruments) interfaced with a MS (Fisons Instruments Trio 2000). Ulberth (147) simultaneously assayed $\alpha$-, $\beta$-, $\alpha$-, and $\alpha$-T with cholesterol in standard preparations after silyation with Sylon HTP (Supelco) or acylation with heptafluorobutyrylimidazol. Chromatography used a fused silica column (20 m) coated with DB-5 and FID. Initial oven temperature was 260°C, programmed to increase to 300°C at 4°C/min after 1 min. Acylation improved resolution of $\alpha$-T and cholesterol compared to that of the trimethylsilyl derivatives. Botsoglou et al. (148) simultaneously assayed cholesterol and $\alpha$-T in eggs without derivatizing the analytes. The study used a simple one-tube sample preparation involving saponification, addition of hexane to the digest, centrifugation, and direct injection of the hexane onto the GC column. Chromatography was on a 15-m fused silica column coated with SPB-1. Oven temperature was programmed from 250°C to 275°C at 2°C/min and held for 12 min. Use of the shorter, thick film column did not result in peak tailing. The method showed good accuracy and precision with recoveries approaching 100% for both analytes. Ballesteros et al. (149) used a continuous system to transesterify triglycerides from edible oils and fats before the GC resolution of $\alpha$-T, *all-rac-$\alpha$-*tocopheryl acetate, and cholesterol. By transesterification, the volatility of the potentially interfering triglycerides was increased, allowing direct injection of the transesterified sample onto the GC column. Elimination of derivatization of the analytes provided an assay with high precision that is applicable to high-fat samples.

In an earlier study, Smidt et al. (153) reported the simultaneous assay of retinol and $\alpha$-T by use of cold on-column injection of nonderivatized analytes. In most prior GC methods, retinol and $\alpha$-T were derivatized to prevent decomposition in hot injectors. Extracts of various biological samples were prepared by fat extraction, saponification, extraction on nonsaponifiable lipids, and use of digitonin-impregnated celite column chromatography to remove sterol interferences. The GC system included a 15-m- by 0.25-mm-id column coated with a 0.25-μm film of methylsilicone and temperature programming from 220°C to 270°C at 3°/min with a 20-min hold. The FID temperature was 290°C. Recoveries for the analytes were above 90%.

## 7.3. HIGH-PERFORMANCE LIQUID CHROMATOGRAPHY

High-performance liquid chromatography (HPLC) was first applied to the resolution of vitamin E and other fat-soluble vitamins in 1971 by Schmit et al. (106) and in a follow-up publication in 1972 (154). Two reversed-phase packing materials, Permaphase ODS and Zipax HCP, introduced by DuPont in the early stages of HPLC, were used to study resolution of the fat-soluble vitamins, including $\alpha$-T and $\alpha$-tocopheryl acetate. Permaphase ODS was a $C_{18}$ column and Zipax HCP was a hydrocarbon coating on Zipax support. Good resolution of the tocopherols in a mixed tocopherol concentrate was obtained with the ODS column, although the peaks other than $\alpha$-T were not identified because the only standard available to the research group was $\alpha$-T. $\alpha$-Tocopherol and *all-rac-$\alpha$*-tocopheryl acetate could be resolved from other fat-soluble vitamins. The mobile phases studied included methanol : water combinations with either isocratic or gradient elution. Ultraviolet (UV) detection at 254 nm was sufficient to detect the fat-soluble vitamins for the quite concentrated preparations used in the study. The work by Schmit and colleagues(106,153) and a study by Van Niekerk(107) published in 1973 showed the power of HPLC for vitamin analysis and led the way for its rapid advance in the next few years. Van Niekerk's work was the first published HPLC paper dealing with food analysis of vitamin E. Also, this study used normal-phase chromatography on Corasil II with a mobile phase of isopropanol ether:hexane (5 : 95). Van Niekerk's work set important principles for the application of HPLC to vitamin E analysis that eased the work of later vitamin E analysts. These included the following:

1. Oils could be injected directly onto a silica column; therefore, no sample preparation other than dilution of the oil was required.
2. Fluorescence provided an ideal, sensitive, and specific detection mode.
3. Positional isomers, $\beta$- and $\gamma$-T, could be resolved.
4. Good reproducibility was possible.
5. Recoveries of added tocopherols to oils were high, approaching 100%.
6. The procedure was "fast and easy." Van Niekerk predicted that HPLC would find wide application for the routine assay of vitamin E in foods.

Other early applications of HPLC to vitamin E analysis of food included that of Cavins and Inglett (108), who resolved the tocopherols and tocotrienols in hexane. These authors applied the method to corn oil and wheat bran, obtaining clean chromatograms with direct injection of the oil diluted in cyclohexane with UV detection at 254 nm. No quantitation was attempted. The study was significant in that it showed that the eight vitamin E homologues could be resolved from plant oils without cleanup or derivatization and that retention time could be a valuable parameter for analyte identification, considering the resolving power of the technique.

In the next year, (1975) Abe et al. (110) also applied HPLC to the quantitation of tocopherols in vegetable oils. They used normal-phase chromatography on JASCO-PACK WC-03 with a mobile phase of diisopropyl ether in hexane (2:98) and fluorescence detection. They quantitated $\alpha$-, $\beta$-, $\gamma$-, and $\delta$-T in soybean, cottonseed, and wheat germ oil, thus providing some of the first quantitative data on the vitamin E content of food determined by HPLC. Additionally, Abe et al. (110) showed that the HPLC data compared closely with GC data and that direct oil injection provided data very comparable to data obtained by saponification of the oils before HPLC resolution. Unlike with GC, $\beta$- and $\gamma$-T were resolved by the HPLC system. They clearly demonstrated the superiority of fluorescence detection to UV detection in terms of sensitivity. After 1975, HPLC coupled with fluorescence detection became the method of choice for vitamin E assay of foods and other biological samples.

Because of the large number of publications dealing with HPLC applications to the analysis of vitamin E in food within the last decade, we do not attempt to provide a comprehensive literature review of methodology. We discuss details of various aspects of significance to the successful use of HPLC to assay vitamin E in food. Some newer approaches to food analysis of specific matrices are covered. Table 7.4 gives summaries of selected references.

### 7.3.1. Extraction of Vitamin E Before Quantification by High-Performance Liquid Chromatography

Because of the possibility of oxidative degradation, all extractions, whatever the approach, need to ensure the stability of the vitamin E analytes as a primary factor influencing the success of the procedure. Depending on the sample matrix, extraction of tocopherols and tocotrienols is usually performed by direct solvent extraction or saponification (alkali hydrolysis). Most oils that contain higher levels of vitamin E than other foods can be diluted with hexane or mobile phase and directly injected onto a normal-phase column. This straightforward approach works well unless a component of the oil has low solubility in the

**TABLE 7.4** Selected High-Performance Liquid Chromatography Methods for the Analysis of Vitamin E in Foods[a]

| | | Sample preparation | High-performance liquid chromatography parameters | | | | |
|---|---|---|---|---|---|---|---|
| Sample matrix | Analyte | Sample extraction and cleanup | Column | Mobile phase | Detection | Quality assurance | References |
| **Oils and fats** | | | | | | | |
| 1. Seed oils | α-, β-, γ-, δ-T<br>α-T3 | Dilute with Hex<br>Direct injection | Polygosil 60–5,<br>5 μm,<br>4.6 × 250 mm | Isocratic Hex DIPE (90 : 10),<br>1.8 mL/min | Fluorescence<br>*Ex* $\lambda = 296$<br>*Em* $\lambda = 320$ | QL 4 μg/g<br>CV% 2.9–8.4<br>%Recovery<br>93–95 | Speek et al., 1985 (155) |
| 2. Vegetable oils, cod liver oil, margarine, butter, dairy spread | α-, β-, γ-, δ-T<br>α-, β-, γ-, δ-T3 | Dilute with Hex<br>Direct injection | LiChrosorb Si60<br>5 μm,<br>4.0 × 250 mm,<br>30°C | Gradient 8% to 17% DIEP in Hex | Fluorescence<br>*Ex* $\lambda = 290$<br>*Em* $\lambda = 325$ | QL 0.25 mg/100 g | Syväoja et al., 1986 (156) |
| 3. Vegetable oils | α-, β-, γ-, δ-T | Dilute with Hex<br>Direct injection | LiChrosorb Si60<br>5 μm,<br>4.6 × 250 mm | Isocratic 3% dioxane in Hex,<br>1 mL/min | Fluorescence<br>*Ex* $\lambda = 295$<br>*Em* $\lambda = 330$ | — | Desai et al., 1988 (157) |
| 4. Rice bran oil | α-, β-, γ-, δ-T<br>α-, β-, γ-, δ-T3<br>γ-Oxyzanol | Dilute with MeCN : MeOH : IPA (50 : 45 : 5)<br>Direct injection | Hypersil ODS<br>5 μm,<br>2.1 × 200 mm | Gradient<br>a. 0–5 min, MeCN : MeOH : IPA : water (45 : 45 : 5 : 5)<br>b. 5–10 min, MeCN : MeOH : IPA (50 : 45 : 5), 1 mL/min | Fluorescence<br>a. Vitamin E<br>*Ex* $\lambda = 290$<br>*Em* $\lambda = 320$<br>b. Oxyzanol<br>325 nm | — | Rogers et al., 1993 (158) |

(*continued*)

**Table 7.4** *Continued*

| | | Sample preparation | High-performance liquid chromatography parameters | | | | |
|---|---|---|---|---|---|---|---|
| Sample matrix | Analyte | Sample extraction and cleanup | Column | Mobile phase | Detection | Quality assurance | References |
| 5. Vegetable oils | α-, β-, γ-, δ-T | Add tocol (IS)<br>Dilute with $CH_2Cl_2$<br>GPC Cleanup<br>Four columns in series<br>1. Ultrasphere 1000 Å<br>2. Ultrasphere 500 Å<br>3. μStyragel 100 Å<br>4. μStyragel 500 Å<br>Collect vitamin fraction, evaporate, and redissolve in mobile phase | Ultrasphere silica 5 μm, 4.6 × 250 mm | Hex : IPA (99.3 : 0.7), 1 mL/min | 1. Evaporative light scattering (ELSD)<br>2. Fluorescence<br>*Ex* λ = 290<br>*Em* λ = 330 | DL On-column (ng)<br>ELSD 250<br>Fluorescence 25 | Chase et al., 1994 (159) |
| 6. Olive oil | α-β-, γ-, δ-T<br>α-, β-, γ-, δ-T3 | a. NP-HPLC<br>Dilute with Hex<br>Direct injection<br>b. RP-HPLC<br>Dilute with THF<br>Dilute with MeOH<br>Direct injection | a. LiChrosorb Si60 5 μm, 4 × 250 mm<br>b. Spherisorb ODS 5μm 4.6 × 250 mm | Isocratic NP-HPLC Hex : IPA (99.7 : 0.3), 1.7 mL/min<br>RP-HPLC 0.05 M $NaClO_4$ : MeOH (10 : 90), 2.0 mL/min | NP-HPLC<br>a. Fluorescence<br>*Ex* λ = 290<br>*Em* λ = 330<br>b. PDA 280 nm<br>RP-HPLC<br>Amperometric 0.6 V | QL<br>γ-T3 1.9 mg/100 g<br>$RSD_R$ (%)<br>α-T 0.5<br>α-T3 0.9<br>β-T3 6.8<br>γ-T3 1.5<br>δ-T3 5.3 | Dionisi et al., 1995 (160) |

| | | | | | | | |
|---|---|---|---|---|---|---|---|
| 7. Rapeseed oil w/wo added antioxidants | α-, β-, γ-, δ-T | Dilute with Hex<br>Direct injection | Apex silica 5 μm, 4.6 × 250 mm | Isocratic Hex : IPA (98.5 : 1.5), 1 mL/min | Fluorescence<br>*Ex* λ = 290<br>*Em* λ = 330 | | Gordan and Kourjmska 1995 (161) |
| 8. Vegetable oils | α-, (β- + γ-), δ-T | Dilute with Hex<br>Direct injection | ODS-2 5 μm, 4.4 × 150 mm | Isocratic MeOH : water (96 : 4), 2 mL/min | PDA 292 nm<br>IS-α-TA | DL<br>On-column (ng)<br>α-T 11.5<br>δ-T 12<br>QL (ng)<br>α-T 23<br>δ-T 25<br>Recovery<br>>92% | Gimeno et al., 2000 (162) |
| 9. Olive oil | α-T, β-carotene | Saponification 70°C, 30 min<br>Extract with Hex : EtOAC (85 : 15)<br>Evaporate<br>Redissolve in MeOH | ODS-2 5 μm, 4.0 × 150 mm | Gradient<br>A, MeOH<br>B, Water<br>C, Butanol<br>A : B : C (92 : 3 : 5) 3 min<br>A : C (92 : 8) in 1 min<br>Hold 5 min, 45°C | PDA<br>α 292<br>β-carotene 450 nm | DL<br>On-column (ng)<br>α-T 11.5<br>β-carotene 15.5<br>QL (ng)<br>α-T 23<br>β-carotene 31<br>Recovery<br>>85% | Gimeno et al., 2000 (163) |
| 10. Vegetable oils | α-, γ-, δ-T | Continuous extraction from oils dissolved in Triton X-114 : MeOH : Hex<br>74% oil in 6% Triton X-114, 10% MeOH, 10% Hex | OD-224 RP-18 5 μm, 4.6 × 220 mm | Isocratic 2.5 mM HAC/NaOAC in MeOH : water (97 : 3) | EC<br>a. Porous graphite −1000 mV<br>b. Reference +500 mV<br>IS-PMC | RSD (%)<br>α-T 6.65<br>γ-T 6.35<br>δ-T 6.35 | Sanchez-Perez et al., 2000 (164) |

*(continued)*

**Table 7.4** *Continued*

| Sample matrix | Analyte | Sample preparation | High-performance liquid chromatography parameters | | | | |
|---|---|---|---|---|---|---|---|
| | | Sample extraction and cleanup | Column | Mobile phase | Detection | Quality assurance | References |
| 11. Olive oil | α-, β-T phenols | MEOH<br>MEOH : IPA (80 : 20)<br>Evaporate, 40°C<br>Redissolve in<br>MEOH : IPA : Hex<br>(1 : 3 : 1) | Apex octadecyl<br>C18<br>4 × 250 mm<br>5 μm | Gradient<br>A, HAC (2%)<br>B, MeOH<br>C, MeCN<br>D, IPA<br>95% A/5% B in 2 min; 60%<br>A/10% B/30%<br>C in 8 min; 25% B/75% C in<br>22 min; maintain for 10 min<br>40% C/60% D in 10 min;<br>maintain for 15 min<br>25% B/75% C in 2 min<br>95% A/5% B in 3 min<br>1 mL/min<br>Run time = 70 min | 280 nm | Recovery 79–87% | Tasioula-Margari et al., 2001 (165) |
| **Margarine** | | | | | | | |
| 1. Full-fat | α-, β-, γ-, δ-T | Dissolve in Hex<br>Direct injection | Hypersil 5 μm,<br>2.1 × 100 mm | Isocratic Hex : IPA (99.8 : 0.2) | Fluorescence<br>*Ex* λ = 290<br>*Em* λ = 330 | Recoveries >96% | Micali et al., 1993 (166) |
| 2. Full-fat<br>Reduced-fat | α-T | Saponification<br>Reflux 60 min<br>Extract with PE | μ-Bondapak C18<br>10 μm<br>4 × 250 mm | Isocratic MeOH : water (93 : 7) or (92 : 8), 1.5 mL/min | 280 nm | %Recovery<br>94.3 ± 7.4 | Rader et al., 1997 (167) |

| | | | | | | | |
|---|---|---|---|---|---|---|---|
| 3. Full-fat<br>Reduced-fat | α-, γ-, δ-T | Extract with<br>Hex + BHT<br>Remove water with $MgSO_4$<br>Direct injection | LiChrosorb Si60<br>5 μm<br>4.6 × 250 mm | Isocratic Hex : IPA (99.1 : 0.9), 1 mL/min | Fluorescence<br>*Ex* $\lambda = 290$<br>*Em* $\lambda = 330$ | Recoveries > 96%<br>RSD (%)<br>Intraday 0.8–3.5<br>Interday 1.4–4.1 | Ye et al., 1998 (168), 2000 (214) |
| **Infant formula, milk, medical foods** | | | | | | | |
| 1. Margarine oils, infant formula, cereals | α-T acetate, retinyl palmitate, β-carotene, vitamin $D_2$ or $D_3$, vitamin $K_1$ | Homogenization in mixture of IPA and $CH_2Cl_2$ with $MgSO_4$ added to remove water<br>Fractionate vitamins from lipids by HP-GPC<br>Four μStyragel columns in series, 100 Å | Zorbax ODS 6 μm<br>4.6 × 250 mm | Isocratic<br>$CH_2Cl_2$ : MeCN : MeOH (300 : 700 : 2), 1 mL/min | Retinyl palmitate 321 nm<br>β-carotene 436 nm<br>$D_2$ or $D_3$ 280 nm<br>Vitamin E 280 nm<br>Vitamin K 280 nm | — | Landen 1982 (169)<br>Landen et al., 1985 (170) |
| 2. Human milk, infant formula | α-, β-, γ-, δ-T<br>α-, β-, γ-, δ-T3 | Saponification, overnight, ambient | LiChrosorb Si60<br>5 μm<br>4 × 250 mm | Isocratic Hex : DIEP (93 : 7) 2.1–2.5 mL/min | Fluorescence<br>*Ex* $\lambda = 290$<br>*Em* $\lambda = 325$ | Recovery 80–90%<br>CV% 3.8–7.2 | Syväoja et al., 1985 (171) |
| 3. Infant formula, milk powder, milk | α-T acetate | Extract with dimethylsulfoxide : dimethylformamide : $CHCl_3$ (200 : 200 : 100); partition with Hex; clarify Hex layer by centrifugation | Rad-Pak silica cartridge 5 μm, 8 mm, id, Z-Module compression unit | Isocratic Hex : IPA (99.92 : 0.08), 2 mL/min | 280 nm | QL<br>0.7 IU/100 g<br>%Recovery<br>92–93 | Woollard and Blott, 1986 (172)<br>Woollard et al., 1987 (173) |

*(continued)*

**Table 7.4** *Continued*

| | | Sample preparation | High-performance liquid chromatography parameters | | | | |
|---|---|---|---|---|---|---|---|
| Sample matrix | Analyte | Sample extraction and cleanup | Column | Mobile phase | Detection | Quality assurance | References |
| 4. Milk, human | α-T, γ-T retinyl esters | Add α-T acetate (IS); dilute with EtOH; extract with Hex; evaporate; dissolve in Hex containing 0.1% BHT | Rad-Pak silica cartridge 5 μm, 8 mm, id | Isocratic Hex : DIPE (95 : 5), 2.5 ml/min | 280 nm | — | Chappell et al., 1986 (174) |
| 5. Infant formula, milk, various foods | α-, β-, γ-, δ-T | Saponify<br>Extract with light petroleum DIEP (2 : 1)<br>Centrifuge<br>Inject 10 μL of upper layer | a. Rad-Pak silica cartridge 5 μm RCM-100<br>b. Rad-Pak silica cartridge 5 μm RCM-100 | Isocratic<br>a. NP-HPLC Hex : IPA (99 : 1) 1 mL/min<br>b. RP-HPLC 100% MeOH 1 mL/min | Fluorescence<br>*Ex* λ = 295<br>*Em* λ = 330 | QL<br>0.4 mg/100 g<br>Recovery<br>93–97%<br>CV% within run<br>1.9–5.7 | Indyk 1988 (175) |
| 6. Infant formula | α-T acetate, α-T | Extract fat by Ross-Gottlieb procedure; saponify lipid fraction; extract with Hex; evaporate; redissolve in IPA : EtOH : Hex (1 : 0.5 : 98.5) | LiChrosorb Si60 4.6 × 120 mm | Isocratic IPA : EtOH : Hex (1 : 0.5 : 98.5), 1 mL/min | Fluorescence<br>*Ex* λ = 292<br>*Em* λ = 320 | Recovery<br>96–108% | Tuan et al., 1989 (176) |

| | | | | | | | |
|---|---|---|---|---|---|---|---|
| 7. Milk, milk powder | α-T, all-*trans*-retinol, vitamin $K_1$ | a. α-T, retinol saponification; overnight, ambient; extract with Hex; evaporate; dissolve in MeOH<br>b. Lipase hydrolysis: add alcoholic sodium hydroxide; immediately extract with Hex<br>Cleanup<br>b. Sep-Pak silica | a. OD-224 RP 18 5 μm 4.6 × 250 mm<br>b. Brownless OD-224 RP 18 | a. Isocratic MeOH : water (99 : 1) containing 2.5 mmol/L HAC 1.25 mL/min<br>b. Isocratic MeOH : water (99 : 1) containing 2.5 mmol/L HAC-NaOAC, 1.25 mL/min | EC Dual-amperometric<br>Glassy carbon<br>− 1100 mV<br>+ 700 mV vs Ag/AgCl | DL (ng)<br>On-column<br>α-T 0.19<br>Retinol 0.06<br>$K_1$ 3.1 | Zamarreno et al., 1992 (177) |
| 8. Infant formula | α-T, retinol | Various<br>Interlaboratory study | Various | Various | Fluorescence | $RSD_R$ 16% | Hollman et al., 1993 (178) |
| 9. Infant formula | α-T | Saponification, 70°C, 25 min; extract with Hex : $CH_2Cl_2$ (3 : 1); evaporate; redissolve in mobile phase<br>Hex : IPA (99.92 : 0.08) | Hypersil silica 5 μm 4.6 × 250 mm | Isocratic Hex : IPA (99.92 : 0.08), 1 mL/min | 280 nm | — | Tanner et al., 1993 (179) |
| 10. Pediatric parenterals | $K_1$, all-*trans*-retinol, α-T acetate, $D_2$ | Extract with Hex<br>Evaporate<br>Dissolve in EtOH | Spherisorb ODS-2 3 μm | Isocratic 100% MeOH, 0.2 mL/min | Multi-wavelength<br>retinol 325 nm<br>$D_2$ 265 nm<br>E 284 nm<br>$K_1$ 250 nm | DL (ng)<br>On-column<br>retinol 0.75<br>$D_2$ 0.95<br>E 4.86<br>$K_1$ 0.95 | Blanco et al., 1994 (180) |

(*continued*)

**TABLE 7.4** *Continued*

| | | Sample preparation | High-performance liquid chromatography parameters | | | | |
|---|---|---|---|---|---|---|---|
| Sample matrix | Analyte | Sample extraction and cleanup | Column | Mobile phase | Detection | Quality assurance | References |
| 11. Italian cheese | α-, β-, γ-, δ-T<br>β-carotene<br>all-*trans*-retinol | Saponification, 70°C, 30 min<br>Extract with Hex : EtOAC (90 : 10)<br>Evaporate<br>Dissolve in mobile phase | Ultrasphre Si 5 μm 4.6 × 250 mm | a. Isocratic Hex : IPA (99 : 1)<br>b. Gradient multilinear<br>Pump A<br>Hex : IPA (99 : 1)<br>Pump B<br>100% Hex<br>1.5 mL/min | a. Tocopherols<br>Fluorescence<br>*Ex* λ = 290<br>*Em* λ = 330<br>b. Retinol<br>Fluorescence<br>*Ex* λ = 290<br>*Em* λ = 330<br>c. β-carotene<br>450 nm | DL (ng)<br>On-column<br>α-T 0.9<br>β-T 0.73<br>γ-T 0.55<br>δ-T 0.56<br>13-*cis*-retinol-0.09<br>all-*trans*-Retinol 0.32<br>β 0.16 | Panfili et al., 1994 (181) |
| 12. Milk, milk powder | $D_3$, all-*trans*-retinol, α-T | Saponification (on-line)<br>Neutralization (on-line)<br>Sep-Pak Plus $C_{18}$ cartridge (on-line concentration)<br>Clean up<br>Washing of C18 cartridge with water : MeOH (60 : 40) | Brownlee OD-224 RP-18 5 μm 4.6 × 250 mm | Isocratic HAC : NaOAC (2.5 mM) in MeOH : water (99 : 1), 1 mL/min | a. 280 nm<br>b. EC<br>+1300 mV | DL (ng)<br>On-column<br>retinol 0.10<br>$D_2$ 6.8<br>E 1.34 | Zamarreño et al., 1995 (182, 183) |

| | | | | | | | |
|---|---|---|---|---|---|---|---|
| 13. Infant formula | α-T, retinal Vitamin D | Saponification Overnight, ambient | Spherisorb ODS 5 μm, 4.6 × 250 mm | Isocratic Water : MeCN : MeOH (4 : 1 : 95) | 292 nm | Recovery α-T 86% RSD (%) 2.25 | Albala-Hurtado et al, 1997 (184) |
| 14. SRM 1846 Soy-based infant formula | α-T acetate α-, β-, γ-, δ-T retinyl palmitate | IPA, Hex : EtOAC (85 : 15) Dehydrated with $MgSO_4$ | LiChrosorb Si60 5 μm 4.6 × 250 mm | Isocratic Hex : IPA (99.5 : 0.5), 1.0 mL/min | Fluorescence *Ex* λ = 285 *Em* λ = 310 | Recovery >94% | Chase et al, 1997, 1998 (185, 186) |
| 15. Bovine milk | α-, γ-, δ-T retinol, β-carotene | Saponification 7 min, 70°C and Röse-Gottlieb extraction | Alltech Econosphere Silica 3 μm 4.6 × 150 mm | Isocratic IPA 0.5% and HAC 0.01% in Hex containing 0.02 mg α-T/L, 1.5 mL/min | Fluorescence Vitamin E *Ex* λ = 295 *Em* λ = 330 | RSDs (%) saponification 3.5 Röse-Gottlieb 3.1 | Hewavitharana et al, 1998 (187) |
| 16. Powdered milk, flour | α-, β + γ-, δ-T retinol | Saponification 30 min, 80°C | LiChrosorb RP-18 5 μm 4.5 × 125 mm | Isocratic MeCN, 0.8 mL/min | 292 nm | RSD (%) 1.94 milk 1.20 flour | Ake et al, 1998 (188) |
| 17. Soy-, milk-based infant formula, medical foods | α-T acetate retinyl palmitate | Matrix solid-phase extraction, $C_{18}$ | LiChrosorb Si60 5 μm 4.6 × 250 mm | Isocratic IPA : Hex (0.5 : 99.5) for α-T acetate, (0.125 : 99.895) for retinyl palmitate, 1.0 mL/min | Fluorescence α-T acetate *Ex* λ = 285 *Em* λ = 310 Retinyl palmitate *Ex* λ = 325 *Em* λ = 470 | Recoveries >91% | Chase and Long 1998 (189) Chase et al, 1998, 1999 (190, 191) |
| 18. Infant formula | α-, β, γ-T, α-T acetate | Extract with $CH_2Cl_2$ : MeOH (2 : 1) Add $H_2O$; shake; remove $CH_2Cl_2$ phase; dry under $N_2$ | Nova-Pak Silica 5 μm 3.9 × 150 mm | Isocratic Hex : EtOAc (98 : 2) 1 mL/min | Fluorescence Ex λ = 295 Em λ = 330 | RSD (%) 7–9.1 | Rodrigo et al, 2002 (215) |

*(continued)*

**Table 7.4** *Continued*

| | | Sample preparation | High-performance liquid chromatography parameters | | | | |
|---|---|---|---|---|---|---|---|
| Sample matrix | Analyte | Sample extraction and cleanup | Column | Mobile phase | Detection | Quality assurance | References |
| **Miscellaneous** | | | | | | | |
| 1. Vegetable oils, wheat flour, barley, milk, frozen dinners, beef, spinach, infant formula | α-, β-, γ-, δ-T<br>α-, β, γ-, δ-T3 | Extract with boiling IPA Filter<br>Extract with A<br>Add water, Hex<br>Collect Hex layer | LiChrosorb Si60 5 μm<br>3.2 × 250 mm | Isocratic<br>Moist hexane : $Et_2O$ (95 : 5), 2 mL/min | Fluorescence<br>*Ex* λ = 290<br>*Em* λ = 330 | DL<br>On-column<br>4 ng | Thompson and Hatina 1979 (132) |
| 2. Forty food products | α-, β-, γ-, δ-T | Saponification, overnight, ambient<br>Extract with Hex | Zorbax ODS 5 μm<br>4.6 × 250 mm | Isocratic MeCN : $MeCl_2$ : MeOH (700 : 300 : 50), 1 mL/min | Fluorescence<br>*Ex* λ = 290<br>*Em* λ = 330 | DL<br>0.1 mg/100 g | Hogarty et al., 1989 (192) |
| 3. Finnish foods | α-, β-, γ-, δ-T<br>α-, β-, γ-, δ-T3 | Saponification, overnight, ambient | LiChrosorb Si60 5 μm<br>4.6 × 250 mm | Isocratic Hex : DIEP (93 : 7), 2.1–2.5 mL/min | Fluorescence<br>*Ex* λ = 290<br>*Em* λ = 325 | Recovery<br>80–90%<br>%CV 3.8–7.2 | Piironen et al., 1984, 1985, 1986, 1987, 1988 (193–199)<br>Syväoja et al., 1985 (200) |
| 4. Chicken muscle | α-, δ-T | Saponification, overnight, ambient, followed by 2 h at 50°C<br>Extract with Hex; evaporate; redissolve in MeOH | Biosil ODS-5S<br>4 × 250 mm | Isocratic MeOH : 100%, 1 mL/min | Fluorescence<br>*Ex* λ = 296<br>*Em* λ = 330 | Recovery<br>92–93% | Ang et al., 1990 (201) |

| | | | | | | | |
|---|---|---|---|---|---|---|---|
| 5. Rodent feed | α-T, all-*trans*-retinol, all-*trans*-retinyl acetate | Saponification, overnight, ambient<br>Extract with Hex<br>Centrifuge | Supelco LC-CN<br>5 μm<br>4.6 × 250 mm | Isocratic Hex : IPA : HAC (990 : 10 : 0.2), 2 mL/min | 265 nm | — | Rushing et al., 1991 (202) |
| 6. Forty foods of animal origin | all-*trans*-retinol, α-carotene, β-carotene, lycopene | Saponification, heating mantle, 30 min; extract with Hex (4X); dry; $Na_2SO_4$; evaporate; dilute with Hex | μBondapack $C_{18}$<br>10 μm<br>3.9 × 300 mm | Isocratic<br>MeCN : MeOH : EtOAC (88 : 10 : 2), 2 mL/min | Carotenoids 436 nm<br>Retinol 313 nm | — | Tee and Lim 1992 (203) |
| 7. Pecans, peanuts | α-, β-, γ-, δ-T | Soxhlet<br>Hex containing 0.01% BHT, 90°C, 6 h<br>Evaporate<br>Redissolve in Hex containing 0.01% BHT | LiChrosorb Si60<br>5 μm<br>4 × 250 mm | Isocratic Hex : IPA (99 : 1), 1 mL/min | Fluorescence<br>*Ex* λ = 290<br>*Em* λ = 330 | DL (ng)<br>On-column α-T 2, β-T 1, γ-T 2, δ-T 0.6<br>Recovery 84–96% | Yao et al., 1992 (204)<br>Hashim et al., 1993 (205, 206) |
| 8. Grain amaranths | α-, β-, γ-, δ-T<br>α-, β-, γ-, δ-T3 | Extract with MeOH<br>Evaporate<br>Extract with Hex | Waters silica<br>4.0 × 300 mm | Isocratic Hex : IPA (99.8 : 0.2), 1 mL/min | Fluorescence<br>*Ex* λ = 295<br>*Em* λ = 330 | — | Lehmann et al., 1994 (207) |
| 9. Multivitamin juices, isotonic beverages, breakfast cereals, infant formula, human milk | α-, β-, γ-, δ-T<br>α-, β-, γ-, δ-T3<br>α-T acetate<br>plastochromanol-8 | Add water, EtOH Shake and sonicate Add tBME, PE Centrifuge Repeat extraction twice Add EtOH Evaporate | LiChrospher 100 diol 5 μm<br>4 × 250 mm | Gradient<br>1. a. 0–4 min Hex<br>b. 4–5 min up to Hex : tBME (97 : 3)<br>c. 5–41 min Isocratic<br>d. 41–42 min up to Hex : tBME (95 : 5) | Fluorescence<br>*Ex* λ = 280<br>*Em* λ = 335<br>or<br>*Ex* λ = 295<br>*Em* λ = 330 | DL<br>On-column (ng)<br>α-T acetate 2.2–4.6<br>Recovery 100–103%, CV 2% | Balz et al., 1993 (208) |

(*continued*)

**Table 7.4** *Continued*

| | | Sample preparation | High-performance liquid chromatography parameters | | | | |
|---|---|---|---|---|---|---|---|
| Sample matrix | Analyte | Sample extraction and cleanup | Column | Mobile phase | Detection | Quality assurance | References |
| | | Redissolve in Hex For infant formula and human milk, add either 25% ammonia solution or 35% dipotassium oxalate before first addition of EtOH | | e. 42–60 min Isocratic<br>f. 2 min down to Hex<br>g. 10 min Hex<br>2. a. 0–4 min Hex<br>b. 4–5 min up to Hex : tBME (97 : 3)<br>c. 5–23 min Isocratic<br>d. 2 min down to Hex<br>e. 10 min Hex | | | |
| 10. Eggs, feeds, tissues | all-*trans*-retinol, β-carotene, α-T | Extract with Hex : A : T : EtOH (10 : 7 : 7 : 6)<br>Saponify extract, ambient, overnight<br>Extract with Hex<br>Evaporate<br>Dissolve in Hex : EtOAC (85 : 15) | Nova-pak silica 4 μm 3.9 × 150 mm | Gradient 0–10 min, Hex : EtOAC (85 : 15)–(70 : 30), 1–2 mL/min, 11–15 min, Hex : EtOAC (70 : 30), 2 mL/min | Retinol 325 nm<br>β-carotene 450 nm<br>α-T 294 nm | QL (μg/L) retinol 9.4<br>β-carotene 0.1<br>α-T 117 | Jiang et al., 1994 (209)<br>McGeachin and Bailey 1995 (210) |
| 11. Animal and plant foods | Tocopherols, retinoids, carotenoids | Homogenize in IPA : $CH_2Cl_2$ (2 : 1)<br>Store under argon overnight<br>Freeze | Microsorb-MV 3 μm 4.6 × 100 mm | Gradient<br>Solvent A MeOH : Water (3 : 1) containing 10 mM $NH_4OAC$<br>Solvent B MeOH : $CH_2Cl_2$ (4 : 1) | PDA | %Recovery<br>Retinoic acid >98% with HAC added | Barua and Olson 1998 (211) |

| | | | | | | | |
|---|---|---|---|---|---|---|---|
| | | Evaporate supernatant<br>Redissolve in<br>IPA : $CH_2Cl_2$ (2 : 1)<br>Inject | | Linear gradient 100% A to 100% B over 15 to 20 min<br>Isocratic<br>Solvent B for additional 15–20 min<br>Reverse gradient for 5 min, 0.8 mL/min | | | |
| 12. Animal feed | α-T, retinyl acetate cholecalciferol | Extract 1 g with A : $CHCl_3$ (3 : 7)<br>Vortex; centrifuge<br>Evaporate to dryness<br>Redissolve in n-butanol | Nova-pak $C_{18}$ 3.9 × 150 mm | Isocratic MeOH, 1.5 mL/min | 290 nm | Recovery >91% | Qian and Sheng, 1997 (212) |
| 13. Peanuts | α-, β-, γ-, δ-T | Extract with Hex + ethyl acetate (90 : 10) containing 0.01% BHT<br>Remove water with $MgSO_4$<br>Evaporate<br>Dissolve with Hex | LiChrosorb Si60<br>5 μm<br>4.6 × 250 mm | Isocratic Hex : IPA (99.4 : 0.6), 1 mL/min | Fluorescence<br>*Ex* λ = 290<br>*Em* λ = 330 | DL (ng)<br>On-column α-T 0.2, β-T 0.1, γ-T 0.1, δ-T 0.1<br>Recovery 97–102%<br>RSD (%)<br>Intraday 3.0–9.0<br>Interday 3.1–9.3 | Lee et al., 1999 (213) |
| 14. Fortified foods | α-, β-, γ-, δ-T<br>α-T acetate<br>β-carotene<br>retinyl palmitate | To 3 g sample, add 2 mL 80°C water, sonicate<br>Add IPA, then Hex containing 0.003% BHT | LiChrosorb Si60<br>5 μm<br>4.6 × 250 mm | Isocratic 0.27% IPA in Hex<br>Gradient flow 0.9–1.5 mL/min over 5.3 min | Fluorescence (programmable)<br>α-T acetate<br>*Ex* λ = 285<br>*Em* λ = 315 | Recovery 99–101% | Ye et al., 2000 (214) |

(*continued*)

**Table 7.4** *Continued*

| | | Sample preparation | High-performance liquid chromatography parameters | | | | |
|---|---|---|---|---|---|---|---|
| Sample matrix | Analyte | Sample extraction and cleanup | Column | Mobile phase | Detection | Quality assurance | References |
| | | Dehydrate with $MgSO_4$; inject | | | Tocopherol<br>*Ex* λ = 290<br>*Em* λ = 330<br>Retinyl palmitate<br>*Ex* λ = 325<br>*Em* λ = 470<br>β-carotene<br>PDA 450 nm | | |
| 15. Plant tissue | α-, β-, γ-, δ-T<br>α-, β-carotene<br>Lutein, other pigments | Powder with liquid $N_2$<br>Extract with A with addition of $CaCO_3$, centrifuge<br>Resuspend pellet in A | Spherisob ODS-1<br>5 μm<br>4.6 × 250 mm | Gradient<br>A MeCN : MEOH : $H_2O$ (84 : 9 : 7)<br>B MEOH : EtoAc 100% A to 100% B in 12 mm, 10% B for 6 min, 100% B to 100% A in 1 min, 100% A for 6 min | PDA | | Garcia-Plazaola and Becerril 1999 (216) |
| 16. Reduced-fat mayonnaise | α-, β-, γ-, δ-T<br>α-T acetate<br>β-carotene<br>retinyl palmitate | | LiChrosorb Si 60<br>5 μm<br>4.6 × 250 mm | Isocratic gradient-Flow rate<br>0.27% IPA in Hex<br>0 min, 0.9 mL/min<br>4.5 min, 0.9 mL/min<br>5.05 min, 1.35 mL/min<br>5.3 min, 1.50 mL/min | Fluorescence<br>0 min<br>*Ex* λ = 285<br>*Em* λ = 310<br>7 min<br>*Ex* λ = 290<br>*Em* λ = 330<br>PDA<br>200–500 nm | RSD (%)<br>Intraday<br>1.6–7.2<br>Interday<br>3.0–9.8 | Ye et al., 2000 (217) |

| | | | | | | | |
|---|---|---|---|---|---|---|---|
| 17. Coffee | α-, β-, γ-T | Extract coffee oil<br>Soxhlet<br>Hex 8 h<br>Dissolve in A<br>Inject | Lichrosphere<br>Si 60 | Isocratic Hex : IPA (99 : 1),<br>1 mL/min | Fluorescence<br>*Ex* λ = 299<br>*Em* λ = 330 | Recovery >89% | Gonzalez et al., 2001 (218) |
| 18. Rosemary leaves | α-T | Dry leaves<br>Grind<br>Add IS<br>Extract with A | Nucleosil C18<br>5 μm<br>4.6 × 250 mm | Gradient<br>A Water<br>B MeOH : MeCH (30 : 70)<br>with 0.1% HAC, 85% B to<br>100% B in 23 min, 2 mL/min<br>IS ergocalciferol | PDA | RSD (%)<br>Intraday 3–4<br>Interday 6–7<br>Recovery<br>93% ± 7% | Torre et al., 2001 (219) |
| 19. Seeds and nuts | α-, (β- and γ-), δ-T | Saponifcation<br>Saponification coupled with continuous membrane extraction, direct extraction through a silicone membrane | OD 224<br>RP 18<br>5 μm<br>4.6 × 220 mm | Isocractic 2.5 mM<br>HAC-NaOAC in MeOH: $H_2O$<br>(97 : 3) | EC<br>Dual porous graphite working electrodes<br>IS-PMC | Continuous, without saponification<br>RSD (%)<br>Intraday 2.9–4.3<br>Interday 7.5–9.1<br>Recovery<br>97–102% | Delgado-Zamarreño et al., 2001 (220) |
| 20. Malt sprouts | α-, γ-, δ-T | SFE<br>$CO_2$, 250 bar, 80°C, 1 mL/min<br>Trap temperature<br>25°C, 180 min | Zorbax reversed-phase 5 μm,<br>4.6 × 250 mm | Isocratic MeOH : water (98 : 2) | Fluorescence<br>*Ex* λ = 303<br>*Ex* λ = 328 | | Carlucci et al., 2001 (221) |

*(continued)*

**TABLE 7.4** *Continued*

| | | Sample preparation | High-performance liquid chromatography parameters | | | | |
|---|---|---|---|---|---|---|---|
| Sample matrix | Analyte | Sample extraction and cleanup | Column | Mobile phase | Detection | Quality assurance | References |
| 21. Nutrition beverages | α-, β-, γ-, δ-T<br>α-T acetate<br>α-carotene<br>β-carotene<br>9-cis, 13-cis<br>β-carotene | Extract with A : Hex (1 : 1)<br>Wash Hex layer<br>NaCl solution<br>Dry with sodium sulfate<br>Evaporate Hex<br>Dissolve in IPA | C30 reversed-phase, YMC<br>5 μm<br>4.6 × 250 mm | Gradient A:<br>MeOH : MTBE : water (81 : 15 : 4)<br>B: MTBE : MeOH : water (90 : 6 : 4)<br>100% A to 56% B in 50 min, 1 mL/min | PDA | Recovery<br>α-T 97–98%<br>α-T acetate 97–98%<br>β-carotene 97–105% | Schieber et al., 2002 (222) |
| 22. Foods | α-, (β- and γ-T) | Saponification | Reversed-phase C8<br>4.6 × 250 mm | Isocratic MeOH : water (94 : 6) | Fluorescence<br>*Ex* $\lambda = 290$<br>*Ex* $\lambda = 330$ | Recovery<br>63–114%<br>8 labs<br>$RSD_R$ %<br>10.2–18.7%<br>8 labs | DeVries and Silvera 2002 (223) |

mobile phase or impurities exist; then more extensive sample cleanup procedures must be employed. In some samples, slow-eluting compounds may be present and slow sample throughput. Preparation of the vitamin E fraction for injection onto the column from most food matrices requires saponification of the sample matrix or of a concentrated lipid fraction or extraction of total lipid from the sample, which then can be directly injected onto a normal-phase column. Diverse extraction procedures are available to extract vitamin E efficiently from food matrices, and several excellent reviews of extraction procedures exist in the literature. Bourgeois (133) particularly provides detailed information on solvent extractions and saponification procedures from a historical perspective. Other detailed reviews include Ball (127), Eitenmiller and Landen (136), and Ruperez et al. (139).

#### 7.3.1.1. Saponification.

*Saponification* refers to alkaline hydrolysis by KOH or, less commonly, by NaOH. The hydrolysis is used to free fat-soluble vitamins, except vitamin K, which is labile under the alkaline environment, from the sample matrix. In general, protein, lipid, and carbohydrate complexes are destroyed; triacylglycerols and phospholipids are hydrolyzed; tocopherol and tocotrienol esters are hydrolyzed; pigments and other substances that may interfere with the chromatography are removed; and the sample matrix is disrupted, facilitating vitamin extraction (2,127,133). The procedure includes the following general steps:

1. Addition of ethanolic base (KOH) to the sample together with a suitable antioxidant such as pyrogallol or ascorbic acid or combinations of antioxidants
2. Dispersion of the sample to ensure that clumping does not occur to such an extent that the ethanolic KOH cannot penetrate the sample matrix
3. Flushing of the saponification vessel with inert gas ($N_2$)
4. Refluxing with the aid of an air condenser (Figure 7.2) under gold fluorescent lighting or in the dark
5. Cooling of the digest
6. Addition of 1% NaCl or water
7. Partitioning of the digest with ether, hexane, ethyl acetate in hexane, or other suitable solvent mixtures
8. Collection of the organic solvent phase
9. Washing of the organic solvent to remove fatty acid soaps
10. Concentration of the nonsaponifiable fraction (vitamin E fraction)

Many saponification procedures have been used with success for vitamin E analysis. Often exact parameters for a specific matrix must be determined through

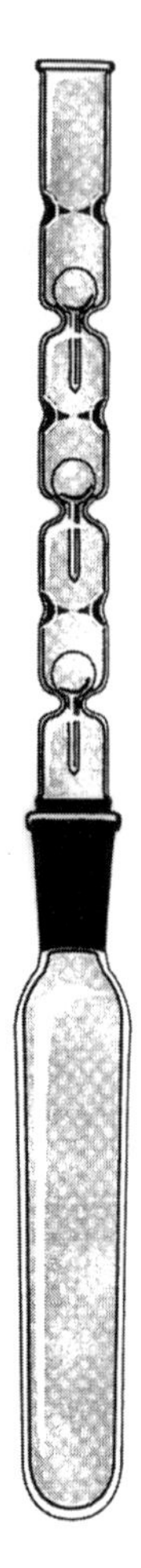

**FIGURE 7.2** Saponification reflux condenser. (From Ref. 136.)

investigation of the effects of the variation of conditions on recovery of vitamin E homologues and analytical values obtained with varying digestion conditions. Ball (127) provides a general guide for the saponification of biologicals, which includes 5 mL of 60% weight-to-volume (w/v) aqueous KOH and 15 mL of ethanol per gram of fat. Temperatures and times used for saponification range from ambient temperature for 12 h or more to 70°C for 30 min or less. Parameters such as sample size, volumes and concentrations of alkali, and time and temperature can be varied to optimize the digestion. It has been our experience that the most efficient saponification and less destructive effects occur, resulting in high recoveries of spiked tocopherols and tocotrienols, when the digestion is completed by reflux. Use of an air condenser simplifies the procedure (Figure 7.2).

In some studies extraction of the food lipid before saponification has been necessary. Tuan et al. (176) extracted lipid from infant formula before saponification to decrease chromatographic interferences. However, if fluorescence detection is coupled with normal-phase chromatography, most samples can be processed with direct saponification without prior fat extraction. Summaries of published saponification procedures are provided in Table 7.5.

From the few studies represented in Table 7.5, recoveries reported for the different vitamin E homologues vary considerably, with lowest recoveries reported for $\delta$-T. Provided necessary precautions have been taken to protect the vitamin E homologues from destruction during digestion, problems can arise in the partitioning of the vitamin E from the aqueous digest into the nonpolar extraction solvent. Ueda and Igarashi (224–227) thoroughly studied this important phase of the assay. They found that ethanol concentration of the digest, composition of the extracting solvent, and level of lipids in the original digest could significantly affect recovery of the vitamin E homologues with hexane as the extractant. Ethanol concentrations must be kept below 30% to extract $\delta$-T or tocol (used as an internal standard) efficiently. For 2,2,5,7,8-pentamethyl-6-chromanol (PMC) internal standard, the upper level of ethanol was 15% for efficient recovery by hexane extraction (226,227). Ethanol concentration did not affect recovery of $\alpha$-T and only slight effects were noted for $\beta$- and $\gamma$-T. Ueda and Igarashi (227) clearly showed that addition of ethyl acetate up to 10% volume-to-volume (v/v) concentration in hexane improved recoveries for $\beta$-, $\gamma$-, and $\delta$-T; tocol; and PMC (227). The more polar nature of the ethyl acetate improves the affinity of the more polar vitamin E homologues for the extracting solvent. At levels above 10%, ethyl acetate causes the volume of the solvent layer to decrease as the mixture becomes more miscible in the aqueous phase. Researchers should note this phenomenon. Addition of ethyl acetate to hexane can greatly improve $\delta$-T recovery and is an easily used corrective approach to vitamin E recovery problems.

In other research, Ueda and Igarashi(225) showed that the fat level in the saponification digest is a significant factor affecting recovery of $\beta$-, $\gamma$-, and $\delta$-T and tocol. Recovery losses were noted at quite low levels of fat (from corn oil); however, $\alpha$-T recovery was not lowered by increasing fat levels. Thompson (228) in discussion of problems with vitamin A analysis explained that use of hexane can lead to low retinol recoveries from saponification digests since ethanol–water–soap mixtures behave similarly to a hydrocarbon solvent. This decreases the affinity of the fat-soluble vitamins to the organic phase. Therefore, $\delta$-T, the most polar of the vitamin E homologues would have greater affinity for the aqueous phase as fatty acid soap content increases. Thompson noted that extraction efficiency of hexane is dependent on the fatty acid concentrations in the digest. Control is achieved by limiting the amount of ingoing fat (sample weight),

**TABLE 7.5** Saponification Conditions Used for Extraction of Vitamin E

| Matrix | Hydrolysis sample size | Conditions | Antioxidant | Internal standard or percentage extractant | Recovery | Reference |
|---|---|---|---|---|---|---|
| Foods | 0.5 g | Ethanolic KOH 70°C, 30 min | Pyrogallol | Hexane diethyl ether petroleum ether | Tocol unsuitable for addition before saponification | 225 |
| Meat | 10 g | Ethanolic KOH ambient overnight | Ascorbic acid | Hexane | α-T 97% β-T 100% γ-T 97% δ-T 68% | 195 |
| Infant formula | 1 g | Ethanolic KOH reflux 30 min | Pyrogallol | Hexane | α-T 96%–109% | 176 |
| Dairy products Foods Tissues | 10 g | Ethanolic KOH 70°C, 7 min | Pyrogallol | Petroleum ether : isopropyl ether (3 : 1) | α-T (IS) added to unfortified sample | 175 |
| Forty foods | 10 g | Ethanolic KOH ambient overnight | Ascorbic acid nitrogen flush | Hexane | >80% For α-T and γ-T in all samples | 192 |
| Infant formula | 10 mL | Ethanolic KOH 70°C, 25 min | Pyrogallol | Hexane : methylene chloride (3 : 1) | None | 179 |
| Human diets | 10–20 g | Ethanolic KOH ambient overnight | Ascorbic acid | Hexane | α-T 99% β-T 95% γ-T 99% δ-T 80% | 193 |
| Seeds oils | 1–5 g | Ethanolic KOH reflux, 30 min | Sodium ascorbate | Diisopropyl ether | α-T 93% γ-T 94% α-T3 95% | 155 |
| Tomato, broccoli | 7.5 g | Ethanolic KOH reflux, variable time | Pyrogallol | Hexane | α-T 102% γ-T 91% | 229 |

α-T, α-tocopherol; IS, internal standard; α-T3, α-tocotrienol.
*Source*: Modified from Ref. 136.

by optimizing the amount of water added before extraction, and by making repeated extractions with small volumes of hexane. Use of small sample weights puts greater stress on sample homogeneity to assure assay reproducibility.

In 2000, Lee et al. (229) used response surface methodology (RSM) to optimize vitamin E extraction from tomato and broccoli by saponification. Variables examined included the amount of 60% KOH, saponification time, and final ethanol concentration. The optimized parameters were obtained by ridge analysis. On the basis of the ridge analysis, optimal saponification conditions were (a) 8.4 to 8.9 mL 60% KOH, (b) 50.7–54.3 min at 70°C, and (c) 30.1–35.0% ethanol. All trials used a sample size of 7.5 g. With the optimized parameters, experimental concentrations agreed closely with values predicted by ridge analysis (Table 7.6). Effects of KOH amount and final ethanol concentration under constant saponification times on response surface plots of γ-T are shown in Figure 7.3.

The RSM technique allows evaluation of the effects of many factors and their interactions on response variables. Advantages of RSM in optimization studies of all types are the reduced number of experimental trials needed to evaluate multiple parameters and their interactions, labor, and time required to obtain the optimized process. The RSM studies have been widely applied for optimization of processes in the food and pharmaceutical industries. They had not been applied to vitamin extraction optimization to any extent before Lee and coworkers' study (229), which shows that RSM can be used to optimize vitamin extraction parameters and may be useful to vitamin chemists.

Protocols to extract vitamin E from biological samples have been designed to decrease time and solvent requirement and to allow for use of small sample weights when samples are limited (175,226).

**TABLE 7.6** Predicted and Experimental Values of the Responses at Optimized Conditions for the Extraction of Tocopherols from Tomato and Broccoli

| | Optimal conditions[a] | | | Value[b] mg/100 g | |
|---|---|---|---|---|---|
| Responses | Amount of 60% KOH mL | Saponification time at 70°C' min | Final ethanol concentration % | Predicted | Experimental |
| α-T Tomato | 8.4 | 54.1 | 33.8 | 0.65 | 0.66 |
| γ-T Tomato | 8.4 | 54.3 | 35.0 | 0.30 | 0.28 |
| α-T Broccoli | 8.9 | 53.5 | 34.0 | 1.06 | 1.06 |
| γ-T Broccoli | 8.9 | 50.7 | 30.1 | 0.39 | 0.33 |

[a]Optimal conditions were obtained from ridge analysis.
[b]Experimental values were obtained by using 8.7 mL (amount of 60% KOH), 53 min (saponification time), and 33% (final ethanol concentration) for both tomato and broccoli.
*Source*: Modified from Ref. 229.

**(A) Saponification time = 15 min**

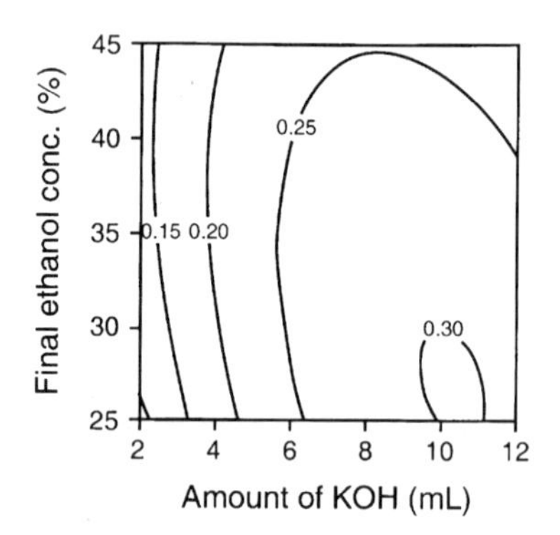


**(B) Saponification time = 35 min**

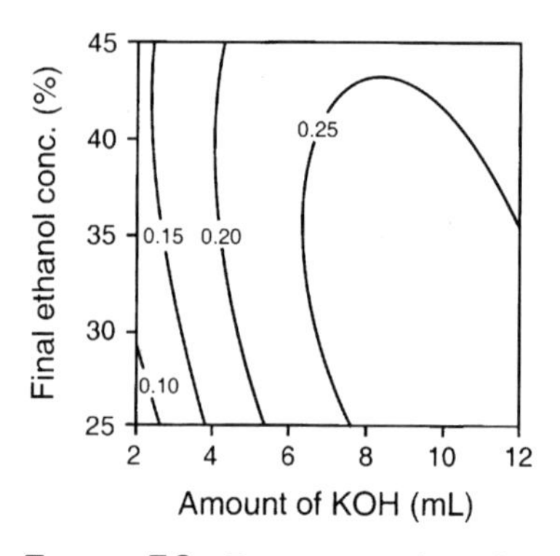


**(C) Saponification time = 55**

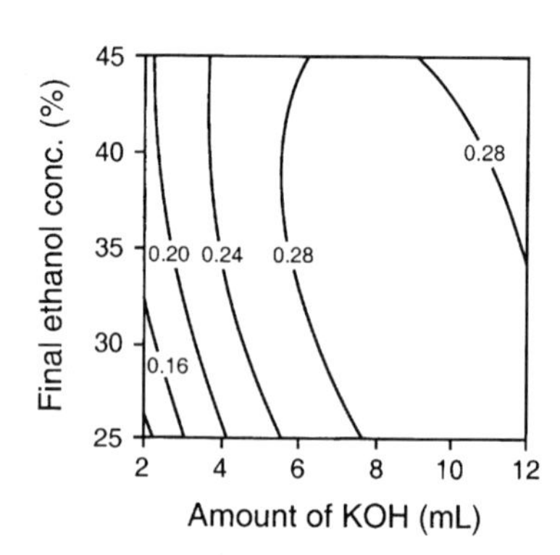


**Figure 7.3** Response surface plots of γ-tocopherol showing effects of the amount of KOH and final ethanol concentration under constant saponification time for saponification of raw tomatoes. The numbers on the surface response plots represent milligrams of tocopherol per 100 grams. (From Ref. 229.)

Eitenmiller and Landen(136) summarized saponification procedures of Indyk(175) and Ueda and Igarashi(226) as follows:

*Procedure Applicable to Dairy Products, Food, and Tissues (Indyk, 175)*

*Sample size*: 0.5 g Whole milk powder, powdered infant formula, freeze-dried organs, fish, cereal, 5.0 g of fluid milk; 0.1–0.2 g butter, margarine, or vegetable oil.

*Procedure*: Weigh sample into test tube and add 10.0 mL ethanol containing 1% pyrogallol. Add α-T standard (200 μL of known concentration) (20 to 30 μg/100 mL absolute ethanol) to the unfortified sample to provide a parallel assay for recovery data. Add 2 mL of 50% KOH and loosely stopper the tubes. Incubate at 70°C for 7 min with periodic agitation. Cool the tubes and add 20 mL of light petroleum ether : diisopropyl ether (3 : 1). Shake mechanically for 5 min. Add 30 mL water, invert 10 times, and centrifuge at 180 × g for 10 min. Inject a 10-μL volume of the clear upper layer directly into an isocratic HPLC system.

*Procedure Applicable to Blood and Tissues* (*Ueda and Igarashi, 226*)

*Blood*: To 200 μL plasma or 400 μL of 50% hematocrit red blood cell (RBC) suspension in two centrifuge tubes with coated (Teflon) screw caps, add 1 mL 6% ethanolic pyrogallol to each tube. Preheat the solution to 70°C for 3 min and to one tube add 1 mL of an ethanolic solution of PMC (0.3 μg) as an internal standard. To the other tube, add 3 mL of an ethanolic solution containing 3.0 μg each of α-, β-, γ-, and δ-T and PMC. Add 0.2 mL of 60% KOH and saponify at 70°C for 30 min. Cool tubes in ice water and add 4.5 mL of 1% NaCl. The saponification mixture is extracted with 3 mL of 10% ethyl acetate in n-hexane. Centrifuge the saponified extracts at 300 rpm for 5 min and pipet 2 mL of n-hexane layer into a 10-mL conical glass tube. Evaporate the n-hexane under a stream of nitrogen. Redissolve the unspiked residue in 200 μL of n-hexane and the residue from the spiked sample in 2.0 mL of n-hexane. For each, inject 10 μL into the HPLC system.

*Tissues*: Weigh 100 mg of tissue into a 10-mL centrifuge tube with coated (Teflon) screw cap. Add 100 μL of 60% KOH. Saponify at 70°C for 60 min. Add 4.5 mL of 1% NaCl to the cooled digest and extract with 3 mL of 10% ethyl acetate in n-hexane. Centrifuge the saponified extracts at 3000 rpm for 5 min and pipet 2 mL of the n-hexane layer into a conical glass tube for concentration under a stream of nitrogen. Redissolve the residue in 200 μL of n-hexane and inject 10 μL into the HPLC. Recoveries can be determined by use of a parallel spike or PMC internal standard.

**7.3.1.2. Direct Solvent Extraction.** Methods applicable to total lipid extraction from foods can be used to extract vitamin E before assay by HPLC. Such methods can yield an extract that can be directly injected onto the LC column without additional cleanup. Many organic solvents and solvent mixtures efficiently extract vitamin E from the sample matrix. Ball (127–129) summarized solvent requirements to include effective penetration of the sample matrix while stabilizing the vitamin E. Under most circumstances, complete lipid extraction must be assured to accomplish complete removal of vitamin E from the sample matrix. Most physiological fluids can be extracted with simple direct solvent extraction procedures. These procedures usually have the following sequence:

1. Addition of a protein denaturing solvent such as isopropanol, ethanol, methanol, or acetonitrile
2. Addition of water or buffer to improve the extraction efficiency of the solvent
3. Addition of the organic phase to extract the vitamin E
4. Centrifugation
5. Solvent evaporation if required to concentrate the analytes

The protocol fits requirements for the extraction of retinoids and carotenoids in addition to vitamin E (136).

Solvents commonly used for vitamin E extraction include the Folch extraction with chloroform : methanol (2 : 1), acetone, diethyl ether, hexane, hexane : ethyl acetate (90 : 10), and Soxhlet extraction with a variety of solvents (127–129). Soxhlet extraction can provide a convenient and simple approach to vitamin E extraction. Wet samples can be ground with magnesium or sodium sulfate to produce a dry powder necessary for Soxhlet extraction. An antioxidant must be added to the organic solvent, and the Soxhlet apparatus must be protected from light throughout the often long (hours) extraction procedure. The presence of polar lipids in the sample can lead to low vitamin E recovery if hexane is used as the extractant (136). An example of a Soxhlet-based procedure is that used by Håkansson et al. (230) to extract vitamin E from wheat products. These authors used hexane containing 1 mg butylated hydroxytoluene (BHT)/125 mL to extract 5 to 15 g of ground cereal samples. A 4-h extraction was used at 90°C. Recoveries were above 95% for $\alpha$- and $\beta$-T. As part of the study, the Soxhlet procedure was compared to a more laborious procedure developed by Thompson and Hatina (132). The Soxhlet procedure provided higher recoveries and higher measured levels for $\alpha$-T, $\alpha$-T3, $\beta$-T, and $\beta$-T3.

The solvent extraction procedure for tocopherols and tocotrienols developed by Thompson and Hatina (132) has been a standard for vitamin E analysts for many years with successful application to many different food matrices (136). The procedure uses isopropanol and acetone extraction combined with partitioning of the vitamin E into hexane. The following steps are included in the somewhat tedious but effective procedure:

1. Homogenize a 10-g sample with 100 mL boiling isopropanol in the cup of a homogenizer (Virtis).
2. After 1 min, add 50 mL of acetone.
3. Filter the mixture through glass fiber paper (Whatman GF/A) into a 500-mL separatory funnel.
4. Homogenize the filter paper and its contents with 100 mL of acetone.
5. Filter the extract into the separatory funnel.
6. Wash the residue with 50 mL of acetone.
7. Add 100 mL hexane to the pooled extracts and mix the contents.

8. Add 100 mL water and swirl to mix the phases.
9. After phase separation, transfer the hexane epiphase to a second funnel.
10. Extract the water phase twice more with 10 mL hexane.
11. Wash the pooled hexane fraction twice with 100-mL portions of water.
12. Evaporate under vacuum.

The recoveries were high (97%), but the large solvent volumes and labor-intensiveness led others to develop more streamlined solvent extractions such as the Håkansson et al. (230) Soxhlet procedure.

Another solvent extraction, developed by Landen (169) for general application to fat-soluble vitamin extraction of fortified foods, has seen much recent use for analysis of vitamin E and *all-rac-α*-tocopheryl acetate from a variety of foods. Landen originally developed the procedure to extract fat-soluble vitamins from infant formula. The extraction uses ispropanol to denature the food protein matrix, extraction with methylene chloride, and addition of magnesium sulfate to dehydrate the extract. The fat-soluble vitamins were fractionated from lipids by high-performance gel permeation chromatography (HP-GPC) before determinative chromatography by nonaqueous reversed-phase chromatography. Landen's extraction has been adapted by several investigators in development of methods for vitamin E analysis from various matrices. For vitamin E assay, it is not necessary to fractionate the analytes from the lipid because of the almost universal use of normal-phase chromatography on silica, so the HP-GPC step is not necessary. Recent studies that have used modification of Landen's extraction include Chase et al.,(185,186) Ye et al. (168,214,217) and Lee et al. (213). The procedures of Chase and coworkers and Ye and associates use modified extractions from Landen's original procedure and are discussed in detail in Sec. 7.4.

Lee et al. (213) developed an extraction based on the Landen extraction specifically for use on peanuts, peanut butter, and other nuts and compared the direct solvent extraction to saponification for general utility. The Lee et al. (213) procedure included the following steps:

1. Weigh 0.4-g sample into a 125-mL round-bottom flask.
2. Add 4 mL of hot (80°C) water.
3. Mix with a spatula.
4. Add 10 mL isopropanol, 5 g magnesium sulfate, and 25 mL of hexane:ethyl acetate (90 : 10) containing 0.01% BHT.
5. Homogenize for 1 min with a homogenizer (Polytron) rinse the tip with 5 mL of extracting solvent.
6. Filter the mixture through a medium-porosity glass filter using a vacuum bell jar filtration unit.

7. Break up filter cake and wash with 5 mL extracting solvent.
8. Transfer the filter cake to the 125-mL flask and reextract with homogenization with 5 mL of isopropanol and 30 mL of extracting solvent.
9. Transfer the combined filtrates to a 100-mL volumetric flask and dilute to volume with extracting solvent.
10. Aliquots of the extract can be concentrated under $N_2$ if required before injection.

Comparison of the direct solvent extraction to saponification and Soxhlet extraction (Table 7.7) showed that the procedure gave higher values for each of the vitamin E homologues when compared to the other procedures. When it was coupled to normal-phase chromatography, highly reproducible results were obtained from peanuts, peanut butter, and several other nuts. Recoveries from peanut butter approached 100% for each of the vitamin E homologues. When used on a routine basis, the extraction is fast with low solvent requirements. It is also applicable to studies requiring the

**TABLE 7.7** Assay Values of Tocopherols in Peanuts and Peanut Butter Using Three Different Extraction Methods

| | Extraction method[a] | | |
|---|---|---|---|
| | Saponification | Direct solvent | Soxhlet |
| | mg/100 g[b] (% recovery) | | |
| **Peanut** | | | |
| α-T[c] | 2.59[a] (87) | 3.55[b] (97) | 2.94[c] (91) |
| β-T | 0.13[a] (117) | 0.14[a] (91) | 0.12[a] (102) |
| γ-T | 6.10[a] (98) | 8.04[b] (99) | 6.94[c] (101) |
| δ-T | 0.46[a] (87) | 0.59[b] (102) | 0.54[b] (106) |
| α-TE | 3.27[a] | 4.44[b] | 3.70[c] |
| **Peanut butter** | | | |
| α-T | 7.92[a] (89) | 9.54[b] (97) | 9.34[b] (100) |
| β-T | 0.19[a] (97) | 0.38[b] (105) | 0.21[a] (106) |
| γ-T | 7.85[a] (94) | 9.78[b] (97) | 9.36[c] (102) |
| δ-T | 0.68[a] (93) | 0.85[b] (103) | 0.78[c] (102) |
| α-TE | 8.82[a] | 10.74[b] | 10.40[c] |

[a]Values in the same row that are followed by the different letter are significantly different ($P < 0.01$).
[b]Data represent a mean ($n = 3$).
[c]Corresponding tocopherols.
*Source*: Modified from Ref. [213].
α-T, α-tocopherol; α-TE, α-tocopherol equivalent.

assay of *all-rac-α*-tocopheryl acetate together with natural vitamin E in fortified products.

Delgado-Zamarreño et al. (220) compared traditional saponification to newer methods of extraction for the analysis of vitamin E in nuts and seeds. Methods compared to saponification included saponification followed by continuous membrane extraction coupled to the LC and direct extraction of tocopherols through a silicone membrane coupled on-line with the LC. Each procedure gave good extraction results. The authors considered that the direct extraction with application of the membrane filtration offered significant porential for food analysis because of the speed and precision of the analysis. The complete assay of a sample including extraction required 40 min. The extraction would require validation before application to other matrices.

**7.3.1.3. Matrix Solid-Phase Dispersion.** In 1998, Chase and Long and Chase et al. (189–191) introduced matrix solid-phase dispersion (MSPD) as an extraction procedure for tocopherols, *all-rac-α*-tocopheryl acetate, and retinyl palmitate in infant formula and medical foods. Previously MSPD has been to isolate drugs from milk and tissue; it is a patented procedure. The technique is based on the dispersion of the sample onto $C_{18}$ to form a powder that is subsequently eluted with a solvent capable of eluting the analytes of interest. The stepwise procedure applied to infant formula and medical foods follows:

1. Weigh 2 g of $C_{18}$ (Bondesil) into a mortar.
2. Add 100 μL of isopropyl palmitate and gently blend the isopropyl palmitate onto the $C_{18}$ with a pestle.
3. Accurately weigh 0.5 g of reconstituted sample (10 g of infant formula powder was mixed with 50 g of 80°C water) onto the $C_{18}$/ isopropyl palmitate mixture.
4. Gently blend the mixture into a fluffy, slightly sticky powder.
5. Transfer the mixture into a 15-mL reservoir tube with a frit at the bottom, and insert the top frit on top of the powdery mix.
6. Tightly compress the reservoir contents with a 10-mL syringe plunger.
7. Pass 7 mL of isopropyl alcohol : hexane (0.5 : 99.5), followed by 7 mL of methylene chloride for infant formula or 7 mL of methylene chloride : ethyl acetate : 0.5% isopropyl alcohol in hexane (3 + 3 + 4 v/v) for medical foods through the reservoir, collecting both eluents into a 50-mL vessel (Turbovap).
8. Evaporate to near-dryness at 45°C in a Turbovap under 5 psi nitrogen.
9. Dilute residue to 1.0 mL with hexane.
10. Inject.

This procedure provides an alternative to traditional saponification and direct solvent extraction procedures used for infant formula and medical foods.

een peer-collaborated for AOAC International, but no approval
forthcoming at the present. The procedure greatly reduces use of
, is amenable to further automation, and is very rapid. Published
coefficients of variation and recoveries above 90% for assay of *all-rac-α*-tocopheryl acetate and retinyl palmitate. No problems were found with the assay of native tocopherols together with the synthetic fortificants. However, the presence of encapsulated vitamins can pose a problem for the method. Addition of isopropyl palmitate as a modifier was necessary for efficient elution of retinyl palmitate from the MSPD column. It was theorized that the isopropyl palmitate competes for binding sites on the $C_{18}$. The presence of the isopropyl palmitate in the final extract increases the viscosity of the extract and must be considered with use of autoinjectors to ensure reproducibility of injection volumes.

## 7.3.2. Chromatography

**7.3.2.1. Supports and Mobile Phases.** Because normal-phase chromatography can resolve β- and γ-T and T3 positional isomers, most studies quantifying vitamin E in foods rely on this chromatographic approach. Additionally, use of normal-phase silica supports allows direct injection of oil, which greatly simplifies assay of fats and oils. Up to 2 mg of oil can be directly injected per injection without influencing resolution, detection, or column life (132). This generality holds unless the fat or oil contains large amounts of polar lipids, which can precipitate out of the nonpolar mobile phase. Studies conducted with reversed-phase chromatography report the combined peaks of the positional isomers as (β- + γ-T). For many foods, this is of little consequence to the calculation of α-tocopherol equivalents (α-TE units), since β-T in most foods is usually present at low or nondetectable levels.

Tan and Brzuskiewicz(231) presented an in-depth comparison of normal- and reversed-phase chromatography for the resolution of the eight vitamin E homologues present in foods. With normal-phase chromatography, the homologues eluted in order of increasing polarity, and separation was based on the number and position of the methyl subsituents on the chromanol ring. Reversed-phase chromatography could not resolve positional isomers (β- and γ-T, β- and γ-T3). Resolution of the other homologues followed class separation based on saturation of the phytyl side chain with the more saturated tocopherols remaining on the column longer. The less polar but more saturated tocopherols were retained in the stationary phase longer, and the order of elution within each class of compounds was from higher polarity to lower polarity. Interaction of the phytyl side chain with the $C_{18}$ was theorized to cause the more saturated tocopherols to remain on the column longer than the unsaturated tocotrienols. Chromatograms for the different systems are shown in Figure 7.4.

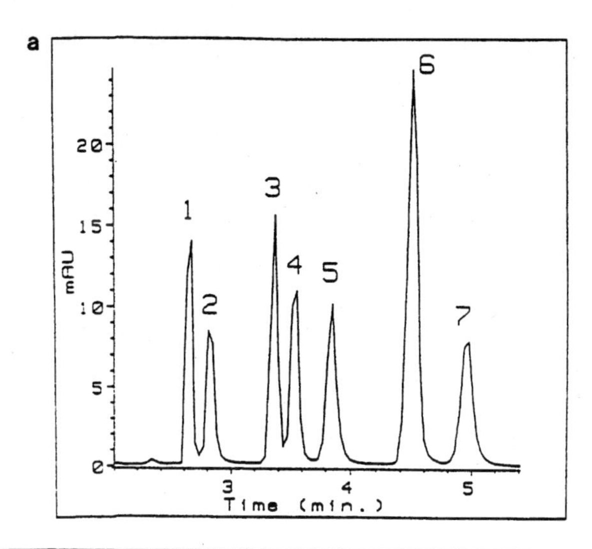


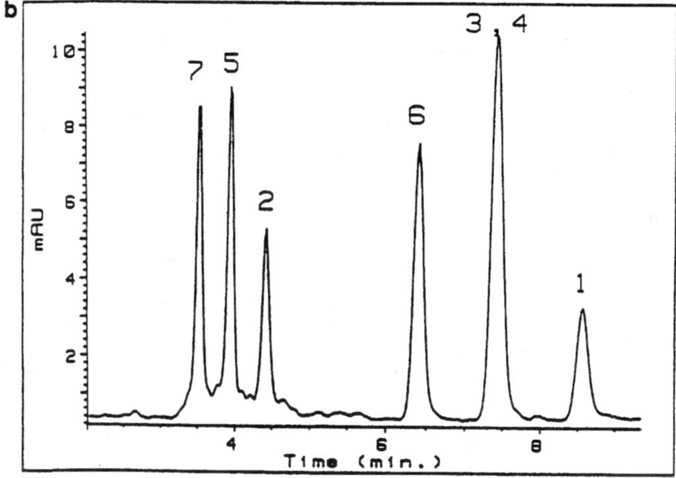


**FIGURE 7.4** Chromatography of tocopherols and tocotrienols on normal and reversed-phase systems. (a) Normal-phase Zorbax SIL with a 99 : 1 (hexane : 2-propanol) mobile phase. (b) Reversed-phase, Zorbax ODS with a 60 : 35 : 5 (acetonitrile : methanol : dichloromethane) mobile phase. 1 = $\alpha$-T, 2 = $\alpha$-T3, 3 = $\beta$-T, 4 = $\gamma$-T, 5 = $\gamma$-T3, 6 = $\delta$-T, 7 = $\delta$-T3. $\alpha$-T, $\alpha$-tocopherol; $\alpha$-T3, $\alpha$-tocotrienol. (From Ref. (231).)

**TABLE 7.8** Chromatographic Optimization of Various Normal-Phase Columns and Polar Modifiers[a]

| Column[c] | 2-Propanol $\alpha$ | n-Butanol $\alpha$ | THF[b] $\alpha$ | $CH_2Cl_2^b$ $\alpha$ |
|---|---|---|---|---|
| Cyano[d] | | | | |
| (1,2) | 1.29 [1.4] | 1.28 [1.8] | 1.29 [1.5] | 1.28 [1.8] |
| (6,7) | 1.23 [1.4] | 1.22 [1.8] | 1.23 [1.5] | 1.23 [1.7] |
| Amino | | | | |
| (1,2) | 1.19 [1.7] | 1.17 [1.4] | 1.18 [1.2] | — |
| (3,4) | 1.14 [2.0] | 1.12 [1.7] | 1.21 [1.6] | — |
| (6,7) | 1.20 [2.8] | 1.17 [2.2] | 1.45 [2.2] | — |
| Silica | | | | |
| (1,2) | 1.17 [1.9] | 1.16 [1.3] | — | — |
| (3,4) | 1.11 [1.2] | 1.09 [1.1] | — | — |
| (6,7) | 1.16 [2.0] | 1.14 [2.1] | — | — |

[a]Values are based on the average of duplicate runs, and all mobile phases consisted of 99% hexane and 1% modifier.
[b]—, the solvent gave no peaks after 15 min or results were not reproducible.
[c]Peak numbers in parentheses refer to those in the legend to Fig. 3a: 1, $\alpha$-T; 2, $\alpha$-T3; 3, $\beta$-T; 4, $\gamma$-T; 6, $\delta$-T; 7, $\delta$-T3. $\alpha$-T, $\alpha$-tocopherol; $\alpha$-T3, $\alpha$-tocotrienol; THF,; $\alpha$, Selectivity; number in [], resolution.
[d]Peak pairs 3 and 4 were not included because $\beta$- and $\gamma$-T coeluted.
*Source*: Modified from Ref. 231.

Tan and Brzuskiewicz (231) optimized solvent systems for cyano-, amino-, and silica-normal-phase columns with mobile phases consisting of 99% hexane and 1% of a variety of polar modifiers. The modifiers were isopropanol, n-butanol, THF, and methylene chloride. Selectivity and resolution of the systems are given in Table 7.8. Column efficiencies with isopropanol as the modifier with the silica column were superior to those of any of the other chromatography systems. Resolution between $\beta$- and $\gamma$-T was lower than for the amino-column but could be improved by addition of the modifier at levels below 1%. The optimal solvent system for normal-phase chromatography on Zorbax-SIL was 1% isopropanol in hexane. This solvent system for vitamin E chromatography on silica is almost universally used, providing reliable and highly reproducible chromatography. For reversed-phase chromatography on Zorbax ODS, acetonitrile : methanol : methylene chloride (60 : 35 : 5) gave excellent resolution of all homologs except $\beta$- and $\gamma$-T.

More recently, Abidi and Mounts(232) studied vitamin E resolution on the more polar aminopropyl-silica and diol-silica supports. Their work showed that the ability of mobile phases containing a weakly polar modifier such as an ester (ethyl acetate) or a monofunctional ether (t-butyl methyl ether) had significantly greater ability to resolve $\beta$- and $\gamma$-T compared to mobile phases containing more polar alcohol or polar ether modifiers, such as dioxane. Vitamin E mixtures were highly resolved on an amino-Si column with hexane : t-butyl ether (90 : 10) or on a diol-Si column with hexane : t-methyl ether (95 : 5). Mobile phases modified with such monofunctional ethers were highly recommended by the researchers to improve tocopherol and tocotrienol resolution. Chromatograms in Figures 7.5 and 7.6 compare resolution of vitamin E mixtures on diol-Si. Baseline resolution of $\beta$- and $\gamma$-T was obtained with the weakly polar modifiers (Figure 7.6).

Kamel-Eldin et al. (233) reported retention factors ($k$), separation factors ($\alpha$), theoretical plates ($N$), and resolution ($RS$) for normal-phase supports including seven silica columns, two amine columns, and a diol column. Chromatography was compared by using a mixture of oat extract, palm oil, and standards to produce a balanced mixture of tocopherols and tocotrienols. Variation exists in the ability of different silica supports to resolve the eight natural vitamin E forms efficiently. Of the seven silica columns, only three effectively resolved the vitamin E mixture. Good separations were also obtained on the amino and diol supports. The results generally agreed with Abidi and Mounts's(232) conclusion that weakly polar modifiers provided better selectivity than stronger modifiers for resolution of $\beta$- and $\gamma$-T. Use of dioxane (4%–5%) in

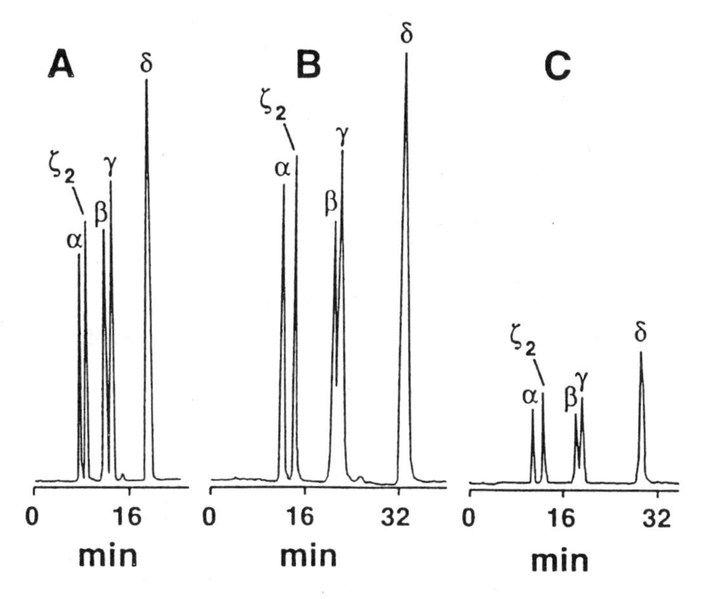


**FIGURE 7.5** Vitamin E chromatography with strongly polar modifiers. A, Amino-Si, hexane : dioxane (90 : 10); B, diol-Si (10 μm), hexane : dioxane (95 : 5); C, diol-Si (5 μm), cyclohexane : dioxane (97.3). (From Ref. 232.)

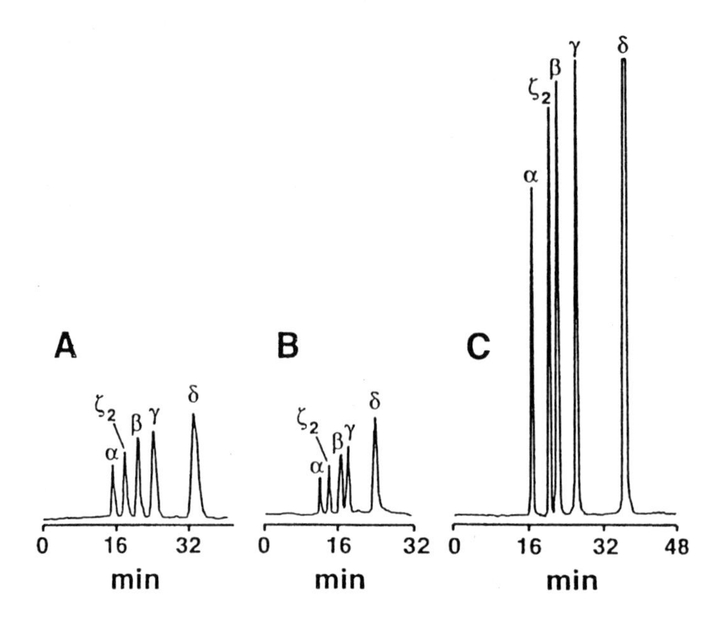


**FIGURE 7.6** Vitamin E chromatography with weakly polar modifiers. A, Amino-Si, cyclohexane : t-butyl methyl ether (90 : 10); B, diol-Si (10 μm), hexane : t-butyl methyl ether (90 : 10); C, diol-Si (5 μm), hexane : diisopropyl ether (90 : 10). (From Ref. 232.)

hexane provided good resolution on three of the silica columns examined in the study (Figure 7.7). Normal-phase diol columns have been successfully used to assay tissue and diet levels of tocopherols and tocotrienols (234).

Ye et al. (235) compared the ability of narrow-bore (2.1-mm id) silica columns to standard-bore (4.6-mm id) silica columns for chromatography of tocopherols. Narrow-bore columns have some combined characteristics of microbore and standard-bore columns but without the specialized hardware requirements of microbore chromatography. Narrow-bore chromatography can be easily implemented on newer, conventional LCs with pumps capable of handling lower flow rates than 1.0 mL/min. Advantages of microbore columns over standard-bore that carry over to narrow-bore columns include less solvent consumption, reduction in stationary phase amount, and higher mass sensitivity (236). Conditions used by Ye et al. (235) included mobile phase of 0.8% isopropanol in hexane pumped at 1.0 mL/min for standard-bore chromatography. Column temperature was controlled at 29°C ± 1°C.

A comparison of column performance statistics is provided in Table 7.9. Notable differences between the two columns include higher theoretical plates, lower back pressure, and better resolution for the standard-bore compared to the narrow-bore column. Narrow-bore gave higher sensitivity and lower solvent

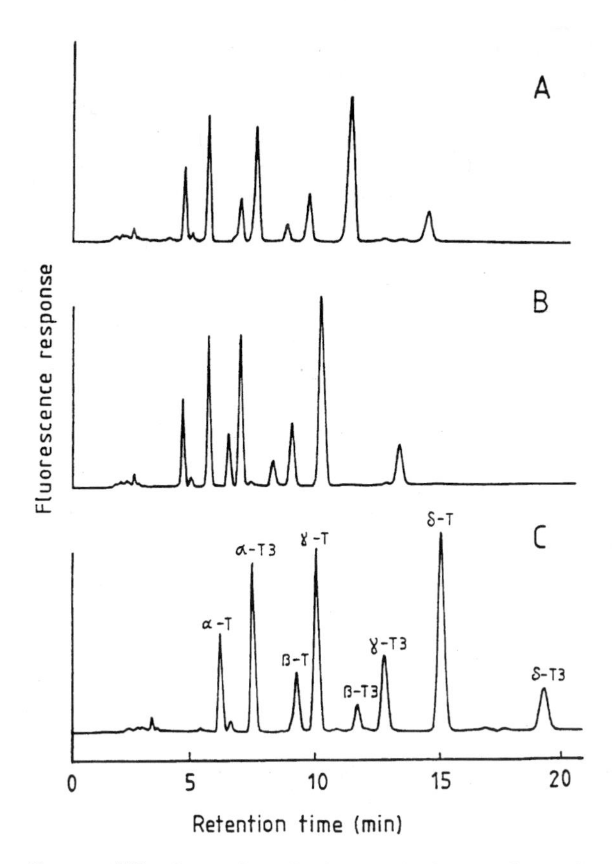


**FIGURE 7.7** Separation of a balanced mixture of tocopherols on three silica columns. A. Alltima SI, 5 m, 25 cm × 4.6 mm [Alltech] using Hex : Dioxane (96 : 4), 2 mL/min; B, Intersil SI, 5 μm, 25 cm × 4.6 mm (Chrompack) using Hex : Dioxane (95 : 5), 2 mL/min; C, Genesis silica, 4 μm, 25 cm × 4.6 mm (Jones) using Hex : Dioxane (96 : 4), 1.5 mL/min. α-T, α-tocopherol; α-T3, α-tocotrienol. (From Ref. 233.)

consumption than standard-bore. Limits of detection (LOD) and limits of quantitation (LOQ) values for the tocopherols are shown in Table 7.10. Peaks elute from the narrow-bore column in much smaller volume with less dispersion; therefore, detector signals are of higher intensity because of higher concentration in the detector flow cell. The LOD values for the vitamin E homologs were four to seven times lower for the narrow-bore column and up to eight times lower for the LOQ (Table 7.10). Narrow-bore chromatography could result in significant solvent savings with the loss of some resolution. Figure 7.8 shows resolution of the tocopherols and differences in detector response of eluting peaks.

**TABLE 7.9** Analytical Figures of Merit for Chromatography of α-, β-, γ-, and δ-Tocopherol on Narrow-Bore and Standard-Bore Columns[a,b]

| Analytes | $r^2$ | $k'$ | $N$ | $T$ | $S$ | α | $R_S$ |
|---|---|---|---|---|---|---|---|
| α-T | 0.9996 | 0.78 | 6,036 | 1.0 | 1.0 | | |
| | (0.9999) | (1.0) | (8,236) | (0.9) | (0.5) | 2.0 | 6.71 |
| β-T | 0.9998 | 1.57 | 5,182 | 1.1 | 0.8 | (2.0) | (10.3) |
| | (0.9999) | (2.0) | (11,274) | (1.1) | (0.5) | 1.1 | 1.4 |
| γ-T | 0.9998 | 1.77 | 5,560 | 1.1 | 0.9 | (1.1) | (2.2) |
| | (0.9999) | (2.2) | (12,777) | (0.9) | (0.5) | 1.8 | 7.72 |
| δ-T | 0.9998 | 3.19 | 5,905 | 1.1 | 1.0 | (1.8) | (11.5) |
| | (0.9999) | (4.0) | (10,630) | (1.0) | (0.5) | | |

[a]10-μL Injection volume and 0.8% IPA in hexane as mobile phase.
[b]Values in brackets are values from standard-bore. $r^2$, Linearity, range 0.33–16.37, 0.15–7.72, 0.31–15.52, 0.34–17.19 ng/injection ($n = 5$) for α-T, β-T, γ-T and δ-T in narrow-bore column, respectively; 0.65–32.74, 0.31–15.43, 0.62–31.03, 0.69–34.38 ng/injection ($n = 5$) for α-T, β-T, γ-T, and δ-T in standard-bore column, respectively. α-T, α-tocopherol. $k'$, Retention factor; $N$, theoretical plates; $T$, tailing factor; $S$, system suitability, RSD% of 5 replicate injections at 3.27, 1.54, 3.10, and 3.44 ng/injection in narrow-bore column for α-T, β-T, γ-T, and δ-T, respectively; at 6.55, 3.09, 6.21, and 6.88 ng/injection in standard-bore column for α-T, β-T, γ-T, and δ-T, respectively. α, separation factor; $R_S$, resolution.
*Source*: Modified from Ref. 235.

Reversed-phase LC has not been used for the analysis of vitamin E in foods to the extent that normal-phase LC has been used. Its inability to provide complete resolution of tocopherols and tocotrienols in complex samples is a powerful negative factor. Abidi (137) in 2000 in a review of applications of reversed-phase LC to vitamin E analysis cited the successful resolution of β and γ-T on pentafluorophenyl silica (237), long-chain alkylsilica (238,239), and non-silica-based octadecanoyl polyvinyl alcohol (240,241). In general, octadecylsilica (ODS) supports cannot achieve resolution of β- and γ-T. The positional isomers were resolved in the alcohol and acetate ester forms on octadecanoyl polyvinyl alcohol (ODPVA); however, only the ester forms were resolved on ODS (240). In a later study, Abidi(241) applied the ODPVA support to studies on the reversed-phase LC of the tocotrienols. Complete resolution of 16 tocotrienols, representing sets of cis/cis, cis/trans, trans/cis, and trans/trans geometrical isomers, was achieved (Figure 7.9). Reversed-phase systems provide compatibility with electrochemical (EC) detection and, as shown by Abidi's work (241), excellent resolution power for the geometrical isomers of the tocotrienols. Therefore, reversed-phase LC provides an important tool for tocotrienol quantification requiring resolution of the geometric isomers.

**Table 7.10** Limit of Detection (ng), Limit of Quantitation (ng) for the Chromatography of α-, β-, γ-, and δ-Tocopherol on Standard-Bore and Narrow-Bore Columns

| | Narrow-bore | | Standard-bore | | | |
|---|---|---|---|---|---|---|
| Analytes | LOD | LOQ | LOD | LOQ | LOD | LOQ |
| α-T | 0.032 | 0.094 | 0.021 | 0.051 | 0.119 | 0.307 |
| β-T | 0.016 | 0.046 | 0.006 | 0.014 | 0.029 | 0.072 |
| γ-T | 0.025 | 0.075 | 0.012 | 0.028 | 0.049 | 0.119 |
| δ-T | 0.039 | 0.113 | 0.011 | 0.024 | 0.075 | 0.200 |
| Column | LiChrosorb Si60, 25 cm × 2.1 mm 5 μm | | LiChrosorb Si60, 25 cm × 2.1 mm 5 μm | | LiChrosorb Si60, 25 cm × 4.6 mm 5 μm | |
| Flow rate | 0.32 mL/min | | 0.32 mL/min | | 1.0 mL/min | |
| MP | 0.6% IPA in hexane | | 0.8% IPA in hexane | | 0.8% IPA in hexane | |

LOD, limit of detection; LOQ, limit of quantitation; α-T, α-tocopherol; MP, mobile phase; IPA, isopropyl alcohol..
*Source*: Modified from Ref. 235.

**7.3.2.2. Detection.** Detection of tocopherols and tocotrienols after LC resolution can be accomplished by UV, fluorescence (FLD), electrochemical (EC) or evaporative light scattering (ELSD) detectors. By far, the most commonly used detector for vitamin E analysis is FLD, which is considerably more sensitive and selective than UV but less sensitive than EC. Fluorescence intensity of the eluted vitamin E peaks depends upon many factors; thus, comparison of fluorescence response to UV or EC measures of detector sensitivity is somewhat dependent on equipment and the chemical environment of the mobile phase passing through the detector. Lang(131) in a review of detection methods for vitamin E reported that one study showed that sensitivity of fluorescence was 2.5-to 3.3-fold greater than absorbance at 292 nm. This sensitivity is probably too low if comparable measurements were performed with new-generation fluorescence detectors with improved engineering and higher-intensity lamps for excitation.

In a 1998 study, Hoehler et al. (242) reported 150-to 340-fold increases in sensitivity of FLD compared to UV at 280 nm for the tocopherols. Sensitivity of FLD depends a great deal upon the composition of the mobile phase. For example, α-T and retinol have a five to sixfold decrease in fluorescence intensity when the mobile phase is changed from hexane to acetonitrile:water (1 : 1) (128). Many reversed-phase mobile phase components lead to decreased fluorescence of

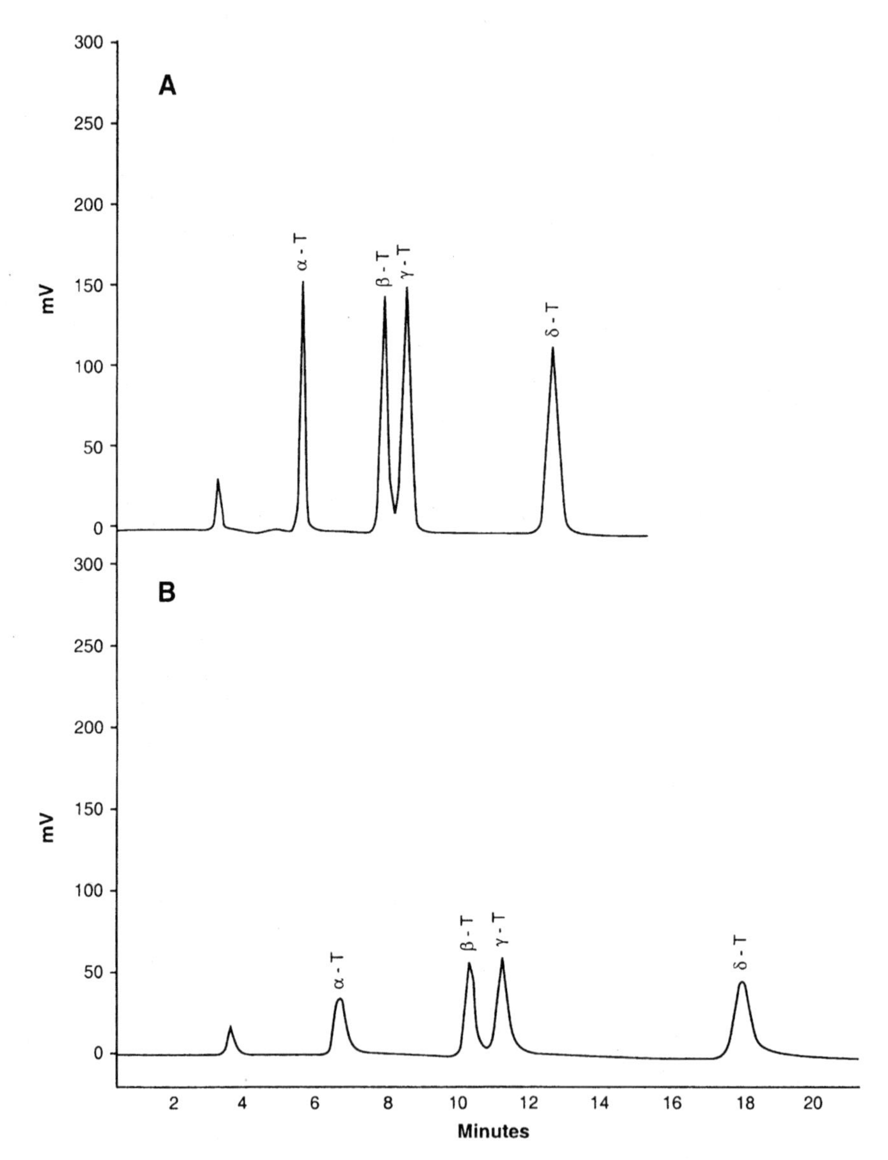


**FIGURE 7.8** Chromatography of tocopherols on (A) 250 × 2.1 mm id LiChrosorb Si60, flow rate 0.32 mL/min, and (B) 250 × 4.6 mm id LiChrosorb Si60, flow rate 1.0 mL/min. Mobile phase was 0.8% isopropanol in hexane; injection volume was 10 mL. $\alpha$-T, $\alpha$-tocopherol. (From Ref. 235.)

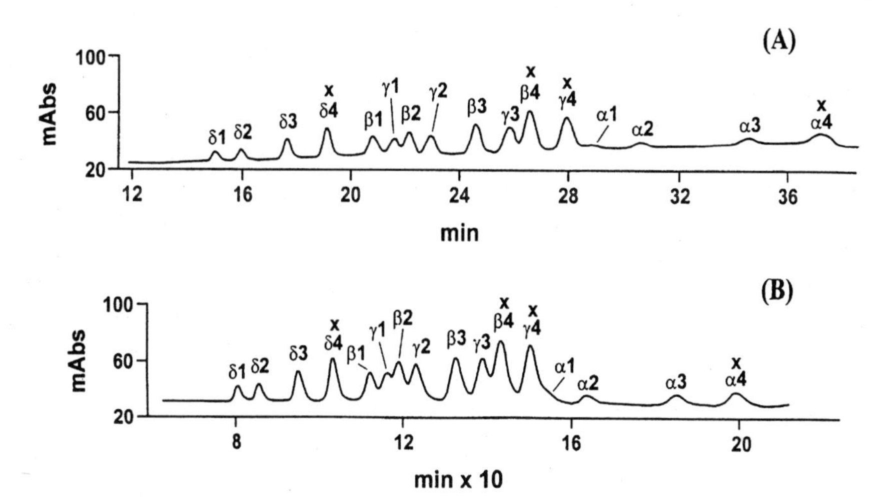


**FIGURE 7.9** Reversed-phase liquid chromatography (LC) of synthetic tocotrienols on octadecanoyl polyvinyl alcohol support column, AsahiPak ODP. Mobile phase, acetonitriles : water (70 : 30, v/v). Flow rates: (A) 0.5 mL/min; (B) 1 mL/min. Detector, fluorescence. 1 = cic/cis, 2 = cis/trans, 3 = trans/cis, 4 = trans/trans. *m*Abs. (From Ref. 241.)

vitamin E components compared to fluorescence intensity possible in normal-phase systems (243). Chen(244) showed that the polarity of the solvent greatly influences fluorescence intensity of many organic compounds. Caution has to be used to prevent fluorescence quenching (reduced fluorescence intensity) when FLD is used. Factors producing quenching include dissociation of the molecule by the light energy necessary for excitation, absorbance of emitted light by other molecular species or by the analyte itself, and dissipation of energy from collisions of molecules.

Selectivity of FLD results from the fact that two wavelengths are used in the measurement compared to one for ultraviolet/visible (UV/VIS) detection. Also, structural features necessary for a molecule to fluoresce are limited in nature, whereas UV/VIS absorbance is common to most organics. The chromanol ring structure of the tocopherols and tocotrienols with fluorescence properties of maximal emission at 345 nm with excitation at 210 or 290 nm(131) provides a highly selective detection system readily noted from clean fluorescence chromatograms from complex matrices, produced with minimal sample cleanup. Most lipids do not fluoresce (127); therefore, lipids can be injected directly onto silica columns and little fluorescence interference will be apparent.

Older literature states that tocopheryl esters such as $\alpha$-tocopheryl acetate do not fluoresce, thereby limiting the detection of such compounds to UV. However, with the availability of high-intensity excitation sources and new FLD design, fluorescence of α-tocopheryl acetate is readily measurable. Reports by Woollard et al. (173) and Baltz et al. (208) were the first to document the ability to measure α-tocopheryl acetate by fluorescence in the assay of infant formula. Since these reports, several methods for determination of α-tocopheryl acetate in fortified foods have been presented (185,186,189,190,196,214). In this respect FLD has improved assay of vitamin E levels in fortified foods since direct solvent extraction can be employed in place of saponification, allowing biological activity to be more accurately assessed.

Electrochemical detection in combination with HPLC resolution is an effective analytical approach. A 1985 review by Ueda and Igarashi(224) indicates that EC is 20 times more sensitive than FLD for the detection of tocopherols. However, EC is limited to reversed-phase chromatography because of the need for electrolyte in the mobile phase for electrical conductance. Electrochemical detection has been used to assay tocopherols in olive oil (160,220).

Evaporation light scattering detection has been suggested as a potential detection mode for vitamin E. However, FLD is at least 10 times more sensitive than ELSD.(159,245) Few studies using evaporative light scattering have been completed because of operational cost and instrument complexity.

**7.3.2.3. Internal Standards.** Internal standards (IS) for vitamin E analysis are not frequently used in analytical studies on foods. Most investigators, including the authors, rely on spiked recoveries to ensure that each tocopherol is efficiently extracted. As previously discussed (Sec. 7.3.1.1), differences in polarities of the homologues can cause recovery problems from saponification digests or from the food matrix by direct solvent extraction when hexane is used as the extracting solvent. Tocol, used in some studies as an IS, was shown to be unsuitable for use with saponification because of low recovery in relation to the tocopherols (225). Ueda and Igarashi (226) then introduced 2,2,5,7,8-pentamethyl-6-chromanol (PMC) as an IS; however, PMC has not been widely used. For serum and plasma, δ-T is normally not detectable and can serve as an IS for either UV- or fluorescence-based methods (136).

## 7.4. ANALYTICAL APPLICATIONS

### 7.4.1. Fats, Oils, and Margarine

Several methods for fats and oils are summarized in Table 7.4. Margarine represents one of the most significant sources of vitamin E in the American diet, representing more than 6% of the total vitamin E available from the food supply (246). Margarine represents a relatively simple food matrix and can be prepared for analysis by a direct solvent extraction of tocopherols and tocotrienols (present if palm oil is an ingredient) or by saponification. The direct solvent extraction developed by Thompson and Hatina (132) (Sec. 7.3.1.2) is effective for the matrix. Syvoja et al. (156) simply diluted margarine samples in hexane and allowed solids to settle. Examples of studies using saponification include Hogarty et al. (192) and Rader et al. (167). Ye et al. (168) published a simple direct solvent extraction for margarine based on a modification of Landen's(169) solvent extraction procedure. Steps in the extraction follow:

1. Accurately weigh 5.0 g margarine or spread into three 125-mL Erlenmeyer flasks for duplicates and spike recovery.
2. Add 40 mL of hexane-BHT solution (0.1% BHT).
3. Sonicate with intermittent mixing until the sample has dissolved.
4. Rinse sides of flask with 10 mL hexane-BHT solution and add 3 drops of Tween 80.
5. Add 3 g $MgSO_4$ (or more, depending water content of the sample: 1 g for each milliliter of water plus 1 g extra).
6. Mix; let stand for $\geq$2 h.
7. Filter through medium-porosity fritted glass filter using a bell jar filtration unit.
8. Wash filter with hexane-BHT solution.
9. Transfer filtrate to 100 mL volumetric and dilute to volume with the extraction solution. Further dilutions are most likely necessary depending on the quality of the FLD.

The HPLC system for the Ye et al. (168) method used a LiChrosorb Si60 column, 0.9% isopropyl alcohol in hexane as the mobile phase, and fluorescence detection ($Ex\lambda = 290$, $Em\lambda = 330$). The chromatography was thoroughly verified and column performance criteria are given in Table 7.11. Recoveries for the tocopherols were higher than 97% and for RSD (%) values were low (intraday, 0.8–3.5; interday, 1.4–4.1).

## 7.4.2. Infant Formula and Medical Foods

Because of the significance of infant formula as the sole source of nutrition to formula-fed infants, many method development efforts have centered on improving methods to assay the fat-soluble vitamins in these products. Included in the analytes of interest are the native tocopherols and *all-rac-α*-tocopheryl acetate, which is the primary source of vitamin E in the formulated products. Most of the procedures developed for analysis of infant formula are multianalyte methods for the simultaneous assay of two or more fat-soluble vitamins in the formula. Barnett et al. (247) reported a nonaqueous reversed-phase method for the simultaneous analysis of retinol, retinyl palmitate, vitamin $D_2$ and $D_3$, $\alpha$-T, *all-rac-α*-tocopheryl acetate, and vitamin $K_1$. The procedure proved applicable to

**TABLE 7.11** Analytical Figures of Merit for Assay of Vitamin E in Margarine

| Homologue | Linearity[a] $R^2$ | Capacity factor $K'$ | Theoretical plates[b] $N$ | Tailing factor[c] $T$ | Selectivity[d] $\alpha$ | Resolution[e] $RS$ |
|---|---|---|---|---|---|---|
| $\alpha$-T | 0.9999 | 1.0 | 4956 | 1.1 | | |
| | | | | | 1.5 | 7.9 |
| $\gamma$-T | 0.9999 | 2.1 | 6815 | 0.9 | | |
| | | | | | 1.4 | 7.8 |
| $\delta$-T | 0.9999 | 3.4 | 7530 | 1.1 | | |

[a]Range 13.91–1159 ng/mL $\alpha$-T ($n = 5$), 16.15–1346 ng/mL $\gamma$-T ($n = 5$), and 16.04–1337 ng/mL $\delta$-T ($n = 5$).
[b]Calculated as $n = 16\,(t/w)^2$.
[c]Calculated at 5% peak height, $T = w_{0.05}/2f$ (Ref. 23).
[d]$\alpha = t_2/t_1$.
[e]$RS = 2(t_2 - t_1)/(w_1 + w_2)$.
$\alpha$-T, $\alpha$-tocopherol.
*Source*: Modified from Ref. 168.

analysis of milk and soy-based infant formulas as well as many types of dairy products. The extraction eliminated saponification to prevent isomerization of $D_2$ and $D_3$ and alkaline destruction of vitamin $K_1$. Lipid removal was through hydrolysis with lipase from *Candida cyclindraccae*, and free fatty acids were removed from the digest by a rapid alkali precipitation. The digest was then extracted with n-pentane. The n-pentane extract was evaporated to dryness, redissolved in ethyl ether, and diluted with acetonitrile:ethyl acetate (1 : 1). Cholesterol phenylacetate was used as an IS. The lipase digestion partially hydrolyzed retinyl palmitate and *all-rac-α*-tocopheryl acetate, so it was necessary to quantify retinol and $\alpha$-T along with the ester forms of these vitamins. Chromatography used gradient elution with methanol : ethyl acetate (86 : 14) against acetonitrile, a variable-wavelength UV detector (retinol, 325 nm; retinyl palmitate, 365 nm; $D_2$, $D_3$, K, $\alpha$-T, *all-rac-α*-tocopheryl acetate, IS, 265 nm), and two Zorbax ODS columns in series.

Several studies on the analysis of infant formula have been conducted at the Atlanta Center for Nutrient Analysis (ACNA), U.S. Food and Drug Administration, Atlanta, Georgia. Landen and colleagues developed an integrated approach to fat-soluble vitamin assay in infant formula that was amenable to the assay of many fortified foods(169,170,248) and included assay of tocopherols and *all-rac-α*-tocopheryl acetate. The method was a nondestructive technique that incorporated a cleanup and concentration step using high-performance gel permeation chromatography (HP-GPC) to fractionate the fat-soluble vitamins from lipids before reversed-phase chromatography. The method also introduced the direct solvent extraction procedure for fat-soluble vitamins developed by

Landen (Sec. 7.3.1.2). The success of the procedure using nonaqueous reversed-phase chromatography as the determinative step depended on the development of a lipid extraction method that would effectively extract the fat-soluble vitamins and be amenable to the further determinative step. The relatively simple extraction has found extensive use in the analysis of natural vitamin E homologues, *all-rac-α*-tocopheryl acetate, retinyl palmitate, and retinyl acetate from fortified foods.

Chase et al. (185,186,189–191) at ACNA published several procedures for the simultaneous analysis of fat-soluble vitamins in infant formula and medical foods that rely on a modification of the original extraction procedure developed by Landen (169,248). The procedures quantitate tocopherols, *all-rac-α*-tocopheryl acetate, and retinyl palmitate and use direct solvent extraction(185,186) or matrix solid-phase dispersion(189,190,191) for simple but effective extraction of the analytes before LC assay. Rodrigo et al. (215) compared several direct solvent extraction procedures to prepare extracts suitable for simultaneous assay of α-, β-, and γ-T and *all-rac-α*-tocopheryl acetate in reconstituted, powdered infant formula. The study indicated that chloroform-methanol extraction (Folch) followed by normal-phase chromatography was well suited for the assay. Because of the rapidity of sample handling (2-h assay time), the extraction steps are summarized here. Excellent analytical parameters were obtained for linearity, precision, and accuracy through asssay of Standard Reference Material (SRM) 1846, Powdered Infant Formula.

1. Mix 1 mL of reconstituted formula (10% w/w) with 5 mL of chloroform : methanol (2 : 1 v/v).
2. Mechanically stir for 3 min.
3. Allow to stand for 5 min.
4. Add 1 mL of water.
5. Manually invert two to three times.
6. Centrifuge at 1500 × g for 10 min at 15°C.
7. Remove chloroform phase and dry under $N_2$.
8. Reconstitute with 1 mL of hexane.
9. Filter (0.20 μm); dilute; inject.

Other methods for the analysis of vitamin E infant formula are summarized in Table 7.4.

Various approaches have been used to determine vitamin E levels in human and bovine milk. Syväoja et al. (171) used the solvent extraction procedure of Thompson and Hatina(132) followed by determinative normal-phase chromatography and fluorescence detection. For infant formula and other infant foods, these authors used saponification for extraction of the tocopherols. Chappell et al. (174) developed a simultaneous analysis of tocopherols and retinyl esters in human milk using direct solvent extraction with hexane and normal-phase chroma-tography on silica. Zamarreño et al. (177,182,183) used lipase hydrolysis and saponification, depending on the matrix and whether or not vitamin $K_1$ was included in the analysis, to assay fat-soluble vitamins in milk and milk powder. Their method was adapted to an on-line system for the simultaneous analysis of retinol, $\alpha$-T, and vitamin $D_3$ from milk and powdered milk. The on-line system linked saponification, preconcentration, and sample cleanup on $C_{18}$ (Sep Pak). Panfilli et al. (181) used the extraction developed by Ueda and Igarashi (225), which included saponification and extraction of the digest with hexane : ethyl acetate (9 : 1) to assay tocopherols, $\beta$-carotene, and *cis*- and *trans*-isomers of retinol in cheese. Gradient elution from Ultrasphere Si was with 1% isopropanol in hexane and hexane. The detection system included programmable UV/VIS and fluorescence detectors in series. Absorbance at 450 nm was used for the carotenoids and fluorescence for tocopherols ($Ex\lambda = 280$, $Em\lambda = 325$) and the retinol isomers ($Ex\lambda = 325$, $Em\lambda = 475$).

### 7.4.3. Miscellaneous Foods

**7.4.3.1. Cereals.** Widicus and Kirk (249) introduced one of the first simultaneous LC methods for analysis of *all-rac-α*-tocopheryl acetate and retinyl palmitate in fortified foods. The method was specific for cereal products and used direct solvent extraction with methylene chloride and 95% ethanol, and normal-phase chromatography with injection of the lipid-containing extract onto μPorasil. This work showed the importance of simultaneous vitamin assays with LC as a labor- and cost-saving approach to routine vitamin analysis programs.

**7.4.3.2. Eggs.** Jiang et al. (209) and McGeachin and Bailey (210) showed the potential of newer, more sensitive diode array detectors for simultaneous analysis of fortified foods and feeds. These authors quantified $\alpha$-T, several carotenoids, and retinol in eggs and fortified feeds. Detection was at 294 nm for $\alpha$-T, 325 nm for retinol, and 445 nm for the carotenoids. Peak identities were verified by comparison to published maxima for carotenoids in hexane.

**7.4.3.3. Mayonnaise.** Ye et al. (217) published a simplified method for the analysis of vitamin E and $\beta$-carotene in reduced-fat mayonnaise that is also applicable to full-fat mayonnaise. Analytes included tocopherols, *all-rac-α*-tocopheryl acetate, and $\beta$-carotene. Extraction is a modification of Landen's extraction (169) and closely follows the extraction of Lee et al. (229) with modifications to sample weights and solvent volumes to adjust for requirements of the sample matrix. The extraction procedure follows:

1. Weigh 3.0-g sample into a 125-mL Erlenmeyer flask.
2. Add 2.0 mL of 80°C water.
3. Sonicate for 5 min to facilitate dissolution.
4. Add 5 mL of isopropanol and approximately 5 g of $MgSO_4$.

5. Mix with a spatula and add 20 mL of hexane containing 0.003% BHT diluted with hexane : ethyl acetate (90 : 10) (30 mL diluted with 470 mL).
6. Homogenize for 1 min with a Polytron.
7. Rinse generator tip with isopropanol.
8. Filter the extract through a 60-mL coarse-porosity fritted glass filter into a 125-mL Phillips beaker. Use a vacuum bell jar filtration unit.
9. Break up material on fritted glass filter and wash twice with 5 mL of hexane (0.003% BHT).
10. Repeat extraction by transferring material on filter to the original extraction container. Use 5 mL isopropanol and 20 mL of the hexane with BHT.
11. Combine filtrates and dilute to 100 mL.
12. Evaporate 4 mL and dilute with mobile phase.

Parameters of the LC determination follow:

| | |
|---|---|
| Column | LiChrosorb Si60, 5 μm, 25 cm × 4.6 mm<br>Guard column Perisorb A, 30–40 μm |
| Mobile phase | 0.27% isopropanol in hexane |
| Flow gradient | 0.9 to 1.5 mL/min over 5.3 min |
| Detectors | Diode array and fluorescence in series, program wavelengths for fluorescence<br>Time 0: $Ex\lambda = 285$, $Em\lambda = 310$<br>7 min: $Ex\lambda = 290$, $Em\lambda = 330$ |

The method provides excellent overall quality parameters as detailed in Table 7.12. Chromatography (Figure 7.10) shows the ability of coupling photo diode array detection and fluorescence detection to handle multianalytes from the same injection.

**7.4.3.4. Peanuts, Peanut Products, Other Nuts.** In 1999 Lee et al. (213) presented a method for analysis of tocopherols in peanuts, peanut butter, and other high-fat nuts. The extraction procedure was discussed in Sec. 7.3.1.2. As an example of a routine chromatographic procedure for the tocopherols, column performance criteria are provided in Table 7.13. Chromatography conditions included a column (LiChrosorb Si60), isopropanol in hexane as the mobile phase, and fluorescence detection at $Ex\lambda = 290$, $Em\lambda = 330$.

### 7.4.4. Multianalyte Procedures

Barua and Olson(211) introduced a multianalyte procedure based on reversed-phase LC to assay very polar to nonpolar retinoids, carotenoids, and tocopherols

**TABLE 7.12** Analytical Figures of Merit for the Chromatography of α-, γ-, and δ-Tocopherol, α-Tocopherol Acetate, and β-Carotene in Mayonnaise

| Analytes | Linearity[a] $R^2$ | Theoretical plates[b] $N$ | Tailing factor[c] $T$ | System suitability[d] $S$ | Resolution[e] $RS$ |
|---|---|---|---|---|---|
| α-TAC | 0.999 | 17,929 | 1.0 | 1.2 | |
| | | | | | 6.0 |
| α-T | 0.999 | 15,974 | 1.0 | 1.0 | |
| | | | | | 18.1 |
| γ-T | 0.999 | 11,026 | 1.0 | 0.8 | |
| | | | | | 14.5 |
| δ-T | 0.999 | 10,574 | 1.0 | 1.7 | |
| β-Carotene | 0.999 | 3,185 | 1.0 | 0.5 | |

[a]Range 6.17–154.3, 3.14–78.57, 8.28–206.9, 12.38–309.4, and 0.11–12.88 ng/injection for α-TAC, α-T, γ-T, δ-T, and β-carotene ($n = 5$), respectively.
[b]Calculated as $N = 16\,(t/w)^2$.
[c]Calculated at 5% peak height, $T = w_{0.05}/2f$ (USP 23, 1995).
[d]RSD% of 5 replicate injections at 30.85, 15.7, 41.4, 61.9, and 1.09 ng/injection for α-TAC, α-T, γ-T, δ-T, and β-carotene, respectively. RSD%,.
[e]$RS = 2(t_2 - t_1)/(w_1 + w_2)$.
α-T, α-tocopherol; α-TAC, α-tocopherol acetate.
*Source*: Modified from Ref. 217.

simultaneously in animal and plant products. Included in the analysis were 18 analytes given in Table 7.14. Various other analytes were identified in the course of the study, including 3, 4-didehydroretinyl ester in human liver, 5,6,5′,6′-diepoxy-β-carotene in mango, and lycopene in papaya. Because of the utility of this procedure, it is outlined here:

| Extraction of animal and plant tissue |
|---|

1. Finely mince tissue and grind in isopropanol : dichloromethane (2 : 1).
2. Transfer mixture to a 20-mL vial and increase volume to 10 mL with the extracting solvent.
3. Stopper and vortex the mixture.
4. Layer with argon and store at −20°C overnight.
5. Vortex; return to freezer.
6. On the third day, vortex, centrifuge or filter, and evaporate supernantant to dryness.
7. Redissolve residue in 200 μL of the isopropanol : dichloromethane solvent.
8. Inject 20–40 μL.

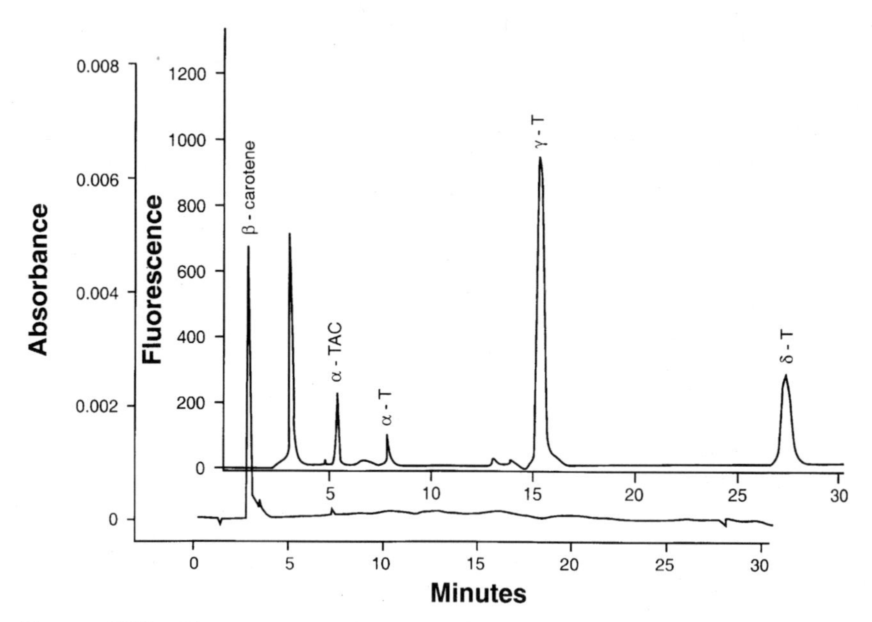


**FIGURE 7.10** Chromatogram of mayonnaise extract. LiChrosorb Si60 (5 μm, 4.6 × 250 mm). Mobile phase: 0.27% isopropanol in hexane with a gradient flow. Detection: tocopherols (fluorescence $Ex\lambda = 290$, $Em\lambda = 330$) α-tocopherol acetate (fluorescence $Ex\lambda = 285$, $Em\lambda = 310$); β-carotene, 450 nm. α-T, α-tocopherol; α-TAC, α-tocopherol acetate. (From Ref. 217.)

| HPLC parameters | |
|---|---|
| Column | Microsorb-MV, 3 μm<br>10 cm × 4.6 mm Preceded by a $C_{18}$ guard column |
| Mobile phase | Solvent A: methanol : water (3 : 1) containing 10 mM ammonium acetate<br>Solvent B: methanol : dichloromethane (4 : 1) |
| Gradient | 100% A to 100% B over 15–20 min, isocratic with solvent B for 15–20 min<br>Reverse gradient to initial conditions over 5 min<br>Equilibrate column with solvent A for 10 min |
| Detection | Photodiode array<br>Retinoids 330 mm<br>Tocopherols 290 mm<br>Carotenoids 445 mm |
| Elution (see Figure 7.11) | |

**TABLE 7.13** Precision and Accuracy of the Assay of Tocopherols in Peanut Butter

| Homologue | Parameters | Precision: Repeatability[b] | Precision: Reproducibility[c] | Accuracy[a] Recovery |
|---|---|---|---|---|
| | | mg/100 g | | % |
| α-T | Mean[d] | 7.7 | 7.3 | 98.2 |
| | SD[e] | 0.2 | 0.2 | 1.2 |
| | CV[f], % | 3.0 | 3.1 | 1.2 |
| β-T | Mean | 0.2 | 0.2 | 102.0 |
| | SD | 0.02 | 0.02 | 11.8 |
| | CV, % | 9.0 | 9.3 | 11.5 |
| γ-T | Mean | 11.6 | 11.1 | 96.6 |
| | SD | 0.6 | 0.4 | 1.5 |
| | CV, % | 5.1 | 3.7 | 1.6 |
| δ-T | Mean | 0.8 | 0.9 | 100.8 |
| | SD | 0.1 | 0.1 | 2.7 |
| | CV, % | 7.0 | 6.0 | 2.7 |

[a]Accuracy is a measure of the closeness of the analytical result to the true value evaluated by analyzing a spiked sample.
[b]Repeatability refers to the results of independent determinations carried out on a sample by analyzing five replicates of the sample on the same day.
[c]Reproducibility refers to the results of independent determinations carried out on a sample by analyzing five replicates of the sample at different periods.
[d]$n = 5$. [e]Standard deviation. [f]Coefficient of variation.
α-T, α-tocopherol.
*Source*: Modified from Ref. 213.

Advantages of the method are its ability to resolve very polar to nonpolar classes of compounds. The PDA detector permitted detection of the compounds from one injection. Use of the ammonium acetate in the mobile phase reduced tailing of carboxyl (very polar) compounds such as retinoic acid without salt precipitation in the mobile phase, which can be problematic in reversed-phase systems. Column regeneration was easy because of the elution of different-polarity substances during the chromatographic run. The authors state that the procedure is a compromise of published procedures specific for single classes of compounds with similar polarities; however, its overall usefulness to vitamin analysts is readily apparent as an advancement because of the coupling of PDA and LC capabilities.

Ye et al. developed methods to assay tocopherols, *all-rac-α*-tocopheryl acetate, retinyl palmitate, and β-carotene in fortified foods and mayonnaise.(214, 217) Again, as seen with Barua and Olson's work (211), coupling of PDA with excellent chromatographic resolution greatly simplifies

**TABLE 7.14** Retention Times ($t_r$) of Selected Retinoids, Carotenoids, and Tocopherols[a]

| Analyte | $t_r$ (min) |
|---|---|
| All-*trans* 4-oxoretinoyl β-glucuronide | 2.1 |
| 13-*cis* Retinoic acid | 9.9 |
| 9-*cis* Retinoic acid | 10.2 |
| All-*trans* retinoic acid | 10.5 |
| All-*trans* retinol | 12.9 |
| All-*trans* retinal | 13.8 |
| All-*trans* retinyl acetate | 15.7 |
| All-*trans* lutein | 16.1 |
| γ-Tocopherol | 18.2 |
| α-Tocopherol | 18.7 |
| All-*trans* retinyl palmitate | 24.1 |
| All-*trans* lycopene | 26.5 |
| All-*trans* β-carotene | 27.1 |

[a]High-performance liquid chromatography was carried out on a Rainin 3-μm Microsorb-MV column (100 × 4.6 mm) by use of PDA 991 system and a linear gradient of methanol–water (75 : 25, v/v) containing 10 mM ammonium acetate) to methanol-dichloromethane (4 : 1, v/v) in 15 min, followed by isocratic elution with the later solvent mixture for an additional 15 min at a flow rate of 0.8 mL/min.
*Source*: Modified from Ref. 211.

simultaneous analysis of several fat-soluble vitamins. The procedure for mayonnaise(217) used gradient flow and fluorescence detection and PDA detection. Figure 7.12 shows resolution of six analytes from a fortified margarine. The method was successfully applied to products containing encapsulated or nonencapsulated vitamins (214).

## 7.5. PREPARATIVE PROCEDURES FOR THE TOCOPHEROLS AND TOCOTRIENOLS

The great interest in vitamin E from a clinical perspective and from a functional perspective in food processing because of its antioxidant properties increased the need for pure standards in relatively large quantities to support feeding or processing trials. Pure standards, particularly for the tocotrienols, are expensive and have limited availability. For these reasons, preparative methods have been published. Such methods published before the 1970s used thin-layer or open-column chromatography to isolate the natural vitamin E homologues. More

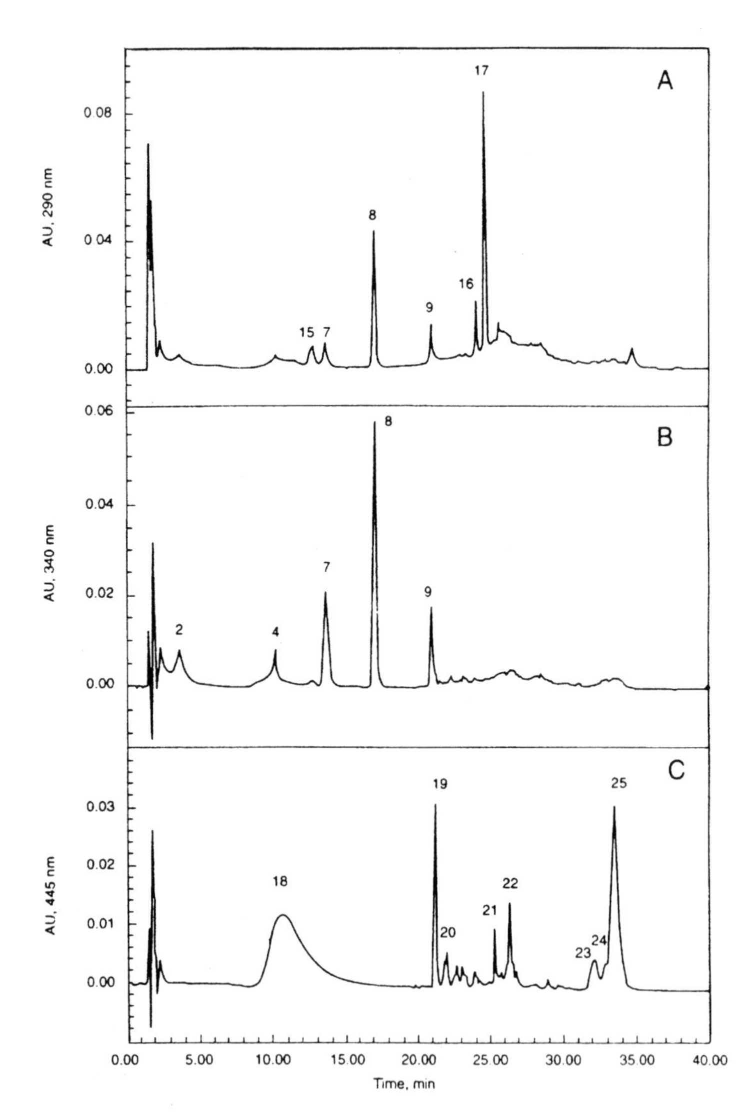


**FIGURE 7.11** Reversed-phase high-performance liquid chromatography (HPLC) elution profiles of tocopherols (A), retinoids (B), and carotenoids (C) present in human plasma (200 μL). Blood was collected 3 h after an oral dose of retinoic acid. The chromatogram was obtained by use of the PDA 996 System and a gradient time of 20 min. Peak identification: 2,4-oxo-retinoic acid; 4, retinoyl β-glucuronide; 7, retinoic acid; 8, retinol; 9, retinyl acetate; 15, butylated hydroxytoluene (BHT); 16, γ-tocopherol; 17, α-tocopherol; 18, free bilirubin; 19, lutein; 20, zeaxanthin; 21, 2′3′-anhydrolutein; 22, β-cryptoxanthin; 23, lycopene; 24, α-carotene; 25, β-carotene. α-T, α-tocopherol; α-TAC, α-tocopherol acetate. (From Ref. 211.)

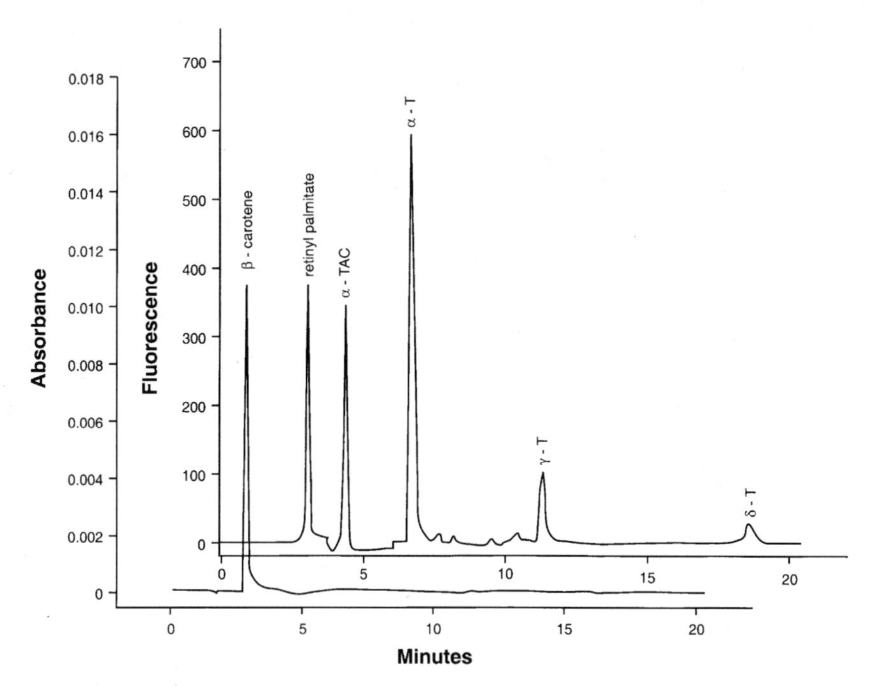


**FIGURE 7.12** Chromatogram of margarine extract. LiChrosorb Si60 (5 μm, 4.6 × 250 mm). Mobile phase: 0.5% isopropanol in hexane with a gradient flow. Detection: tocopherols (fluorescence $Ex\lambda = 290$, $Em\lambda = 330$); $\alpha$-tocopheryl acetate (fluorescence $Ex\lambda = 285$, $Em\lambda = 310$), retinyl palmitate (fluorescence $Ex\lambda = 325$, $Em\lambda = 470$); $\beta$-carotene, 450 nm. $\alpha$-T, $\alpha$-tocopherol; $\alpha$-TAC, $\alpha$-tocopherol acetate. (From Ref. 214.)

recent preparative methods have used flash chromatography, preparatory HPLC (Prep-LC), or combinations of these methods to concentrate and partially purify the vitamin E compounds.

Flash chromatography was first proposed by Still et al. (250) as a simple absorption chromatography technique for the routine purification of organic compounds traditionally carried out by tedious long-column chromatography. The technique was described by Still et al. (250) as a hybrid of medium-pressure and short-column chromatography using gas pressure for rapid solvent flow through the column. Although resolution capability is moderate, the system is simple and inexpensive. Samples from 0.01 to 10 g can be fractionated in 10 to 15 min depending on column size and the solvent system.

Pearce et al. (251) isolated $\alpha$-T, $\alpha$-T3, $\gamma$-T3, and $\delta$-T3 from a tocotrienol-rich fraction (TRF) of palm oil using flash chromatography. The chromatography system included a 60-by-90-mm column of 230–400 mesh silica gel and gradient elution from 40 : 1 to 30 : 1 hexane : ethyl ether. Nine major fractions were recovered from the TRF, and $\alpha$-T, $\alpha$-T3, $\gamma$-T3, and $\delta$-T3 were >90% pure by the one pass. In order to purify larger quantities of the homologues, the TRF was silylated under conditions that preferentially silylated $\delta$-T3 followed by $\gamma$-T3. These homologues were isolated by flash chromatography as a colorless oil after ether extraction from water. The free phenolic forms were regenerated from the silylated forms by treatment of the silyl ethers with tetra-n-butylammonium fluoride.

Bruns et al. (252) were the first to apply Prep-LC to the purification of natural tocopherol from vegetable oil. The starting material for injection onto the preparative column was a 70% (w/w) tocopherol concentrate that was 60% *RRR*-$\gamma$-T. Chromatography used a chromatograph (Merck Prepbar 100) with a 40-by-10-cm column (LiChroprep Si60) with 3% t-butylmethyl ether in hexane as the mobile phase (flow rate = 450 mL/min). Fifty milliliters, representing 15 g of the tocopherol concentrate, was injected. A chromatogram showing fraction cuts to obtain $\gamma$-T at >95% purity is shown in Figure 7.13. Up to 4 g of *RRR*-$\gamma$-T could be obtained per injection. Other tocopherols were not purified to the extent

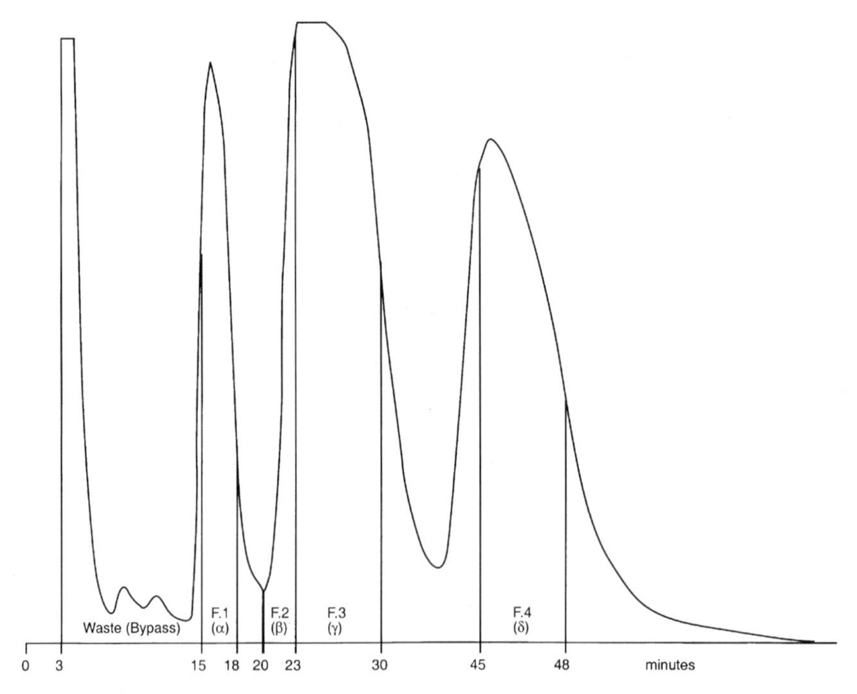


**FIGURE 7.13** Preparative chromatogram with time marks for the cuts of the various tocopherol fractions. (From Ref. 252.)

of γ-T, but the procedure could have easily produced purified α- and δ-T with repeated injections.

Shin and Godber(253) purified α-, β-, γ-, and δ-T from a mixture of soybean oil and wheat germ and α-, β-, γ-, and δ-T3 from a mixture of wheat bran and rubber latex with a semiprep LC procedure. Preconcentration of the toco-pherol and tocotrienols from wheat bran oil and wheat germ incorporated a saponification step to remove saponfiables. Before injection, the crude nonsaponifiable fraction was dissolved in methanol and allowed to stand overnight at −20°C to crystallize waxes and sterols. Saponification was also used to concentrate the tocotrienols from latex oil and tocopherols from soybean oil. The semiprep LC system included pumps, (Waters M-45 and 510), a gradient controller (Waters 680), a fluorescence detector (Waters 470), and a 25-by-10-cm (10-μm) silica column (Alltech Econosil). Gradient elution was 0–15% THF in hexane at a flow rate of 8–9 mL/min. The eight vitamin E homologues were isolated to >99% purity with recoveries ranging from 54–83%. Identification of the purified vitamin E homologues was confirmed by mass spectrometry.

Feng (254) coupled short path distillation, flash chromatography, and Prep-LC to purify α-T and α-T3 and γ-T and γ-T3 from palm oil distillate. Summaries of the various procedures follow:

---

Short path distillation

---

Equipment
  Unit: KDL-4 single-unit glass distillation unit (UIC, Joliet, IL).
Procedure
  1. Place 100–200 g of distillate into the sample feed vessel.
  2. Distill fatty acid fraction at 168°C, 1 torr.
  3. Distill vitamin E fraction at 220°C, 0.1 torr.
  4. Redistill vitamin E fraction.
Same priority as short path distillation
  1. Saponify 2 g of the vitamin E short path distillation fraction and extract the digest with 30 mL of 5% ethyl acetate in hexane.
  2. Apply the entire extract to the flash chromatography column.
  3. Chromatography
    a. Column: 46-by-2.0-cm glass equipped with a flow controller with needle valve and nitrogen tank.
    b. Column packing
      (1) 1/8-in Layer of sea sand
      (2) Glass wool packing
      (3) 6-in Layer of dry silica gel
      (4) 1/8-in Layer of sea sand
Elution (see Table 7.15)

---

**Table 7.15** Parameters for Gradient Elution of Tocopherols and Tocotrienols with Various Solvent Systems

| Fraction | Presence of specific homologues | Solvent volume per 50 mL[a] | | | Total mL |
|---|---|---|---|---|---|
| | | A | B | C | |
| 1 | — | 10 | 40 | 0 | 50 |
| 2 | — | 5 | 45 | 0 | 50 |
| 3 | α-T | 0 | 50 | 0 | 100 |
| 4 | α-T | 0 | 46 | 4 | 100 |
| 5 | α-T, α-T3 | 0 | 42 | 8 | 200 |
| 6 | α-T | 0 | 38 | 12 | 250 |
| 7 | — | 0 | 32 | 18 | 100 |
| 8 | — | 0 | 28 | 22 | 50 |
| 9 | γ-T3 | 0 | 25 | 25 | 150 |
| 10 | γ-T3 | 0 | 20 | 30 | 100 |
| 11 | γ-T3 | 0 | 15 | 35 | 100 |
| 12 | γ-T3 | 0 | 10 | 40 | 50 |
| 13 | δ-T3 | 0 | 5 | 45 | 50 |
| 14 | δ-T3 | 0 | 0 | 50 | 200 |

[a]A, 40 : 1; B, 30 : 1; C, 30 : 4 of hexane : diethyl ether (v/v). α-T, α-tocopherol; α-T3, α-tocotrienol.
*Source*: Modified from Ref. 254.

Solvent system I: Vitamin E homologues were eluted with hexane : diethyl ether in ratios of 40 : 1 (A), 30 : 1 (B), and 30 : 4 (C). Fifty- to 250-milliliter fractions were eluted to obtain good resolution. Five vitamin E fractions, containing α-T, α-T + α-T3, α-T3, γ-T3, and δ-T3, were obtained. Single homologs were approximately 90% pure.

Solvent system II: A 550-mL gradient was run in 50-mL fractions progressing from 40 : 1 to 30 : 1 hexane : diethyl ether. After the gradient, 300 mL of 30 : 5 hexane : diethyl ether and 200 mL of 30 : 6 hexane : diethyl ether were passed through the column in 50-mL increments. In the gradient stage, the final two 50-mL fractions contained α-T. The fractions eluted with 30 : 5 solvent contained α-T, α-T3, and γ-T3. The fraction eluted with 30 : 6 hexane : diethyl ether contained primarily δ-T3. All fractions were evaporated under vacuum and stored under nitrogen.

Preparative chromatography
- Apparatus
  - Waters Delta Prep 4000
  - Waters 486 UV/VIS detector
  - Waters 746 Data Module

At the outlet of the detector, a three-way valve flow adapter was connected to control the direction of the eluate flow from the detector. Two 25-by-100-mm (10-μm) μPorasil cartridge columns were used in series.

Mobile phase: isopropanol in hexane gradient (see Table 7.16)
A: 0.25% isopropanol in hexane
B: 0.1% isopropanol in hexane
C: 1% isopropanol in hexane

For resolution of α-T and α-T3 the injection had to be less than 50 mg total tocopherols and tocotrienols. A representative chromatogram is shown in Figure 7.14. Feng's procedure(254) provided purity greater than 99% for the four homologues. Structural identity was confirmed by direct mass spectroscopy.

## 7.6. ADDITIONAL ANALYTICAL APPROACHES TO VITAMIN E AND OTHER FAT-SOLUBLE VITAMINS

### 7.6.1. Resolution of Stereoisomers of *all-rac*-α-Tocopherol

Methods to resolve the eight stereoisomers of *all-rac*-α-T have been developed to facilitate the study of absorption, transport, and distribution of the stereoisomers in mammals. Vecchi and associates(255) separated the stereosiomers into four stereoisomer pairs (RSR + RSS, *RRR* + RRS, SSS + SSR, and SRS + *SRR*) by chiral LC. The chiral pairs were derivatized to α-T-methyl ethers and resolved by capillary GC. The method was later simplified through use of a commercially available chiral LC column and omission of an acetylation step early in the assay

**TABLE 7.16** Mobile-Phase Gradient Program in Prep-LC for Isolation of Tocotrienols

| Time (min) | Flow rate (mL/min) | %A[a] | %B[a] | %C[b] | %D[c] |
|---|---|---|---|---|---|
| Initial | 25 | 0 | 0 | 100 | 0 |
| 20 | 25 | 50 | 50 | 0 | 0 |
| 22 | 40 | 50 | 50 | 0 | 0 |
| 30 | 40 | 50 | 50 | 0 | 0 |
| 35 | 40 | 40 | 40 | 0 | 20 |
| 50 | 40 | 40 | 40 | 0 | 20 |
| 51 | 2 | 40 | 40 | 0 | 20 |

[a]0.25% Isopropanol in hexane.
[b]0.1% Isopropanol in hexane.
[c]1%Isopropanol in hexane.
*Source*: Modified from Ref. 254.

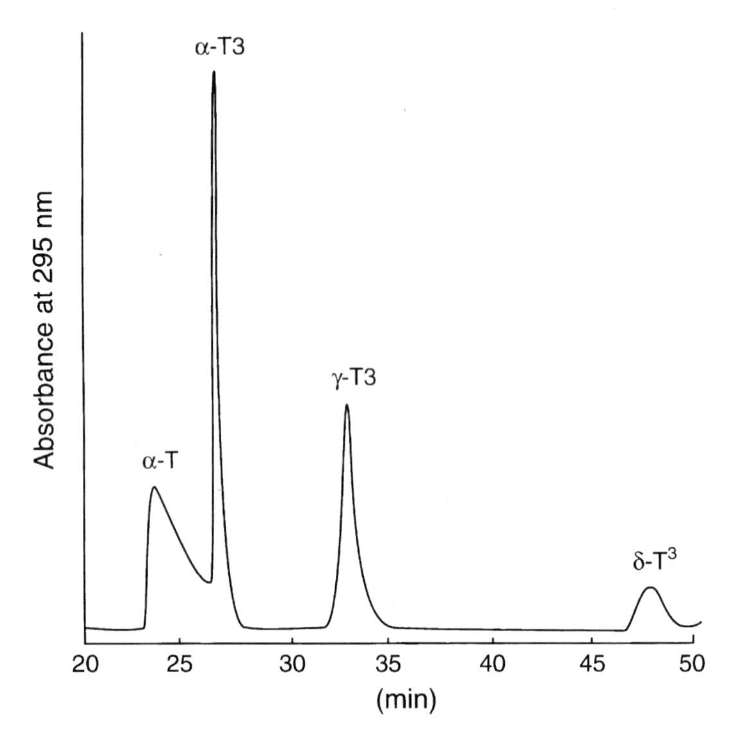


**FIGURE 7.14** Preparative chromatogram of tocopherols and tocotrienols. *α*-T, *α*-tocopherol; *α*-T3, *α*-tocotrienol. (From Ref. 254.)

procedure (256). The refined method utilizes semipreparative LC to purify and concentrate extracts before conversion of the *α*-T stereoisomers to the methyl ethers. The *α*-T methyl ether stereoisomers were resolved by chiral LC on a chiral column (Spherisorb S3-W) into five peaks with the *2S* isomers eluting as a single peak. The *2R* isomers were resolved into four homogeneous peaks. Capillary GC then resolved the *2S* isomers. Procedural steps for the method include the following:

1. Extract *α*-T from tissue or plasma with SDS and methanol containing 0.01% BHT. Centrifuge the extract.
2. Wash the supernatant with n-heptane and centrifuge.
3. Dry the n-heptane fractions with sodium sulfate and evaporate under nitrogen.
4. Dissolve the residue in methanol : THF (1 : 1 v/v).
5. Purify and concentrate the extract by semipreparative HPLC on a Radial-Pak $C_{18}$, 10-μm, 0.8-by-10-cm column with methanol as the mobile phase.

6. Collect the $\alpha$-T peaks and evaporate under nitrogen.
7. Derivatize the purified $\alpha$-T to $\alpha$-T methyl ether.
8. Resolve the derivatized stereoisomers by chiral phase HPLC on a column (Sperisorb S3-W), 0.4 $\times$ 25 cm, with a mobile phase of hexane containing 0.5% methyl tert-butyl ether. This separation resolves *2R* isomers with a single peak containing the *2S* isomers.
9. Resolve the *2S* isomers by GC on a 100-m silanized glass column $\times$ 0.3 mm i.d.

Ueda et al. and Kiyose et al.(257,258) developed a chiral LC method that resolves the eight stereoisomers into four peaks (*2R* isomers, SSS + SSR, *SRR*, and SRS). The overall procedure included acetylation and LC on Chiralpak (OP) (+) with methanol : water (96 : 4, v/v) as the mobile phase. Procedural steps include the following:

1. Saponify tissue, plasma, or red blood cells in ethanolic KOH at 70°C for 30 min.
2. Extract the saponification mixture with 10% ethyl acetate in hexane.
3. Collect and evaporate the hexane layer under nitrogen.
4. Acetylate the residue with dry pyridine and acetic anhydride.
5. Extract the acetylated residue with hexane; evaporate the hexane under nitrogen.
6. Dissolve the residue in methanol : water (96 : 4, v/v).
7. Chromatograph the *all-rac-$\alpha$*-tocopheryl acetate esters on a Chiralpak (OP) (+), 4.6 $\times$ 250 mm, with methanol : water (96 : 4) as the mobile phase. This resolves the esters into a single peak containing the *2R* isomers and three peaks containing the *2S* isomers (SSS + SSR, SSR, and SRS).

## 7.6.2. Electrophoretic Methods

Capillary electrophoresis (CE) applied as capillary zone electrophoresis (CZE) or micellar electrokinetic capillary chromatography (MEKC) is an established method to quantify vitamins in pharmaceutical products (259). Unfortunately, the methods are of limited value for food analysis. Trenerry(259) stated that CE is faster, more efficient, and cost-effective compared to more traditional methods but lacks the sensitivity of LC. Other problems associated with food analysis by CE include incompatibility of sample extracts with buffers used in CE and column fouling by macromolecular components in the food extract (259). Normally MEKC is used to separate neutral molecules on the basis of partitioning between an aqueous electrolyte and a pseudostationary phase of charged micelles (260). Although MEKC is more amenable to fat-soluble vitamin analysis than CZE, hydrophobic characteristic of the fat-soluble vitamins cause strong interactions with the micelles, resulting in increased resolution times (259).

Pedersen-Bjergaard et al. (260) noted that most hydrophobic vitamins including retinyl palmitate can precipitate during electrophoresis because of poor solubility in aqueous MEKC buffers. Applications of MEKC to the electrophoretic resolution of fat-soluble vitamins include studies on retinyl palmitate and various vitamin A metabolites (261–265), vitamin E ($\alpha$-T) (261,263,266–268), and vitamins $D_2$ and $D_3$ (268). Such work has mainly been limited to high-concentration pharmaceuticals or standards.

In order to overcome deficiencies of MEKC with hydrophobic analytes, microemulsion electrokinetic chromatography (MEEKC) was developed.(260, 269) This CE technique partitions solutes with moving oil droplets in a microemulsion buffer and by electrophoretic mobility. Solubilization of the fat-soluble vitamins is significantly improved with the microemulsion in the buffer (260). Pedersen-Bjergaard et al. (260) applied MEEKC to resolution of retinyl palmitate, *all-rac-$\alpha$-*tocopheryl acetate, and vitamin $D_3$ and quantification of vitamin E from vitamin tablets.

Electrokinetic chromatography (EKC) with tetradecylammonium ions ($TDA^+$) as the pseudostationary phase is useful for resolution of retinyl palmitate, *all-rac-$\alpha$*-tocopheryl acetate, and vitamin $D_3$ (270–271), and of vitamin $K_1$ from methylparaben and propylparaben in pharmaceuticals (272). Acetonitrile in the separation medium keeps the fat-soluble vitamins soluble, and the $TDA^+$ ions serve as the pseudostationary phase. The method was quantitative for *all-rac-$\alpha$*-tocopheryl acetate in vitamin tablets (271).

Capillary electrochromatography (CEC) combines chromatographic separation provided by LC supports and the high efficiency of CZE. The technique has been successfully used to quantify tocopherols and tocotrienols in vegetable oil(273) and tocopherols in human serum (274). Abidi and Rennick(273) compared CEC on $C_8$, $C_{18}$, and phenyl reversed-phase supports with various mobile phases. Optimal résolution was on $C_8$ with acetonitrile : - methanol (64 : 36), 25 mM Tris (hydroxymethyl) amino methane, pH 8.0 (95 : 5) as the mobile phase. Separation voltage and column temperature were maintained at 25 kV and 30°C. Baseline separation of tocopherols and tocotrienols was in the order normally observed on reversed-phase LC. The authors noted that optimization of the CEC conditions provided a fast and sensitive analytical method for analysis of vitamin E in edible oils as an alternative to LC.

### 7.6.3. Gas Chromatography/Mass Spectrometry

Availability of stable isotopes of *RRR*- and *all-rac-$\alpha$*-tocopherol and their esters, $\beta$-carotene, retinol, and vitamin $K_1$ (phylloquinone) has greatly expanded knowledge of the absorption, deposition, and metabolism of these fat-soluble vitamins in humans. Specific gas chromatography/mass spectrometry (GC/MS) techniques were developed to study $\beta$-carotene conversion to retinol (275–278), absorption and deposition of *RRR*- and *all-rac-$\alpha$*-T (279–281), quantification of $\alpha$-T and major oxidation products (282,283), and uptake and metabolism of vitamin $K_1$ (284,285). Each of these methods involves careful concentration, and in most cases, purification of the analytes before derivatization to their trimethylsilyl derivatives and GC/MS analysis of vitamin $K_1$ have been accomplished without derivatization (285). Melchert and Pabel (286) showed in 2000 that GC/MS could be used as an alternative method to LC for quantification of $\alpha$-, $\beta$-, $\gamma$-, and $\delta$-T in serum. This procedure was based on a simple extraction of serum using SPE (Extrelut) and chromatography on silica gel before trimethylsilyl derivative formation.

### 7.6.4. Liquid Chromatography/Mass Spectrometry

Interfacing of liquid chromatography (LC) and mass spectrometry (MS) produced a powerful analytical tool for quantification and structural confirmation of the fat-soluble vitamins. Usually GC/MS cannot be used for analysis of carotenoids because of their instability at temperatures necessary for GC/MS. van Breemen(287) traced the evolution of LC/MS to carotenoid analysis, showing technological advances in methodology with improvement in analysis results. In general chronological order, particle beam (288–289) fast atom bombardment (290–292), electrospray ionization (293–294), and atmospheric pressure chemical ioniz-ation (295–298) have been successfully applied. Development of electrospray and atmospheric chemical ionization techniques substantially improved the ability of LC/MS to quantify analyte levels present in LC eluents of extracts of biological samples. Solvent removal and ionization take place at atmospheric pressure, and solvent splitting is not required (287). Coupling LC/MS with the resolution power of the $C_{30}$ reversed-phase column for carotenoids greatly increased ability to resolve and unambiguously identify components of complex carotenoid mixtures encountered in nature.

Application of LC/MS to analysis of vitamin E has been achieved with particle beam (289), electrospray (294), coordination ion spray (299), and, more recently, liquid chromatography–tandem mass spectrometry (LC-MS/MS) (300–302). Rentel et al. (294) increased sensitivity of MS for tocopherols and carotenoids by addition of silver ions to the LC eluant to form $Ag^+$-tocopherol and $Ag^+$-carotenoid adducts that facilitated ionization. The technique was called *coordination ion spray* (294,299). Rentel et al. (294) resolved the fat-soluble vitamins on a $C_{30}$ stationary phase (Sec. 7.6.6) to facilitate identification further. Deuterated and unlabeled $\alpha$-T and deuterated tocopherolquinone were quantified by LC-MS/MS (300–302). The technique uses selective multiple reaction monitoring, which is a tandem mass spectrometric method designed to measure parent/product ions. Lauridsen et al. (300) successfully applied LC-MS/MS to follow uptake and retention of deuterated *RRR*-$\alpha$-T and deuterated *all-rac*-$\alpha$-T in human serum after oral doses of the deuterated tocopheryl acetates. The LC-MS/MS procedures are more sensitive and faster than GC/MS methods available for vitamin E. Derivatization, necessary for GC/MS analysis, is not required.

### 7.6.5. Supercritical Fluid Chromatography

Instrumentation for application of supercritical fluid chromatography (SFC) to resolution of analytes in complex extracts of biological samples became available in the early 1980s. As a separation science SFC was reviewed in depth by Anton and Berger (303). Specific applications to nonsaponifiable lipids from biological samples were reviewed by Lesellier (304). Some of the earliest and successful applications of SFC dealt with resolution of tocopherols and carotenoids. Snyder, Taylor, and King's research group at the National Center for Agricultural Utilization, USDA, showed that SFC or SFC/MS systems provided excellent quantification procedures for tocopherols in complex lipid mixtures (305). Other work combined supercritical fluid extraction (SFE) with preparative SFC to produce tocopherol concentrates from soybean flakes (306). Triacylglycerols and tocopherols were characterized in milk fat, fish oil, sea buckthorn, and cloudberry seed oil by SFC (307). Supercritical fluid extraction was used to extract tocopherols from olive by-products (308), olive leaves (309), and malt sprouts (310). Resolution of eight fat-soluble vitamins including $\alpha$-T and *all-rac-$\alpha$-*tocopheryl acetate was achieved on pure silica coated with Carbowax, 20M (311).

Shen et al. (312) resolved a mixture of $\alpha$-T, all-*trans*-retinol, vitamins $K_1$ and $K_2$, and vitamins $D_2$ and $D_3$ on liquid crystal polysiloxane-coated particles with supercritical $CO_2$. Ibáñez and coworkers (313) coupled SFE and SFC and resolved the specified fat-soluble vitamins and *all-rac-$\alpha$-*tocopheryl acetate and *all-trans*-retinyl acetate on two micropacked columns in series packed with SE-54 and carbowax 20M, respectively. This system was used to resolve tocopherol standards from a mixture of n-alkanes (314). Tocopherols and *all-trans*-retinyl palmitate were quantified from vitamin A-fortified vegetable oils using SFC with a column packed with $C_{18}$ (315).

Supercritical fluid chromatography is highly effective for the study of complex mixtures of carotenoids. Early studies successfully resolved *cis-* and *trans-*isomers of $\alpha$- and $\beta$-carotene (316–320). Lesellier et al. (321) reviewed SFC separation science of the carotenoids through 1991. More recent research defined the retention behavior of $\beta$-carotene on polar and nonpolar stationary phases (322) and the resolution of $\beta$-carotene and lycopene (323). Lesellier et al. (324) improved the resolution of *cis-* and *trans-* isomers of $\beta$-carotene by coupling columns packed with various $C_{18}$ stationary phases. Optimal resolution was obtained with a four-column system consisting of three columns (UBS225) connected to a column (Hypersil ODS). The SFC parameters were $CO_2$:-acetonitrile : methanol (94 : 5.6 : 0.4, v/v/v), 45°C, flow rate of 3.0 mL/min, outlet pressure of 10 MPa with detection at 450 nm. The SFC resolved 10 peaks from a highly isomerized β-carotene solution. *all-trans-*, 9-*cis-*, 13-*cis-*, 15-*cis-*, β-Carotene, and 9-9′-di-cis β-carotene were identifiable. Five additional isomers were resolved but not identified.

### 7.6.6. Liquid Chromatography on Polymeric $C_{30}$

In 1994, a new dimension was added to the resolution of fat-soluble vitamins by reversed-phase chromatography. Sanders et al. (325) developed a polymeric stationary phase to provide high absolute retention, enhanced shape recognition, and moderate silanol activity to aid in resolution of complex mixtures of carotenoid isomers. The polymeric support was quickly accepted by the scientific community, and through 1999 more than 50 publications reported the application of the $C_{30}$ support to various separations involving biological samples (326). An early application resolved 39 carotenoids from orange juice (327). Since initial success with carotenoid analysis, LC on the $C_{30}$ has been highly successful with other fat-soluble vitamins including vitamin E and vitamin K. Specific applications to resolution of tocopherols and tocotrienols include research by Danko et al. (328) demonstrating the simultaneous resolution of 13 carotenoids and five tocopherols and tocotrienols from red palm oil. Earlier, the separation of γ- and β-T was demonstrated on the $C_{30}$ support, a demonstration that usually is not possible on commonly used $C_{18}$ stationary phases (329). Use of the $C_{30}$ stationary phase increases the power of LC/MS for identification and quantification of tocopherols and carotenoids (294).

Routine use of the $C_{30}$ support is increasing. A major advantage is the ability to resolve β- and γ-T under reversed-phase conditions. As shown in Figure 7.15, excellent resolution of the positional isomers is obtainable (330). Undoubtedly, development of the $C_{30}$ stationary phase was a major advance in LC analysis of the fat-soluble vitamins.

## 7.7. REGULATORY AND COMPENDIUM METHODS

As shown in Table 7.2, methods for the analysis of tocopherols and tocotrienols matured rapidly from their beginnings in the 1930s as colorimetric and early chromatographic procedures were largely replaced in the 1960s by GC. In the next 15 years, many collaborated GC-based procedures were put into regulatory handbooks, such as the AOAC International Official Methods of Analysis (331), for routine use in situations requiring validated methodology. These methods, along with colorimetric and other assay methods, are still considered valid methods and maintain their proper place in accepted regulatory handbooks and method compendiums. Such methods that are available internationally are summarized in Table 7.17.

AOAC International methods include AOAC Official Method 971.30 (45.1.24) "alpha Tocopherol and alpha Tocopheryl Acetate in Foods and Feeds" and AOAC Official Method 948.26 (45.1.26) "alpha-Tocopherol Acetate

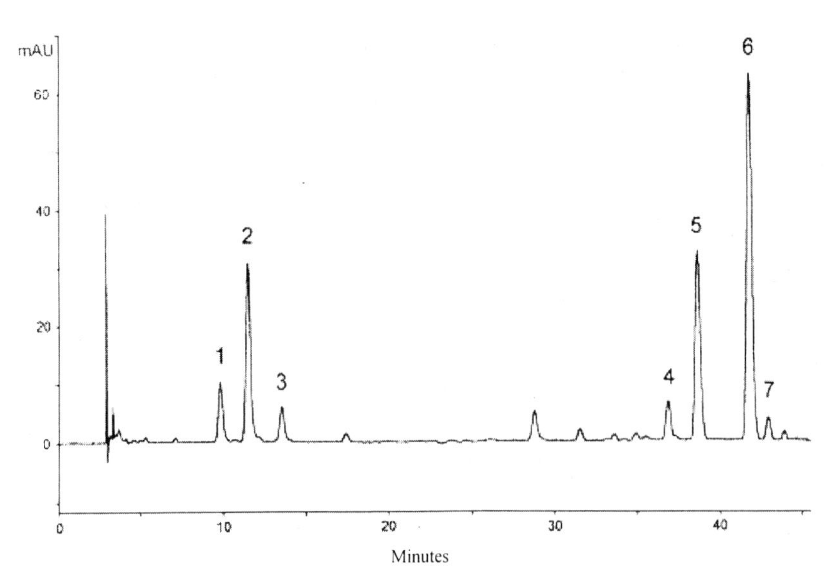


**FIGURE 7.15** Separation of tocopherols and carotenoids from a nutrition drink. 1 = $\delta$-T, 2 = $\gamma$-T, 3 = $\beta$-T, 4 = 13-*cis*-$\beta$-carotene, 5 = all-*trans*-$\alpha$-carotene, 6 = all-*trans*-$\beta$-carotene, 7 = 9-*cis*-$\beta$-carotene. $\delta$-T, $\delta$-tocopherol. (From Ref. 330.)

(supplemental) in Foods and Feeds." In both methods, the products are saponified and $\alpha$-T is quantified after thin-layer chromatography (971.30) or after open-column chromatography (948.26) colorimetrically with bathophenanthroline solution. When the isomeric form of $\alpha$-tocopheryl acetate is unknown, AOAC Method 975.43 (45.1.25) "Identification of *RRR*- or *all-rac*-alpha-Tocopherol in Drugs" can be used to determine the isomeric form of the added $\alpha$-tocopheryl acetate by polarimetry. The optical rotation of the ferricyanide oxidation product of $\alpha$-T is measured after saponification of the product. Optical rotation is negligible for *all-rac*-$\alpha$-T and positive for *RRR*-$\alpha$-T. This procedure, after identification of the isomeric form of the supplemental $\alpha$-tocopheryl acetate, allows correct calculation of the biological activity in IUs or $\alpha$-TE units. Method 975.43 can be used only on concentrated extracts containing $\geq$200 mg $\alpha$-T/g before the ferricyanide oxidation step. The procedures described are cumbersome and subject to analytical error because of their complexity (136).

AOAC International offers straightforward GC procedures for mixed tocopherols in concentrates, $\alpha$-tocopheryl acetate in supplements and concentrates, and tocopherols in drugs. These methods are AOAC Official Method 988.14 (45.1.27) "Tocopherol Isomers in Mixed Tocopherols Concentrate," AOAC Official Method 989.09 (45.1.28) "$\alpha$-Tocopheryl Acetate in Supplemental Vitamin E Concentrates," and AOAC Official Method 969.40 (45.1.29) "Vitamin E in Drugs." Desai and Machlin(130) give a thorough

**Table 7.17** Compendium of Regulatory, and Handbook Methods for Vitamin E Analysis

| Source | Form | Methods and applications | Approach |
|---|---|---|---|
| *AOAC Official Methods of Analysis*, 2000 (Ref. [331]) | | | |
| 1. 45.1.24 | *all-rac-* or *RRR*-α-tocopherol<br>*all-rac-* or *RRR*-α-tocopheryl acetate | AOAC Official Method 971.30<br>α-Tocopherol and α-Tocopherol Acetate in Foods and Feeds Colorimetric Method | Colorimetric 534 nm |
| 2. 45.1.25 | *all-rac-* or *RRR*-α-tocopherol<br>*all-rac-* or *RRR*-α-tocopheryl acetate | AOAC Official Method 975.43<br>Identification of *RRR-* or *all-rac-* α-Tocopherol in Drugs and Food or Feed Supplements (≥200 mg/g) | Polarimetric |
| 3. 45.1.26 | *all-rac-* or *RRR*-α-tocopherol<br>*all-rac-* or *RRR*-α-tocopheryl acetate | AOAC Official Method 948.26<br>α-Tocopherol Acetate (Supplemental) in Foods and Feeds | Colorimetric 534 nm |
| 4. 45.1.27 | *RRR*-tocopherol<br>*RRR*-β-tocopherol + *RRR* γ-tocopherol<br>*RRR*-δ-tocopherol | AOAC Official Method 988.14<br>Tocopherol Isomers in Mixed Tocopherols Concentrate | GC flame ionization |

(*continued*)

**Table 7.17** *Continued*

| Source | Form | Methods and applications | Approach |
|---|---|---|---|
| 5. 45.1.28 | *all-rac*-α-tocopheryl acetate | AOAC Official Method 989.09 α-Tocopheryl Acetate in Supplemental Vitamin E Concentrates | GC flame ionization |
| 6. 45.1.29 | *all-rac*- or *RRR*-α-tocopherol<br>*all-rac*- or *RRR*-α-tocopheryl acetate<br>*all-rac*- or *RRR*-α-tocopheryl succinate | AOAC Official Method 969.40 Vitamin E in Drugs | GC flame ionization |
| 7. 50.1.04 | *all-rac*-α-tocopheryl acetate as α-tocopherol | AOAC Official Method 992.03 Vitamin E Activity (*all-rac*-α-tocopherol) in Milk-Based Infant Formula | HPLC 280 nm |
| *Official Methods and Recommended Practices of AOCS* (Ref. [141]) | | | |
| 1. Ce 7-87 | *RRR*-tocopherols | Total Tocopherols in Deodorizer Distillate | Capillary GC |
| 2. Ce 8-89 | *RRR*-tocopherols<br>*RRR*-tocotrienols | Tocopherols and Tocotrienols in Vegetable Oils and Fats by HPLC | Normal-phase LC |
| *U.S. Pharmacopeia National Formulary*, 2002, USP 25/NF 20; Nutritional Supplements Official Monograph (Ref. [334]) | | | |
| 1. Pages 1804–1806 | *all-rac*- or *RRR*-α-tocopherol<br>*all-rac*- or *RRR*-α-tocopheryl acetate<br>*all-rac*- or *RRR*-α-tocopheryl succinate | Vitamin E<br>Vitamin E in preparation and capsules | GC flame ionization |
| 2. Pages 2427, 2429 | *all-rac*- or *RRR*-α-tocopherol<br>*all-rac*- or *RRR*-α-tocopheryl acetate<br>*all-rac*- or *RRR*-α-tocopheryl succinate | Vitamin E in oil-soluble vitamin capsules/tablets | HPLC 254 nm |

| | | | |
|---|---|---|---|
| 3. Pages 2430, 2435, 2437, 2450–2451 | *all-rac-* or *RRR*-α-tocopherol<br>*all-rac-* or *RRR*-α-tocopheryl acetate<br>*all-rac-* or *RRR*-α-tocopheryl succinate | Vitamin E in oil- and water-soluble capsules/tablets with/without minerals | HPLC |
| 4. Pages 2633–2634 | *RRR*-α-tocopherol<br>*RRR*-β-tocopherol<br>*RRR*-γ-tocopherol<br>*RRR*-δ-tocopherol | Tocopherols<br>Excipient | GC flame ionization |
| *British Pharmacopoeia*, 1993 (Ref. [335]) | | | |
| 1. Pages 1519–1521, vol. I | α-Tocopherol | α-Tocopherol | GC flame ionization |
| 2. Pages 1521–1522, vol. I | *RRR*-α-tocopherol | α-Tocopherol | GC flame ionization |
| 3. Pages 1522–1524, vol. I | α-Tocopheryl acetate | α-Tocopherol acetate | GC flame ionization |
| 4. Pages 1524–1525, vol. I | α-Tocopheryl acetate | α-Tocopherol acetate concentrate (powder form) | GC flame ionization |
| 5. Pages 1525–1527, vol. I | *RRR*-α-tocopheryl acetate | α-Tocopheryl acetate | GC flame ionization |
| 6. Pages 1527–1529, vol. I | α-Tocopheryl hydrogen succinate | α-Tocopheryl succinate | GC flame ionization |
| 7. Pages 1529–1531, vol. I | *RRR*-α-tocopheryl succinate | α-Tocopheryl succinate tablets | GC flame ionization |
| American Feed Ingredients Association, *Laboratory Methods Compendium*, 1991, vol. I (Ref. [336]) | | | |
| 1. Pages 197–200 | *all-rac*-α-tocopheryl acetate | Vitamin $D_3$, vitamin E in concentrates and premixes (≥50 IU/g) | HPLC 292 nm |

*(continued)*

**Table 7.17** *Continued*

| Source | Form | Methods and applications | Approach |
|---|---|---|---|
| 2. Pages 201–202 | *all-rac*-α-tocopheryl acetate as α-tocopherol | Vitamin E (coated) in powders containing no other vitamins | Colorimetric 520 nm |
| 3. Pages 203–205 | *all-rac*-α-tocopheryl acetate as tocopherol | Determination of vitamin E in feeds, supplements, and premixes (>1 mg/kg) | HPLC 284 nm or fluorescence $\lambda_{ex}$ 290 $\lambda_{em}$ 325 |
| 4. Pages 207–209 | α-, β, γ-, δ-Tocopherol (*all-rac*- or *RRR*-tocopherols or esters) | Method for the determination of vitamin E in feed and tissue by HPLC | HPLC fluorescence $\lambda_{ex}$ 254 $\lambda_{em}$ 325 |
| 5. Pages 221–213 | *all-rac*- or *RRR*-α-tocopherol | Determination of vitamin E in premixes by HPLC (1–20 mg/g) | HPLC 292 nm |
| Hoffman-LaRoche, *Analytical Methods for Vitamins and Carotenoids, in Feeds*, 1988 (Ref. [337]) | | | |
| 1. Pages 12–14 | *RRR*-α-tocopherol and added esters as α-tocopherol; applicable to other homologues | Determination of α-tocopherol in complete feeds, premixes, and vitamin concentrates with the aid of HPLC (>1 mg/kg) | HPLC fluorescence $\lambda_{ex}$ 293 $\lambda_{em}$ 326 |
| 2. Page 418 | *all-rac*-α-tocopheryl acetate | Determination of α-tocopheryl acetate in feed premixes with HPLC (>1000 mg/kg) | HPLC 280 nm |
| *Food Chemicals Codex*, 1996 (Ref. [338]) | | | |
| 1. Pages 417–418 | *all-rac*-α-Tocopherol | *all-rac*-α-tocopherol (NLT 96.0%, NMT 102.0%) | GC flame ionization |

| | | | |
|---|---|---|---|
| 2. Page 418 | *RRR*-α-Tocopherol | *all-rac*-α-Tocopherol concentrate (concentrates from edible oil deodorizer distillate) | GC flame ionization |
| 3. Pages 419–420 | *RRR*-α-tocopherol<br>*RRR*-β-tocopherol<br>*RRR*-γ-tocopherol<br>*RRR*-δ-tocopherol | Tocopherols concentrate, mixed (concentrate from edible oil deodorizer distillate) | GC flame ionization |
| 4. Pages 420–421 | α-Tocopheryl acetate (NLT 96.0%, NMT 102.0%) | *RRR*-α-tocopheryl acetate (acetylization of α-tocopherol from edible oil) | GC flame ionization |
| 5. Pages 421–422 | *RRR*-α-tocopheryl acetate (NLT 96.0%, NMT 102.0%) | *all-rac*-α-Tocopheryl acetate | GC flame ionization |
| 6. Page 422 | *RRR*-α-tocopheryl acetate | *RRR*-α-Tocopheryl acetate concentrate | GC flame ionization |
| 7. Pages 422–424 | *RRR*-α-tocopheryl succinate | *all-rac*-α-Tocopheryl acid succinate | GC flame ionization |
| *Methods for the Determination of Vitamins in Foods*, COST 91 (Ref. [339]) | | | |
| 1. Page 91 | *RRR*-α-tocopherol or *all-rac*-α-tocopheryl acetate | Foods | HPLC fluorescence<br>$\lambda_{ex}$ 293<br>$\lambda_{em}$ 326 |
| 2. Page 107 | *RRR*-tocopherols<br>*RRR*-tocotrienols | Fats and oils | HPLC fluorescence<br>$\lambda_{ex}$ 293<br>$\lambda_{em}$ 326 |

GC, gas chromatography; HPLC, high-performance liquid chromatography; LC, liquid chromatography; NLT, no less than; NMT, no more than.

procedural guide to Method 969.40. They stress that the method is limited to pharmaceutical products without interfering material. The method resolves *RRR*- and *all-rac-α*-tocopherols and the acetate and succinate esters. Either internal or external standard methodology can be used.

AOAC International (331) provides one HPLC-based procedure for the assay of vitamin E activity in milk-based infant formula, AOAC Official Method 992.03 (50.1.04) "Vitamin E Activity (*all-rac-α*-tocopherol) in Milk-Based Infant Formula." The method, collaborated in 1993 (179), utilizes saponification and chromatography on silica with hexane : isopropanol (99.92 : 0.08) with UV detection at 280 nm. Collaboration of AOAC Method 992.03 was recommended for use with other matrices by the AOAC Task Force on Methods for Nutrition Labeling (332). However, such studies have not been completed. We note that the use of fluorescence detection and better instructions to prevent vitamin E decomposition during saponification would improve the method and help novice analysts not well versed in controlling saponification parameters.

The International Union of Pure and Applied Chemistry (IUPAC) and the American Oil Chemists' Society (AOCS) provide detailed HPLC procedures for vitamin E assay of oils and fats (141,333). The AOCS handbook also provides a capillary GC procedure for total tocopherol analysis of deodorizer distillate (Method Ce 7-87)(140,141). Parameters of the IUPAC and AOCS methods for vitamin E in fats and oils are the same; the AOCS method originated in the IUPAC standard method. Details of the procedure include the following:

---

Apparatus
  HPLC equipped with a fluorescence detector
    UV spectrometer
    Rotary evaporator
Reagents
  α-, β-, α, and α-T standards
  Methanol
  Dichloromethane
  Hexane
  Isopropanol
Chromatography
  Column: 25 cm × 4.6 mm
  Stationary phase: microparticulate silica, 5 μm
  Mobile phase: isopropanol in hexane (0.5 : 99.5)
  Column temperature: ambient
  Flow: 1 mL/min (0.7–1.5 mL/min)
  Injection: 20 μL
  Detection: Fluorescence, $Ex\lambda = 290$
    $Em\lambda = 330$ or UV at 292 nm (not preferred)
  Calculation: external standard, peak area

---

These method guides are easy to follow and include discussions of procedural steps in enough detail to lead one not well versed in vitamin E assay by HPLC to a successful analysis of fats and oils without trouble. Therefore, anyone beginning vitamin E assay of foods or any other sample matrix should obtain the procedures from AOCS or the cited IUPAC reference.

## REFERENCES


1. Bunnell, R.H. Modern procedures for the analysis of tocopherols. Lipids **1971**, *6*, 245–253.
2. Parrish, D.B. Determination of vitamin E in foods—a review. CRC Crit. Rev. Food Sci. Nutr. **1980**, 161–187.
3. Lehman, R.W. Determination of vitamin E. In *Methods of Biochemical Analysis*, Vol. 2; Glick, D., Ed.; Interscience: New York, 1955.
4. Kofler, M.; Sommer, P.F.; Bollinger, H.R.; Schmidli, B.; Vecchi, M. Physiochemical properties and assay of the tocopherols. In *Vitamins and Hormones*, Vol. 20; Harris, R.S., Wool, I.G., Eds.; Academic Press: New York, 1962.
5. Bunnell, R.H. Vitamin E assay by chemical methods. In *The Vitamins*, Vol. 6; György, P., Pearson, W.N.; Eds.; Academic Press: New York, 1967.
6. Bliss, C.I.; György, P. Bioassays of vitamin E. In *The Vitamins*, Vol. 6; György, P., Pearson, W.N., Eds.; Academic Press: New York, 1967.
7. Brubacher, G. The determination of vitamins and carotenoids in fats. In *Analysis and Characterization of Oils, Fats and Fat Products*, Vol. 2; Boekenoogen, H.A., Ed.; Interscience: New York, 1968.
8. Vogel, P.; Wieske, T. Paper and thin-layer chromatography in fat chemistry. XIV. Tocopherols. In *Analysis and Characterization of Oils, Fats and Fat Products*, Vol. 2; Interscience: New York, 1968.
9. Bieri, J.G. Chromatography of Tocopherols. In *Lipid Chromatographic Analysis*; Marinetti, G.V., Ed.; Marcel Dekker: New York, 1969.
10. Sheppard, A.J.; Prosser, A.R.; Hubbard, W.D. Gas chromatography of vitamin E. In *Methods in Enzymology, Vitamins and Coenzymes*, Part C; McCormick, D.B., Wright, L.D., Eds.; Academic Press: New York, 1971.
11. Ames, S.R. Tocopherols. IV. Estimation in foods and food supplements. In *The Vitamins*, Vol 5; Sebrell, W.H., Jr., Harris, R.S., Eds.; Academic Press: New York, 1972.
12. Sheppard, A.J.; Prosser, A.R.; Hubbard, W.D. Gas chromatography of the fat-soluble vitamins: A review. JAOCS **1972**, *11*, 619–633.
13. Green, J. Distribution of fat-soluble vitamins and their standardization and assay by biological methods. In *Fat-Soluble Vitamins*; Morton, R.A., Ed.; Pergamon Press: Oxford, 1970.

14. Draper, H.H. Chemical assays of vitamin E. In *Fat-Soluble Vitamins*; Morton, R.A., Ed.; 1970.
15. Laidman, D.L.; Hall, G.S. Adsorption column chromatography of tocopherols. In *Methods in Enzymology, Vitamins and Coenzymes*, Part C; McCormick, D.B., Wright, L.D., Eds.; Academic Press: New York, 1971.
16. Desai, I.D. Assay methods. In *Vitamin E: A Comprehensive Treatise*; Macklin, L.J., Ed.; Marcel Dekker: New York, 1980.
17. Joffe, M.; Harris, P.L. The biological potency of natural tocopherols and certain derivatives. J. Am. Chem. Soc. **1943**, *65*, 925–927.
18. Mason, K.E.; Harris, P.L. Bioassay of vitamin E. Biol. Symp. **1947**, *12*, 459–483.
19. Harris, P.L.; Ludwig, M.I. Relative vitamin E potency of natural and synthetic $\alpha$-tocopherol. J. Biol. Chem. **1949**, *179*, 1111–1115.
20. Bunyan, J.; McHale, D.; Green, J.; Marcinkiewicz, S. Biological potencies of $\xi$- and $\delta$-tocoperhol and 5-methyl tocopherol. Br. J. Nutr. **1961**, *15*, 253–257.
21. Ames, S.R.; Ludwig, M.I.; Nelan, D.R.; Robeson, C.D. Biological activitiy of an 1-epimer of d-$\alpha$-tocopheroyl acetate. Biochemistry **1963**, *2*, 188–190.
22. Dam, H.; Sondergaard, E. Comparisons of the activities of the acetates of d-, d, 1- and 1-$\alpha$-tocopherols against encephalomalacia in chicks. Z. Ernahrungwiss **1964**, *5*, 73–79.
23. Hakkarainen, R.V.G.; Työppoönen, J.T.; Hassan, S.; Bengtsson, S.G.; Jönsson, S.R.L.; Lindberg, P.O. Biopotency of vitamin E in barley. Br. J. Nutr. **1984**, *52*, 335–349.
24. Hove, E.L.; Harris, P.L. Relative activity of the tocopherols in curing muscular dystrophy in rabbits. J. Nutr. **1947**, *33*, 95–106.
25. Fitch, C.D.; Diehl, J.F. Metabolism of 1-alpha-tocopherol by the vitamin E-deficient rabbit. Proc. Soc. Exp. Biol. Med. **1965**, *119*, 553–557.
26. Rose, C.S.; György, P. Specificity of hemolytic reaction in vitamin E-deficient erythrocytes. Am. J. Physiol. **1952**, *168*, 414–420.
27. Horwitt, M.K.; Harvey, C.C.; Duncan, G.D.; Wilson, W.C. Effects of limited tocopherol intake in man with relationships to erythrocyte hemolysis and lipid oxidations. Am. J. Clin. Nutr. **1956**, *4*, 408–419.
28. Friedman, L.; Weiss, L.; Wherry, W.; Kline, O.L. Bioassay of vitamin E by the dialuric acid hemolysis method. J. Nutr. **1958**, *65*, 143–160.
29. Mason, K.E. Distribution of vitamin E in tissues of the rat. J. Nutr. **1942**, *23*, 71–81.
30. Bunnell, R.H. The vitamin E potency of alfalfa as measured by the tocopherol content of the liver of the chick. Poult. Sci. **1957**, *36*, 413–416.
31. Pudelkiwicz, W.J.; Matterson, L.D.; Potter, L.M.; Webster, L.; Singsen, E.P. Chick tissue storage bioassay of alpha tocopherol: Chemical analytical techniques and relative biopotency of natural and synthetic alpha-tocopherol. J. Nutr. **1960**, *71*, 115–121.
32. Dicks, M.W.; Matterson, L.D. Chick liver storage bioassay of alpha-tocopherol: Methods. J. Nutr. **1961**, *75*, 165–174.
33. Lambertsen, G.; Braekkan, O.R. The spectrophotometric determination of $\alpha$-tocopherol. Analyst. **1959**, *84*, 706–711.

34. Emmerie, A.; Engel, C. Colorimetric determination of α-tocopherol (vitamin E ). Rec. Trav. Chim. **1938**, *57*, 1351–1355.
35. Emmerie, A.; Engel, C. Colorimetric determination of tocopherol (vitamin E). II. Adsorption experiments. Rec. Trav. Chem. **1939**, *58*, 283–289.
36. Emmerie, A.; Engel, C. Colorimetric determination of tocopherol (vitamin E). III. Estimation of tocoperhol in blood serum. Rec. Trav. Chem. **1940**, *59*, 895–902.
37. Emmerie, A. Colorimetric determination of tocopherol (vitamin E). IV. The quantitative determination of tocopherol in oils after saponification. Rec. Trav. Chem. **1940**, *59*, 246–248.
38. Emmerie, A. Colorimetric determination of tocopherol (vitamin E). V. The estimation of vitamin E in butter. Rec. Trav. Chem. **1941**, *60*, 104–105.
39. Smith, G.F.; McCurdy, W.H.; Diehl, H. The colorimetric determination of iron in raw and treated municipal water supplies by use of 4:7 diphenyl-1:10-phenanthroline. Analyst. **1952**, *77*, 418–422.
40. Tsen, C.C. An improved spectrophotometric method for the determination of tocopherols using 4,7-diphenyl-1,10-phenanthroline. Anal. Chem. **1961**, *33*, 849–851.
41. Duggan, D.E. Spectrofluorometric determination of tocopherols. Arch. Biochem. Biophys. **1959**, *84*, 116–122.
42. Thompson, J.N.; Erdody, P.; Maxwell, W.B. Chromatographic separation and spectrophotofluorometric determination of tocopherols using hydroxyalkoxypropyl sephadex. Anal. Biochem. **1972**, *50*, 267–280.
43. Brown, F. The estimation of vitamin E. 1. Separation of tocopherol mixtures occurring in natural products by paper chromatography. Biochem. J. **1952**, *51*, 237–239.
44. Brown, F. The estimation of vitamin E. 2. Quantitative analysis of tocoperhol mixtures by paper chromatography. Biochem. J. **1952**, *52*, 523–526.
45. Eggitt, P.W.R.; Ward, L.D. The estimation of vitamin-E activity by paper chromatography. J. Sci. Food Agric. **1953**, *4*, 176–179.
46. Eggitt, P.W.R.; Ward, L.D. The chemical estimation of vitamin-E activity in cereal products. I. The tocopherol pattern of wheat-germ oil. J. Sci. Food Agric. **1953**, *4*, 569–579.
47. Green, J.; Marcinkiewicz, S.; Watt, P.R. The determination of tocopherols by paper chromatography. J. Sci. Food Agric. **1955**, *6*, 274–282.
48. Green, J. The distribution of tocopherols during the life-cycle of some plants. J. Sci. Food Agric. **1958**, *9*, 801–812.
49. Booth, V.H. Spurious recovery tests in tocopherol determination. Anal. Chem. **1961**, *33*, 1224–1226.
50. Seher, A. Die analyse von tocopherolgemischen mit hilfe der dunnschichtchromatographie. Acta **1961**, *2*, 308–313.
51. Dilley, R.A.; Crane, F.L. A specific assay of tocopherols in plant tissue. Anal. Biochem. **1963**, *5*, 531–541.
52. Stowe, H.D. Separation of beta- and gamma tocopherol. Arch, Biochem, Biophys. **1963**, *103*, 42–44.

53. Rao, M.K.G.; Rao, S.V.; Acharya, K.T. Separation and estimation of tocopherols in vegetable oils by thin-layer chromatography. J. Sci. Food Agric. **1965**, *16*, 121–124.
54. Sturm, P.A.; Parkhurst, R.M.; Skinner, W.A. Quantitative determination of individual tocopherols by thin-layer chromatographic separation and spectrophotometry. Anal. Chem. **1966**, *38*, 1244–1247.
55. Whittle, K.J.; Pennock, J.F. The examination of tocopherols by two-dimensional thin-layer chromatography and subsequent colorimetric determination. Analyst. **1967**, *92*, 423–430.
56. Chow, C.K.; Draper, H.H.; Csallany, A.S. Method for the assay of free and esterified tocopherols Anal. Biochem. **1969**, *32*, 81–90.
57. Ames, S.R. Vitamins and other nutrients: Determination of vitamin E in foods and feeds—a collaborative study. JAOAC **1971**, *54*, 1–12.
58. Lovelady, H.G. Separation of beta- and gamma-tocopherols in the presence of alpha- and delta- tocopherols and vitamin A acetate. J. Chromatogr. **1973**, *78*, 449–452.
59. Drummond, J.C.; Singer, E.; McWalter, R.J.. A study of the unsaponifiable fraction of wheat germ oil with special reference to vitamin E. Biochem. J. **1935**, *29*, 456–471.
60. Kjolhede, K.T. The elimination of the "vitamin A and carotenoid error" in the chemical determination of tocopherol. Z. Vitaminforsch. **1942**, *12*, 138–145.
61. Devlin, H.B.; Mattill, H.A. The chemical determination of tocopherols in muscle tissue. J. Biol. Chem. **1942**, *146*, 123–130.
62. Meunier, P.; Vinet, A. Chromatographie des extraits lipoidiques totaux des tissus en vue de la determination de leur teneur en vitamine E. Bull. Soc. Chem. Biol. **1942**, *24*, 365–370.
63. Tosic, J.; Moore, T. The chemical estimation of vitamin E in vegetable oils. Biochem. J. **1945**, *39*, 498–507.
64. Kofler, M. Die getrennte bestimmung der tocopherole. Helv. Chim. Acta **1947**, *30*, 1053–1072.
65. Emmerie, A. The chromatographic separation of the tocopherols. Ann. N Y Acad. Sci. **1949**, *52*, 309–311.
66. Eggitt, P.W.R.; Norris, F.W. The chemical estimation of vitamin E activity in cereal products. III. The application of partition chromatography to the isolation of $\xi$-tocopherol from bran and to the determination of the individual tocopherols of cereals. J. Sci. Food Agric. **1955**, *6*, 689–696.
67. Bro-Rasmussen, F.; Hjarde, W. Determination of $\alpha$-tocopherol by chromatography on secondary magnesium phosphate (with collaborative tests by four laboratories). Acta Chem. Scand. **1957**, *11*, 34–43.
68. Pudelkiewicz, W.J.; Matterson, L.D. Effect of coenzyme $Q_{10}$ on the determination of tocopherhol in animal tissue. J. Biol. Chem. **1960**, *235*, 496–498.
69. Bieri, J.G.; Pollard, C.J.; Prange, I.; Dam, H. The determination of $\alpha$-tocopherol in animal tissues by column chromatography. Acta Chem. Scand. **1961**, *15*, 783–790.

70. Herting, D.C.; Drury, E.-J.E. Vitamin E content of vegetable oils and fats. J. Nutr. **1963**, *81*, 335–342.
71. Dicks-Bushnell, M.W. Column chromatography in the determination of tocopherols: Florisil, silicic acid and secondary magnesium phosphate. J. Chromatogr. **1967**, *27*, 96–103.
72. Strong, J.W. Combined assay for vitamins A, D (ergocalciferol), and E in multivitamins preparations with separation by reversed-phase partition chromatography. J. Pharm. Sci. **1976**, *65*, 968–974.
73. Nicolaides, N. The use of silicone rubber gums or grease in low concentration as stationary phase for the high temperature gas chromatographic separation of lipids. J. Chromatogr. **1960**, *4*, 496–499.
74. Wilson, P.W.; Kodicek, E.; Booth, V.H. Separation of tocopherols by gas-liquid chromatography. Biochem. J. **1962**, *84*, 524–531.
75. Nair, P.P.; Turner, D.A. The application of gas-liquid chromatography to the determination of vitamins A and K. JAOCS **1963**, *40*, 353–356.
76. Sweeley, C.C.; Bentley, R.; Makita, M.; Wells, W.W. Gas-liquid chromatography of trimethylsilyl derivatives of sugars and related substances. J. Am. Chem. Soc. **1963**, *85*, 2497–2507.
77. Carroll, K.K.; Herting, D.C. Gas-liquid chromatography of fat-soluble vitamins. JAOCS **1964**, *41*, 473–474.
78. Libby, D.A.; Sheppard, A.J. Gas-liquid chromatographic method for the determination of fat-soluble vitamins. I. Application to vitamin E. JAOAC **1964**, *47*, 371–376.
79. Bieri, J.G.; Prival, E.L. Serum vitamin E determined by thin-layer chromatgraphy. Proc. Soc. Exp. Biol. Med. **1965**, *120*, 554–557.
80. Nair, P.P.; Sarlos, I.; Machiz, J. Microquanitative separation of isomeric dimethyltocols by gas-liquid chromatography. Arch. Biochem. Biophys. **1966**, *114*, 488–493.
81. Ishikawa, S.; Katsui, G. Separation and determination of tocopherols by gas chromatography. J. Vitaminol. **1966**, *12*, 106–111.
82. Eisner, J.; Iverson, J.I.; Firestone, D. Gas chromatography of unsaponifiable matter. IV. Aliphatic alcohols, tocopherols, and triterpenoid alcohols in butter and vegetable oils. JAOAC **1966**, *49*, 580–590.
83. Slover, H.T.; Shelley, L.M.; Burks, T.L. Identification and estimation of tocopherols by gas-liquid chromatography. JAOCS **1967**, *44*, 161–166.
84. Slover, H.T.; Valis, R.J.; Lehmann, J.J. Gas chromatographic separation of tocotrienols: validation of predicted retention data. JAOCS **1968**, *45*, 580.
85. Slover, H.T.; Lehman, J.; Valis, R.J. Vitamin E in foods: Determination of tocols and tocotrienols. JAOCS **1969**, *46*, 417–420.
86. Slover, H.T.; Lehmann, J.; Valis, R.J. Nutrient composition of selected wheats and wheat products. III. Tocopherols. Cereal. Chem. **1969**, *46*, 635–641.
87. Slover, H.T.; Thompson, R.H.; Merola, G.V. Determination of tocoperhols and sterols by capillary gas chromatography JAOAC **1983**, *60*, 1524–1528.
88. Slover, H.T.; Thompson, R.H.; Davis, C.S.; Merola, G.V. Lipids in margarines and margarine like foods. JAOCS **1985**, *62*, 775–786.

89. Nair, P.P.; Machiz, J. Gas-liquid chromatography of isomeric methyltocols and their derivatives. Biochim. Biophys. Acta **1967**, *144*, 446–451.
90. Nair, P.P.; Luna, Z. Identification of α-tocopherol from tissues by combined gas-liquid chromatography, mass spectrometry and infrared spectroscopy. Arch. Biochem. Biophys. **1968**, *127*, 413–418.
91. Mann, F.P.; Viswanthan, V.; Plinton, C.; Menyharth, A.; Senkowski, B.Z. Determination of vitamin E in multivitamin products by gas-liquid chromatography. J. Pharm. Sci. **1968**, *57*, 2149–2153.
92. Nelson, J.P.; Milun, A.J. Gas chromatographic determination of tocopherols and sterols in soya sludges and residues. JAOCS **1968**, *45*, 848–851.
93. Sheppard, A.J.; Hubbard, W.D.; Prosser, A.R. Collaborative study comparing gas-liquid chromatographic and chemical methods for quantitatively determining vitamin E content of pharmaceutical products. JAOAC **1969**, *52*, 442–448.
94. Nelson, J.P.; Milun, A.J.; Fisher, H.D. Gas chromatographic determination of tocopherols and sterols in soya sludges and residues—an improved method. JAOCS **1970**, *47*, 259–261.
95. Bieri, J.G.; Poukka, R.K.H.; Prival, E.L. Determination of α-tocopherol in erythrocytes by gas-liquid chromatography. J. Lipid Res. **1970**, *11*, 118–123.
96. Lehmann, J.; Slover, H.T. Determination of plasma tocopherols by gas liquid chromatography. Lipids **1971**, *6*, 35–39.
97. Slover, H.T. Tocopherols in foods and fats. Lipids **1971**, *6*, 291–296.
98. Dasilva, E.J.; Jensen, A. Content of α-tocopherol in some blue-green algae. Biochim. Biophys. Acta **1971**, *239*, 345–347.
99. Rudy, B.C.; Mann, F.P.; Senkowski, B.Z.; Sheppard, A.J.; Hubbard, W.D. Collaborative study of the gas-liquid assay for vitamin E. JAOAC **1972**, *55*, 1211–1218.
100. Lovelady, H.G. Separation of individual tocopherols from human plasma and red blood cells by thin-layer and gas-liquid chromatography. J. Chromatogr. **1973**, *85*, 81–92.
101. Feeter, D.K. Determination of tocopherols, sterols, and steryl esters in vegetable oil distillates and residues. JAOCS **1974**, *51*, 184–187.
102. Hartman, K.T. A simplied gas liquid chromatographic determination for vitamin E in vegetable oils. JAOCS **1977**, *54*, 421–423.
103. Slover, H.T.; Lanza, E. Quantitative analysis of food fatty acids by capillary gas chromatography. JAOCS **1979**, *56*, 933–943, 1979.
104. Sheppard, A.J.; Hubbard, W.D. Collaborative study of GLC method for vitamin E. J. Pharm. Sci. **1979**, *68*, 115–120.
105. Slover, H.T.; Thompson, R.H. Chromatographic separation of the stereoisomers of alpha-tocopherol. Lipids **1981**, *16*, 268–275.
106. Schmit, J.A.; Henry, R.A.; Williams, R.C.; Diekman, J.F. Applications of high speed reversed phase chromatography. J. Chromatogr. Sci. **1971**, *9*, 645–651.
107. Van Niekerk, P.J. The direct determination of free tocopherols in plant oils by liquid-solid chromatography. Anal. Biochem. **1973**, *52*, 533–537.

108. Cavins, J.F.; Inglett, G.E. High-resolution liquid chromatography of vitamin E isomers. Cereal Chem. **1974**, *51*, 605–609.
109. Carr, C.D. Use of a new variable wavelength detector in high performance liquid chromatography. Anal. Chem. **1974**, *46*, 743–746.
110. Abe, K.; Yaguchi, Y.; Katsui, G. Quanitative determination of tocopherols by high-speed liquid chromatography. J. Nutr. Sci. Vitaminol. **1975**, *21*, 183–188.
111. Matsuo, M.; Tahara, Y. High performance liquid chromatography of tocopherols and their model compounds. Chem. Pharm. Bull. **1977**, *25*, 3381–3384.
112. Eriksson, T.; Sörensen, B. High performance liquid chromatography of vitamin E. Acta Pharm. Suecica. **1977**, *14*, 475–484.
113. Vatassery, G.T.; Maynard, V.R.; Hagen, D.F. High performance liquid chromatography of various tocopherols. J. Chromatogr. **1978**, *161*, 299–302.
114. Nilsson, B.; Johansson, B.; Jansson, L.; Holmberg, L. Determination of plasma $\alpha$-tocopherol by high-performance liquid chromatography. J. Chromatogr. **1978**, *145*, 169–172.
115. Söderhjelm, P.; Andersson, B. Simultaneous determination of vitamins A and E in foods and foods by reversed phase high-pressure liquid chromatography. J. Sci. Food Agric. **1978**, *29*, 697–702.
116. De Leenheer, A.P.; De Bevere, V.O.; Cruyl, A.A.; Claeys, A.E. Determination of serum $\alpha$-tocopherol (vitamin E) by high-performance liquid chromatography. Clin. Chem. **1978**, *24*, 585–590.
117. Cohen, H.; Lapointe, M. Method for the extraction and clean up of animal feed for the determination of liposoluble viatmins D, A, and E by high-pressure liquid chromatography. J. Agric. Food Chem. **1978**, *26*, 1210–1213.
118. Barnett, S.A.; Frick, L.W. Simultaneous determination of vitamin A acetate, Vitamin $D_2$, and vitamin E acetate in multivitamin mineral tablets by high performance liquid chromatography with coupled columns. Anal. Chem. **1979**, *51*, 641–645.
119. Ikenoya, S.; Abe, K.; Tsuda, T.; Yamano, Y.; Hiroshima, O.; Ohmae, M.; Kawabe, K. Electrochemical detector for high-perforance liquid chromatography. II. Determination of tocopherols, ubiquinones and phylloquinone in blood. Chem. Pharm. Bull. **1979**, *27*, 1237–1244.
120. Tagney, C.C.; Driskell, J.A.; McNair, H.M. Separation of vitamin E isomers by high-performance liquid chromatography. J. Chromatogr. **1979**, *176*, 513–515.
121. Bieri, J.G.; Tolliver, T.J.; Catignani, G.L. Simultaneous determination of $\alpha$-tocopherol and retinol in plasma or red cells by high pressure liquid chromatography. Am. J. Clin. Nutr. **1979**, *32*, 2143–2149.
122. Carpenter, A.P., Jr. Determination of tocopherols in vegetable oils. JAOCS **1979**, *56*, 668–671.
123. McMurray, C.H.; Blanchflower, W.J. Determination of $\alpha$-tocopherol in animal feedstuffs using high-performance liquid chromatography with spectrofluorescence detection. J. Chromatogr. **1979**, *176*, 488–492.

124. Barnes, P.J.; Taylor, P.W. The composition of acyl lipds and tocopherols in wheat germ oils from various sources. J. Sci. Food Agric. **1980**, *31*, 997–1006.
125. Ruggeri, B.A.; Watkins, T.R.; Grey, R.J.H.; Tomlins, R.I. Comparative analysis of tocopherols by thin-lay chromatography and high-performance liquid chromatography. J. Chromatogr. **1984**, *291*, 377–383.
126. Nelis, H.J.; De Bevere, V.O.R.C.; De Leenheer, A.P. Vitamin E: Tocopherols and tocotrienols. In *Modern Chromatographic Analysis of the Vitamins*; De Leenheer, A.P., Lambert, W.E., DeRuyter, M.G.M., Eds.; Marcel Dekker: New York, 1985.
127. Ball, G.F.M. *Fat Soluble Vitamin Assays in Food Analysis*. Elsevier Applied Science: New York, 1988; 7–56, 142–291 pp.
128. Ball, G.F.M. Applications of HPLC to the determination of fat-soluble vitamins in foods and animal feeds. J. Micronutr. Anal. **1988**, *4*, 255–283.
129. Ball, G.F.M. *Bioavailability and Analysis of Vitamins in Foods*. Chapman and Hall: London, 1998; 195–239 pp.
130. Desai, I.D.; Machlin, L.J. Vitamin E. In *Methods of Vitamin Assay*, 4th ed.; Augustin, J., Klein, B.P., Becker, D.A., Venugopal, P.B., Eds.; John Wiley & Sons: New York, 1985.
131. Lang, J.K.; Schillaci, M.; Irvin, B. Vitamin E. In *Modern Chromatographic Analysis of Vitamins*, 2nd ed.; De Leenheer, A.P., Lambert, W.E., Nelis, H.J., Eds.; Marcel Dekker: New York, 1992.
132. Thompson, J.N.; Hatina, G. Determination of tocopherols and tocotrienols in foods and tissues by high performance liquid chromatography. J. Liq. Chromatogr. **1979**, *2*, 327–344.
133. Bourgeois, C. *Determination of Vitamin E: Tocopherols and Tocotrienols*. Elsevier Applied Science: London, 1992; 21–131 pp.
134. Lumley, I.D. Vitamin analysis in foods. In *The Technology of Vitamins in Food*; Ottaway, P.B., Ed.; Chapman & Hall: New York, 1993.
135. Eitenmiller, R.R.; Landen, W.O., Jr. Vitamins. In *Analyzing Food for Nutrition Labeling and Hazardous Contaminants*; Jeon, I.J., Ikins, W.G., Eds.; Marcel Dekker: New York, 1995.
136. Eitenmiller, R.R.; Landen, W.O., Jr. Vitamin E: Tocopherols and Tocotrienols. In *Vitamin Analysis for the Health and Food Sciences*. CRC Press: Boca Raton, FL, 1999.
137. Abidi, S.L. Chromatographic analysis of tocol-derived lipid antioxidants. J. Chromatogr. **2000**, *A881*, 197–216.
138. Piironen, V.I. Determination of tocopherols and tocotrienols. Chemical Analysis. In *Modern Analytical Methodologies in Fat- and Water-Soluble Vitamins*, Vol. 154; Song, W.O., Beecher, G.R., Eitenmiller, R.R., Eds.; John Wiley & Sons, New York, 2000.
139. Ruperez, F.J.; Marin, D.; Herrera, E.; Barbas, C. Chromatographic analysis of $\alpha$-tocopherol and related compounds in various matrices. J. Chromatogr. **2001**, *A935*, 45–69.
140. Marks, C. Determination of free tocopherols in deodorizer distillate by capillary gas chromatography. JAOCS **1988**, *65*, 1936–1939.

141. American Oil Chemists' Society. Official Methods and Recommended Practices of the AOCS. 5th ed. American Oil Chemists' Society: Champaign, IL, 1998; Ce 7-87, Ce 8-89.
142. Berner, D. Tocopherols in deodorizer distillate. JAOCS **1988**, *65*, 881–882.
143. Frega, N.; Mozzon, M.; Bocci, F. Indentification and estimation of tocotrienols in the Annatto lipd fraction by gas chromatography-mass spectrometry. JAOCS **1988**, *75*, 1723–1727.
144. Liebler, D.C.; Burr, J.A.; Philips, L.; Ham, A.J.L. Gas chromatography-mass spectrometry analysis of vitamin E and its oxidation products. Anal. Biochem. **1996**, *236*, 27–34.
145. Melchert, H.U.; Pabel, E. Quantitative determination of $\alpha$-, $\beta$-, $\gamma$- and $\delta$-tocopherols in human serum by high-performance liquid chromatography and gas chromatography-mass spectrometry as trimethylsilyl derivatives with a two-step sample preparation. J. Chromatogr. **2000**, *A896*, 209–215.
146. Maraschiello, C.; Garcia Regueiro, J.A. Procedure for the determination of retinol and $\alpha$-tocopherol in poultry tissues using capillary gas chromatography with solvent venting injection. J. Chromatogr. **1998**, *A818*, 109–121.
147. Ulberth, F. Simultaneous determination of vitamin E isomers and cholesterol by GLC. J. High Resol. Chromatogr. **1998**, *14*, 343–344.
148. Botsoglou, N.; Fletouris, D.; Psomas, I.; Mantis, A. Rapid gas chromatographic method for simultaneous determination of cholesterol and $\alpha$-tocopherol in eggs. JAOAC **1998**, *81*, 1177–1183.
149. Ballesteros, E.; Gallego, M.; Valcarcel, M. Gas chromatographic determination of cholesterol and tocopherols in edible oils and fats with automatic removal of interfering triglycerides. J. Chromatogr. **1996**, *A719*, 221–227.
150. Lechner, M.; Reiter, B.; Lorbeer, E. Determination of tocopherols and sterols in vegetable oils by solid-phase extraction and subsequent capillary gas chromatographic analysis. J. Chromatogr. **1999**, *A857*, 231–238.
151. Parcerisa, J.; Casals, I.; Boatella, J.; Codony, R.; Rafecas, M. Analysis of olive and hazelnut oil mixtures by high-performance liquid chromatography-atmospheric pressure chemical ionisation mass spectrometry of triacylglycerols and gas-liquid chromatography of non-saponifiable compounds (tocopherols and sterols). J. Chromatogr. **2000**, *A881*, 149–158.
152. Du, M.; Ahn, D.U. Simultaneous analysis of tocopherols, cholesterol, and phytosterols using gas chromatography. J. Food Sci. **2002**, *67*, 1696–1700.
153. Smidt, C.R.; Jones, A.D.; Clifford, A.J. Gas chromatography of retinol and $\alpha$-tocopherol without derivatization. J. Chromatogr. **1988**, *434*, 21–29.
154. Williams, R.C.; Schmit, J.A.; Henry, R.A. Quantitative analysis of fat-soluble vitamins by high-speed liquid chromatography. J. Chromatogr. Sci. **1972**, *10*, 4984–501.
155. Speek, A.J.; Schrijuer, J.; Schreurs, W.H.P. Vitamin E composition of some seed oils as determined by high-performance liquid chromatography with fluorescence detection. J. Food Sci. **1985**, *50*, 121–124.
156. Syväoja, E.L.; Piironen, V.; Varo, P.; Koivistoinen, P.; Salminen, K. Tocopherols and tocotrienols in Finnish foods: oils and fats. JAOCS **1986**, *63*, 328–329.

157. Desai, I.D.; Bhagavan, H.; Salkeld, R.; Dutra De Oliveira, J.E. Vitamin E content of crude and refined vegetable oils in southern Brazil. J. Food Comp. Anal. **1998**, *1*, 231–238.
158. Rogers, E.; Rice, S.M.; Nicolosi, R.J.; Carpenter, D.R.; McClelland, C.A.; Romanczyk, L.J. Identification and quantitation of $\alpha$-oryzanol components and simultaneous assessment of tocols in rice bran oil JAOCS **1993**, *70*, 301–307.
159. Chase, G.W., Jr.; Akoh, C.C.; Eitenmiller, R.R. Analysis of tocopherols in vegetable oils by high-performance liquid chromatography: Comparison of fluorescence and evaporative light-scattering detection. JAOCS **1994**, *71*, 877–881.
160. Dionisi, F.; Prodolliet, J.; Tagliaferri, E. Assessment of olive oil adulteration by reversed-phase high performance liquid chromatography/amperometric detection of tocopherols and tocotrienols. JAOCS **1995**, *72*, 1505–1511.
161. Gordan, M.H.; Kourjmska, L. Effect of antioxidants on losses of tocopherols during deep-fat frying. Food Chem. **1995**, *52*, 175–177.
162. Gimeno, E.; Casellote, A.I.; Lamuela-Raventós, R.M.; de la Torre, M.C.; López-Sabater, M.C. Rapid determination of vitamin E in vegetable oils by reversed-phase high-performance liquid chromatography. J. Chromatogr. **2000**, *A881*, 251–254.
163. Gimeno, E.; Calero, E.; Castellote, A.I.; Lamuela-Raventós, R.M.; de la Torre, M.C.; López-Sabater, M.C. Simultaneous determination of $\alpha$-tocopherol and $\beta$-carotene in olive oil by reversed-phase high-performance liquid chromatography. J. Chromatogr. **2000**, *A881*, 255–259.
164. Sanchez-Pérez, A.; Delgado-Zamarreño, M.M.; Bustamante-Rangel, M.; Hernán-dez-Méndez, J. Automated analysis of vitamin E isomers in vegetable oils by continuous membrane extraction and liquid chromatography-electrochemical detection. J. Chromatogr. **2000**, *A881*, 229–241.
165. Tasioula-Margari, M.; Okogeri, O. Simultaneous determination of phenolic compounds and tocopherols in virgin olive oil using HPLC and UV detection. Food Chem. **2001**, *74*, 377–383.
166. Micali, G.; Lanuzza, F.; Carro, P. Analysis of tocopherols in margarine by on-line HPLC-HRGC coupling. J. High Resol. Chromatogr. **1993**, *16*, 536–538.
167. Rader, J.I.; Weaver, C.M.; Patrascu, L.; Ali, L.H.; Angyal, G. $\alpha$-Tocopherol, total vitamin A and total fat in margarines and margarine-like products. Food Chem. **1997**, *58*, 373–379.
168. Ye, L.; Landen, W.O., Jr.; Lee, J.; Eitenmiller, R.R. Vitamin E content of margarine and reduced fat products using a simplified extraction procedure and HPLC determination. J. Liq. Chromatogr. Rel. Technol. **1998**, *21*, 1227–1238.
169. Landen, W.O., Jr. Application of gel permeation chromatography and nonaqueous reverse phase chromatography to high performance liquid chromatographic determination of retinyl palmitate and $\alpha$-tocopheryl acetate in infant formula. JAOAC **1982**, *65*, 810–816.
170. Landen, W.O., Jr.; Hines, D.; Hamill, T.; Martin, J.; Young, E.; Eitenmiller, R.; Soliman, A. Vitamin A and Vitamin E content of infant formulas produced in the United States. JAOAC **1985**, *68*, 509–511.

171. Syväoja, E.L.; Piironen, V.; Varo, P.; Koivistoinen, P.; Salminen, K. Tocopherols and tocotrienols in Finnish foods: Human milk and infant formulas. Int. J. Vit. Nutr. Res. **1985**, *55*, 159–166.
172. Woollard, D.C.; Blott, A.D. The routine determiation of vitamin E acetate in milk powder formulations using high-performance liquid chromatography. J. Micronutr. Anal. **1986**, *2*, 97–115.
173. Woollard, D.C.; Blott, A.D.; Indyk, H. Fluorometric detection of tocopheryl acetate and its use in the analysis of infant formulas. J. Micronutr. Anal. **1987**, *3*, 1–14.
174. Chappell, J.E.; Francis, T.; Clandinin, M.T. Simultaneous high performance liquid chromatography analysis of retinol esters and tocopherol isomers in human milk. Nutr. Res. **1986**, *6*, 849–852.
175. Indyk, H.E. Simplified saponification procedure for the routine determination of total vitamin E in dairy products, foods, and tissues by high-performance liquid chromatography. Analyst. **1988**, *113*, 1217–1221.
176. Tuan, S.; Lee, T.F.; Chou, C.C.; Wei, Q.K. Determination of vitamin E homologues in infant formulas by HPLC using fluorometric detection. J. Micronutr. Anal. **1989**, *6*, 35–45.
177. Zamarreño, M.; Perez, A.; Perez, M.; Mendez, J. High performance liquid chromatography with electrochemical detection for the simultaneous determination of vitamin A, $D_3$, and E in milk. J. Chromatogr. **1992**, *623*, 69–74.
178. Hollman, P.; Slangen, J.; Wagstaffe, P.; Faure, U.; Southgate, D.T.; Finglas, P.M. Intercomparison of methods for the determination of vitamins in foods. Part 1. Fat-soluble vitamins. Analyst. **1993**, *118*, 475–118.
179. Tanner, J.T.; Barnett, S.A.; Mountford, M.K. Analysis of milk-based infant formula. Phase V. Vitamins A and E, folic acid, and pantothonic acid: Food and Drug Administration—Infant Formula Council: Collaborative study. JAOAC Int. **1993**, *76*, 399–413.
180. Blanco, D.; Pajares, M.; Escotet, V.; Gutierrez, M. Determination of fat-soluble vitamins by liquid chromatography in pediatric parenteral nutritionals. J. Liq. Chromatogr. **1994**, *17*, 4513–4521.
181. Panfili, G.; Manzi, P.; Pizzoferrato, C. High performance liquid chromatographic method for the simultaneous determination of tocopherols, carotenes, and retinol and its geometric isomers in Italian cheeses. Analyst. **1994**, *119*, 1161–1164.
182. Zamarreño, M.; Perez, A.; Perez, M.; Moro, M.; Mendez, J. Determination of vitamins A, E, and K in milk by high performance liquid chromatography with dual amperometeric detection. Analyst. **1995**, *120*, 2489–2492.
183. Zamarreño, M.; Perez, A.; Perez, M.; Mendez, J. Directly coupled sample treatment-high performance liquid chromatography for on-line automatic determination of lipsoluble vitamins in milk. J. Chromatogr. **1995**, *A694*, 399–406.
184. Albala-Hurtado, S.; Rodriguez, S.; Nogues, M.T.; Marine-Font, A. Determination of vitamins A and E in infant milk formulae by high performance liquid chromatography. J. Chromatogr. **1997**, *A778*, 243–246.

185. Chase, G.W., Jr.; Eitenmiller, R.; Long, A.R. Liquid chromatographic analysis of *all-rac-α*-tocopheryl acetate, tocopherols, and retinyl palmitate in SRM 1846. J. Liq. Chromatogr. Rel. Technol. **1997**, *20*, 3317–3327.
186. GW Chase, Jr.; Long, A.R.; Eitenmiller, R. Liquid chromatographic method for analysis of *all-rac-α*-tocopheryl acetate and retinyl palmitate in soy-based infant formula using a zero-control reference material (ZRM) as a method development tool. JAOAC Int. **1998**, *81*, 577–581.
187. Hewavitharana, A.K.; Van Brakel, A.S. A rapid saponification procedure for the simultaneous determination of the natural levels of vitamins A, E and *β*-carotene in milk. Milchwissenschaft. **1998**, *53*, 1–15.
188. Ake, M.; Fabre, H.; Malan, A.K.; Mandrou, B. Column chromatography determination of vitamins A and E in powdered milk and local flour: a validation procedure. J. Chromatogr. **1998**, *A826*, 183–189.
189. Chase, G.W., Jr.; Long, A.R. Liquid chromatographic method for analysis of all-rac-*α*-tocopheryl acetate and retinyl palmitate in milk-based infant formula using matrix solid-phase dispersion. JAOAC Int. **1998**, *81*, 582–586.
190. Chase, G.W., Jr.; Eitenmiller, R.; Long, A.R. Liquid chromatographic method for the analysis of *all-rac-α*-tocopheryl acetate and retinyl palmitate in soy-based infant formula using matrix solid phase dispersion. J. Liq. Chromatogr. Rel. Technol. **1998**, *21*, 2853–2861.
191. Chase, G.W., Jr.; Eitenmiller, R.; Long, A.R. A liquid chromatographic method for analysis of *all-rac-α*-tocopheryl acetate and retinyl palmitate in medical food using matrix solid-phase dispersion in conjunction with a zero reference material as a method development tool. JAOAC Int. **1999**, *82*, 107–111.
192. Hogarty, C.J.; Ang, C.; Eitenmiller, R.R. Tocopherol content of selected foods by HPLC/fluorescence quantitation. J. Food Comp. Anal. **1989**, *2*, 200–209.
193. Piironen, V.; Varo, P.; Syväoja, E.L.; Salminen, K.; Koivistoinen, P. High performance liquid chromatographic determination of tocopherols and tocotrienols and its application to diets and plasma of Finnish men. I. Analytical method. Int. J. Vit. Nutr. Res. **1984**, *53*, 35–40.
194. Piironen, V.; Varo, P.; Salminen, E.L.; Koivistoinen, P.; Arvilommi, H. High performance liquid chromatographic determination of tocopherols and its application to diets and plasma of Finnish men. II. Applications. Int. J. Vitam. Nutr. Res. **1984**, *53*, 41–46.
195. Piironen, V.; Syväoja, E.L.; Varo, P.; Salminen, K.; Koivistoinen, P. Tocopherols and tocotrienols in Finnish foods: meat and meat products. J. Agric. Food Chem. **1985**, *33*, 1215–1218.
196. Piironen, V.; Syväoja, E.L.; Varo, P.; Salminen, K.; Koivistoinen, P. Tocopherols and tocotrienols in ceral products from Finland. Cereal Chem. **1986**, *63*, 78–81.
197. Piironen, V.; Syväoja, E.L.; Varo, P.; Salminen, K.; Koivistoinen, P. Tocopherols and tocotrienols in Finnish foods: vegetables, fruits and berries. J. Agric. Food Chem. **1986**, *34*, 742–746.
198. Piironen, V.; Varo, P.; Koivistoinen, P. Stability of tocopherols and tocotrienols in food preparation procedures. J. Food Comp. Anal. **1987**, *1*, 53–58.

199. Piironen, V.; Varo, P.; Koivistoinen, P. Stability of tocopherols and tocotrienols during storage of foods. J. Food Comp. Anal. **1988**, *1*, 124–131.
200. Syväoja, E.L.; Salminen, K.; Piironen, V.; Varo, P.; Kerojoki, D.; Koivistoinen, P. Tocopherols and tocotrienols in Finnish foods: Fish and fish products. JAOCS **1985**, *62*, 1245–1248.
201. Ang, C.Y.W.; Seancy, G.K.; Eitenmiller, R.R. Tocopherols in chicken breast and leg muscles determined by reverse phase liquid chromatography. J. Food Sci. **1990**, *55*, 1536–1539.
202. Rushing, L.G.; Cooper, W.M.; Thompson, H.C. Simultaneous analysis of vitamins A and E in rodent feed by high performance liquid chromatography. J. Agric. Food Chem. **1991**, *39*, 296–299.
203. Tee, E.-S.; Lim, C.L. Re-analysis of vitamin A values of selected Malaysian foods of animal origin by the AOAC and HPLC methods. Food Chem. **1992**, *45*, 289–296.
204. Yao, F.; Dull, G.; Eitenmiller, R.R. Tocopherol quantification by HPLC in pecans and relationship to kernel quality during storage. J. Food Sci. **1992**, *57*, 1194–1197.
205. Hashim, I.B.; Koehler, P.E.; Eitenmiller, R.R.; Kvien, C.K. Fatty acid composition and tocopherols content of drought stressed florunner peanuts. Peanut Sci. **1993**, *20*, 21–24.
206. Hashim, I.B.; Koehler, P.E.; Eitenmiller, R.R. Tocopherols in Runner and Virginia peanut cultivars at various maturity stages. JAOCS **1993**, *70*, 633–635.
207. Lehmann, J.W.; Putnam, D.H.; Qureshi, A.A. Vitamin E isomers in grain Amaranths (*Amaranthus* spp.). Lipids **1994**, *29*, 177–181.
208. Balz, M.K.; Schulte, E.; Thier, H.P. Simultaneous determination of $\alpha$-tocopheryl acetate, tocopherols and tocotrienols by HPLC with fluorescence detection in foods. Fat Sci. Technol. **1993**, *95*, 215–220.
209. Jiang, Y.H.; McGeachin, R.B.; Bailey, C.A. $\alpha$-Tocopherol, $\beta$-carotene, and retinol enrichment of chicken eggs. Poult. Sci. **1994**, *73*, 1137–1143.
210. McGeachin, R.B.; Bailey, C.A. Determination of carotenoid pigments, retinol, and $\alpha$-tocopherol in feeds, tissues, and blood serum by normal phase high performance liquid chromatography. Poult. Sci. **1995**, *74*, 407–411.
211. Barua, A.B.; Olson, J.A. Reversed-phase gradient high-performance liquid chromatographic procedure for simultaneous analysis of very polar to nonpolar retinoids, carotenoids and tocopherols in animal and plant samples. J. Chromatogr. **1998**, *B707*, 69–79.
212. Qian, H.; Sheng, M. Simultaneous determination of fat-soluble vitamins A, D and E and pro-vitamin $D_2$ in animal feeds by one-step extraction and high-performance liquid chromatography analysis. J. Chromatogr. **1998**, *A825*, 127–133.
213. Lee, J.; Landen, W.O., Jr.; Phillips, R.D.; Eitenmiller, R.R. Application of direct solvent extraction to the LC quantificiation of vitamin E in peanuts, peanut butter, and selected nuts. Peanut Sci. **1999**, *25*, 123–128.
214. Ye, L.; Landen, W.O., Jr.; Eitenmiller, R.R. Liquid chromatographic analysis of *all-trans* retinyl palmitate, $\beta$-carotene and vitamin E in fortified foods and the extraction of encapsulated and nonencapsulated retinyl palmitate. J. Agric. Food Chem. **2000**, *48*, 4003–4008.

215. Rodrigo, N.; Alegria, A.; Barbera, R.; Farre, R. High-performance liquid chromatographic determination of tocopherols in infant formulas. J. Chromatogr. **2002**, *A947*, 97–102.
216. Garcia-Plazaola, J.I.; Becerril, J.M. A rapid high-performance liquid chromatography method to measure lipophilic antioxidants in stressed plants: simultaneous determination of carotenoids and tocopherols. Phytochem. Anal. **1999**, *10*, 307–313.
217. Ye, L.; Landen, W.O., Jr.; Eitenmiller, R.R. Simplified extraction procedure and HPLC determination for total vitamin E and β-carotene of reduced-fat mayonnaise. J. Food Sci. **2000**, *65*, 1–5.
218. Gonzalez, A.G.; Pablos, F.; Martin, M.J.; Leon-Camacho, M.; Valdenebro, M.S. HPLC analysis of tocopherols and triglycerides in coffee and their use as authentication parameters. Food Chem. **2001**, *73*, 93–101.
219. Torre, J.; Lorenzo, M.P.; Martinez-Alcazar, M.P.; Barbas, C. Simple high-performance liquid chromatography method for α-tocopherol measurement in *Rosmarinus officinalis* leaves: New data on α-tocopherol content. J. Chromatogr. **2001**, *A919*, 305–311.
220. Delgado-Zamarreño, M.M.; Bustamante-Rangel, M.; Sanchez-Perez, A.; Hernandez-Mendez, J. Analysis of vitamin E isomers in seeds and nuts with and without coupled hydrolysis by liquid chromatography and coulometric detection. J. Chromatogr. **2001**, *A935*, 77–86.
221. Carlucci, G.; Mazzeo, P.; Governatore, S.D.; Giacomo, G.D.; Re, G.D. Liquid chromatographic method for the analysis of tocopherols in nalt sprouts with supercritical fluid extraction. J. Chromatogr. **2001**, *A935*, 87–91.
222. Schieber, A.; Marx, M.; Carle, R. Simultaneous determination of carotenes and tocopherols in ATBC drinks by high-performance liquid chromatography. Food Chem. **2002**, *76*, 357–362.
223. DeVries, J.W.; Silvera, K.R. Determination of vitamins A (Retinol) and E (alpha-tocopherol) in foods by liquid chromatography: collaborative study. JAOAC Int. **2002**, *85*, 424–434.
224. Ueda, T.; Igarashi, O. Evaluation of the electrochemical detector for the determination of tocopherols in feeds by high performance liquid chromatography. J. Micronutr. Anal. **1985**, *1*, 31–38.
225. Ueda, T.; Igarashi, O. Effect of coexisting fat on the extraction of tocopherols from tissues after saponification as a pretreatment for HPLC determination. J. Micronutr. Anal. **1987**, *3*, 15–25.
226. Ueda, T.; Igarashi, O. New solvent for extraction of tocopherols from biological specimans for HPLC determination and the evaluation of 2,2,5,7,8-pentamethyl-6-chromanol as an internal standard. J. Micronutr. Anal. **1987**, *3*, 185–198.
227. Ueda, T.; Igarashi, D. Determination of vitamin E in biological specimens and foods by HPLC: Pretreatment of samples and extraction of tocopherols. J. Micronutr. Anal. **1990**, *7*, 79–96.
228. Thompson, J.N. Review: Official methods for measurement of vitamin A: Problems of official methods and new techniques for analysis of foods and feeds for vitamin A. JAOAC **1986**, *69*, 727–738.

229. Lee, J.; Ye, L.; Landen, W.O., Jr.; Eitenmiller, R.R. Optimization of an analysis procedure for the quanitification of vitamin E in tomato and broccoli using response surface methodology with potential for application to other food matrices. J. Food Comp. Anal. **2000**, *13*, 45–57.
230. Håkansson, B.; Jägerstad, M.; Öste, R. Determination of vitamin E in wheat products by HPLC. J. Micronutr. Anal. **1987**, *3*, 307–318.
231. Tan, B.; Brzuskiewicz, L. Separation of tocopherol and tocotrienol isomers using normal- and reverse-phase chromatography. Anal. Biochem. **1988**, *180*, 368–373.
232. Abidi, S.L.; Mounts, T.L. Normal phase high performance liquid chromatography of tocopherols on polar phases. J. Liq. Chromatogr. Rel. Technol. **1996**, *19*, 509–520.
233. Kamal-Eldin, A.; Görgen, S.; Pettersson, J.; Lampi, A.-M. Normal phase high-performance liquid chromatography of tocopherols and tocotrienols: Comparison of different chromatographic columns. J. Chromatogr. **2000**, *A881*, 217–227.
234. Kramer, J.K.G.; Blais, L.; Fouchard, R.C.; Melnyk, R.A.; Kallury, K.M.R. A rapid method for the determination of vitamin E forms in tissues and diet by high-performance liquid chromatography using a normal-phase diol column. Lipids **1997**, *32*, 323–330.
235. Ye, L.; Landen, W.O., Jr.; Eitenmiller, R.R. Comparison of the column performance of narrow-bore and standard-bore column for the chromatographic determination of $\alpha$-, $\beta$-, $\gamma$- and $\delta$-tocopherol. J. Chromatogr. Sci. **2001**, *39*, 1–6.
236. Scott, R.P.W. An introduction to small-bore columns. J. Chromatogr. Sci. **1985**, *23*, 233–237.
237. Richheimer, S.L.; Kent, M.C.; Bernart, M.W. Reversed-phase high-performance liquid chromatographic method using a pentafluorophenyl bonded phase for analysis of tocopherols. J. Chromatogr. **1994**, *A677*, 75–80.
238. Rentel, C.; Strohschein, S.; Albert, K.; Bayer, E. Silver-plated vitamins: A method for detecting tocopherols and carotenoids in LC/ESI-MS coupling. Anal. Chem. **1998**, *70*, 4394–4400.
239. Strohschein, S.; Rentel, C.; Laker, T.; Bayer, E.; Albert, K. Separation and identification of tocotrienol isomers by HPLC-MS and HPLC-NMR coupling. Anal. Chem. **1999**, *71*, 1780–1785.
240. Abidi, S.L.; Mounts, T.L. Reversed-phase high-performance liquid chromatographic separation of tocopherols. J. Chromatogr. **1997**, *A782*, 25–52.
241. Abidi, S.L. Reversed-phase retention characteristics of tocotrienol antioxidants. J. Chromatogr. **1999**, *A844*, 67–75.
242. Hoehler, D.; Frohlich, A.A.; Marquardt, R.R.; Stelsovsky, H. Extraction of $\alpha$-tocopherol from serum prior to reversed-phase liquid chromatography. J. Agric. Food Chem. **1998**, *46*, 973–978.
243. Rhys-Williams, A.T. Simultaneous determination of serum vitamin A and E by liquid chromatography with fluorescence detection. J. Chromatogr. **1985**, *341*, 198–201.
244. Chen, R.F. Fluorescence of dansyl amino acids in organic solvents and protein solutions. Arch. Biochem. Biophys. **1967**, *120*, 6092–62.

245. Warner, K.; Mounts, T.L. Analysis of tocopherols and phytosterols in vegetable oils by HPLC with evaporative light-scattering detection. JAOCS **1990**, *67*, 827–831.
246. Eitenmiller, R.R. Vitamin E content of fats and oils—nutritional implications. Food Technol. **1997**, *51*, 78–81.
247. Barnett, S.A.; Frick, L.W.; Baine, H.M. Simultaneous determination of vitamins A, $D_2$, $D_3$, E and $K_1$ in infant formulas and dairy products by reversed-phase liquid chromatography. Anal. Chem. **1980**, *52*, 610–614.
248. Landen, W.O., Jr.; Eitenmiller, R.R. Application of gel permeation chromatography and nonaqueous reverse phase chromatography to high pressure liquid chromatographic determination of retinyl palmitate and $\beta$-carotene in oil and margarine. JAOAC **1979**, *62*, 283–289.
249. Widicus, W.A.; Kirk, J.R. High pressure liquid chromatographic determination of vitamins A and E in cereal products. JAOAC **1979**, *62*, 637–641.
250. Still, W.C.; Kahn, M.; Mitra, A. Rapid chromatographic technique for prepartive separation with moderate resolution. J. Org. Chem. **1978**, *43*, 2923–2925.
251. Pearce, B.C.; Parker, R.A.; Deason, M.E.; Qureshi, A.A.; Wright, J.J. Hypocholesterolemic activity of synthetic and natural tocotrienols. J. Med. Chem. **1992**, *35*, 3595–3606.
252. Bruns, A.; Berg, D.; Werner-Busse, A. Isolation of tocopherol homologs by preparative high performance liquid chromatography. J. Chromatogr. **1988**, *450*, 111–113.
253. Shin, T.S.; Godber, J.S. Isolation of four tocopherols and four tocotrienols from a variety of natural sources by semi-preparative high performance liquid chromatography. J. Chromatogr. **1994**, *A678*, 49–58.
254. Feng, H.-P. Preparative techniques for isolation of vitamin E homologs and evaluation of their antioxidant activities. PhD dissertation. Athens: University of Georgia, 1995.
255. Vecchi, M.; Walther, W.; Glinz, E.; Netscher, T.; Schmid, R.; Lalonde, M.; Vetter, W. Separation and quantntitation of all 8 stereoisomers of $\alpha$-tocopherol by chromatography. Helv. Chim. Acta **1990**, *73*, 782–789.
256. Riss, G.; Kormann, A.W.; Glinz, E.; Walther, W.; Ranalder, U.B. Separation of the eight stereoisomers of *all rac*-$\alpha$-tocopherol from tissue and plasma: Chiral phase high-performance liquid chromatography and capillary gas chromatography. Methods Enzymol. **1994**, *234*, 302–310.
257. Ueda, T.; Ichikawa, H.; Igarashi, O. Determination of $\alpha$-tocopherol stereoisomers in biological specimens using chiral phase high-performance liquid chromatography. J. Nutr. Sci. Vitaminol. **1993**, *39*, 207–219.
258. Kiyose, C.; Muramatsu, R.; Kameyama, Y.; Ueda, T.; Igarashi, O. Biodiscrimination of $\alpha$-tocopherol stereoisomers in humans after oral administration. Am. J. Clin. Nutr. **1997**, *65*, 785–789.
259. Trenerry, V.C. The application of capillary electrophoresis to the analysis of vitamins in food and beverages. Electrophoresis **2001**, *22*, 1466–1476.
260. Pedersen-Bjergaard, S.; Næss, Ø; Moestue, S.; Rasmussen, K.E. Microemulsion electrokinetic chromatography in suppressed electroosmotic flow environment separation of fat-soluble vitamins. J. Chromatogr. **2000**, *A876*, 201–211.

261. Ong, C.P.; Ng, C.L.; Lee, H.K.; Li, S.F.Y. Separation of water- and fat-soluble vitamins by micellar electrokinetic chromatography. J. Chromatogr. **1991**, *547*, 419–428.
262. Chan, K.C.; Lewis, K.C.; Phang, J.M.; Issaq, H.J. Separation of retinoic acid isomers using micellar electrokinetic chromatography. J. High Resol. Chromatogr. **1993**, *16*, 560–561.
263. Boso, R.L.; Bellini, M.S.; Mikšík, I.; Deyl, Z. Microemulsion electrokinetic chromatography with different organic modifiers: Separation of water- and lipid-soluble vitamins. J. Chromatogr. **1995**, *A709*, 11–19.
264. Profumo, A.; Profumo, V.; Vidali, G. Micellar electrokinetic capillary chromatography of three natural vitamin A derivatives. Electrophoresis **1996**, *17*, 1617–1621.
265. Hsieh, Y.Z.; Kuo, K.L. Separation of retinoids by micellar electrokinetic capillary chromatography. J. Chromatogr. **1997**, *A761*, 307–313.
266. Boyce, M.C.; Spickett, E.E. Separation of food grade antioxidants (synthetic and natural) using mixed micellar electokinetic capillary chromatography. J. Agric. Food Chem. **1999**, *47*, 1970–1975.
267. Zhao, J.; Yang, G.; Duan, H.; Li, J. Determination of synthesized $\alpha$-vitamin E by micellar electrokinetic chromatography. Electrophoresis **2001**, *22*, 151–154.
268. Spencer, B.J.; Purdy, W.C. Comparison of the separation of fat-soluble vitamins using $\beta$-cyclodextrins in high-performance liquid chromatography and micellar electrokinetic chromatography. J. Chromatogr. **1997**, *A782*, 227–235.
269. Altria, K.D. Application of microemulsion electrokinetic chromatography to the analysis of a wide range of pharmaceuticals and excipients. J. Chromatogr. **1999**, *A844*, 371–386.
270. Pedersen-Bjergaard, S.; Rasmussen, K.E.; Tilander, J. Separation of fat-soluble vitamins by hydrophobic interaction electrokinetic chromatography with tetradecylammonium ions as pseudostationary phase. J. Chromatogr. **1998**, *A807*, 285–295.
271. Næss, Ø; Tilander, T.; Pedersen-Bjergaard, S.; Rasmussen, K.E. Analysis of vitamin formulations by electrokinetic chromatography utilizing tetradecylammonium ions as the pseudostationary phase. Electrophoresis **1998**, *19*, 2912–2917.
272. Tjørnelund, T.; Hansen, S.H. Separation of neutral substances by non-aqueous capillary electrophoresis through interactions with cationic additives. J. Chromatogr. **1997**, *A792*, 475–482.
273. Abidi, S.L.; Rennick, K.A. Capillary elctrochromatographic evaluation of vitamin E-active oil constituents: Tocopherols and tocotrienols. J. Chromatogr. **2001**, *A913*, 379–386.
274. Fanali, S.; Catarcini, P.; Quaglia, M.G.; Camera, E.; Rinaldi, M.; Picardo, m. Separation of $\delta$-, $\gamma$- and $\alpha$-tocopherols by CEC. J. Pharm. Biomed. Anal. **2002**, *29*, 973–979.
275. Dueker, S.R.; Jones, A.D.; Smith, M.; Clifford, A.J. Stable isotope methods for the study of $\beta$-carotene-$d_8$ metabolism in humans utilizing tandem mass spectrometry and high-performance liquid chromatography. Anal. Chem. **1994**, *66*, 4177–4185.

276. Tang, G.; Andrien, B.A.; Dolnikowski, G.G.; Russell, R.M. Atmospheric pressure chemical ionization and electron capture negative chemical ionization mass spectrometry in studying $\beta$-carotene conversion to retinol in humans. Methods Enzymol. **1997**, *282*, 140–154.
277. Tang, G.; Qin, J.; Dolnikowski, G.G. Deuterium enrichment of retinol in humans determined by gas chromatography electron capture negative chemical ionization mass spectrometry. J. Nutr. Biochem. **1998**, *9*, 408–414.
278. Tang, G.; Qin, J.; Dolnikowski, G.G.; Russell, R.M. Vitamin A equivalence of $\beta$-carotene in a woman as determined by a stable isotope reference method. Eur. J. Nutr. **2000**, *39*, 7–11.
279. Traber, M.G.; Rader, D.; Acuff, R.V.; Ramakrishnan, R.; Brewer, H.B.; Kayden, H.J. Vitamin E dose-response studies in humans with use of deuterated *RRR*-$\alpha$-tocopherol. Am. J. Clin. Nutr. **1998**, *68*, 847–853.
280. Acuff, R.V.; Dunworth, R.G.; Webb, L.W.; Lane, J.R. Transport of deuterium-labeled tocopherols during pregnancy. Am. J. Clin. Nutr. **1998**, *67*, 459–464.
281. Roxborough, H.E.; Burton, G.W.; Kelly, F.J. Inter and intra-individual variation in plasma and red blood cell vitamin E after supplementation. Free Radic. Res. **2000**, *33*, 437–445.
282. Liebler, D.C.; Burr, J.A.; Philips, L.; Ham, A.J.L. Gas chromatography-mass spectrometry analysis of vitamin E and its oxidation products. Anal. Biochem. **1996**, *236*, 27–34.
283. Liebler, D.C.; Burr, J.A.; Ham, A.J.L. Gas chromatography-mass spectrometry analysis of vitamin E and its oxidation products. Methods Enzymol. **1999**, *299*, 309–348.
284. Fauler, G.; Leis, H.J.; Schalamon, J.; Muntean, W.; Gleispach, H. Method for the determination of vitamin K1(20) in human plasma by stable isotope dilution/gas chromatography/mass spectrometry. J. Mass. Spectrom. **1996**, *31*, 655–660.
285. Dolnikowski, G.G.; Sun, Z.; Grusak, M.A.; Peterson, J.W.; Booth, S.L. HPLC and GC/MS determination of deuterated vitamin K (phylloquinone) in human serum after ingestion of deuterium-labeled broccoli. J. Nutr. Biochem. **2002**, *13*, 168–174.
286. Melchert, H.U.; Pabel, E. Quantitative determination of $\alpha$-, $\beta$-, $\gamma$- and $\delta$-tocopherols in human serum by high-performance liquid chromatography and gas chromatography-mass spectrometry as trimethylsilyl derivatives with a two-step sample preparation. J. Chromatogr. **2000**, *A896*, 209–215.
287. van Breemen, R.B. Innovations in carotenoid analysis using LC/MS. Anal. Chem. **1996**, *68*, A299–A304.
288. Khachik, F.; Beecher, G.R.; Goli, M.B.; Lusby, W.R.; Smith, J.C., Jr. Separation and identification of carotenoids and their oxidation products in the extracts of human plasma. Anal. Chem. **1992**, *64*, 2111–2122.
289. Andreoli, R.; Careri, M.; Manini, P.; Mori, G.; Musci, M. HPLC analysis of fat-soluble vitamins on standard and narrow bore columns with UV, electrochemical and particle beam MS detection. Chromatographia **1997**, *44*, 605–612.
290. Vetter, W.; Meister, W. Fast atom bombardment mass spectrum of $\beta$-carotene. Org. Mass. Spectrom. **1985**, *20*, 266–267.

291. Caccamese, S.; Garozzo, D. Odd-electron molecular ion and loss of toluene in fast atom bombardment mass spectra of some carotenoids. Org. Mass. Spectrom. **1990**, *25*, 137–140.
292. van Breemen, R.B.; Schmitz, H.H.; Schwartz, S.J. Continuous-flow fast atom bombardment liquid chromatography/mass spectrometry of carotenoids. Anal. Chem. **1993**, *65*, 965–969.
293. van Breemen, R.B. Electrospray liquid chromatography—mass spectrometry of carotenoids. Anal. Chem. **1995**, *67*, 2004–2009.
294. Rentel, C.; Strohschein, S.; Albert, K.; Bayer, E. Silver-plated vitamins: A method of detecting tocopherols and carotenoids in LC/ESI-MS coupling. Anal. Chem. **1998**, *70*, 4394–4400.
295. van Breemen, R.B.; Huang, C.R.; Tan, Y.; Sander, L.C.; Schilling, A.B. Liquid chromatography/mass spectrometry of carotenoids using atmospheric pressure chemical ionization. J. Mass. Spectrom. **1996**, *31*, 975–981.
296. Breithaupt, D.E.; Schwack, W. Determination of free and bound carotenoids in paprika (*Capsicum annuum* L.) by LC/MS. Eur. Food Res. Technol. **2000**, *211*, 52–55.
297. van Breemen, R.B.; Xu, X.; Viana, M.A.; Chen, L.; Stacewicz-Sapuntzakis, M.; Duncan, C.; Bowen, P.E.; Sharifi, R. Liquid chromatography-mass spectrometry of *cis* and *all-trans*-lycopene in human serum and prostate tissue after dietary supplementation with tomato sauce. J. Agric. Food Chem. **2002**, *50*, 2214–2219.
298. Breithaupt, D.E.; Wirt, U.; Bamedi, A. Differentiation between lutein monoester regioisomers and detection of lutein diesters from marigold flowers (*Tagetes erecta* L.) and several fruits by liquid chromatography-mass spectrometry. J. Agric. Food Chem. **2002**, *50*, 66–70.
299. Strohschein, S.; Rentel, C.; Lacker, T.; Bayer, E.; Albert, K. Separation and identification of tocotrienol isomers by HPLC-MS and HPLC-NMR coupling. Anal. Chem. **1999**, *71*, 1780–1785.
300. Lauridsen, C.; Leonard, S.W.; Griffin, D.A.; Liebler, D.C.; McClure, T.D.; Traber, M.C. Quantitative analysis by liquid chromatography-tandem mass spectrometry of deuterium-labeled and unlabeled vitamin E in biological samples. Anal. Biochem. **2001**, *289*, 89–95.
301. Gautier, J.C.; Holzhaeuser, D.; Markovic, J.; Gremaud, E.; Schilter, B.; Turesky, R.J. Oxidative damage and stress response from ochratoxin A exposure in rats. Free Radic. Biol. Med. **2001**, *30*, 1089–1098.
302. Mottier, P.; Gremaud, E.; Guy, P.A.; Turesky, R.J. Comparison of gas chromatography-mass spectrometry and liquid chromatography-tandem mass spectrometry methods to quantify $\alpha$-tocopherol and $\alpha$-tocopherolquinone levels in human plasma. Anal. Biochem. **2002**, *301*, 128–135.
303. Anton, K.; Berger, C. *Supercritical Fluid Chromatography with Packed Columns: Techniques and Applications*. Marcel Dekker: New York, 1997.
304. Lesellier, E. Analysis of non-saponifiable lipids by super-/subcritical-fluid chromatography. J. Chromatogr. **2001**, *A936*, 201–214.
305. Snyder, J.M.; Taylor, S.L.; King, J.W. Analysis of tocopherols by capillary supercritical fluid chromatography and mass spectrometry. JAOCS **1993**, *70*, 349–354.

306. King, J.W.; Favati, F.; Taylor, S.L. Production of tocopherol concentrates by supercritical fluid extraction and chromatography. Sep. Sci. Technol. **1996**, *31*, 1843–1857.
307. Manninen, P.; Laakso, P.; Kallio, H. Method for characterization of triacylglycerols and fat-soluble vitamins in edible oils and fats by supercritical fluid chromatography. JAOCS **1995**, *72*, 1001–1008.
308. Ibáñez, E.; Palacios, J.; Señoráns, F.J.; Santa-Maria, G.; Tabera, J.; Reglero, G. Isolation and separation of tocopherols from olive by-products with supercritical fluids. JACOS **2000**, *77*, 187–190.
309. de Lucas, A.; de la Ossa, E.M.; Rincón, J.; Blanco, M.A.; Graca, I. Supercritical fluid extraction of tocopherol concentrates from olive tree leaves. J. Supercrit. Fluids **2002**, *22*, 221–228.
310. Carlucci, G.; Mazzeo, P.; Governatore, S.D.; Giacomo, G.D.; Re, G.D. Liquid chromatographic method for the analysis of tocopherols in malt sprouts with supercritical fluid extraction. J. Chromatogr. **2001**, *A935*, 87–91.
311. Ibáñez, E.; Tabera, J.; Reglero, G.; Herraiz, M. Optimization of fat-soluble vitamin separation by supercritical fluid chromatography. Chromatographia **1995**, *40*, 448–452.
312. Shen, Y.; Bradshaw, J.S.; Lee, M.L. Packed capillary column supercritical fluid chromatography of fat-soluble vitamins using liquid crystal polysiloxane coated particles. Chromatographia **1996**, *43*, 53–58.
313. Ibáñez, E.; Herraiz, M.; Reglero, G. On-line SFE-SFC coupling using micropacked columns. J. High Resol. Chromatogr. **1995**, *18*, 507–509.
314. Ibáñez, E.; Palacios, J.; Reglero, G. Analysis of tocopherols by on-line coupling supercritical fluid extraction-supercritical fluid chromatography. J. Microclumn. Sep. **1999**, *11*, 605–611.
315. Señoráns, F.J.; Markides, K.E.; Nyholm, L. Determination of tocopherols and vitamin A in vegetable oils using packed capillary column supercritical fluid chromatography with electrochemical detection. J. Microcolumn. Sep. **1999**, *11*, 385–391.
316. Schmitz, J.J.; Artz, W.E.; Poor, C.L.; Dietz, J.M.; Erdman, J.W., Jr. High-performance liquid chromatography and capillary supercritical-fluid chromatography separation of vegetable carotenoids and carotenoid isomers. J. Chromatogr. **1989**, *479*, 261–268.
317. Aubert, M.C.; Lee, C.R.; Krstulović, A.M.; Lesellier, E.; Pèchard, M.R.; Tchapla, A. Separation of *trans/cis* $\alpha$- and $\beta$-carotenes by supercritical fluid chromatography. J. Chromatogr. **1991**, *557*, 47–67.
318. Lesellier, E.; Krstulović, A.M.; Tchapla, A. Specific effects of modifiers in subcritical fluid chromatography of carotenoid pigments. J. Chromatogr. **1993**, *641*, 137–145.
319. Lesellier, E.; Krstulović, A.M.; Tchapla, A. Influence of the modifiers on the nature of the stationary phase and the separation of carotenes in sub-critical fluid chromatography. Chromatographia **1993**, *36*, 275–282.
320. Lesellier, E.; Tchapla, A.; Krstulović, A.M. Use of carotenoids in the characterization of octadecylsilane bonded columns and mechanism of retention of carotenoids on monomeric and polymeric stationary phases. J. Chromatogr. **1993**, *645*, 29–39.

321. Lesellier, E.; Tchapla, A.; Marty, C.; Lebert, A. Analysis of carotenoids by high-performance liquid chromatography and supercritical fluid chromatography. J. Chromatogr. **1993**, *633*, 9–23.
322. Sakaki, K.; Shinbo, T.; Kawamura, M. Retention behavior of β-carotene on polar and nonpolar stationary phases in supercritical fluid chromatography. J. Chromatogr. Sci. **1994**, *32*, 172–178.
323. Ibáñez, E.; Lopez-Sebastian, S.; Tabera, J.; Reglero, G. Separation of carotenoids by subcritical fluid chromatography with coated, packed capillary columns and neat carbon dioxide. J. Chromatogr. **1998**, *A823*, 313–319.
324. Lesellier, E.; Gurdale, K.; Tchapla, A. Separation of *cis/trans* isomers of β-carotene by supercritical fluid chromatography. J. Chromatogr. **1999**, *A844*, 307–320.
325. Sander, L.C.; Sharpless, K.E.; Craft, N.E.; Wise, S.A. Development of engineered stationary phases for the separation of carotenoid isomers. Anal. Chem. **1994**, *66*, 1667–1674.
326. Sander, L.C.; Sharpless, K.E.; Pursch, M. $C_{30}$ stationary phases for the analysis of food by liquid chromatography. J. Chromatogr. **2000**, *A880*, 189–202.
327. Rouseff, R.; Raley, L. Application of diode array detection with a C-30 reversed phase column for the separation and identification of saponified orange juice carotenoids. J. Agric. Food Chem. **1996**, *44*, 2176–2181.
328. Darnoko, D.; Cheryan, M.; Moros, E.; Jerrel, J.; Perkins, E.G. Simutaneous HPLC analysis of palm carotenoids and tocopherols using a C-30 column and photodiode array detector. J. Liq. Chromatogr. Rel. Technol. **2000**, *23*, 1873–1885.
329. Strohschein, S.; Pursch, M.; Lubda, D.; Albert, K. Shape selectivity of C-30 phases for RP-HPLC separation of tocophenol isomers and correlation with MAS NMR data from suspended stationary phases. Anal. Chem. **1988**, *70*, 13–18.
330. Schieber, A.; Marx, M.; Carle, R. Simultaneous determination of carotenes and tocopherols in ATBC drinks by high-performance liquid chromatography. Food Chem. **2002**, *76*, 357–362.
331. AOAC International. *Official Methods of Analysis*, 17th ed., Chaps. 45, 50. AOAC International: Arlington, VA, 2000.
332. AOAC International. Report of the AOAC International Task Force on Methods for Nutrient Labeling Analyses. JAOAC Int. **1993**, *76*, 108A–201A.
333. Pocklington, W.D.; Dieffenbacher, A. Determination of tocopherols and tocotrienols in vegetable oils and fats by high performance liquid chromatography: Results of a colloboration study and the standardized method. Pure Appl. Chem. **1988**, *60*, 877–892.
334. United States Pharmacopeial Convention. U.S. Pharmacopeia National Formulary, USP25N/F20, Nutritional Supplements, Official Monographs. United States Pharmacopeial Convention: Rockville, MD, 2002; 1804–1806, 2427–2429, 2450–2451, 2430, 2435, 2437 pp.
335. Scottish Home and Health Department. *British Pharmacopoeia*, 15th ed. British Pharmacopoeic Convention:, 1993; 675–677, 1394, 1464 pp.

336. American Feed Ingredients Association. *Laboratory Methods Compendium*, Vol. I. Vitamins and Minerals. American Feed Ingredients Association: West Des Moines, 1991; 197–213 pp.
337. Keller, H.E. *Analytical Methods for Vitamins and Carotenoids*. Hoffmann-LaRoche: Basel, 1988; 12–16.
338. *Food Chemicals Codex*, 4th ed. National Academy Press: Washington DC, 1996; 417–424.
339. Brubacher, G.; Müller-Mulot, W.; Southgate, D.A.T. *Methods for the Determination of Vitamins in Foods Recommended by COST 91*. Elsevier Applied Science: New York, 1985.

# 8

# Food Composition—Vitamin E

## 8.1. INTRODUCTION

Over the past two decades, general interest in the vitamin E content of the human diet dramatically increased as knowledge of the interrelationships of vitamin E to the cure and/or prevention of chronic diseases developed. As is the case for many other nutrients and food components that are gaining increased interest among consumers, reliable data on food composition and guides to intake are fragmented in the scientific literature or largely undeveloped. This is certainly the present situation for vitamin E. Although substantial data are available, they are spread throughout the scientific literature. Our goal in this chapter is to provide an organized guide to the vitamin E content of food based on reliable data obtained with gas and liquid chromatographic methods that are currently acceptable for the analysis and reporting of vitamin E levels in the food supply.

## 8.2. FOOD COMPOSITION DATABASES AND VITAMIN E

Availability and access to food composition information are improving with the development and/or expansion of food composition databases provided by governmental and international agencies involved with the dissemination of nutrition information to the public. Currently, more than 150 food composition or nutrient databases are in existence (1). These databases widely vary in the foods represented, methods of presentation, format, currentness, nutrients included, units used, and general worth. The International Network of Food Data Systems (INFOODS) (2) under the auspices of the Food and Agriculture Organization has the goal of harmonizing international procedures for better interchange and comparability of nutrient data (3). Additionally, guidelines are provided on organization and content of food composition data-bases, food descriptions and classifications, analytical methods, units, and nutrient terminology. INFOODS tagnames (4,5) provide harmonization in nomenclature of foods and nutrients. The tagnames are significant to global harmonization of nutrient data and define the units on a nutrient data-base. This advance is particularly important for exchange of data on an inter-national basis (6). INFOODS (2) provides a complete guide to available food composition tables on its website (http://www.fao.org/infoods/index-em.stm). The following are brief descriptions of significant food composition sources together with a discussion of their treatment of vitamin E data.

## 8.2.1. National Nutrient Databases

1. United States—The USDA's *Composition of Foods: Raw, Processed Prepared*, Agricultural Handbook, 8-1–8-21, with additional supplements. [7–31] The USDA handbook represents the most comprehensive nutrient database available. All data in the printed version have been converted to electronic data files available over the World Wide Web, http://www.nal.usda.gov/fnic/foodcomp (32). The latest version, USDA Nutrient Database for Standard Reference, Release 16 (32), represents more than three decades of efforts to upgrade the availability and reliability of compositional information pertinent to the United States consumer's diet. It is available at no cost on the Internet, providing compositional information on 6661 food items. Up to 125 components are covered for each food. Vitamin E values are provided for 3567 food items. Data files are rapidly revised as new compositional information becomes available. Emphasis has been placed on improving available information on vitamin E through contract analysis supported by the USDA Nutrient Data Laboratory. References for the data are not provided, but, on request, original sources of the analytical values can be obtained. The vitamin E values were given as milligram $\alpha$-tocopherol equivalents (mg $\alpha$-TEs) calculated from the following accepted conversion factors (see Chapter 2) through Release 15 (33–35):

| | mg $\alpha$-TE |
|---|---|
| 1 mg *RRR*-$\alpha$-T | = 1 |
| 1 mg *RRR*-$\beta$-T | = 0.5 |
| 1 mg *RRR*-$\gamma$-T | = 0.1 |
| 1 mg *RRR*-$\delta$-T | = 0.01 |
| 1 mg *RRR*-$\alpha$-T3 | = 0.3 |
| 1 mg *RRR*-$\beta$-T3 | = 0.05 |
| 1 mg *RRR*-$\gamma$-T3 | = Unknown |
| 1 mg *RRR*-$\delta$-T3 | = Unknown |
| 1 mg *all-rac*-$\alpha$-T | = 0.74 |
| 1 mg *all-rac*-$\alpha$-T acetate | = 0.67 |
| 1 mg *all-rac*-$\alpha$-T succinate | = 0.6 |

$\alpha$-Tocopherol ($\alpha$-T) concentrations and levels of other tocopherols and tocotrienols are provided when available. Beginning with Release 16, the USDA Nutrient Database for Standard Reference reports only $\alpha$-T values and mg $\alpha$-TE are no longer used. This change reflects the recommendation of the Institute of Medicine Dietary Reference Intake (DRI) report[36] that recommended intakes of vitamin E for the human be based only on *2R*-stereoisomeric forms of $\alpha$-T (see Chapter 2). It is assumed that quantitative data for all tocopherols and tocotrienols will be reported when reliable data are available.

2. United Kingdom—*McCance and Widdowson's The Composition of Foods, 6th Edition* (37), and its supplements form the basis of the UK Nutrient Database (http://www.rsc.org/is/database/nutsabou.htm) (38). The database is accessible through licensing agreements with the copyright office of Her Majesty's Stationery Office (HMSO). *McCance and Widdowson's The Composition of Foods* tabulates nutrients on more than 1200 common food items consumed in the United Kingdom. Vitamin E values are given for approximately 700 food items in 13 food categories as milligram $\alpha$-TE units. Many of the analytical values were obtained through studies commissioned by the UK Ministry of Agriculture, Fisheries and Food. Literature sources are not provided for the analytical values given in the text.

3. Australia—The Australian nutrient database, *The Composition of Foods, Australia*, is based on several publications published in handbook format from 1989 to 1993 (39–45). The database has not been introduced to the World Wide Web. The database covers more than 2500 food items but does not include vitamin E data. Vitamin E analysis is part of studies commissioned by the Australian Government Analytical Laboratories (46), but, at this time, such data are not included in the published database. Lewis and associates[46] and Cashel

and Greenfield[47] give detailed descriptions of the plans for use of the database, largely sponsored by the Australian National Food Authority.

4. New Zealand—The New Zealand food composition database is rapidly expanding and currently contains data on more than 2000 food items. It is a compilation of data obtained from Australia, the United Kingdom, United States Department of Agriculture, and New Zealand analytical studies and various other international sources. The primary compilation, containing information on 28 nutrients, is The Concise New Zealand Food Composition Tables (48), which is a subset of the New Zealand Food Composition Database. Other publications arising from the database include *Composition of New Zealand Foods*: Volumes 1, *Characteristic Fruits and Vegetables*;[49] 2, *Export Fruits and Vegetables*;[50] 3, *Dairy Products*;[51] 4, *Poultry*;[52] and 5, *Bread and Flour* (53). Vitamin E is not included in the published information but is included for some food items in the complete New Zealand Food Composition Database, which can be obtained from the New Zealand Institute for Crop and Food Research.

5. Pacific Islands—The Pacific Islands Food Composition Tables[54] represent data compiled from several databases on 800 foods common to the Pacific Islands. Data are provided for 22 nutrients including vitamin E on 800 food items. However, vitamin E values are not available for all foods in the composition table (55).

## 8.2.2. Books

1. *Bowes and Church's Food Values of Portions Commonly Used*, 17th ed (56).

This source, representing one of the oldest food composition sources, provides vitamin E values for more than 2000 foods on the basis of international units. The data in the 17th edition were obtained from 92 food companies and trade associations and from the United States Department of Agriculture, Nutrient Data Base for Standard Reference, Release 11 (SR11). The vitamin E table provides a quick guide to approximate vitamin E levels in 34 food classifications. Individual food values are not referenced by source.

2. SW Souci, W Fachmann, H Kraut. *Food Composition and Nutrition Tables*. 6th ed. Boca Raton: CRC Press, 2000 (57).

This excellent compilation of nutrient values of European foods provides composition information on approximately 1100 food items with vitamin E values for more than 200 of the foods. The Souci and colleagues (57) tables treat vitamin E data more comprehensively than previously mentioned sources, in that values are given in milligrams per 100 g for the specific tocopherols and tocotrienols in the foods and as total vitamin E (milligrams per 100 g), representing milligrams of $\alpha$-TE calculated according to McLaughlin and

Weihrauch (33). Some confusion can arise in interpretation of the meaning of the total tocopherol value, since it is a representation of the milligrams of $\alpha$-TE and not mg/100 g of total tocopherols on a weight basis. The definition of total vitamin E is clearly stated in the introductory description of the methodology; however, the milligrams of $\alpha$-TE designation is not provided on the table. Sources for the analytical values are not referenced by the authors. The 6th edition is now on-line[58] (www.sfk-online.net).

### 8.2.3. Book Chapters, Reviews, and Historically Significant Journal Articles

Slover[59] published a review of the literature covering vitamin E composition papers published between 1964 and 1970. Slover's review represents the first compilation of vitamin E that provides comprehensive information on the specific forms of tocopherols and tocotrienols present in common dietary sources largely determined by gas chromatographic (GC) methods. Up until this time, vitamin E compositional tables reported vitamin E as total tocopherols or were limited to values for $\alpha$-T. Two reviews cited by Slover have historical significance. The first large compilation of vitamin E compositional data, published by Harris and coworkers[60] in 1962, considered the retention of vitamin E in processed and stored foods. The Harris and associates compilation clearly showed that a strong correlation existed between total tocopherol level in oils and degree of unsaturation, indicating the role of vitamin E as an antioxidant (61). Dicks[62] in 1965 published a large review citing more than 400 publications on the vitamin E content of foods. Slover[59] stated that about 5% of the data cited by Dicks included information on the individual tocopherols or tocotrienols that were present in the individual foods.

As late as 1970, Draper[61] in an extensive treatment of the tocopherols used data from Harris and associates (63), 1950; Brown (64), 1953; Mahon and Chapman (65), 1954; Green (66), 1958; Mason and Jones (67), 1958; Booth and Bradford (68), 1963; and Hertig and Drury (69), 1963, to report $\alpha$-T levels. All of these data were obtained by methods other than GC.

Slover's review[59] on work up through 1969 was based on 23 citations including several studies completed in the 1950s by thin-layer chromatography that quantitated the tocopherols and tocotrienols. Values were provided for 15 oils, 13 seeds, seven grains, and seven fruits and vegetables. In summarizing the data, Slover noted that for seeds and oils

> consistent patterns are beginning to emerge. Refined and prepared foods are less predictable. These have tocopherol contents that depend on processing, treatment and formulation, and both identities and amounts vary greatly. The accumulation of a body of useful data will depend on

> the use of specific reproducible methods applied to adequately described samples. There is still much work to be done in this field.

Indeed, we are still trying to meet the challenge of providing accurate vitamin E data, as alluded to by Slover in 1970. Slover's tabulation clearly showed the variability to be expected in natural vitamin E sources and the uniqueness of vitamin E profiles of specific food sources.

Shortly after the publication of Slover's (59) compilation, Ames (70) published $\alpha$-T values for 178 foods based on 23 references published from 1950 to 1967. At the time of publication of Ames's review (1972), significant data of a much more specific nature, collected largely by GC methods, were available. Ames's objective was to provide data on the availability of $\alpha$-T in the U.S. food supply, which was known to be the primary provider of vitamin E activity to the consumer on the basis of surveys completed before the compilation of the data. Ames's data showed that in the United States in 1960, approximately 10 mg per day $\alpha$-T was available for consumption from fats and oils and 5 mg per day from other food fats including dairy products, eggs, meats, legumes, nuts, fruits, vegetables, and grains. Although Ames's review did not improve the availability of information on the specific vitamin E profiles of the food supply, it did create a significantly clearer picture of where the U.S. consumer obtained dietary $\alpha$-T.

In 1977, Bauernfeind (71) presented a quite comprehensive compilation of vitamin E food composition values, which was later published in book chapter format (72). The data were organized into 15 food categories for 472 food items. Bauernfeind cited 26 references covering the period 1965–1975. Examination of the tabular data shows that most vitamin E values were based on assay of one sample and few values were determined from 10 or more samples. Although the data were limited in many instances to very low sample numbers, Bauernfeind's compilation of vitamin E food values has been useful to many investigators as the best available guide to vitamin E food composition. Data were provided on the basis of milligrams per 100 g for the tocopherols and tocotrienols, and the sum of their values was reported as milligrams total tocopherols/100 g. Bauernfeind stated that an unrealized objective of those involved with vitamin E food composition should be the "complete understanding of the distribution and significance of the known tocopherols in our commonly used food products." He recognized the lack of knowledge on vitamin E composition in 1977 and clearly stated its shortcomings:

> the table must be used with caution as the data have been obtained by different methodologies and by different investigators. Added to variation in natural content of food are further influences of harvesting, processing, and storage variables. Hence, while reference to food composition tables may give one a relative concept of tocopherol values, the best estimate of tocopherol content will be an analysis of the food sample in question (71).

Bauernfeind (71) certainly put shortcomings of all food composition tables—shortcomings that we still face—in perspective with that statement. Bauernfeind's treatment of the available data were particularly helpful to investigators wishing to access the literature, since all data were referenced to the original source.

McLaughlin and Weihrauch (33) published the first compilation of the U.S. Department of Agriculture of the vitamin E content of food in 1979. Data were provided on 506 food items and reported tocopherol, tocotrienols, and total vitamin E on a milligrams per 100 g basis. The data were compiled from more than 300 scientific articles, but values were not referenced to the sources, because the values were reported as averages of all data judged to be reliable by the authors. Deficiencies of available studies noted by McLaughlin and Weihrauch (33) included the following: (a) Many sources reported only total vitamin E or $\alpha$-T; (b) for some foods, partial reports were available with only a few analyses of all the vitamin E homologues; (c) variation among samples was high, requiring the data to be reported as a range for total vitamin E; (d) $\beta$-T and $\gamma$-T were often reported as a sum because of the inability of various methods to resolve the positional isomers.

Of major significance, McLaughlin and Weihrauch (33) presented the factors to calculate milligrams $\alpha$-TE to include the participation of tocopherols and tocotrienols other than $\alpha$-T in a measure of the biological activity of vitamin E. It was clear from calculations presented by the authors that consideration of only $\alpha$-T content of a food, or of only total vitamin E content, does not always provide complete information about the vitamin E biological activity based on biological activity as understood at the time. The use of milligrams $\alpha$-TE was first accepted by the Food and Nutrition Board as the accepted way to express vitamin E activity of the diet with publication of the 9th edition of the Recommended Dietary Allowances (34) in 1980. Factors were the same as given by McLaughlin and Weihrauch (33), except the factor to convert $\beta$-T (mg) to mg $\alpha$-TE was 0.5 instead of the 0.4 factor used originally. In 2000, the Institute of Medicine, Panel on Dietary Antioxidants and Related Compounds (36) recommended that only *2R*-stereoisomeric forms of $\alpha$-T be considered as sources of vitamin E for the human. On the basis of the quite clear specificity of the $\alpha$-T transfer protein for the *2R*-stereoisomers, Dietary Reference Intakes (DRIs) were set by using only $\alpha$-T (see Chapter 2). This major change in view of the DRI panel compared to the earlier Recommended Dietary Allowance discussions on the role of other tocopherols and tocotrienols in human nutrition will undoubtedly decrease the use of $\alpha$-TE in relation to human vitamin E requirements and will most likely change vitamin E labeling of foods and pharmaceuticals.

Despite plans promulgated by McLaughlin and Weihrauch (33) to include vitamin E values in revised and updated sections of Agricultural Handbook No. 8,[7–31] vitamin E information was not included in United States Department of

Agriculture databases until computerized versions of the USDA Database for Standard Reference were released.

In 1990, USDA personnel together with Food and Drug Administration personnel summarized vitamin E levels from several studies (73) and unpublished USDA contract work. The vitamin E values were presented on 85 food items in eight food categories. At this point in time, Sheppard (73) noted that vitamin E levels in vegetable oils, nuts, seeds, and other unprocessed foods tend to present predictable quantitative and qualitative patterns. However, such patterns are not discernible in processed and highly refined foods. These authors also stated that the tabular data should be used with caution because of the many variables recognized to cause large deviations in analytical values for vitamin E content of specific foods. They further suggested that when precise vitamin E intake data are required, they should be obtained by analysis of the foods in the form consumed. The recommendations follow those presented by Bauernfeind in 1977 (71).

## 8.3. VITAMIN E FOOD COMPOSITION TABLES

As food scientists working in the nutritional quality area, we have been extensively involved with the generation of vitamin E food compositional data over a good part of our careers. We know that excellent data exist on the tocopherol and tocotrienol content of the food supply and that, at the same time, it is increasingly difficult to gain fast access to verifiable data. We also know that access to literature sources pertaining to specific food matrices is often required in food analysis laboratories. One of the primary objectives of the completion this book was to compile the more recent vitamin E composition data, primarily those quantified by liquid chromatographic (LC) methodology, into a usable reference source for those in all areas of science needing access to values and to the original literature on which the vitamin E data were obtained. We included data from studies through the 1970s that Bauernfeind published as the chapter "Tocopherols in Foods" in L. J. Machlin's *Vitamin E: A Comprehensive Treatise* (72). Indeed, we have personally relied heavily on this excellent source as a ready guide to vitamin E food composition information and to the studies behind the "numbers." The facts that we appreciate Bauernfeind's effort and that this compilation is now more than 20 years old convinced us to develop the following food composition tables referenced to the original research.

### 8.3.1. Developmental Aspects of the Vitamin E Tables

It is often difficult when using databases of food composition information to make high-quality judgments of the values. Indeed, the user may be looking at imputed values (values determined from samples of similar nature but not of the exact sample) or at values obtained through poorly conducted studies. For each cited reference used in the tables, we have provided a quality evaluation of the data based on a system developed by United States Department of Agriculture personnel for application to the USDA Nutrient Database.[74–79] The evaluation system evaluates data in five general categories: the suitability of the analytical method, quality control applied to the assay, number of samples, sample handling, and the sampling plan used to ensure representative samples. Details of the evaluation criteria along with relative scores for the five evaluation categories are provided in Table 8.1. Specific criteria pertain to each category and ratings range from 0 (unacceptable) to 3 (highly acceptable). A quality index was calculated on the basis of overall data quality of each referenced vitamin E value. According to the USDA evaluation system, the mean of the five ratings determines the quality index (QI).

The USDA evaluation includes the determination of a quality sum and the assignment of a confidence code to indicate the relative strength of a dataset for a food. We applied the USDA confidence code as explained in Table 8.2 to the foods included in our compilation. A confidence code of A indicates considerable confidence because of the existence of either a few high-quality studies or a larger number of studies of varying quality (74). Codes of B or C indicate lesser confidence in the vitamin E value.

The system as we used it was first designed by USDA as a manual system to assess the analytical data for copper, selenium, and the carotenoids.[74–79] In 2002, a new data evaluation system that expands the rating scales of the evaluation criteria was developed by the USDA Nutrient Data Laboratory. The expanded data evaluation system was created as a module for the recently redesigned USDA Nutrient Databank, Architecture and Integration Management, Nutrient Data Bank System (AIM-NDBS) (80).

In addition to the original USDA data quality evaluation, we applied the following procedures to compilation of the data on vitamin E:

1. All data were obtained from the scientific literature or, in some instances, contract reports to USDA originating in the authors' laboratory. None was retrieved from existing handbook compilations, databases, or review articles.
2. Data for the most part represent values determined by LC and GC. In a few cases, data were obtained by two-dimensional thin-layer-chromatography (TLC) or other analytical methods. These studies are denoted in Table 8.3 by footnote h on the reference number.
3. Means were calculated from analyses of like samples, if not provided by the original authors.
4. All values for the vitamin E homologues were converted to milligrams per 100 g if not reported as such.

**TABLE 8.1** Generic Description of Food Composition Data Evaluation Criteria

| Criteria categories | Relative scores 3 | 2 | 1 | 0 |
|---|---|---|---|---|
| Analytical method | Published documentation with validation for foods analyzed, including use of appropriate reference material with results within acceptable range or 95%–105% recoveries on similar food and use of other method or laboratory on same sample with excellent agreement; acceptable repeatability; exemplary processing of sample; detailed identification of analyte(s) | Some documentation; incomplete validation studies, including 90%–110% recoveries on similar foods or use of other method or laboratory on same sample with good agreement; acceptable repeatability; adequate processing of sample; adequate identification of analyte(s) | Some documentation; minimal validation, including 80%–120% recoveries on food similar to sample or use of other method or laboratory on related food with acceptable agreement; acceptable repeatability; minimally acceptable processing of sample; limited identification of analyte(s) | No documentation of method, no reference or inaccessible reference given; no validation studies or failure to achieve acceptable results with reference material, lack of acceptable repeatability, recovery (<80% or 120%), or comparison method or laboratory; inadequate processing of sample; inadequate identification of analyte(s) |
| Analytical quality control | Optimal accuracy and precision of method monitored and indicated explicitly by data | Documentation of assessment of both accuracy and precision of method; acceptable accuracy and precision | Some description of minimally acceptable accuracy and/or precision | No documentation of accuracy or precision; unacceptable accuracy and/or precision |

| Number of samples | Extensive | Adequate | Limited | — |
|---|---|---|---|---|
| Sampling handling | Complete documentation of procedures including analysis of edible portion only, validation of homogenization method, details of food preparation, and storage and moisture changes monitored | Pertinent procedures documented including analysis of edible portion only; procedures that seem reasonable but some unreported details | Limited description of procedures including evidence of analysis of edible portion only | Totally inappropriate procedures or no documentation of criteria pertinent to food analyzed |
| Sampling plan | Multiple geographical sampling with description of and statistical basis for sampling, sample representative of brands/varieties consumed or commercially used; comprehensive sampling of wholesale locations, or special or ethnic foods with limited distribution | At least two geographic regions sample; sample representative; representative sampling of wholesale locations, or special or ethnic foods with limited distribution | One geographical area sampled; sample representative of what some eat; limited sampling of wholesale locations, or special or ethnic foods with limited distribution | Not described or unrepresentative sample |

*Source*: Modified from Refs. 74–77.

**Table 8.2** Assignment and Meaning of Confidence Codes

| Sum of quality indexes | Confidence code | Meaning of confidence code |
|---|---|---|
| >6.0 | A | The user can have considerable confidence in this value. |
| 3.4 to 6.0 | B | The user can have confidence in this value; however, some problems regarding the data on which the value is based exist. |
| 1.0 to <3.4 | C | The user can have less confidence in this value because of limited quantity and/or quality of data. |

*Source*: Modified from Refs. 74–77.

5. Milligrams $\alpha$-tocopherol equivalent values were calculated from the data if not provided in the original report.
6. If a study was rated as zero by evaluation of the analytical method or if any three ratings were zero, the data were not included in the mean or range reported for the specific food matrices. A quality index of 1 or greater indicated an acceptable value for use in the table (74).

## 8.3.2. Vitamin E Composition of Food

Table 8.3 represents data compiled from 111 research publications and from USDA contracts completed in the authors' laboratory from 1988 to 2001. Data used for the compilation appeared in the literature from 1970 through 2002. Publications appearing after 1980 represent data collected almost exclusively by high-performance liquid chromatography (HPLC) analysis. Studies from 1970 through 1979 include most of the meaningful reports on the vitamin E content of food assayed by gas chromatographic techniques. These data were included in previous compilations of vitamin E food composition (33,71–72). For the majority of the food items, data published before 1970 were not included in the tabulation. In the case of fats and oils, a few significant composition papers published in the 1960s were included. Although we have attempted over the years to compile all of the available literature on vitamin E in foods, undoubtedly some pertinent data have been omitted. To those authors, we apologize and ask to be informed of such omissions so that the data will be included in future revisions of the table.

**8.3.2.1. Oils and Fats.** Not surprisingly, the largest body of food composition data on vitamin E exists for oils and fats. Since all natural forms of vitamin E are plant-derived, vegetable oils are the single most important and concentrated source of vitamin E to the human. Early studies (63,167,168) as compiled by Ames (70) showed that in the average human diet in the United States more than 50% of the vitamin E was obtained from oilseeds and vegetable sources. Carpenter et al. (81) reported the rapid increase in vegetable oil consumption in the United States during the mid-1900s. Consumption of liquid vegetable oils increased from 6.5% of all fat consumed (1947–49) to 16.3% in 1973. Margarine and dairy products at this point contributed 6.8% and 10%, respectively, of total fat consumed.

During this period, increased emphasis was placed on method development and the completion of studies to delineate the content of vitamin E in specific foods. Research emphasis on food composition was due to the following factors: (a) increased understanding of human and animal vitamin E requirements, (b) understanding of the relationship of requirements to the level of intake of polyunsaturated fatty acids, and (c) clearer understanding of oxidative aspects of oil stability and the oil's vitamin E content.

Data collected before 1970 were extensive enough in the identification and quantification of vitamin E profiles of oils and fats to show that consistent patterns existed for tocopherols and tocotrienols by food source. Slover (59) first recognized this aspect of food composition. Data on fats and oils in Table 8.3 include several studies completed during the 1960s (91–92,101,106) by thin-layer or early gas chromatographic techniques. These data are quite comparable to data provided by later studies using more refined GC and HPLC methods.

The vitamin E content of a specific plant oil is quite variable because of cultivar variation and above all variation induced by oxidative changes that occur throughout the harvesting, processing, marketing, and utilization stages. Because of the natural antioxidant activity of the vitamin E homologues, oxidative events can lead to large losses in biological activity (see Chapters 3 and 5). The differences in biological activity of the vitamin E homologues led to the development of the milligram $\alpha$-TE calculation and its acceptance by the nutrition community as a measure of the biological activity of vitamin E in a food source from all forms of the vitamin (34). Biological activity reported as milligrams $\alpha$-TE is largely influenced by the amount of $\alpha$-T in the fat or oil. However, for some oils, such as soybean, quite large amounts of other homologues can significantly contribute to the milligram $\alpha$-TE value. In the future, use of milligram $\alpha$-T will be less emphasized as a result of better understanding of the role of $\alpha$-T in human nutrition (see Sec. 8.2.1) (36). However, for comparative purposes, milligram $\alpha$-TE is included in the vitamin E composition table. Table 8.4 summarizes some of the data on fats and oils with regard to $\alpha$-T, total vitamin E, milligram $\alpha$-TE levels, and primary forms of vitamin E. Mean values from Table 8.3 were used to formulate Table 8.4. The oils and fats are ordered from the highest to lowest

**TABLE 8.3** Tocopherols and Tocotrienols in Selected Food Products (mg/100 g)

| Product | CC[a] | QI[b] | α-T[c] | β-T | γ-T | δ-T | α-T3[d] | β-T3 | γ-T3 | δ-T3 | Total | α-TE[e] mg | Ref. |
|---|---|---|---|---|---|---|---|---|---|---|---|---|---|
| **Oils and fats** | | | | | | | | | | | | | |
| Apricot kernel oil | C | 1.4 | 1.0 | — | 17.0 | 2.0 | — | — | — | — | 20.0 | 2.7 | 81 |
| Avocado oil | C | 1.4 | 6.4 | — | 1.9 | — | — | — | — | — | 8.3 | 6.6 | 82 |
| Barley oil | C | 1.8 | 0.3 | 0.1 | 0.1 | Tr | 1.2 | 0.3 | 0.1 | — | 2.1 | 0.7 | 83 |
| | | 1.2 | 14.2 | 0.6 | 10.4 | 0.1 | 55.8 | — | 8.5 | 0.5 | 90.1 | 32.3 | 166 |
| Canbra oil | C | 1.2 | 24.0 | — | 69.0 | 2.0 | — | — | — | — | 95.0 | 31.0 | 84 |
| Castor oil | B | 2.2 | 0.9 | 0.9 | 45.8 | 34.3 | — | — | — | — | 82.0 | 7.0 | 85 |
| | | 1.2 | — | 1.6 | 29.2 | 50.2 | — | Tr | — | — | 81.0 | 5.2 | 86 |
| | | 1.4 | 2.8 | 2.9 | 11.1 | 31.0 | — | — | — | — | 47.8 | 5.4 | 82 |
| **Castor oil mean ± SD** | | | 1.2 ± 1.2 | 1.8 ± 0.8 | 28.7 ± 14.2 | 38.5 ± 8.4 | — | Tr | — | — | 70.3 ± 15.9 | 5.9 ± 0.8 | |
| Canola and rapeseed oil | A | 2.2 | 20.9 | 0.1 | 42.2 | 1.2 | 0.2 | — | Tr | — | 64.6 | 25.3 | 87 |
| | | 2.8 | 16.4 | Tr | 28.4 | 0.9 | — | — | — | — | 45.8 | 19.3 | 88 |
| | | 1.4 | 17.2 | — | 21.3 | 2.0 | — | — | — | — | 40.5 | 19.4 | 89 |
| | | 2.2 | 18.9 | — | 48.6 | 1.2 | — | — | — | — | 68.7 | 23.8 | 85 |
| | | 1.0 | 23.8 | — | 42.4 | 1.1 | — | — | — | — | 67.3 | 28.5 | 89 |
| | | 1.2 | 33.5 | — | 55.0 | — | — | — | — | — | 88.5 | 39.0 | 84 |
| | | 1.2 | 22.5 | 1.5 | 59.2 | 4.1 | — | — | — | — | 87.3 | 29.3 | 167 |
| | | 2.0 | 19.7 | — | 58.6 | — | — | — | — | — | 78.3 | 25.6 | 206 |
| | | 2.0 | 9.9 | — | 15.1 | — | — | — | — | — | 12.5 | 11.4 | 208 |
| | | 2.0 | 19.7 | — | 36.9 | — | — | — | — | — | 56.6 | 23.4 | 209 |
| High-oleic | | 2.0 | 18.0 | — | 42.1 | — | — | — | — | — | 60.1 | 22.2 | 209 |
| High-oleic, low-linolenic | | 2.0 | 29.0 | — | 60.3 | — | — | — | — | — | 89.3 | 35.0 | 209 |
| Low-linolenic | | 2.0 | 15.2 | — | 37.4 | — | — | — | — | — | 52.6 | 18.9 | 209 |
| Rapeseed oil, crude | | 2.2 | 22.0 | — | 32.3 | 1.2 | — | — | — | — | 55.5 | 25.3 | 202 |
| bleached | | 2.0 | 19.9 | — | 29.1 | 0.9 | — | — | — | — | 49.9 | 22.8 | 202 |

| | | | | | | | | | | | | | |
|---|---|---|---|---|---|---|---|---|---|---|---|---|---|
| refined | | 2.0 | 15.4 | — | 22.4 | 0.7 | — | — | — | — | 38.5 | 17.6 | 202 |
| **Canola and rapeseed oil mean ± SD** | | | 21.9 ± 6.3 | Tr | 37.6 ± 11.3 | 1.3 ± 0.6 | Tr | — | Tr | — | 63.6 ± 17.3 | 26.7 ± 7.3 | |
| Cocoa butter | C | 1.4 | 0.6 | 0.2 | 17.8 | 0.3 | 0.3 | — | 0.9 | — | 20.2 | 2.7 | 90 |
| | | 2.0 | 1.2 | — | 20.6 | 3.4 | 0.8 | — | — | — | 26.0 | 3.5 | 199 |
| Cocoa butter, nonalkalized, deodorized | C | 1.4 | 1.8 | 0.4 | 19.6 | 1.4 | — | — | — | — | 23.2 | 4.0 | 82 |
| Cocoa butter, nonalkalized, nondeodorized | C | 1.4 | 1.0 | — | 17.0 | 1.7 | — | — | — | — | 19.8 | 2.8 | 82 |
| Coconut oil | B | 2.2 | 0.1 | — | 0.2 | — | 0.6 | — | 0.1 | — | 1.0 | 0.3 | 87 |
| | | 1.8 | 0.4 | — | 0.5 | — | 0.3 | 0.2 | 1.5 | — | 2.8 | 0.5 | 83 |
| | | 1.2 | 0.5 | — | — | 0.6 | 0.5 | 0.1 | 1.9 | — | 3.6 | 0.8 | 91 |
| | | 2.0 | 0.4 | — | — | 1.4 | 1.0 | — | 3.0 | — | 5.7 | 0.7 | 199 |
| **Coconut oil mean ± SD** | | | 0.3 ± 0.2 | — | 0.2 ± 0.2 | 0.2 ± 0.3 | 0.5 ± 0.1 | 0.1 ± 0.1 | 1.2 ± 0.8 | — | 2.5 ± 1.1 | 0.5 ± 0.2 | |
| Coconut oil, hardened | C | 2.2 | 1.8 | 0.3 | Tr | 0.4 | 1.1 | — | 0.3 | — | 3.9 | 2.3 | 85 |
| Cod liver oil | C | 2.2 | 20.3 | — | — | — | — | — | — | — | 20.3 | 20.3 | 85 |
| Corn oil | A | 2.2 | 25.7 | 1.0 | 75.2 | 3.3 | 1.5 | — | 2.0 | — | 108.7 | 34.2 | 85 |
| | | 1.4 | 17.3 | — | 62.3 | 4.5 | — | — | — | — | 84.2 | 23.6 | 81 |
| | | 1.2 | 20.8 | 1.4 | 105.6 | 3.7 | 1.0 | — | 1.3 | — | 133.8 | 32.4 | 86 |
| | | 1.2 | 12.1 | — | 52.5 | 0.4 | — | — | — | — | 65.0 | 17.3 | 91 |
| | | 1.2 | 17.0 | — | 66.0 | 5.0 | — | — | — | — | 88.0 | 23.8 | 84 |
| | | 1.0 | 26.0 | — | 89.5 | Tr | — | — | — | — | 115.5 | 34.0 | 93 |
| | | 1.0 | 11.9 | — | 39.5 | — | — | — | — | — | 51.4 | 15.9 | 94 |
| | | 1.4 | 12.3 | 0.5 | 58.5 | 2.6 | 1.2 | — | 1.1 | — | 76.7 | 18.8 | 95 |

*(continued)*

**TABLE 8.3** *Continued*

| Product | CC[a] | QI[b] | α-T[c] | β-T | γ-T | δ-T | α-T3[d] | β-T3 | γ-T3 | δ-T3 | Total | α-TE[e] mg | Ref. |
|---|---|---|---|---|---|---|---|---|---|---|---|---|---|
| | | 1.8 | 18.8 | 1.1 | 54.0 | 2.6 | — | — | — | — | 76.5 | 24.8 | 96 |
| | | 2.0 | 27.2 | 0.2 | 56.6 | 2.5 | 5.4 | 1.1 | 6.2 | — | 99.2 | 34.7 | 97 |
| | | 1.6 | 32.4 | 1.3 | 74.9 | 4.1 | 2.1 | — | — | — | 112.7 | 40.7 | 98 |
| | | 1.2 | 13.4 | 1.8 | 41.2 | 3.9 | — | — | — | — | 60.3 | 18.5 | 84 |
| | | 1.2 | 11.6 | 0.8 | 37.5 | 1.3 | 2.3 | — | 0.5 | — | 54.0 | 16.5 | 166 |
| | | 1.2 | 10.6 | 1.7 | 61.5 | 2.9 | 2.1 | — | 4.0 | — | 82.8 | 18.3 | 166 |
| | | 2.0 | 25.4 | — | 134.2 | 7.6 | — | — | — | — | 167.2 | 38.9 | 199 |
| | | 2.5 | 15.1 | 0.7 | 77.6 | 2.9 | 6.9 | — | 8.3 | — | 111.5 | 25.7 | 214 |
| **Corn oil mean ± SD** | | | 18.6 ± 6.9 | 1.1 ± 0.5 | 67.9 ± 25.4 | 3.1 ± 1.8 | 2.9 ± 2.3 | | 3.3 ± 3.0 | — | 93.0 ± 31.1 | 26.1 ± 8.5 | |
| Cottonseed oil | A | 2.0 | 40.3 | 0.2 | 38.3 | 0.5 | Tr | 0.8 | 0.1 | — | 80.2 | 44.3 | 97 |
| | | 1.4 | 57.3 | 4.0 | 31.7 | Tr | — | — | — | — | 93.0 | 62.5 | 99 |
| | | 1.2 | 31.0 | — | 33.0 | — | — | — | — | — | 64.0 | 34.3 | 100 |
| | | 1.2 | 40.2 | 0.2 | 57.2 | 0.8 | — | — | — | — | 98.3 | 46.0 | 84 |
| | | 2.0 | 32.0 | — | 31.3 | — | — | — | — | — | 63.3 | 35.1 | 101 |
| | | 1.2 | 32.0 | — | 31.3 | — | — | — | — | — | 63.3 | 35.1 | 91 |
| | | 1.0 | 48.9 | — | 29.6 | — | — | — | — | — | 78.5 | 51.9 | 92[h] |
| | | 1.2 | 34.0 | — | 27.0 | — | — | — | — | — | 61.0 | 36.7 | 84 |
| | | 1.0 | 56.0 | — | 38.0 | Tr | — | — | — | — | 94.0 | 59.8 | 93 |
| | | 1.0 | 42.6 | — | 36.9 | Tr | — | — | — | — | 79.5 | 46.3 | 102 |
| | | 1.8 | 30.5 | 0.3 | 10.5 | Tr | — | — | — | — | 41.3 | 31.7 | 96 |
| **Cottonseed oil mean ± SD** | | | 40.4 ± 9.4 | 0.4 ± 1.1 | 33.2 ± 10.5 | 0.1 ± 0.3 | Tr | Tr | Tr | — | 74.2 ± 16.5 | 44.0 ± 10.1 | |
| Grapefruit oil | <C | 0.8 | 26.5 | — | — | — | — | — | — | — | 26.5 | 26.5 | 103 |
| Grapeseed oil, virgin | C | 2.6 | 6.0 | — | 2.0 | — | 9.2 | — | 27.8 | 0.8 | 45.8 | 9.0 | 168 |
| Grapeseed oil, refined | C | 2.6 | 14.4 | — | — | — | 7.0 | — | 16.1 | — | 37.5 | 16.5 | 168 |
| Hazelnut oil | | 2.0 | 45.2 | — | 7.1 | 1.6 | — | — | — | — | 53.8 | 45.9 | 199 |
| Hazelnut oil, virgin | C | 2.6 | 36.0 | — | 5.6 | Tr | — | — | — | — | 41.6 | 36.6 | 168 |
| Lard | B | 2.2 | 0.6 | — | — | — | — | — | — | — | 0.6 | 0.6 | 87 |
| | | 2.0 | 1.2 | — | 0.1 | — | Tr | — | — | — | 1.3 | 1.2 | 101 |

| | | | | | | | | | | | | | |
|---|---|---|---|---|---|---|---|---|---|---|---|---|---|
| Lard | | 1.0 | 1.2 | — | 0.1 | — | 0.1 | — | — | — | 1.4 | 1.3 | 92[h] |
| **Lard mean ± SD** | | | 1.0 ± 0.3 | — | 0.1 ± 0.1 | — | Tr | — | — | — | 1.1 ± 0.4 | 1.0 ± 0.3 | |
| Linseed oil | B | 2.2 | 0.5 | — | 57.3 | 0.8 | — | — | — | — | 58.6 | 6.3 | 85 |
| | | 1.2 | 1.8 | 0.6 | 53.1 | 1.8 | — | — | — | — | 57.4 | 7.5 | 86 |
| Mustardseed, crude oil | C | 1.2 | 7.5 | — | 49.4 | 3.1 | — | — | — | — | 60.0 | 12.5 | 84 |
| Oats oil | C | 1.8 | 0.3 | 0.1 | — | — | 1.0 | 0.3 | — | — | 1.7 | 0.7 | 83 |
| Olive oil | A | 2.2 | 11.9 | — | 1.3 | — | — | — | — | — | 13.3 | 12.0 | 85 |
| | | 1.6 | 17.9 | 0.2 | 1.1 | Tr | Tr | — | — | — | 19.1 | 18.1 | 98 |
| | | 2.0 | 9.0 | 0.2 | 0.5 | Tr | — | 0.4 | Tr | — | 10.1 | 9.2 | 97 |
| | | 1.4 | 7.0 | — | 2.0 | Tr | — | — | — | — | 9.0 | 7.2 | 99 |
| | | 1.4 | 14.0 | — | — | — | — | — | — | — | 14.0 | 14.0 | 81 |
| | | 1.2 | 9.3 | — | 0.7 | — | — | — | — | — | 10.0 | 9.4 | 84 |
| | | 1.8 | 9.3 | — | 0.8 | — | — | — | — | — | 10.1 | 9.4 | 104 |
| | | 1.0 | 24.0 | — | Tr | Tr | — | — | — | — | 24.0 | 24.0 | 93 |
| | | 1.0 | 10.4 | — | — | — | — | — | — | — | 10.4 | 10.4 | 94 |
| | | 1.0 | 7.6 | 0.4 | 0.9 | — | — | — | — | — | 8.8 | 7.8 | 105 |
| | | 2.8 | 14.4 | 0.1 | 0.8 | — | — | — | — | — | 15.3 | 14.5 | 88 |
| | | 1.0 | 13.0 | Tr | 2.9 | Tr | — | — | — | — | 15.9 | 13.3 | 96 |
| | | 2.5 | 14.7 | — | — | — | — | — | — | — | 14.7 | 14.7 | 205 |
| | | 2.0 | 20.5 | — | — | — | — | — | — | — | 20.5 | 20.5 | 206 |
| Olive oil, extra virgin, Italy origin | | 2.6 | 19.9 | — | 1.4 | — | — | — | — | — | 21.3 | 20.0 | 168 |
| Spain origin | | 2.6 | 17.7 | — | 1.6 | — | — | — | — | — | 19.3 | 17.9 | 168 |
| Greece origin | | 2.6 | 20.9 | — | 1.6 | — | — | — | — | — | 22.5 | 21.1 | 168 |

*(continued)*

**Table 8.3** *Continued*

| Product | CC[a] | QI[b] | α-T[c] | β-T | γ-T | δ-T | α-T3[d] | β-T3 | γ-T3 | δ-T3 | Total | α-TE[e] mg | Ref. |
|---|---|---|---|---|---|---|---|---|---|---|---|---|---|
| Olive oil, virgin lampante, Italy origin | | 2.6 | 10.1 | — | 1.1 | — | — | — | — | — | 11.2 | 10.2 | 168 |
| Spain origin | | 2.6 | 12.5 | — | 0.5 | — | — | — | — | — | 13.0 | 12.6 | 168 |
| Tunisia origin | | 2.6 | 13.6 | — | 1.0 | — | — | — | — | — | 14.6 | 13.7 | 168 |
| **Olive oil mean ± SD** | | | 13.5 ± 4.7 | 0.1 ± 0.1 | 1.0 ± 0.7 | Tr | — | — | — | — | 14.6 ± 4.7 | 13.6 ± 4.7 | |
| Orange oil | <C | 0.8 | 11.9 | — | — | — | — | — | — | — | 11.9 | 11.9 | 103 |
| Palm oil | A | 2.2 | 12.8 | — | — | — | 22.3 | — | 15.3 | 2.1 | 52.5 | 19.5 | 87 |
| | | 2.2 | 6.1 | — | Tr | — | 5.7 | 0.8 | 11.3 | 3.3 | 27.2 | 7.8 | 85 |
| | | 2.0 | 9.1 | 0.2 | 0.8 | Tr | 5.2 | 0.4 | 13.2 | — | 28.9 | 10.8 | 97 |
| | | 1.2 | 13.1 | — | 0.8 | — | 15.3 | 1.6 | 34.3 | 4.9 | 70.1 | 17.9 | 86 |
| | | 1.0 | 20.7 | — | — | — | 14.3 | 2.9 | 28.6 | 6.9 | 73.3 | 25.1 | 92[h] |
| | | 1.0 | 22.0 | — | Tr | — | 13.0 | — | 21.5 | 2.2 | 58.7 | 25.9 | 102 |
| | | 2.6 | 19.7 | — | — | — | 9.4 | 1.4 | 26.3 | 6.8 | 63.6 | 22.6 | 168 |
| | | 2.0 | 21.5 | — | — | 1.0 | 22.4 | — | 41.7 | 8.3 | 94.8 | 28.2 | 198 |
| **Palm oil mean ± SD** | | | 14.8 ± 5.7 | Tr | 0.2 ± 0.4 | Tr | 12.2 ± 5.6 | 1.0 ± 1.0 | 21.5 ± 8.0 | 3.7 ± 2.4 | 53.5 ± 17.3 | 18.5 ± 6.4 | |
| Palm kernel oil | C | 2.0 | 1.3 | — | — | — | 2.1 | — | — | — | 3.4 | 2.1 | 183 |
| Palm olein | C | 1.4 | 15.5 | — | — | 1.5 | 16.5 | 1.4 | 20.7 | 4.2 | 59.6 | 19.4 | 95 |
| Peanut oil | A | 2.0 | 14.1 | 0.4 | 0.2 | 0.9 | Tr | Tr | Tr | — | 15.6 | 14.3 | 97 |
| | | 2.2 | 8.9 | 0.4 | 3.5 | 0.9 | — | — | — | — | 13.6 | 9.4 | 85 |
| | | 1.4 | 30.4 | — | 19.2 | 3.1 | — | — | — | — | 52.7 | 32.3 | 99 |
| | | 1.4 | 21.0 | — | 15.0 | — | — | — | — | — | 36.0 | 22.5 | 81 |
| | | 1.2 | 16.9 | 0.5 | 14.4 | 1.3 | — | — | — | — | 33.1 | 18.6 | 84 |
| | | 1.2 | 18.6 | — | 13.8 | — | — | — | — | — | 32.4 | 20.0 | 91 |
| | | 1.2 | 15.6 | — | 18.2 | 14.2 | — | — | — | — | 48.0 | 17.4 | 106[h] |
| | | 1.0 | 23.0 | — | 31.0 | Tr | — | — | — | — | 54.0 | 26.1 | 93 |
| | | 2.8 | 15.7 | 0.5 | 15.9 | 1.4 | — | — | — | — | 33.4 | 17.6 | 88 |
| | | 1.8 | 19.7 | 0.8 | 17.8 | 2.7 | — | — | — | — | 41.0 | 22.0 | 96 |
| | | 2.8 | 12.6 | 0.4 | 11.8 | 1.0 | — | — | — | — | 25.8 | 14.0 | 156 |
| **Peanut oil Mean ± SD** | | | 17.9 ± 5.5 | 0.3 ± 0.3 | 14.6 ± 7.7 | 2.3 ± 3.9 | Tr | Tr | Tr | — | 34.1 ± 13.4 | 19.5 ± 6.0 | |

| | | | | | | | | | | | | | |
|---|---|---|---|---|---|---|---|---|---|---|---|---|---|
| Pecan oil | | 1.5 | 0.6 | — | 31.9 | 0.3 | — | — | — | — | 32.8 | 3.8 | 204 |
| Rice bran oil | B | 1.8 | 8.2 | — | 12.8 | 1.3 | 3.7 | — | 34.3 | 3.5 | 68.8 | 10.6 | 107 |
| | | 2.4 | 56.1 | Tr | 5.5 | 1.0 | 29.8 | — | 32.1 | 2.0 | 126.5 | 65.6 | 108 |
| Safflower oil | A | 2.2 | 35.8 | 0.7 | 0.9 | — | — | — | — | — | 37.4 | 36.2 | 87 |
| | | 2.2 | 44.9 | 1.2 | 2.6 | 0.7 | — | — | — | — | 49.3 | 45.8 | 85 |
| | | 1.6 | 57.5 | 1.8 | 1.6 | Tr | Tr | — | — | — | 60.9 | 58.6 | 98 |
| | | 1.4 | 42.2 | — | 2.2 | Tr | — | — | — | — | 44.4 | 42.4 | 99 |
| | | 1.4 | 54.0 | — | — | — | — | — | — | — | 54.0 | 54.0 | 81 |
| | | 1.4 | 22.3 | 0.7 | 3.3 | 0.4 | — | — | — | — | 26.7 | 23.5 | 82 |
| | | 1.2 | 34.2 | — | 7.1 | — | — | — | — | — | 41.3 | 34.9 | 91 |
| | | 1.8 | 52.2 | — | 4.2 | — | — | — | — | — | 56.4 | 52.6 | 104 |
| **Safflower oil mean ± SD** | | | 42.9 ± 11.1 | 0.5 ± 0.7 | 3.0 ± 2.2 | 0.2 ± 0.3 | — | — | — | — | 46.3 ± 10.5 | 43.5 ± 10.9 | |
| Sesame oil | C | 1.6 | 0.9 | Tr | 51.7 | 0.2 | Tr | — | — | — | 52.8 | 6.1 | 98 |
| | | 1.2 | 1.2 | 0.6 | 24.4 | 3.2 | — | — | — | — | 29.4 | 4.0 | 84 |
| Soybean oil | A | 2.2 | 7.5 | 1.5 | 79.7 | 26.6 | 0.2 | 0.1 | — | Tr | 115.5 | 17.0 | 87 |
| | | 1.6 | 2.5 | 2.5 | 95.4 | 48.9 | — | — | — | — | 149.3 | 14.8 | 109 |
| | | 2.2 | 9.5 | 1.3 | 69.9 | 23.8 | — | — | — | — | 104.6 | 17.9 | 85 |
| | | 1.6 | 10.7 | 2.7 | 74.3 | 35.6 | — | — | — | — | 123.3 | 20.6 | 98 |
| | | 2.0 | 17.9 | 2.8 | 60.4 | 37.1 | Tr | 0.4 | 0.1 | — | 118.7 | 26.5 | 97 |
| | | 2.2 | 7.5 | 1.2 | 77.6 | 25.7 | Tr | Tr | — | — | 112.0 | 15.9 | 110 |
| | | 1.4 | 5.5 | Tr | 76.2 | 30.3 | — | — | — | — | 111.9 | 13.1 | 99 |
| | | 1.4 | 9.5 | — | 73.0 | 23.3 | — | — | — | — | 105.8 | 16.9 | 81 |
| | | 1.2 | 6.0 | — | 42.0 | 14.0 | — | — | — | — | 62.0 | 10.3 | 100 |

*(continued)*

**TABLE 8.3** *Continued*

| Product | CC[a] | QI[b] | α-T[c] | β-T | γ-T | δ-T | α-T3[d] | β-T3 | γ-T3 | δ-T3 | Total | α-TE[e] mg | Ref. |
|---|---|---|---|---|---|---|---|---|---|---|---|---|---|
| | | 1.8 | 10.3 | — | 55.5 | 23.9 | — | — | — | — | 89.7 | 15.9 | 83 |
| | | 1.4 | 11.6 | 3.4 | 73.7 | 27.5 | — | — | — | — | 116.2 | 21.5 | 82 |
| | | 2.0 | 6.8 | — | 44.1 | 14.3 | — | — | — | — | 65.2 | 11.3 | 101 |
| | | 1.2 | 6.8 | — | 45.7 | 14.2 | — | — | — | — | 66.7 | 11.4 | 91 |
| | | 1.2 | 12.0 | — | 86.0 | 26.5 | — | — | — | — | 124.5 | 21.4 | 82 |
| | | 1.0 | 6.5 | — | 69.5 | 25.0 | — | — | — | — | 101.0 | 14.2 | 93 |
| | | 2.8 | 7.4 | 1.0 | 67.0 | 23.4 | — | — | — | — | 98.8 | 15.4 | 88 |
| | | 1.4 | 7.9 | 1.1 | 47.4 | 12.0 | — | — | — | — | 68.3 | 12.7 | 95 |
| | | 1.4 | 7.8 | 3.3 | 87.6 | 44.5 | — | — | — | — | 142.4 | 18.8 | 89 |
| | | 1.2 | 12.8 | — | 72.8 | 22.2 | — | — | — | — | 107.8 | 20.7 | 111 |
| | | 1.8 | 17.8 | 3.2 | 77.2 | 33.3 | — | — | — | — | 131.4 | 28.1 | 96 |
| | | 1.6 | 3.2 | — | 80.0 | 49.0 | — | — | — | — | 132.2 | 12.7 | 112 |
| | | 1.8 | 7.4 | — | 73.6 | 40.3 | — | — | — | — | 121.3 | 16.0 | 113 |
| | | 1.4 | 9.6 | — | 65.5 | 24.9 | — | — | — | — | 100.0 | 16.9 | 114 |
| **Soybean oil mean ± SD** | | | 8.2 ± 4.2 | 1.0 ± 1.3 | 69.3 ± 14.3 | 28.1 ± 10.5 | Tr | Tr | Tr | — | 107.3 ± 24.1 | 17.0 ± 4.6 | |
| Sunflower oil | A | 2.2 | 33.3 | 1.5 | 9.4 | 1.8 | — | — | — | — | 46.0 | 35.1 | 87 |
| | | 2.2 | 62.2 | 2.3 | 2.7 | — | — | — | — | — | 67.1 | 63.7 | 85 |
| | | 1.6 | 78.3 | 2.5 | 1.9 | 0.7 | Tr | — | — | — | 83.4 | 79.8 | 98 |
| | | 1.4 | 73.7 | — | 4.4 | Tr | — | — | — | — | 78.1 | 74.1 | 99 |
| | | 1.2 | 60.8 | 1.7 | 1.1 | — | — | — | — | — | 63.6 | 61.8 | 84 |
| | | 1.8 | 49.2 | — | 17.6 | — | — | — | — | — | 66.8 | 51.0 | 104 |
| | | 1.0 | 52.0 | — | 11.9 | — | — | — | — | — | 63.9 | 53.1 | 102 |
| | | 1.8 | 32.7 | Tr | 4.5 | 0.5 | — | — | — | — | 37.7 | 33.2 | 96 |
| | | 2.0 | 56.4 | 2.5 | 0.4 | 0.1 | Tr | 0.2 | Tr | — | 59.6 | 57.7 | 97 |
| | | 2.6 | 55.7 | — | 4.5 | 0.7 | — | — | — | — | 60.9 | 56.2 | 168 |
| | | 2.0 | 73.8 | — | — | — | — | — | — | — | 73.8 | 73.8 | 199 |
| | | 2.2 | 6.1 | — | 1.5 | — | — | — | — | — | 7.6 | 6.3 | 202 |
| Physical refined | | 2.5 | 55.1 | 1.6 | 0.2 | — | — | — | — | — | 56.9 | 55.9 | 211 |

| | | | | | | | | | | | | | |
|---|---|---|---|---|---|---|---|---|---|---|---|---|---|
| Chemical refined | | 2.5 | 61.2 | 0.9 | 0.1 | — | — | — | — | — | 62.1 | 61.6 | 211 |
| Soft column deodorized | | 2.5 | 72.1 | 1.4 | 1.0 | — | — | — | — | — | 74.5 | 72.9 | 211 |
| **Sunflower oil mean ± SD** | | | 55.4 ± 14.1 | 1.1 ± 1.1 | 5.8 ± 5.2 | 0.5 ± 0.7 | Tr | Tr | Tr | — | 62.8 ± 12.9 | 56.6 ± 14.1 | |
| Tomato seed oil | C | | 20.2 | — | 105.9 | — | — | — | — | — | 126.1 | 30.8 | 201 |
| Walnut oil | C | | 1.4 | — | 54.3 | 6.7 | — | — | — | — | 62.3 | 6.8 | 199 |
| | | | 0.3 | — | 4.9 | 0.3 | — | — | — | — | 5.5 | 0.8 | 204 |
| Walnut oil, cold pressed | C | 1.4 | — | — | 26.3 | 4.6 | — | — | — | — | 30.9 | 2.8 | 82 |
| Wheat bran oil | C | 2.2 | 90.0 | 34.9 | Tr | Tr | 21.4 | 78.4 | — | — | 224.7 | 117.8 | 110 |
| Wheat germ oil | A | 1.6 | 156.4 | 91.9 | 22.3 | 1.9 | — | — | — | — | 272.5 | 204.6 | 109 |
| | | 2.2 | 150.8 | 31.2 | 52.7 | — | 3.6 | — | 1.9 | — | 240.2 | 172.7 | 85 |
| | | 2.2 | 155.2 | 55.2 | 23.3 | 2.3 | 2.2 | 12.7 | — | — | 250.8 | 186.4 | 110 |
| | | 1.2 | 180.0 | 74.0 | 10.0 | — | — | — | — | — | 264.0 | 218.0 | 100 |
| | | 1.8 | 110.0 | 80.8 | — | — | 8.5 | 12.7 | — | — | 212.0 | 153.6 | 83 |
| | | 1.2 | 117.9 | 39.8 | 49.3 | 11.8 | Tr | — | — | — | 218.8 | 143.1 | 84 |
| | | 1.2 | 115.3 | 66.0 | — | — | 2.6 | 8.1 | — | — | 192.0 | 149.5 | 91 |
| | | 1.4 | 140.2 | 63.3 | 40.00 | 6.5 | 3.7 | 12.3 | — | — | 265.9 | 177.5 | 90 |
| | | 2.2 | 217.0 | 18.0 | 4.00 | — | — | 3.2 | — | — | 242.2 | 226.6 | 85 |
| **Wheat germ oil mean ± SD** | | | 149.2 ± 34.2 | 57.8 ± 24.2 | 22.4 ± 19.6 | 2.5 ± 3.9 | 2.3 ± 2.7 | 5.4 ± 5.6 | 0.2 ± 0.6 | — | 239.8 ± 27.3 | 175.7 ± 26.7 | |
| Margarines, salad oils, spreads, shortening, peanut butter | | | | | | | | | | | | | |
| Margarine[g] | | | | | | | | | | | | | |
| C | A | 2.4 | 19.3 | — | 48.0 | 2.4 | — | — | — | — | 69.7 | 24.2 | 115 |
| | | 2.4 | 10.8 | — | 37.4 | 2.0 | — | — | — | — | 50.1 | 14.6 | 116 |
| | | 3.0 | 9.6 | — | 37.1 | 2.4 | — | — | — | — | 48.7 | 13.3 | 117 |
| | | 2.4 | 30.5 | — | — | — | — | — | — | — | — | 30.5 | 118 |

(*continued*)

**Table 8.3** *Continued*

| Product | CC[a] | QI[b] | α-T[c] | β-T | γ-T | δ-T | α-T3[d] | β-T3 | γ-T3 | δ-T3 | Total | α-TE[e] mg | Ref. |
|---|---|---|---|---|---|---|---|---|---|---|---|---|---|
| | | 2.4 | 23.9 | — | — | — | — | — | — | — | — | 23.9 | 118 |
| | | 2.8 | 17.4 | — | 46.5 | 2.5 | — | — | — | — | 66.4 | 22.1 | 88 |
| **mean ± SD** | | | 18.6 ± 7.2 | — | 42.3 ± 5.0 | 2.3 ± 0.2 | — | — | — | — | 58.7 ± 9.4 | 21.4 ± 5.9 | |
| SB | A | 2.4 | 4.4 | — | 54.3 | 20.0 | — | — | — | — | 78.7 | 10.5 | 115 |
| | | 3.0 | 4.5 | — | 34.5 | 12.7 | — | — | — | — | 51.8 | 8.4 | 117 |
| | | 2.4 | 5.2 | — | — | — | — | — | — | — | — | 5.2 | 118 |
| SB | | 2.8 | 4.1 | — | 53.6 | 23.3 | — | — | — | — | 81.0 | 10.1 | 88 |
| **mean ± SD** | | | 4.6 ± 0.4 | — | 47.5 ± 9.2 | 18.7 ± 4.4 | — | — | — | — | 70.5 ± 13.3 | 8.6 ± 2.1 | |
| C/SB | B | 3.0 | 9.3 | — | 37.4 | 6.6 | — | — | — | — | 53.3 | 13.2 | 117 |
| | | 2.4 | 10.5 | — | — | — | — | — | — | — | — | 10.5 | 118 |
| CS/SB | B | 2.4 | 4.7 | — | 19.7 | 5.1 | — | — | — | — | 29.5 | 6.8 | 116 |
| | | 3.0 | 5.0 | — | 19.2 | 8.3 | — | — | — | — | 31.6 | 7.1 | 117 |
| P/SB | C | 3.0 | 6.5 | — | 49.7 | 17.1 | — | — | — | — | 73.3 | 12.0 | 117 |
| SB/SF | C | 2.4 | 11.7 | — | 29.0 | 8.1 | — | — | — | — | 48.8 | 14.8 | 116 |
| C/CA/SB | B | 2.4 | 7.6 | — | — | — | — | — | — | — | — | 7.6 | 118 |
| | | 2.4 | 4.3 | — | — | — | — | — | — | — | — | 4.3 | 118 |
| C/CS/SB | C | 2.4 | 6.9 | — | 22.7 | 3.5 | — | — | — | — | 33.1 | 9.3 | 116 |
| CS/SB/SF | C | 3.0 | 5.2 | — | 39.1 | 14.6 | — | — | — | — | 58.9 | 9.5 | 117 |
| CS/SB/SN | B | 3.0 | 11.7 | — | 9.8 | 4.5 | — | — | — | — | 26.0 | 12.8 | 117 |
| | | 2.4 | 15.1 | — | — | — | — | — | — | — | — | 15.1 | 118 |
| C/CS/SB/SN | C | 3.0 | 4.4 | — | 14.6 | 8.3 | — | — | — | — | 27.3 | 6.1 | 117 |
| C/CS/P/SB/SN | C | 3.0 | 4.4 | — | 27.5 | 12.6 | — | — | — | — | 44.5 | 7.5 | 117 |
| Margarine, unspecified | A | 1.6 | 8.4 | 0.6 | 22.3 | 7.1 | 1.9 | 0.7 | 3.2 | 0.9 | 45.1 | 11.7 | 119 |
| | | 2.2 | 12.5 | 1.7 | 46.0 | 1.8 | — | — | — | — | 60.2 | 17.4 | 87 |
| | | 2.4 | 8.2 | — | 23.8 | 2.2 | — | — | — | — | 34.2 | 10.6 | 120 |
| | | 1.6 | 27.5 | 2.5 | 27.4 | 13.9 | — | — | — | — | 71.3 | 31.9 | 109 |
| | | 2.2 | 14.9 | 0.8 | 25.1 | 6.8 | Tr | — | 0.4 | 0.3 | 48.3 | 18.0 | 85 |

| | | | | | | | | | | | | | |
|---|---|---|---|---|---|---|---|---|---|---|---|---|---|
| Margarine, unspecified | | 2.2 | 19.0 | — | 45.0 | 9.0 | — | — | — | — | 73.0 | 23.8 | 121 |
| | | 2.2 | 5.2 | — | 9.6 | 0.4 | Tr | — | — | — | 15.2 | 6.2 | 85 |
| **Overall margarine mean ± SD** | | | 10.7 ± 7.0 | Tr | 32.4 ± 13.2 | 7.8 ± 6.2 | Tr | Tr | Tr | Tr | 50.8 ± 18.0 | 13.5 ± 7.2 | |
| Margarine, reduced-fat | | | | | | | | | | | | | |
| C (50%) | C | 2.4 | 12.5 | — | — | — | — | — | — | — | — | 12.5 | 118 |
| C (60%) | C | 3.0 | 1.1 | — | 3.3 | 3.0 | — | — | — | — | 7.4 | 1.5 | 117 |
| SB (40%) | A | 3.0 | 1.2 | — | 11.8 | 2.4 | — | — | — | — | 15.4 | 2.5 | 113 |
| | | 2.4 | 4.3 | — | — | — | — | — | — | — | — | 4.3 | 118 |
| | | 2.8 | 3.3 | — | 26.0 | 10.8 | — | — | — | — | 40.4 | 6.2 | 88 |
| **SB reduced-fat mean ± SD** | | | 2.9 ± 1.3 | — | 18.9 ± 7.1 | 6.6 ± 4.2 | — | — | — | — | 27.9 ± 12.5 | 4.3 ± 1.5 | |
| SB (50%) | B | 2.4 | 5.5 | — | — | — | — | — | — | — | — | 5.5 | 118 |
| | | 2.4 | 3.5 | — | — | — | — | — | — | — | — | 3.5 | 118 |
| SB (60%) | C | 3.0 | 3.4 | — | 29.3 | 9.6 | — | — | — | — | 42.3 | 6.6 | 117 |
| SB (64%) | C | 2.4 | 3.6 | — | 23.8 | 7.7 | — | — | — | — | 35.1 | 6.2 | 115 |
| SB (70%) | C | 2.4 | 6.9 | — | — | — | — | — | — | — | — | 6.9 | 118 |
| C/CA (30%) | C | 2.4 | 3.1 | — | — | — | — | — | — | — | — | 3.1 | 118 |
| CA/SB (20%) | C | 2.4 | 4.5 | — | — | — | — | — | — | — | — | 4.5 | 118 |
| CS/SB (40%) | C | 3.0 | 2.0 | — | 11.5 | 5.9 | — | — | — | — | 19.4 | 3.3 | 117 |
| P/SB (60%) | C | 3.0 | 2.9 | — | 26.6 | 10.5 | — | — | — | — | 39.9 | 5.9 | 117 |
| CA/P/SB (64%) | C | 2.4 | 1.9 | — | 25.2 | 9.1 | 3.0 | — | 2.2 | 1.3 | 42.7 | 5.6 | 115 |
| CA/SB/SF (43%) | C | **2.4** | 8.3 | — | 4.6 | 1.9 | — | — | — | — | 19.4 | 3.3 | 115 |
| CA/SB/SN (30%) | C | 2.4 | 4.0 | — | — | — | — | — | — | — | — | 4.0 | 118 |

*(continued)*

**TABLE 8.3** *Continued*

| Product | CC[a] | QI[b] | α-T[c] | β-T | γ-T | δ-T | α-T3[d] | β-T3 | γ-T3 | δ-T3 | Total | α-TE[e] mg | Ref. |
|---|---|---|---|---|---|---|---|---|---|---|---|---|---|
| CS/SB/SN (50%) | C | 2.8 | 4.6 | — | 26.0 | 9.6 | — | — | — | — | 40.2 | 7.5 | 88 |
| CS/SB/SN (70%) | C | 2.4 | 23.1 | — | — | — | — | — | — | — | — | 23.1 | 118 |
| Margarine, fat-free | | | | | | | | | | | | | |
| | C | 2.4 | 0.6 | — | — | — | — | — | — | — | — | 0.6 | 118 |
| | C | 2.4 | 0.5 | — | — | — | — | — | — | — | — | 0.5 | 118 |
| Mayonnaise | C | 2.8 | 3.2 | — | 48.2 | 17.0 | — | — | — | — | 65.2 | 5.3 | 88 |
| **Mayonnaise, reduced-fat** | C | 2.2 | Tr | — | Tr | — | — | — | — | — | 0.1 | Tr | 87 |
| **Salad dressing** | | | | | | | | | | | | | |
| Blue cheese | C | 2.4 | 3.8 | — | 53.3 | 19.9 | — | — | — | — | 76.9 | 9.7 | 120 |
| Roquefort cheese | C | 1.8 | 2.9 | — | 37.9 | — | — | — | — | — | 40.8 | 6.7 | 104 |
| French | B | 2.4 | 3.1 | — | 64.4 | 23.0 | — | — | — | — | 90.4 | 10.2 | 120 |
| | | 2.8 | — | — | 34.4 | 14.1 | — | — | — | — | 48.5 | 3.9 | 88 |
| French, reduced-fat | C | 2.2 | 0.3 | — | 0.8 | — | — | — | — | — | 1.1 | 0.4 | 87 |
| French cottonseed oil | C | 1.8 | 34.8 | — | 38.1 | — | — | — | — | — | 72.9 | 38.6 | 104 |
| Italian | B | 2.4 | 4.2 | — | 61.7 | 23.9 | — | — | — | — | 89.8 | 11.1 | 120 |
| | | 2.8 | — | — | 16.9 | 8.5 | — | — | — | — | 25.4 | 2.0 | 88 |
| Italian, reduced-fat | C | 2.2 | Tr | — | 0.1 | Tr | — | — | — | — | 0.1 | Tr | 87 |
| Thousand island, reduced-fat | C | 2.2 | 0.3 | — | — | — | — | — | — | — | 0.3 | 0.3 | 87 |
| Shortening | A | 2.4 | 5.6 | — | 25.2 | 5.4 | — | — | — | — | 36.2 | 8.3 | 120 |
| Shortening | | 1.2 | 9.9 | — | 66.2 | 23.0 | — | — | — | — | 99.1 | 16.9 | 91 |
| | | 2.8 | — | — | 30.2 | 18.6 | — | — | — | — | 48.7 | 3.6 | 88 |
| **Shortening mean ± SD** | | | 5.2 ± 4.9 | — | 40.5 ± 18.3 | 15.7 ± 7.5 | — | — | — | — | 61.3 ± 33.3 | 9.6 ± 6.7 | |
| Butter | C | 1.0 | 3.2 | — | — | — | — | — | — | — | 3.2 | 3.2 | 94 |
| **Peanut butter** | A | 2.2 | 10.4 | 0.3 | 7.7 | — | — | — | — | — | 18.4 | 11.3 | 87 |
| | | 2.8 | 9.5 | 0.2 | 9.8 | 0.5 | — | — | — | — | 20.0 | 10.6 | 88 |

| | | | | | | | | | | | | |
|---|---|---|---|---|---|---|---|---|---|---|---|---|
| | | 2.2 | 9.9 | 0.4 | 10.1 | 0.7 | — | — | — | — | 21.1 | 11.1 | 122 |
| | | 2.8 | 10.2 | 0.4 | 9.7 | 0.8 | — | — | — | — | 21.1 | 11.4 | 156 |
| **Peanut butter mean ± SD** | | | 10.0 ± 0.3 | 0.3 ± 0.1 | 9.3 ± 0.9 | 0.5 ± 0.3 | — | — | — | — | 20.2 ± 1.1 | 11.1 ± 0.3 | |
| Peanut butter, reduced-fat | C | 2.2 | 6.6 | 0.2 | 7.4 | 0.5 | — | — | — | — | 14.7 | 7.5 | 122 |
| **Cereals and cereal products** | | | | | | | | | | | | | |
| Amaranth | C | 1.8 | 1.7 | 2.2 | 0.3 | 0.8 | Tr | — | — | — | 5.0 | 2.8 | 123 |
| Barley | A | 1.2 | 0.2 | Tr | Tr | Tr | 1.1 | 0.3 | 0.2 | — | 1.9 | 0.6 | 91 |
| | | 1.8 | 0.9 | 0.2 | 0.4 | Tr | 0.8 | — | 0.4 | — | 2.6 | 1.3 | 123 |
| | | 1.2 | 0.6 | — | Tr | Tr | 2.0 | 0.5 | 0.6 | 0.1 | 3.8 | 1.2 | 124 |
| | | 1.2 | 1.2 | 0.1 | 0.5 | — | 4.0 | 1.0 | — | — | 6.7 | 2.5 | 127 |
| | | 2.0 | 0.7 | 0.1 | 0.3 | Tr | 1.9 | — | 0.3 | — | 3.3 | 1.4 | 126 |
| **Barley mean ± SD** | | | 0.7 ± 0.4 | 0.1 ± 0.1 | 0.2 ± 0.2 | Tr | 2.0 ± 1.3 | 0.4 ± 0.4 | 0.3 ± 0.2 | Tr | 3.7 ± 1.8 | 1.4 ± 0.7 | |
| Barley, endosperm | C | 1.2 | 0.1 | Tr | — | Tr | 2.3 | 0.5 | 0.4 | Tr | 3.3 | 0.8 | 124 |
| Barley, hull | C | 1.2 | 1.0 | 0.1 | Tr | Tr | 1.4 | 0.2 | 0.2 | Tr | 2.9 | 1.5 | 124 |
| Barley, germ | C | 1.2 | 17.5 | — | 1.0 | 0.2 | — | 2.0 | — | — | 20.7 | 17.7 | 124 |
| Barley meal | C | 2.8 | 0.3 | Tr | 0.1 | Tr | 1.6 | 0.6 | 0.5 | — | 3.2 | 0.8 | 125 |
| Buckwheat, whole grain | B | 2.8 | 0.2 | Tr | 5.8 | 0.3 | Tr | — | Tr | — | 6.3 | 0.8 | 125 |
| | | 1.8 | 0.5 | — | 2.9 | 0.2 | Tr | — | — | — | 3.5 | 0.8 | 123 |
| Corn | B | 2.0 | 1.0 | 0.1 | 3.5 | — | 0.7 | — | 1.3 | — | 6.6 | 1.6 | 126 |
| | | 1.2 | 0.1 | — | 0.4 | — | 0.2 | — | 0.4 | — | 1.1 | 0.2 | 91 |
| | | 1.8 | 0.9 | 0.2 | 2.9 | 0.1 | 0.2 | — | 0.5 | — | 4.7 | 1.3 | 123 |
| **Corn mean ± SD** | | | 0.7 ± 0.5 | 0.1 ± 0.1 | 2.3 ± 1.6 | Tr | 0.4 ± 0.3 | — | 0.7 ± 0.5 | — | 4.1 ± 2.8 | 1.0 ± 0.7 | |
| Corn meal, whole | C | 2.2 | 0.4 | — | 1.9 | — | 0.2 | — | 0.1 | — | 2.6 | 0.7 | 87 |

*(continued)*

**TABLE 8.3** *Continued*

| Product | CC[a] | QI[b] | α-T[c] | β-T | γ-T | δ-T | α-T3[d] | β-T3 | γ-T3 | δ-T3 | Total | α-TE[e] mg | Ref. |
|---|---|---|---|---|---|---|---|---|---|---|---|---|---|
| Corn flaked | C | 2.8 | Tr | — | 0.1 | Tr | 0.2 | — | 0.4 | — | 0.7 | 0.1 | 125 |
| Durum | B | 2.0 | 1.0 | 0.5 | — | — | 0.7 | 3.7 | — | — | 5.8 | 1.6 | 101 |
| | | 1.8 | 1.6 | — | 0.6 | 0.7 | — | — | — | — | 2.9 | 1.7 | 128 |
| Durum flour | C | 2.0 | 0.3 | 0.15 | — | — | 0.3 | 1.8 | — | — | 2.5 | 0.5 | 101 |
| Lupin | C | 1.8 | 0.6 | 0.3 | 6.1 | 0.2 | 0.1 | — | 0.2 | — | 7.5 | 1.4 | 123 |
| Macaroni | A | 2.2 | Tr | Tr | 0.3 | Tr | Tr | 0.1 | — | — | 0.4 | 0.1 | 87 |
| | | 2.8 | 0.1 | 0.1 | — | — | 0.1 | 0.8 | — | — | 1.1 | 0.2 | 125 |
| | | 2.0 | Tr | Tr | — | — | Tr | 0.2 | — | — | 0.3 | 0.0 | 101 |
| **Macaroni mean ± SD** | | | Tr | Tr | 0.1 ± 0.2 | Tr | Tr | 0.4 ± 0.4 | — | — | 0.6 ± 0.4 | 0.1 ± 0.1 | |
| Millet, whole grain | C | 2.8 | 0.1 | 0.1 | 1.7 | 0.6 | Tr | — | Tr | — | 2.5 | 0.3 | 125 |
| Milo | C | 2.0 | 0.5 | 0.1 | 1.1 | 0.3 | — | — | 0.5 | — | 2.5 | 0.7 | 126 |
| Oats | A | 1.2 | 0.5 | 0.1 | — | — | 1.1 | 0.2 | — | — | 1.9 | 0.9 | 91 |
| | | 1.8 | 1.0 | 0.2 | 0.4 | Tr | 0.5 | — | — | — | 2.1 | 1.3 | 123 |
| | | 1.2 | 0.9 | 0.1 | — | — | 1.9 | 0.3 | — | — | 3.2 | 1.6 | 127 |
| | | 2.0 | 0.9 | — | 2.5 | 0.1 | 3.6 | — | 2.4 | — | 9.5 | 2.2 | 126 |
| **Oats mean ± SD** | | | 0.8 ± 0.2 | 0.6 ± 1.0 | 0.7 ± 1.2 | Tr | 2.0 ± 1.6 | 0.1 ± 0.2 | 0.6 ± 1.2 | — | 4.6 ± 3.4 | 1.7 ± 0.6 | |
| Oat bran | C | 2.2 | 1.0 | 0.1 | — | 0.1 | 2.2 | 0.1 | — | — | 3.5 | 1.7 | 87 |
| | | 1.0 | 0.5 | 0.3 | 0.1 | — | 1.8 | 0.2 | — | 0.1 | 3.0 | 1.3 | 129 |
| Oat flour | C | 1.0 | 0.6 | 0.3 | 0.1 | Tr | 1.5 | 0.1 | — | 0.1 | 2.7 | 1.2 | 129 |
| Oats, instant | C | 1.0 | 0.6 | 0.3 | 0.1 | — | 1.9 | 0.2 | — | 0.1 | 3.2 | 1.3 | 129 |
| Oats, puffed | C | 2.8 | 0.8 | 0.1 | — | Tr | 1.4 | 0.3 | Tr | — | 2.6 | 1.3 | 125 |
| Oats, quick | C | 1.0 | 0.6 | 0.4 | 0.1 | — | 1.7 | 0.2 | 0.1 | 0.1 | 3.2 | 1.3 | 129 |
| Oats, rolled | B | 2.8 | 0.8 | 0.1 | — | — | 2.0 | 0.3 | — | — | 3.2 | 1.5 | 125 |
| | | 1.0 | 0.5 | 0.3 | 0.1 | — | 1.7 | 0.2 | — | 0.1 | 2.9 | 1.2 | 129 |
| Rice | C | 2.2 | 0.6 | — | — | — | 0.9 | 0.2 | 0.6 | — | 1.4 | 0.5 | 87 |
| Rice, polished | C | 2.8 | Tr | Tr | Tr | Tr | 0.1 | Tr | 0.3 | — | 0.4 | 0.1 | 125 |
| Rice, brown | C | 2.8 | 0.6 | Tr | 0.1 | Tr | 0.3 | Tr | 0.7 | — | 1.8 | 0.8 | 125 |
| Rice, brown, cooked | C | 2.2 | Tr | — | — | — | 0.1 | Tr | 0.1 | — | 0.2 | 0.0 | 87 |

| | | | | | | | | | | | | | |
|---|---|---|---|---|---|---|---|---|---|---|---|---|---|
| Rye | C | 1.2 | 1.6 | 0.4 | — | — | 1.5 | 0.8 | — | — | 4.3 | 2.3 | 91 |
| Rye, rolled | C | 2.8 | 0.4 | 0.1 | — | — | 1.5 | 0.9 | — | — | 2.9 | 0.9 | 125 |
| Rye meal | C | 2.8 | 1.0 | 0.3 | — | — | 1.4 | 1.1 | — | — | 3.9 | 1.7 | 125 |
| Rye flour | C | 2.8 | 0.6 | 0.3 | — | — | 0.4 | 0.6 | — | — | 1.9 | 0.8 | 125 |
| Semolina | C | 2.8 | 0.2 | 0.1 | — | — | 0.1 | 1.3 | — | — | 1.7 | 0.3 | 125 |
| Sesame | C | 1.2 | — | — | 22.7 | — | — | — | — | — | 22.7 | 2.3 | 91 |
| Wheat, unspecified | A | 1.2 | 1.0 | 0.7 | — | — | 0.4 | 2.8 | — | — | 4.9 | 1.6 | 91 |
| | | 2.0 | 1.1 | 0.8 | — | — | 0.3 | 2.9 | — | — | 5.1 | 1.7 | 130 |
| | | 1.2 | 1.0 | 0.3 | — | — | 0.5 | 2.8 | — | — | 4.6 | 1.4 | 131 |
| | | 1.8 | 1.1 | 0.4 | 6.2 | — | 0.1 | — | — | — | 7.8 | 2.0 | 123 |
| | | 2.0 | 0.9 | 0.5 | — | — | 0.2 | — | — | — | 1.6 | 1.2 | 126 |
| **Wheat mean ± SD** | | | 1.0 ± 0.1 | 0.5 ± 0.2 | 1.2 ± 2.8 | — | 0.3 ± 0.2 | 1.7 ± 1.6 | — | — | 4.8 ± 2.2 | 1.6 ± 0.3 | |
| Wheat, hard | B | 2.0 | 1.4 | 0.7 | — | — | 0.5 | 3.3 | — | — | 5.8 | 2.0 | 101 |
| | | 1.8 | 1.8 | — | 1.2 | 2.2 | — | — | — | — | 5.2 | 2.0 | 128 |
| Wheat, soft | B | 2.0 | 1.2 | 0.7 | — | — | 0.5 | 3.0 | — | — | 5.4 | 1.9 | 101 |
| | | 1.8 | 1.5 | — | 0.8 | 1.2 | — | — | — | — | 3.5 | 1.6 | 128 |
| Wheat, steam flaked | C | 1.2 | 1.0 | 0.3 | — | — | 0.5 | 2.6 | — | — | 4.4 | 1.4 | 131 |
| Wheat, steam flaked and drum dried | C | 1.2 | 0.4 | 0.2 | — | — | 0.3 | 1.2 | — | — | 2.1 | 0.7 | 131 |
| Wheat bran | A | 2.2 | 0.6 | 0.2 | — | — | 1.3 | 6.8 | — | — | 9.0 | 1.5 | 87 |
| | | 2.8 | 1.6 | 0.8 | — | — | 1.5 | 5.6 | — | — | 9.5 | 2.7 | 125 |
| | | 2.0 | 1.7 | 1.3 | — | — | 1.1 | 6.4 | — | — | 10.5 | 3.0 | 130 |
| **Wheat bran mean ± SD** | | | 1.3 ± 0.5 | 0.8 ± 0.4 | — | — | 1.3 ± 0.2 | 6.3 ± 0.5 | — | — | 9.7 ± 0.6 | 2.4 ± 0.6 | |
| Wheat endosperm | C | 1.0 | 0.4 | Tr | 0.1 | — | 3.8 | 0.2 | Tr | Tr | 4.5 | 1.6 | 129 |
| Wheat flour | A | 2.2 | Tr | Tr | — | Tr | Tr | 0.2 | 1.1 | — | 1.3 | 0.1 | 87 |
| | | 2.0 | Tr | 0.1 | — | — | — | 0.6 | — | — | 0.6 | 0.1 | 101 |

*(continued)*

**Table 8.3** *Continued*

| Product | CC[a] | QI[b] | α-T[c] | β-T | γ-T | δ-T | α-T3[d] | β-T3 | γ-T3 | δ-T3 | Total | α-TE[e] mg | Ref. |
|---|---|---|---|---|---|---|---|---|---|---|---|---|---|
| | | 1.2 | 0.9 | 0.4 | — | — | 0.2 | 1.8 | — | — | 3.3 | 1.3 | 131 |
| | | 2.8 | 0.1 | 0.1 | 0.5 | — | — | — | — | — | 0.7 | 0.2 | 88 |
| | | 2.0 | Tr | Tr | 0.1 | — | — | 0.3 | — | — | 0.4 | 0.1 | 101 |
| | | 2.0 | 0.3 | 0.2 | — | — | 0.1 | 2.2 | — | — | 2.8 | 0.5 | 130 |
| **Wheat flour mean ± SD** | | | 0.2 ± 0.4 | 0.1 ± 0.2 | 0.1 ± 0.2 | Tr | 0.1 ± 0.1 | 0.9 ± 0.9 | 0.2 ± 0.4 | — | 1.5 ± 1.2 | 0.4 ± 0.5 | |
| Wheat flour, drum dried | C | 1.2 | Tr | Tr | — | — | Tr | 0.2 | — | — | 0.2 | 0.0 | 131 |
| Wheat flour, 1.2%–1.4% ash | C | 2.8 | 1.6 | 0.8 | — | — | 0.3 | 1.7 | — | — | 4.5 | 2.2 | 125 |
| Wheat flour, 0.7% ash | C | 2.8 | 0.4 | 0.2 | — | — | 0.2 | 1.5 | — | — | 2.3 | 0.6 | 125 |
| Wheat flour, 0.5% ash | C | 2.8 | 0.2 | 0.1 | — | — | 0.1 | 1.4 | — | — | 1.8 | 0.3 | 125 |
| Wheat flour, wholemeal | C | 2.0 | 1.3 | 0.6 | — | — | 0.5 | 3.5 | — | — | 5.9 | 1.9 | 132 |
| | | 1.2 | 2.1 | 0.7 | — | — | 0.5 | 2.6 | — | — | 5.9 | 2.7 | 131 |
| Wheat flour, wholemeal, drum dried | C | 1.2 | 0.1 | Tr | — | — | Tr | 0.2 | — | — | 0.3 | 0.1 | 131 |
| Wheat germ | A | 2.2 | 16.8 | 8.5 | — | — | 0.4 | — | — | — | 25.7 | 21.2 | 87 |
| | | 2.0 | 11.1 | 4.7 | — | — | 0.5 | 2.7 | — | — | 19.0 | 13.7 | 132 |
| | | 2.8 | 22.1 | 8.6 | — | Tr | 0.3 | 1.0 | — | — | 31.9 | 26.5 | 125 |
| | | 1.0 | 10.8 | — | 2.0 | — | 0.1 | 0.2 | Tr | — | 13.1 | 11.0 | 129 |
| **Wheat germ mean ± SD** | | | 15.2 ± 5.4 | 5.5 ± 4.1 | 0.5 ± 1.0 | Tr | 0.3 ± 0.2 | 1.1 ± 1.2 | Tr | — | 21.3 ± 9.6 | 17.1 ± 8.3 | |
| Wheat hull | C | 1.0 | 0.1 | Tr | — | — | 0.2 | — | Tr | Tr | 0.3 | 0.2 | 129 |
| Wheat meal | C | 2.8 | 1.0 | 0.5 | — | Tr | 0.4 | 2.1 | — | — | 4.1 | 1.5 | 125 |

| | | | | | | | | | | | | | |
|---|---|---|---|---|---|---|---|---|---|---|---|---|---|
| **Bakery products** | | | | | | | | | | | | | |
| Biscuit | C | 2.8 | 0.5 | 0.2 | 1.4 | 0.3 | 0.1 | 0.9 | Tr | — | 3.4 | 0.9 | 125 |
| Bread, brown, seasoned | C | 2.8 | 0.7 | 0.4 | 0.3 | 0.1 | 0.2 | 1.0 | 0.2 | — | 2.8 | 1.0 | 125 |
| Bread, cracked wheat | C | 2.2 | 0.1 | Tr | 0.4 | 0.1 | 0.1 | — | — | — | 0.6 | 0.1 | 87 |
| Bread crumb | C | 2.8 | 0.1 | 0.1 | 3.2 | 0.3 | — | — | — | — | 3.7 | 0.4 | 88 |
| Bread, French | C | 2.2 | 0.1 | 0.1 | 1.8 | 0.3 | Tr | — | — | — | 2.4 | 0.4 | 87 |
| Bread, rye | C | 2.2 | 0.2 | 0.2 | 1.0 | 0.3 | 0.2 | 0.2 | — | — | 2.0 | 0.5 | 87 |
| Bread, rye, sour | C | 2.8 | 0.7 | 0.2 | Tr | Tr | 0.9 | 0.7 | Tr | — | 2.6 | 1.1 | 125 |
| Bread, rye, brown | C | 2.8 | 0.8 | 0.2 | Tr | Tr | 0.9 | 0.8 | Tr | — | 2.7 | 1.2 | 125 |
| Bread, sweet wheat, 7% fat | C | 2.8 | 0.4 | 0.1 | 0.4 | 0.1 | 0.1 | 0.8 | Tr | — | 1.8 | 0.5 | 125 |
| Bread, sweet wheat, 10% fat | C | 2.8 | 0.8 | 0.2 | 1.0 | 0.2 | 0.1 | 0.8 | Tr | — | 3.0 | 1.1 | 125 |
| Bread, wheat | A | 2.8 | 0.4 | 0.2 | 0.3 | 0.1 | 0.1 | 0.9 | — | — | 1.9 | 0.6 | 125 |
| | | 2.0 | 0.1 | 0.1 | 0.6 | 0.4 | 0.2 | 0.5 | — | — | 1.4 | 0.3 | 101 |
| | | 2.8 | 0.3 | 0.3 | 1.5 | 0.4 | — | — | — | — | 2.5 | 0.6 | 88 |
| **Bread, wheat mean ± SD** | | | 0.3 ± 0.1 | 0.2 ± 0.1 | 0.8 ± 0.5 | 0.3 ± 0.1 | 0.1 ± 0.1 | 0.5 ± 0.5 | — | — | 1.9 ± 0.4 | 0.5 ± 0.1 | |
| Bread, wheat, dark | C | 2.8 | 0.6 | 0.3 | 0.2 | 0.1 | 0.1 | 1.0 | — | — | 2.3 | 0.8 | 125 |
| Bread, white | C | 2.2 | Tr | Tr | 0.2 | 0.1 | — | — | — | — | 0.4 | 0.1 | 87 |
| Corn bread mix | C | 2.2 | 0.3 | Tr | 0.1 | 0.1 | — | — | 0.1 | — | 0.5 | 0.3 | 87 |
| Danish pastry | C | 2.8 | 0.9 | 0.1 | 1.1 | 0.1 | 0.1 | 0.6 | Tr | — | 2.9 | 1.1 | 125 |
| Doughnut | B | 2.8 | 1.0 | 0.2 | 1.5 | 0.2 | 0.1 | 0.7 | Tr | — | 3.7 | 1.3 | 125 |
| | | 2.0 | 0.9 | — | 2.9 | 1.0 | — | 0.5 | — | — | 5.3 | 1.3 | 101 |
| Hamburger rolls | A | 2.0 | 0.1 | Tr | 0.4 | 0.2 | — | — | — | — | 0.7 | 0.1 | 101 |
| | | 2.0 | 1.1 | — | 4.9 | 1.7 | 0.3 | 1.2 | — | — | 9.2 | 1.8 | 130 |
| | | 2.8 | 0.1 | 0.1 | 0.8 | 0.3 | — | — | — | — | 1.3 | 0.2 | 88 |

(*continued*)

**TABLE 8.3** *Continued*

| Product | CC[a] | QI[b] | α-T[c] | β-T | γ-T | δ-T | α-T3[d] | β-T3 | γ-T3 | δ-T3 | Total | α-TE[e] mg | Ref. |
|---|---|---|---|---|---|---|---|---|---|---|---|---|---|
| **Hamburger rolls mean ± SD** | | | 0.4 ± 0.5 | Tr | 2.0 ± 2.0 | 0.7 ± 0.7 | 0.1 ± 0.2 | 0.5 ± 0.6 | — | — | 3.8 ± 3.8 | 0.7 ± 0.8 | |
| Hard tack | C | 2.8 | 0.5 | 0.2 | — | — | 0.7 | 0.7 | — | — | 2.1 | 0.8 | 125 |
| Jelly roll | C | 2.8 | 1.0 | 0.1 | 1.9 | 0.4 | 0.2 | 0.3 | Tr | — | 3.8 | 1.3 | 125 |
| Rye crisp | C | 2.8 | 0.7 | 0.2 | — | — | 1.3 | 0.9 | — | — | 3.1 | 1.2 | 125 |
| Sponge cake | C | 2.8 | 1.5 | 0.1 | 1.5 | 0.1 | 0.2 | 0.4 | Tr | — | 3.7 | 1.7 | 125 |
| Sponge cake with fruit filling | C | 2.8 | 1.0 | 0.1 | 0.6 | 0.2 | 0.1 | 0.1 | Tr | — | 2.0 | 1.1 | 125 |
| Sponge cake with cream filling | C | 2.8 | 0.7 | Tr | 0.1 | Tr | 0.1 | 0.1 | — | — | 1.0 | 0.8 | 125 |
| Whole wheat rusk | C | 2.8 | 0.4 | 0.3 | 0.7 | 0.4 | 0.2 | 1.4 | — | — | 3.3 | 0.7 | 125 |
| **Cake mix** | | | | | | | | | | | | | |
| Biscuit mix | C | 2.0 | 0.3 | Tr | 1.8 | 0.6 | — | 0.1 | — | — | 2.7 | 0.5 | 101 |
| Chocolate | C | 2.2 | 0.7 | — | 4.2 | 0.9 | — | — | — | — | 5.8 | 1.1 | 87 |
| Duncan hines, white | C | 2.2 | 1.5 | 0.2 | 8.8 | 1.6 | — | — | — | — | 12.0 | 2.5 | 87 |
| Duncan hines, yellow | C | 2.2 | 0.9 | 0.2 | 12.4 | 2.0 | — | — | — | — | 15.5 | 2.2 | 87 |
| Piggly wiggly, yellow | C | 2.2 | 0.2 | Tr | 1.7 | 1.7 | — | — | — | — | 3.6 | 0.4 | 87 |
| Pilsbury, yellow | C | 2.2 | 1.3 | 0.2 | 6.8 | 1.5 | — | — | — | — | 9.8 | 2.1 | 87 |
| **Breakfast cereals** | | | | | | | | | | | | | |
| All bran | C | 2.2 | 0.4 | 0.2 | — | — | 0.9 | 3.8 | 0.3 | — | 5.5 | 1.0 | 87 |
| Bran flakes | C | 2.2 | 0.4 | — | — | — | 0.4 | 0.8 | — | — | 1.6 | 0.5 | 87 |
| Cheerios | C | 2.2 | 0.4 | — | — | — | 0.8 | — | — | — | 1.1 | 0.6 | 87 |
| Chex multibran | C | 2.2 | 0.3 | — | — | — | 0.6 | 0.8 | 0.3 | — | 2.0 | 0.5 | 87 |
| Fiber one | C | 2.2 | 0.3 | — | — | — | 0.4 | 1.8 | — | — | 2.5 | 0.5 | 87 |
| Four-grain cereals, rolled | C | 2.8 | 0.4 | 0.1 | — | — | 1.4 | 1.0 | 0.1 | — | 3.0 | 0.9 | 125 |

| | | | | | | | | | | | | | |
|---|---|---|---|---|---|---|---|---|---|---|---|---|---|
| Kellogg's corn flakes | C | 2.4 | 1.3 | — | — | — | — | — | — | — | 1.3 | 1.3 | 120 |
| Post natural raisin bran | C | 2.4 | 1.5 | — | — | — | — | — | — | — | 1.5 | 1.5 | 120 |
| Raisin bran | C | 2.2 | 0.4 | 0.1 | 1.3 | 0.4 | — | — | — | — | 2.1 | 0.6 | 87 |
| Rice crispies | C | 2.8 | 0.2 | Tr | Tr | Tr | 0.3 | Tr | 0.5 | — | 1.0 | 0.3 | 125 |
| Rice bran | C | 2.2 | 0.7 | — | 0.3 | — | 0.3 | — | 1.1 | — | 2.4 | 0.9 | 87 |
| Whole wheat | C | 2.0 | 1.2 | 0.6 | 0.3 | — | — | 2.4 | — | — | 4.5 | 1.6 | 101 |
| Shredded wheat | C | 2.0 | 0.4 | 0.3 | 0.3 | — | — | 1.4 | — | — | 2.3 | 0.6 | 101 |
| Wheat flakes | C | 2.0 | 0.4 | 0.3 | 0.3 | — | — | 1.3 | — | — | 2.3 | 0.6 | 101 |
| Six different brands, not specified | C | 1.2 | 0.4 | 0.3 | 0.3 | 0.2 | 0.3 | 1.3 | 0.6 | — | 2.0 | 0.6 | 133 |
| King vitamin, fortified | C | 2.4 | 35.1 | — | — | — | — | — | — | — | 35.1 | 35.1 | 120 |
| Total, fortified | C | 2.4 | 104.5 | — | — | — | — | — | — | — | 104.5 | 104.5 | 120 |
| **Milk, dairy products, and eggs** | | | | | | | | | | | | | |
| Buttermilk | C | 2.2 | 0.1 | Tr | Tr | Tr | — | — | — | — | 0.1 | 0.1 | 87 |
| Cheese | | | | | | | | | | | | | |
| American, low-fat | C | 2.4 | 0.8 | — | — | — | — | — | — | — | 0.8 | 0.8 | 120 |
| Cheddar | C | 2.4 | 0.3 | — | — | — | — | — | — | — | 0.3 | 0.3 | 120 |
| Muenster | C | 2.4 | 0.4 | — | — | — | — | — | — | — | 0.4 | 0.4 | 120 |
| Swiss | C | 2.4 | 0.5 | — | — | — | — | — | — | — | 0.5 | 0.5 | 120 |
| Milk, bovine | | | | | | | | | | | | | |
| Whole | B | 2.2 | 0.1 | — | Tr | — | — | — | — | — | 0.1 | 0.1 | 87 |
| | | 1.6 | 0.1 | — | — | — | — | — | — | — | 0.1 | 0.1 | 134 |
| Whole, dried | C | 1.6 | 0.8 | — | — | — | — | — | — | — | 0.8 | 0.8 | 112 |
| | C | 1.6 | 0.5 | — | Tr | — | — | — | — | — | 0.5 | 0.5 | 109 |
| Freeze dried | C | 1.0 | 0.7 | — | — | — | — | — | — | — | 0.7 | 0.7 | 94 |

*(continued)*

**TABLE 8.3** *Continued*

| Product | CC[a] | QI[b] | α-T[c] | β-T | γ-T | δ-T | α-T3[d] | β-T3 | γ-T3 | δ-T3 | Total | α-TE[e] mg | Ref. |
|---|---|---|---|---|---|---|---|---|---|---|---|---|---|
| Colostrum | C | 1.6 | 0.5 | — | — | — | — | — | — | — | 0.5 | 0.5 | 134 |
| Condensed | C | 1.6 | 0.1 | — | — | — | — | — | — | — | 0.1 | 0.1 | 134 |
| Evaporated | C | 1.6 | 0.1 | — | — | — | — | — | | — | 0.1 | 0.1 | 134 |
| 2% Fat | C | 2.2 | 0.1 | Tr | Tr | Tr | — | — | — | — | 0.1 | 0.1 | 87 |
| Nonfat dry milk | B | 2.2 | — | — | — | — | — | — | — | — | 0.0 | 0.0 | 87 |
| | | 1.6 | Tr | — | — | — | — | — | — | — | 0.0 | 0.0 | 134 |
| Milk fat | C | 2.0 | 1.7 | — | 0.1 | — | — | — | — | — | 1.8 | 1.7 | 135 |
| Milk, human | | | | | | | | | | | | | |
| mature | B | 2.2 | 0.3 | — | 0.1 | — | — | — | — | — | 0.4 | 0.3 | 138 |
| | | 2.6 | 0.5 | Tr | 0.1 | Tr | — | — | — | — | 0.6 | 0.5 | 139 |
| Colostrum | C | 2.6 | 1.9 | 0.1 | 0.1 | Tr | — | — | — | — | 2.1 | 1.9 | 139 |
| Transitional | C | 2.6 | 0.7 | Tr | 0.1 | Tr | — | — | — | — | 0.8 | 0.7 | 139 |
| Frozen fresh | C | 1.6 | Tr | — | — | — | — | — | — | — | 0.0 | 0.0 | 134 |
| Pasteurized | C | 1.6 | 0.2 | — | — | — | — | — | — | — | 0.2 | 0.2 | 134 |
| Lyophilized | C | 1.6 | 1.1 | — | — | — | — | — | — | — | 1.1 | 1.1 | 134 |
| Eggs | | | | | | | | | | | | | |
| Raw | B | 2.2 | 1.9 | 0.1 | 0.6 | Tr | 0.3 | — | — | — | 2.9 | 2.1 | 87 |
| | | 1.2 | 3.2 | — | 1.4 | — | — | — | — | — | 4.6 | 3.3 | 136 |
| Boiled | C | 2.2 | 1.8 | 0.1 | 0.6 | — | 0.2 | — | — | — | 2.7 | 1.9 | 87 |
| Dried | C | 1.0 | 9.6 | — | — | — | — | — | — | — | 9.6 | 9.6 | 94 |
| Egg yolk | B | 1.6 | 2.3 | 1.8 | — | — | — | — | — | — | 4.1 | 3.3 | 112 |
| | | 2.4 | 15.0 | — | — | — | — | — | — | — | 15.0 | 15.0 | 137 |
| **Meat, fish, and seafood** | | | | | | | | | | | | | |
| Baltic herring, deep frozen | C | 2.8 | 2.9 | — | — | — | — | — | — | — | 2.9 | 2.9 | 140 |
| Baltic herring fish fingers | C | 2.8 | 2.6 | — | 3.5 | — | — | — | — | — | 6.1 | 2.9 | 140 |
| Blue crab, canned | C | 2.2 | 1.8 | — | — | Tr | — | — | — | — | 1.9 | 1.8 | 87 |

| | | | | | | | | | | | | | |
|---|---|---|---|---|---|---|---|---|---|---|---|---|---|
| Bream | C | 2.8 | 2.9 | — | — | — | — | — | — | — | 2.9 | 2.9 | 140 |
| Burbot | C | 2.8 | 0.9 | — | Tr | — | — | — | — | — | 0.9 | 0.9 | 140 |
| Burbot, liver | C | 2.8 | 16.1 | — | — | — | — | — | — | — | 16.1 | 16.1 | 140 |
| Catfish, muscle tissue | B | 1.8 | 2.6 | — | 0.3 | — | — | — | — | — | 2.9 | 2.6 | 141 |
| | | 2.6 | 1.3 | — | 0.7 | — | — | — | — | — | 2.0 | 1.4 | 142 |
| Catfish, muscle tissue, cooked | C | 1.8 | 2.6 | — | 0.3 | — | — | — | — | — | 2.9 | 2.6 | 141 |
| Clam | C | 2.2 | 0.3 | — | — | Tr | — | — | — | — | 0.3 | 0.3 | 87 |
| Cod | B | 2.2 | 0.6 | — | — | — | — | — | — | — | 0.6 | 0.6 | 87 |
| | | 2.8 | 1.1 | — | — | — | — | — | — | — | 1.1 | 1.1 | 140 |
| Cod, white tissue | C | 1.4 | 0.2 | — | — | — | — | — | — | — | 0.2 | 0.2 | 143 |
| Cod, dark tissue | C | 1.4 | 1.2 | — | — | — | — | — | — | — | 1.2 | 1.2 | 143 |
| Cod, frozen, uncooked | C | 2.2 | 0.6 | — | — | — | — | — | — | — | 0.6 | 0.6 | 87 |
| Cod, liver | C | 1.4 | 22.0 | — | — | — | — | — | — | — | 22.0 | 22.0 | 143 |
| Dogfish | C | 1.4 | 1.9 | — | — | — | — | — | — | — | 1.9 | 1.9 | 143 |
| Dogwinkle | C | 1.4 | 2.1 | — | — | — | — | — | — | — | 2.1 | 2.1 | 143 |
| Flounder | A | 2.2 | 0.7 | — | — | — | — | — | — | — | 0.7 | 0.7 | 87 |
| | | 1.4 | 0.4 | — | — | — | — | — | — | — | 0.4 | 0.4 | 143 |
| | | 2.8 | 0.5 | — | — | — | — | — | — | — | 0.5 | 0.5 | 88 |
| **Flounder mean ± SD** | | | 0.5 ± 0.1 | — | — | — | — | — | — | — | 0.5 ± 0.1 | 0.5 ± 0.1 | |
| Flounder, frozen, uncooked | C | 2.2 | 0.6 | — | — | — | — | — | — | — | 0.6 | 0.6 | 87 |
| Herring, Baltic | C | 2.8 | 2.5 | Tr | Tr | — | — | — | — | — | 2.5 | 2.5 | 140 |
| Herring, marinated | C | 2.8 | 1.6 | Tr | — | — | — | — | — | — | 1.6 | 1.6 | 140 |
| Lobster, claw and tail meat | C | 1.4 | 1.5 | — | — | — | — | — | — | — | 1.5 | 1.5 | 143 |

*(continued)*

**TABLE 8.3** *Continued*

| Product | CC[a] | QI[b] | α-T[c] | β-T | γ-T | δ-T | α-T3[d] | β-T3 | γ-T3 | δ-T3 | Total | α-TE[e] mg | Ref. |
|---|---|---|---|---|---|---|---|---|---|---|---|---|---|
| Lobster, liver | C | 1.4 | 1.4 | — | — | — | — | — | — | — | 1.4 | 1.4 | 143 |
| Mackerel | C | 1.4 | 1.5 | — | — | — | — | — | — | — | 1.5 | 1.5 | 143 |
| Mackerel, liver | C | 1.4 | 3.1 | — | — | — | — | — | — | — | 3.1 | 3.1 | 143 |
| Mussel | C | 2.2 | 0.6 | — | — | — | — | — | — | — | 0.6 | 0.6 | 87 |
| Mussel, horse | C | 1.4 | 0.6 | — | — | — | — | — | — | — | 0.6 | 0.6 | 143 |
| Mussel, ribbed | C | 1.4 | 0.5 | — | — | — | — | — | — | — | 0.5 | 0.5 | 143 |
| Mussel, blue | C | 1.4 | 0.4 | — | — | — | — | — | — | — | 0.4 | 0.4 | 143 |
| Oyster | C | 1.4 | 0.6 | — | — | — | — | — | — | — | 0.6 | 0.6 | 143 |
| Perch | C | 2.8 | 1.5 | Tr | Tr | — | — | — | — | — | 1.5 | 1.5 | 140 |
| Periwinkle | C | 1.4 | 3.6 | — | — | — | — | — | — | — | 3.6 | 3.6 | 143 |
| Pike | C | 2.8 | 1.0 | — | — | — | — | — | — | — | 1.0 | 1.0 | 140 |
| Pikeperch | C | 2.8 | 1.4 | — | — | — | — | — | — | — | 1.4 | 1.4 | 140 |
| Pollack, deep frozen | C | 2.8 | 0.8 | — | — | — | — | — | — | — | 0.8 | 0.8 | 140 |
| Quahog, bay | C | 1.4 | 0.9 | — | — | — | — | — | — | — | 0.9 | 0.9 | 143 |
| Quahog, ocean | C | 1.4 | 0.2 | — | — | — | — | — | — | — | 0.2 | 0.2 | 143 |
| Rainbow trout | C | 2.8 | 1.9 | Tr | 0.1 | — | — | — | — | — | 2.0 | 1.9 | 140 |
| Redfish, deep frozen | C | 2.8 | 0.9 | — | — | — | — | — | — | — | 0.9 | 0.9 | 140 |
| Roe, vendace | C | 2.8 | 8.9 | — | — | — | — | — | — | — | 8.9 | 8.9 | 140 |
| Roe, whitefish | C | 2.8 | 17.4 | — | — | — | — | — | — | — | 17.4 | 17.4 | 140 |
| Roe, Baltic herring | C | 2.8 | 5.0 | — | — | — | — | — | — | — | 5.0 | 5.0 | 140 |
| Sablefish | C | 1.4 | 4.4 | — | — | — | — | — | — | — | 4.4 | 4.4 | 143 |
| Salmon | C | 2.8 | 2.0 | — | Tr | — | — | — | — | — | 2.0 | 2.0 | 140 |
| Salmon, water packed | C | 2.4 | 0.7 | — | — | — | — | — | — | — | 0.7 | 0.7 | 120 |
| Sardines, canned in tomato sauce | C | 2.4 | 3.8 | — | 0.2 | 0.1 | — | — | — | — | 4.1 | 3.8 | 120 |
| Scallops | C | 2.2 | 0.8 | — | — | — | — | — | — | — | 0.8 | 0.8 | 87 |
| Shrimp | B | 2.2 | 0.8 | — | — | — | — | — | — | — | 0.8 | 0.8 | 87 |
| | | 2.8 | 1.2 | — | 0.1 | — | — | — | — | — | 1.3 | 1.2 | 88 |
| Shrimp, breaded | C | 1.4 | 0.5 | — | 0.1 | — | — | — | — | — | 0.6 | 0.5 | 95 |

| | | | | | | | | | | | | | |
|---|---|---|---|---|---|---|---|---|---|---|---|---|---|
| Sprat, in oil, preserved | C | 2.8 | 2.3 | Tr | 3.8 | 1.2 | — | — | — | — | 7.3 | 2.7 | 140 |
| Sprat, preserved | C | 2.8 | 2.5 | — | — | — | — | — | — | — | 2.5 | 2.5 | 140 |
| Tuna, canned in oil | B | 2.2 | 0.6 | 0.1 | 4.5 | 0.8 | 0.1 | — | — | — | 5.9 | 1.1 | 87 |
| | | 2.4 | 1.0 | — | 3.7 | 1.5 | — | — | — | — | 6.2 | 1.4 | 120 |
| Tuna, canned in water | B | 2.2 | 0.5 | — | 0.1 | Tr | 0.1 | — | — | — | 0.7 | 0.5 | 87 |
| | | 2.8 | 0.4 | — | — | — | — | — | — | — | 0.4 | 0.4 | 88 |
| Tuna, white, canned | C | 2.2 | 0.9 | — | Tr | Tr | 0.1 | — | — | — | 1.0 | 0.9 | 87 |
| Vendace, lake fish | C | 2.8 | 2.0 | — | — | — | — | — | — | — | 2.0 | 2.0 | 140 |
| Vendace, sea fish | C | 2.8 | 1.5 | — | — | — | — | — | — | — | 1.5 | 1.5 | 140 |
| Whitefish | C | 2.8 | 2.7 | Tr | Tr | — | — | — | — | — | 2.7 | 2.7 | 140 |
| Beef, lean | | | | | | | | | | | | | |
| Prime, raw | C | 2.0 | 0.2 | | | | | | | | 0.2 | 0.2 | 198[f,h] |
| Prime, broiled | C | 2.0 | 0.1 | | | | | | | | 0.1 | 0.1 | 198 |
| Prime, roasted | C | 2.0 | 0.1 | | | | | | | | 0.1 | 0.1 | 198 |
| Prime, braised | C | 2.0 | 0.1 | | | | | | | | 0.1 | 0.1 | 198 |
| Choice, raw | C | 2.0 | 0.2 | | | | | | | | 0.2 | 0.2 | 198 |
| Choice, broiled | C | 2.0 | 0.2 | | | | | | | | 0.2 | 0.2 | 198 |
| Choice, roasted | C | 2.0 | 0.2 | | | | | | | | 0.2 | 0.2 | 198 |
| Choice, braised | C | 2.0 | 0.2 | | | | | | | | 0.2 | 0.2 | 198 |
| Good, raw | C | 2.0 | 0.1 | | | | | | | | 0.3 | 0.3 | 198 |
| Good, broiled | C | 2.0 | 0.1 | | | | | | | | 0.1 | 0.1 | 198 |
| Good, roasted | C | 2.0 | 0.1 | | | | | | | | 0.2 | 0.2 | 198 |
| Good, braised | C | 2.0 | 0.1 | | | | | | | | 0.2 | 0.2 | 198 |
| Standard, raw | C | 2.0 | 0.3 | | | | | | | | 0.2 | 0.2 | 198 |
| Standard, broiled | C | 2.0 | 0.1 | | | | | | | | 0.1 | 0.1 | 198 |

(*continued*)

**TABLE 8.3** *Continued*

| Product | CC[a] | QI[b] | α-T[c] | β-T | γ-T | δ-T | α-T3[d] | β-T3 | γ-T3 | δ-T3 | Total | α-TE[e] mg | Ref. |
|---|---|---|---|---|---|---|---|---|---|---|---|---|---|
| Standard, roasted | C | 2.0 | 0.2 | | | | | | | | 0.1 | 0.1 | 198 |
| Standard, braised | C | 2.0 | 0.2 | | | | | | | | 0.2 | 0.2 | 198 |
| Pork sausage, cooked | | | | | | | | | | | | | |
| Prepared with lard | C | 2.0 | 0.1 | — | 0.1 | — | — | — | — | — | 0.2 | 0.1 | 200 |
| Prepared with corn oil | C | 2.0 | 0.1 | — | 0.2 | — | — | — | — | — | 0.3 | 0.1 | 200 |
| Prepared with flaxseed oil | C | 2.0 | 0.2 | — | 2.4 | — | — | — | — | — | 2.6 | 0.4 | 200 |
| Chicken | | | | | | | | | | | | | |
| Breast | B | 2.4 | 0.2 | — | 0.1 | — | — | — | — | — | 0.3 | 0.2 | 145 |
| | | 2.8 | 0.1 | — | 0.1 | — | — | — | — | — | 0.2 | 0.1 | 88 |
| Leg | C | 2.4 | 0.4 | — | 0.2 | — | — | — | — | — | 0.6 | 0.4 | 144 |
| Thigh | C | 2.8 | 0.3 | — | 0.1 | — | — | — | — | — | 0.4 | 0.3 | 88 |
| Breast, cooked | C | 2.4 | 0.2 | — | 0.1 | — | — | — | — | — | 0.3 | 0.2 | 144 |
| Leg, cooked | C | 2.4 | 0.4 | — | 0.2 | — | — | — | — | — | 0.6 | 0.4 | 144 |
| Turkey breast | C | 2.0 | 0.2 | — | 0.1 | — | — | — | — | — | 0.3 | 0.2 | 203 |
| Turkey breast, irradiated | C | 2.0 | 0.1 | — | 0.1 | — | — | — | — | — | 0.2 | 0.1 | 203 |
| Turkey breast, nitrogen packing | C | 2.0 | 0.2 | — | 0.1 | — | — | — | — | — | 0.3 | 0.2 | 203 |
| **Fruits** (fresh weight, unless otherwise specified) | | | | | | | | | | | | | |
| Amazoniam palm fruit | | | | | | | | | | | | | |
| *Maximiliana maripa* pulp oil | C | 1.8 | 9.2 | 2.5 | — | — | 3.6 | 1.2 | 1.0 | 1.0 | 18.5 | 11.6 | 155, 210 |
| *Maximiliana maripa* kernel oil | C | 1.8 | 0.2 | 0.1 | 0.1 | — | 0.7 | 0.2 | 0.2 | — | 1.5 | 0.5 | 210 |
| Apple | A | 2.2 | 0.2 | Tr | Tr | Tr | — | — | — | — | 0.3 | 0.2 | 87 |
| | | 2.6 | 0.2 | — | — | — | — | — | — | — | 0.2 | 0.2 | 145 |
| | | 2.8 | 0.2 | — | — | — | — | — | — | — | 0.2 | 0.2 | 88 |

| | | | | | | | | | | | | |
|---|---|---|---|---|---|---|---|---|---|---|---|---|
| **Apple mean ± SD** | | | 0.2 ± 0.0 | Tr | Tr | Tr | — | — | — | — | 0.2 ± 0.0 | 0.2 ± 0.0 | |
| Apple juice | C | 2.6 | — | — | — | — | — | — | — | — | 0.0 | 0.0 | 145 |
| Applesauce | C | 2.2 | 0.2 | — | — | — | — | — | — | — | 0.2 | 0.2 | 87 |
| Apricot, dried | C | 2.6 | 6.2 | Tr | 0.2 | 0.2 | 0.1 | — | — | — | 6.7 | 6.3 | 145 |
| Avocado | C | 2.2 | 2.0 | 0.1 | 0.4 | Tr | Tr | 0.1 | — | — | 2.5 | 2.1 | 87 |
| Banana | B | 2.6 | 0.2 | Tr | Tr | — | — | — | — | — | 0.2 | 0.2 | 145 |
| | | 2.8 | 0.3 | — | Tr | — | — | — | — | — | 0.3 | 0.3 | 88 |
| Berry juice, mixed | C | 2.6 | Tr | — | — | — | — | — | — | — | 0.0 | 0.0 | 139 |
| Blueberry | C | 2.6 | 1.9 | — | 0.2 | — | Tr | — | 0.7 | — | 2.7 | 1.9 | 145 |
| Blueberry, frozen | C | 2.6 | 1.8 | Tr | 0.2 | Tr | Tr | — | 0.4 | — | 2.5 | 1.9 | 145 |
| Cantaloupe | B | 2.2 | Tr | — | 0.1 | — | — | — | — | — | 0.2 | 0.1 | 87 |
| | | 2.8 | 0.1 | — | 0.1 | — | — | — | — | — | 0.2 | 0.1 | 88 |
| Cherries, canned | C | 2.2 | 0.2 | — | — | — | — | — | — | — | 0.2 | 0.2 | 87 |
| Cherry, Bing | C | 2.2 | 0.1 | Tr | 0.1 | — | 0.1 | — | — | — | 0.2 | 0.1 | 87 |
| Cloudberry | C | 2.6 | 3.0 | 0.2 | 0.5 | Tr | — | — | — | — | 3.6 | 3.1 | 145 |
| Cranberry | C | 2.6 | 0.9 | Tr | 0.3 | Tr | 0.1 | — | 0.4 | — | 1.7 | 1.0 | 145 |
| Currant, black | C | 2.6 | 2.2 | — | 0.8 | Tr | Tr | — | — | — | 3.0 | 2.4 | 145 |
| | C | 2.8 | 1.2 | — | 2.1 | 0.2 | — | — | — | — | 3.5 | 1.4 | 207 |
| Currant, red | C | 2.6 | 0.8 | 0.2 | 0.3 | 0.2 | Tr | — | — | — | 1.5 | 0.9 | 145 |
| Currant, red and black | C | 2.8 | 0.5 | 0.1 | 1.7 | 0.6 | — | — | — | — | 2.7 | 0.7 | 207 |
| Currant juice, black | C | 2.6 | Tr | — | — | — | — | — | — | — | 0.0 | 0.0 | 145 |
| Flavedo | C | 1.4 | 7.2 | — | 4.5 | — | — | — | — | — | 11.7 | 7.7 | 146 |
| Fruit cocktail | B | 2.2 | 0.5 | — | — | — | — | — | — | — | 0.5 | 0.5 | 87 |
| | | 2.6 | 0.9 | Tr | Tr | — | — | — | — | — | 0.9 | 0.9 | 145 |
| Gooseberry | C | 2.2 | 0.7 | Tr | 0.1 | Tr | — | — | — | — | 0.8 | 0.7 | 145 |
| Gooseberry, red–black | C | 2.8 | 0.4 | — | 1.1 | 0.1 | — | — | — | — | 1.6 | 0.5 | 207 |

*(continued)*

**TABLE 8.3** *Continued*

| Product | CC[a] | QI[b] | α-T[c] | β-T | γ-T | δ-T | α-T3[d] | β-T3 | γ-T3 | δ-T3 | Total | α-TE[e] mg | Ref. |
|---|---|---|---|---|---|---|---|---|---|---|---|---|---|
| Grape, unspecified | C | 2.6 | 0.6 | Tr | 0.1 | — | 0.1 | — | 0.1 | — | 0.9 | 0.7 | 145 |
| Grape, white seedless | C | 2.8 | 0.4 | — | 0.2 | — | — | — | — | — | 0.6 | 0.4 | 88 |
| Grapefruit | B | 2.2 | 0.2 | — | — | — | — | — | — | — | 0.2 | 0.2 | 87 |
| | | 2.6 | 0.3 | Tr | Tr | — | — | — | — | — | 0.3 | 0.3 | 145 |
| Jostaberry | | | 1.1 | — | 1.4 | 0.1 | — | — | — | — | 2.5 | 1.2 | 207 |
| Lingonberry | C | 2.6 | 1.5 | Tr | 0.1 | — | 0.1 | — | 0.4 | — | 2.1 | 1.6 | 145 |
| Mandarin | C | 2.6 | 0.3 | Tr | Tr | — | — | — | — | — | 0.3 | 0.3 | 145 |
| Mixed fruit juice | C | 2.6 | Tr | — | — | — | — | — | — | — | 0.0 | 0.0 | 145 |
| Nectarine | C | 2.2 | 1.0 | — | — | — | — | — | — | — | 1.0 | 1.0 | 87 |
| Olive | | | | | | | | | | | | | |
| Black, raw | C | 2.4 | 13.8 | 2.1 | 3.0 | — | 15.4 | — | — | — | 34.3 | 15.6 | 147 |
| Green, raw | C | 2.4 | 13.5 | Tr | 1.58 | Tr | — | — | — | — | 15.1 | 13.7 | 147 |
| Green, bottled | C | 2.2 | 3.8 | — | — | — | — | — | — | — | 3.8 | 3.8 | 87 |
| Ripe, canned | C | 2.2 | 1.7 | — | — | — | — | — | — | — | 1.7 | 1.7 | 87 |
| Oranges, unspecified | B | 2.2 | 0.3 | — | — | — | — | — | — | — | 0.3 | 0.3 | 87 |
| | | 2.6 | 0.4 | Tr | Tr | — | — | — | — | — | 0.4 | 0.4 | 145 |
| Orange juice, fresh | A | 2.2 | 0.1 | — | — | — | — | — | — | — | 0.1 | 0.1 | 87 |
| | | 2.4 | 0.2 | — | 0.1 | — | — | — | — | — | 0.3 | 0.2 | 120 |
| Orange juice, fresh | | 2.6 | 0.2 | Tr | Tr | — | Tr | — | — | — | 0.2 | 0.2 | 145 |
| **Orange juice, fresh mean ± SD** | | | 0.2 ± 0.0 | Tr | Tr | — | Tr | — | — | — | 0.2 ± 0.1 | 0.2 ± 0.0 | |
| Peaches | | | | | | | | | | | | | |
| Unspecified | B | 2.2 | 0.8 | — | — | — | 0.1 | — | — | — | 0.9 | 0.8 | 87 |
| | | 2.6 | 1.0 | Tr | 0.1 | — | — | — | — | — | 1.0 | 1.0 | 145 |
| Canned | B | 2.2 | 0.8 | — | — | — | — | — | — | — | 0.8 | 0.8 | 87 |
| | | 2.6 | 2.0 | Tr | 0.1 | — | Tr | — | — | — | 2.0 | 2.0 | 145 |
| Dried | C | 2.2 | 0.2 | — | — | — | — | — | — | — | 0.2 | 0.2 | 87 |
| Frozen | C | 2.2 | 0.6 | — | — | — | — | — | — | — | 0.6 | 0.6 | 87 |
| Pears | | | | | | | | | | | | | |

| | | | | | | | | | | | | | |
|---|---|---|---|---|---|---|---|---|---|---|---|---|---|
| Unspecified | B | 2.2 | 0.4 | Tr | 0.2 | — | 0.3 | — | — | — | 0.9 | 0.5 | 87 |
| | | 2.6 | 0.1 | Tr | Tr | — | — | — | — | — | 0.1 | 0.1 | 145 |
| Dried | C | 2.2 | 0.1 | — | Tr | — | — | — | — | — | 0.1 | 0.1 | 87 |
| Pineapple, canned | B | 2.6 | Tr | Tr | — | — | — | — | — | — | 0.0 | 0.0 | 145 |
| Plums, unspecified | A | 2.2 | 0.2 | — | 0.2 | — | 0.1 | — | — | — | 0.4 | 0.2 | 87 |
| | | 2.4 | 0.6 | — | 0.1 | — | — | — | — | — | 0.7 | 0.6 | 120 |
| | | 2.6 | 0.9 | Tr | 0.1 | — | Tr | — | — | — | 0.9 | 0.9 | 145 |
| **Plums mean ± SD** | | | 0.6 ± 0.3 | Tr | 0.1 ± 0.0 | — | Tr | — | — | — | 0.7 ± 0.2 | 0.6 ± 0.3 | |
| Prunes | B | 2.2 | 0.5 | — | — | — | Tr | — | — | — | 0.6 | 0.6 | 87 |
| | | 2.6 | 1.8 | Tr | 0.1 | Tr | — | — | — | — | 1.9 | 1.8 | 145 |
| Prune juice | C | 2.2 | 0.1 | — | — | — | — | — | — | — | 0.1 | 0.1 | 87 |
| Raisins | B | 2.2 | 0.1 | — | 0.1 | — | — | — | — | — | 0.2 | 0.1 | 87 |
| | | 2.6 | 0.3 | Tr | 0.1 | Tr | — | — | — | — | 0.4 | 0.3 | 145 |
| Raspberry, unspecified | C | 2.6 | 0.9 | 0.2 | 1.5 | 1.2 | — | — | — | — | 3.7 | 1.1 | 145 |
| Rose hip | C | 2.6 | 4.1 | 0.1 | 0.1 | Tr | — | — | — | — | 4.3 | 4.2 | 145 |
| Rose hip sauce, frozen | C | 2.6 | 1.6 | Tr | 0.9 | 0.1 | — | — | — | — | 2.6 | 1.7 | 145 |
| Sea buckthorn | C | 2.6 | 3.1 | 0.3 | 0.7 | — | — | — | Tr | — | 4.0 | 3.3 | 145 |
| Var. sinensis | C | 2.0 | 7.0 | Tr | Tr | Tr | Tr | Tr | Tr | Tr | 7.0 | 7.0 | 213 |
| Var. mongolica | C | 2.0 | 7.5 | Tr | Tr | Tr | Tr | Tr | Tr | Tr | 7.5 | 7.5 | 213 |
| Strawberry, unspecified | C | 2.6 | 0.6 | Tr | 0.2 | Tr | — | — | — | — | 0.7 | 0.6 | 145 |
| Watermelon, unspecified | C | 2.2 | 0.1 | — | — | — | — | — | — | — | 0.1 | 0.1 | 87 |

(*continued*)

**TABLE 8.3** *Continued*

| Product | CC[a] | QI[b] | α-T[c] | β-T | γ-T | δ-T | α-T3[d] | β-T3 | γ-T3 | δ-T3 | Total | α-TE[e] mg | Ref. |
|---|---|---|---|---|---|---|---|---|---|---|---|---|---|
| Vegetables (Fresh weight, unless otherwise specified) | | | | | | | | | | | | | |
| Asparagus | | | | | | | | | | | | | |
| Fresh | C | 2.4 | 1.2 | — | 0.1 | — | — | — | — | — | 1.3 | 1.2 | 120 |
| Frozen | C | 2.2 | 1.1 | Tr | 0.1 | — | Tr | — | — | — | 1.2 | 1.1 | 87 |
| Frozen, boiled | C | 2.2 | 1.1 | — | 0.1 | — | — | — | — | — | 1.2 | 1.1 | 87 |
| Broccoli | | | | | | | | | | | | | |
| Fresh | A | 2.2 | 1.6 | Tr | 0.4 | — | 0.1 | — | — | — | 2.1 | 1.7 | 87 |
| | | 2.6 | 0.7 | Tr | 0.1 | — | — | — | — | — | 0.8 | 0.7 | 145 |
| | | 2.8 | 1.4 | — | 0.3 | — | — | — | — | — | 1.7 | 1.5 | 88 |
| **Broccoli mean ± SD** | | | 1.2 ± 0.4 | Tr | 0.3 ± 0.1 | — | Tr | — | — | — | 1.5 ± 0.5 | 1.3 ± 0.4 | |
| Freeze dried | C | 1.6 | 6.3 | — | — | — | — | — | — | — | 6.3 | 6.3 | 112 |
| Frozen | B | 2.2 | 1.3 | — | 0.3 | — | — | — | — | — | 1.6 | 1.3 | 87 |
| | | 2.8 | 1.0 | Tr | 0.2 | — | — | — | — | — | 1.2 | 1.0 | 88 |
| Boiled | C | 2.2 | 1.4 | Tr | 0.4 | Tr | 0.1 | — | — | — | 1.8 | 1.4 | 87 |
| Brussels sprouts | | | | | | | | | | | | | |
| Fresh | C | 2.6 | 0.4 | Tr | Tr | — | Tr | — | — | — | 0.4 | 0.4 | 145 |
| Boiled | C | 2.2 | 0.4 | — | — | — | — | — | — | — | 0.4 | 0.4 | 87 |
| Frozen | C | 2.2 | 0.4 | — | — | — | — | — | — | — | 0.4 | 0.4 | 87 |
| Cabbage, unspecified | A | 2.2 | 0.1 | — | — | — | Tr | — | — | — | 0.1 | 0.1 | 87 |
| | | 2.4 | 0.1 | — | — | — | — | — | — | — | 0.1 | 0.1 | 120 |
| | | 2.6 | Tr | — | — | — | — | — | — | — | 0.0 | 0.0 | 145 |
| | | 2.8 | 0.2 | — | Tr | — | — | — | — | — | 0.2 | 0.2 | 88 |
| **Cabbage mean ± SD** | | | 0.1 ± 0.1 | — | Tr | — | Tr | — | — | — | 0.1 ± 0.1 | 0.1 ± 0.1 | |
| Cabbage, Chinese | C | 2.6 | 0.2 | — | Tr | — | — | — | — | — | 0.2 | 0.2 | 145 |
| Cabbage, red | C | 2.6 | 0.1 | — | — | — | — | — | — | — | 0.1 | 0.1 | 145 |
| Cantharelle | C | 2.6 | — | — | — | — | — | — | — | — | 0.0 | 0.0 | 145 |

| | | | | | | | | | | | | | |
|---|---|---|---|---|---|---|---|---|---|---|---|---|---|
| Carrot | A | 2.2 | 0.3 | — | — | — | — | — | — | — | 0.3 | 0.3 | 87 |
| | | 2.6 | 0.4 | Tr | Tr | — | Tr | — | — | — | 0.4 | 0.4 | 145 |
| | | 2.8 | 1.2 | Tr | — | — | — | — | — | — | 1.2 | 1.2 | 88 |
| **Carrot mean ± SD** | | | 0.6 ± 0.4 | Tr | Tr | — | Tr | — | — | — | 0.6 ± 0.4 | 0.6 ± 0.4 | |
| Carrot, boiled | C | 2.2 | 0.2 | — | — | — | — | — | — | — | 0.2 | 0.2 | 87 |
| Carrot, frozen | C | 2.6 | 0.6 | Tr | — | — | 0.1 | — | — | — | 0.7 | 0.6 | 145 |
| Cauliflower, unspecified | B | 2.2 | 0.1 | — | 0.2 | — | 0.1 | — | — | — | 0.3 | 0.1 | 87 |
| | | 2.6 | 0.1 | — | 0.3 | — | — | — | — | — | 0.4 | 0.1 | 145 |
| Celery, unspecified | A | 2.2 | 0.1 | — | — | — | — | — | — | — | 0.1 | 0.1 | 87 |
| | | 2.6 | 0.5 | Tr | 0.1 | — | 0.1 | — | — | — | 0.7 | 0.5 | 145 |
| | | 2.8 | 0.5 | Tr | — | — | — | — | — | — | 0.5 | 0.5 | 88 |
| **Celery mean ± SD** | | | 0.4 ± 0.2 | Tr | Tr | — | Tr | — | — | — | 0.4 ± 0.2 | 0.4 ± 0.2 | |
| Champignon, canned | C | 2.6 | — | — | — | — | — | — | — | — | 0.0 | 0.0 | 145 |
| Corn | | | | | | | | | | | | | |
| Canned | C | 2.2 | Tr | — | — | — | 0.1 | — | 1.3 | — | 1.5 | 0.1 | 87 |
| Frozen | C | 2.2 | 0.1 | — | 0.5 | — | 0.4 | — | 1.0 | — | 2.0 | 0.2 | 87 |
| Frozen, boiled | C | 2.2 | 0.1 | — | 0.1 | — | 0.2 | — | 0.7 | — | 1.1 | 0.1 | 87 |
| Creamed, canned | C | 2.2 | 0.1 | — | 0.1 | — | — | — | 0.2 | — | 0.4 | 0.1 | 87 |
| Cucumber | A | 2.2 | Tr | Tr | Tr | — | 0.1 | — | — | — | 0.2 | 0.1 | 87 |
| | | 2.4 | 0.1 | — | Tr | — | — | — | — | — | 0.1 | 0.1 | 120 |
| | | 2.6 | Tr | Tr | Tr | Tr | — | — | — | — | 0.1 | 0.0 | 145 |
| **Cucumber mean ± SD** | | | Tr | Tr | Tr | Tr | Tr | — | — | — | 0.1 ± 0.0 | 0.1 ± 0.0 | |
| Dill | C | 2.6 | 1.6 | Tr | 0.2 | — | — | — | — | — | 1.8 | 1.6 | 145 |
| Green bean, canned | C | 2.2 | — | — | 1.3 | — | — | — | — | — | 1.3 | 0.1 | 87 |
| Green bean, frozen | C | 2.2 | Tr | — | 0.1 | Tr | — | — | — | — | 0.1 | 0.0 | 87 |
| Leek | C | 2.6 | 0.3 | — | Tr | — | — | — | — | — | 0.4 | 0.3 | 145 |

(*continued*)

**TABLE 8.3** *Continued*

| Product | CC[a] | QI[b] | α-T[c] | β-T | γ-T | δ-T | α-T3[d] | β-T3 | γ-T3 | δ-T3 | Total | α-TE[e] mg | Ref. |
|---|---|---|---|---|---|---|---|---|---|---|---|---|---|
| Lettuce, unspecified | A | 2.2 | 0.4 | Tr | 0.5 | Tr | — | — | — | — | 0.8 | 0.4 | 87 |
| | | 2.6 | 0.6 | Tr | 0.3 | — | — | — | — | — | 0.9 | 0.7 | 145 |
| | | 1.0 | 0.5 | — | 0.7 | — | — | — | — | — | 1.2 | 0.6 | 94 |
| **Lettuce mean ± SD** | | | 0.5 ± 0.1 | Tr | 0.5 ± 0.2 | Tr | — | — | — | — | 1.0 ± 0.2 | 0.6 ± 0.1 | |
| Lettuce, iceberg | B | 2.8 | 0.3 | — | 0.1 | — | — | — | — | — | 0.4 | 0.3 | 88 |
| | | 2.2 | 0.3 | — | 0.3 | Tr | — | — | — | — | 0.6 | 0.3 | 87 |
| Lettuce, leaf | C | 2.2 | 0.3 | Tr | 0.7 | — | — | — | — | — | 1.0 | 0.4 | 87 |
| Lettuce, romaine | C | 2.2 | 0.6 | — | 0.4 | — | — | — | — | — | 1.0 | 0.6 | 87 |
| Nettle | C | 2.6 | 1.6 | 0.1 | 0.2 | — | — | — | — | — | 1.9 | 1.7 | 145 |
| Okra | C | 2.2 | 0.3 | — | 0.2 | — | — | — | — | — | 0.5 | 0.3 | 87 |
| Onion, boiled | C | 2.2 | Tr | — | — | — | — | — | — | — | 0.0 | 0.0 | 87 |
| Onion, white | B | 2.2 | Tr | — | — | — | 0.1 | — | — | — | 0.1 | 0.1 | 87 |
| Onion, yellow | C | 2.6 | Tr | Tr | Tr | — | — | — | — | — | 0.1 | 0.0 | 145 |
| Onion, red | C | 2.6 | Tr | Tr | Tr | — | — | — | — | — | 0.1 | 0.0 | 145 |
| Parsley | B | 2.2 | 0.8 | — | 0.5 | — | — | — | — | — | 1.3 | 0.8 | 87 |
| | | 2.6 | 3.6 | Tr | 1.2 | Tr | Tr | — | Tr | — | 4.8 | 3.7 | 145 |
| Parsnip | C | 2.6 | 0.8 | Tr | Tr | — | Tr | — | — | — | 0.9 | 0.8 | 145 |
| Pepper | C | 2.2 | 0.1 | — | — | — | — | — | — | — | 0.1 | 0.1 | 87 |
| Pepper Vandel, green | C | 2.0 | 1.0 | — | — | — | — | — | — | — | 1.0 | 1.0 | 169 |
| Vandel, red | C | 2.0 | 2.8 | — | — | — | — | — | — | — | 2.8 | 2.8 | 169 |
| Gamba, green | C | 2.0 | 1.0 | — | — | — | — | — | — | — | 1.0 | 1.0 | 169 |
| Gamba, red | C | 2.0 | 3.1 | — | — | — | — | — | — | — | 3.1 | 3.1 | 169 |
| Mild, green | C | 2.0 | 3.2 | — | — | — | — | — | — | — | 3.2 | 3.2 | 169 |
| Mild, green–red | C | 2.0 | 6.6 | — | — | — | — | — | — | — | 6.6 | 6.6 | 169 |
| Mild, red | C | 2.0 | 10.8 | — | — | — | — | — | — | — | 10.8 | 10.8 | 169 |

| | | | | | | | | | | | | | |
|---|---|---|---|---|---|---|---|---|---|---|---|---|---|
| Pepper (*Capsicum annum*, dry weight) | | | | | | | | | | | | | |
| Breaker | C | 2.4 | 7.6 | — | 35.3 | — | — | — | — | — | 42.9 | 11.1 | 164 |
| Mature, green | C | 2.4 | 3.9 | — | 23.6 | — | — | — | — | — | 27.5 | 6.3 | 164 |
| Red, succulent | C | 2.4 | 17.6 | — | 41.7 | — | — | — | — | — | 59.3 | 21.8 | 164 |
| Red, partially dried | C | 2.4 | 12.2 | — | 17.0 | — | — | — | — | — | 29.2 | 13.9 | 164 |
| Red, fully dried | C | 2.4 | 23.8 | — | 7.5 | — | — | — | — | — | 31.3 | 24.6 | 164 |
| Potato | B | 2.2 | Tr | — | — | — | — | — | — | — | 0.0 | 0.0 | 87 |
| | | 2.6 | 0.1 | — | — | — | — | — | — | — | 0.1 | 0.1 | 145 |
| Potato, boiled | C | 2.2 | Tr | — | — | — | — | — | — | — | 0.0 | 0.0 | 87 |
| Potato, sweet | C | 2.2 | 0.3 | Tr | — | — | 0.1 | — | — | — | 0.4 | 0.3 | 87 |
| Potato, sweet, baked | C | 2.2 | 0.2 | — | — | — | Tr | — | — | — | 0.2 | 0.2 | 87 |
| Radish | C | 2.6 | Tr | — | — | — | — | — | — | — | 0.0 | 0.0 | 145 |
| Red beet | C | 2.6 | 0.1 | Tr | — | — | — | — | — | — | 0.1 | 0.1 | 145 |
| Red beet, pickled | C | 2.6 | 0.1 | Tr | — | — | — | — | — | — | 0.1 | 0.1 | 145 |
| Rhubarb | C | 2.6 | 0.3 | Tr | — | — | — | — | — | — | 0.3 | 0.3 | 145 |
| Rutabaga | C | 2.6 | Tr | — | — | — | — | — | — | — | 0.0 | 0.0 | 145 |
| Spinach | A | 2.2 | 1.4 | — | — | — | — | — | — | — | 1.4 | 1.4 | 87 |
| | | 2.6 | 1.2 | — | — | — | — | — | — | — | 1.2 | 1.2 | 145 |
| | | 2.8 | 2.1 | — | 0.2 | — | — | — | — | — | 2.3 | 2.2 | 88 |
| **Spinach mean ± SD** | | | 1.6 ± 0.4 | — | 0.1 ± 0.1 | — | — | — | — | — | 1.6 ± 0.5 | 1.6 ± 0.4 | |
| Spinach, frozen | B | 2.2 | 2.3 | — | 0.1 | — | — | — | — | — | 2.4 | 2.3 | 87 |
| | | 2.6 | 1.3 | Tr | 0.1 | — | — | — | — | — | 1.4 | 1.3 | 145 |
| Tomato | | | | | | | | | | | | | |
| Fresh | A | 2.2 | 0.6 | — | 0.1 | — | — | — | — | — | 0.7 | 0.6 | 87 |
| | | 2.6 | 0.7 | Tr | 0.2 | Tr | — | — | — | — | 0.9 | 0.7 | 145 |
| | | 2.8 | 0.7 | — | 0.1 | — | — | — | — | — | 0.8 | 0.8 | 88 |
| **Tomato mean ± SD** | | | 0.7 ± 0.0 | Tr | 0.1 ± 0.1 | Tr | — | — | — | — | 0.8 ± 0.1 | 0.7 ± 0.1 | |
| Peeled | C | 2.2 | 0.6 | — | 0.1 | — | — | — | — | — | 0.7 | 0.6 | 87 |

(*continued*)

**TABLE 8.3** *Continued*

| Product | CC[a] | QI[b] | α-T[c] | β-T | γ-T | δ-T | α-T3[d] | β-T3 | γ-T3 | δ-T3 | Total | α-TE[e] mg | Ref. |
|---|---|---|---|---|---|---|---|---|---|---|---|---|---|
| Canned, whole | C | 2.8 | 0.9 | Tr | 0.1 | — | — | — | — | — | 1.0 | 0.9 | 88 |
| Barbecue sauce | C | 2.4 | 1.1 | — | 0.6 | 0.1 | — | — | — | — | 1.8 | 1.1 | 120 |
| Ketchup | C | 2.4 | 1.5 | — | 0.2 | — | — | — | — | — | 1.6 | 1.5 | 120 |
| Chili sauce | C | 2.4 | 3.0 | — | 0.3 | — | — | — | — | — | 3.3 | 3.0 | 120 |
| Juice | C | 2.8 | 0.8 | Tr | Tr | — | — | — | — | — | 0.8 | 0.8 | 88 |
| Paste | C | 2.4 | 4.3 | — | 0.5 | — | — | — | — | — | 4.8 | 4.4 | 120 |
| Sauce | B | 2.4 | 1.5 | — | 0.2 | — | — | — | — | — | 1.7 | 1.5 | 120 |
| | | 2.8 | 1.4 | Tr | 0.1 | — | — | — | — | — | 1.5 | 1.4 | 88 |
| Soup | B | 2.4 | 0.7 | — | 0.2 | Tr | — | — | — | — | 0.9 | 0.7 | 120 |
| | | 2.8 | 1.2 | Tr | 0.4 | 0.1 | — | — | — | — | 1.7 | 1.2 | 88 |
| Stewed | C | 2.4 | 0.8 | — | 0.2 | — | — | — | — | — | 1.0 | 0.8 | 120 |
| Turnip, greens | C | 2.4 | 2.9 | — | 0.2 | — | — | — | — | — | 3.1 | 2.9 | 120 |
| Turnip, yellow | C | 2.6 | — | — | — | — | — | — | — | — | 0.0 | 0.0 | 145 |
| Turnip, white | C | 2.6 | — | — | — | — | — | — | — | — | 0.0 | 0.0 | 145 |
| Vegetable juice, canned | C | 2.2 | 0.7 | — | — | — | — | — | — | — | 0.7 | 0.7 | 87 |
| Vegetable, mixed, frozen | C | 2.6 | 0.3 | Tr | 0.5 | Tr | Tr | — | Tr | — | 0.8 | 0.3 | 145 |
| Tropical plants | | | | | | | | | | | | | |
| *Sauropus androgynus*, leaves | C | 2.0 | 42.6 | — | — | — | — | — | — | — | 42.6 | 42.6 | 212[f] |
| *Citrus hystrix*, leaves | C | 2.0 | 39.8 | — | — | — | — | — | — | — | 39.8 | 39.8 | 212 |
| *Calamus scipronum*, leaves | C | 2.0 | 19.4 | — | — | — | — | — | — | — | 19.4 | 19.4 | 212 |
| *Averrhoa belimbi*, leaves | C | 2.0 | 16.8 | — | — | — | — | — | — | — | 16.8 | 16.8 | 212 |

| | | | | | | | | | | | | | |
|---|---|---|---|---|---|---|---|---|---|---|---|---|---|
| *Apium graveolens*, leaves | C | 2.0 | 13.6 | — | — | — | — | — | — | — | 13.6 | 13.6 | 212 |
| *Pandanus odorus*, leaves | C | 2.0 | 13.1 | — | — | — | — | — | — | — | 13.1 | 13.1 | 212 |
| *Oenanthe javanica*, leaves | C | 2.0 | 14.7 | — | — | — | — | — | — | — | 14.7 | 14.7 | 212 |
| *Camellia chinensis*, black, leaves | C | 2.0 | 18.3 | — | — | — | — | — | — | — | 18.3 | 18.3 | 212 |
| *Lycium chinese*, leaves | C | 2.0 | 9.4 | — | — | — | — | — | — | — | 9.4 | 9.4 | 212 |
| *Moringa oleifera*, leaves | C | 2.0 | 9.0 | — | — | — | — | — | — | — | 9.0 | 9.0 | 212 |
| *Allium fistulosum*, leaves | C | 2.0 | 7.5 | — | — | — | — | — | — | — | 7.5 | 7.5 | 212 |
| *Brassica alboglabra*, leaves | C | 2.0 | 7.3 | — | — | — | — | — | — | — | 7.3 | 7.3 | 212 |
| *Piper sarmentosum*, leaves | C | 2.0 | 6.0 | — | — | — | — | — | — | — | 6.0 | 6.0 | 212 |
| *Sesbania grandiflora*, leaves | C | 2.0 | 5.5 | — | — | — | — | — | — | — | 5.5 | 5.5 | 212 |
| *Mentha arvensis*, leaves | C | 2.0 | 4.9 | — | — | — | — | — | — | — | 4.9 | 4.9 | 212 |
| *Piper betel*, leaves | C | 2.0 | 4.3 | — | — | — | — | — | — | — | 4.3 | 4.3 | 212 |
| *Gynandropsis gynandra*, leaves | C | 2.0 | 3.6 | — | — | — | — | — | — | — | 3.6 | 3.6 | 212 |

*(continued)*

**TABLE 8.3** *Continued*

| Product | CC[a] | QI[b] | α-T[c] | β-T | γ-T | δ-T | α-T3[d] | β-T3 | γ-T3 | δ-T3 | Total | α-TE[e] mg | Ref. |
|---|---|---|---|---|---|---|---|---|---|---|---|---|---|
| *Hydrocotyle asiatica*, leaves | C | 2.0 | 3.0 | — | — | — | — | — | — | — | 3.0 | 3.0 | 212 |
| *Allium odorum*, leaves | C | 2.0 | 1.7 | — | — | — | — | — | — | — | 1.7 | 1.7 | 212 |
| *Colocasia esculentum*, leaf stalk | C | 2.0 | 1.6 | — | — | — | — | — | — | — | 1.6 | 1.6 | 212 |
| *Amaranthus spinosus*, leaves | C | 2.0 | 1.6 | — | — | — | — | — | — | — | 1.6 | 1.6 | 212 |
| *Ipomoea aucatica*, leaves | C | 2.0 | 1.4 | — | — | — | — | — | — | — | 1.4 | 1.4 | 212 |
| *Polygonum minus*, leaves | C | 2.0 | 1.4 | — | — | — | — | — | — | — | 1.4 | 1.4 | 212 |
| *Cymbopogon citratus, leaves* | C | 2.0 | 1.3 | — | — | — | — | — | — | — | 1.3 | 1.3 | 212 |
| *Amaranthus gangeticus*, leaves | C | 2.0 | 1.2 | — | — | — | — | — | — | — | 1.2 | 1.2 | 212 |
| *Brassica chinensis*, leaves | C | 2.0 | 0.9 | — | — | — | — | — | — | — | 0.9 | 0.9 | 212 |
| *Brassica oleracea* cabbage, leaves | C | 2.0 | 0.7 | — | — | — | — | — | — | — | 0.7 | 0.7 | 212 |
| *Ipomea batatas*, shoots | C | 2.0 | 13.0 | — | — | — | — | — | — | — | 13.0 | 13.0 | 212 |
| *Carica papaya*, shoots | C | 2.0 | 11.1 | — | — | — | — | — | — | — | 11.1 | 11.1 | 212 |
| *Anacardium occidentale*, shoots | C | 2.0 | 3.1 | — | — | — | — | — | — | — | 3.1 | 3.1 | 212 |

| | | | | | | | | | | | | | |
|---|---|---|---|---|---|---|---|---|---|---|---|---|---|
| *Manihot utilissima*, shoots | C | 2.0 | 2.7 | — | — | — | — | — | — | — | 2.7 | 2.7 | 212 |
| *Diplazium esculentum*, shoots | C | 2.0 | 2.7 | — | — | — | — | — | — | — | 2.7 | 2.7 | 212 |
| *Glycine max*, sprout | C | 2.0 | 1.8 | — | — | — | — | — | — | — | 1.8 | 1.8 | 212 |
| *Phaseolus aureus*, sprout | C | 2.0 | 1.6 | — | — | — | — | — | — | — | 1.6 | 1.6 | 212 |
| *Capsicum annum*, red, fruit | C | 2.0 | 15.5 | — | — | — | — | — | — | — | 15.5 | 15.5 | 212 |
| *Capsicum frutescens*, fruit | C | 2.0 | 9.5 | — | — | — | — | — | — | — | 9.5 | 9.5 | 212 |
| *Capsicum annum*, green, fruit | C | 2.0 | 8.7 | — | — | — | — | — | — | — | 8.7 | 8.7 | 212 |
| *Capsicum annum*, bell pepper, fruit | C | 2.0 | 7.1 | — | — | — | — | — | — | — | 7.1 | 7.1 | 212 |
| *Momordica charantia*, fruit | C | 2.0 | 6.1 | — | — | — | — | — | — | — | 6.1 | 6.1 | 212 |
| *Garcinia atroviridis*, fruit | C | 2.0 | 7.6 | — | — | — | — | — | — | — | 7.6 | 7.6 | 212 |
| *Trichosanthes anguina*, snake gourd | C | 2.0 | 1.7 | — | — | — | — | — | — | — | 1.7 | 1.7 | 212 |
| *Averrhoa belimbi*, starfruit | C | 2.0 | 0.9 | — | — | — | — | — | — | — | 0.9 | 0.9 | 212 |
| *Psidium guajava*, guava, fruit | C | 2.0 | 0.9 | — | — | — | — | — | — | — | 0.9 | 0.9 | 212 |
| *Luffah acutangula*, angular luffa, fruit | C | 2.0 | 0.7 | — | — | — | — | — | — | — | 0.7 | 0.7 | 212 |

*(continued)*

**TABLE 8.3** *Continued*

| Product | CC[a] | QI[b] | α-T[c] | β-T | γ-T | δ-T | α-T3[d] | β-T3 | γ-T3 | δ-T3 | Total | α-TE[e] mg | Ref. |
|---|---|---|---|---|---|---|---|---|---|---|---|---|---|
| *Cucurbita maxima*, pumpkin, fruit | C | 2.0 | 0.7 | — | — | — | — | — | — | — | 0.7 | 0.7 | 212 |
| *Solanum melongena*, brinjal, fruit | C | 2.0 | — | — | — | — | — | — | — | — | — | — | 212 |
| *Psophocarpus tetragonolobus*, beans winged | C | 2.0 | 4.6 | | | | | | | | 4.6 | 4.6 | 212 |
| *Parkia speciosa*, petai beans | C | 2.0 | 4.2 | | | | | | | | 4.2 | 4.2 | 212 |
| *Vigna sinensis*, beans | C | 2.0 | 1.7 | | | | | | | | 1.7 | 1.7 | 212 |
| *Phaseolus vulgaris*, beans | C | 2.0 | 1.7 | | | | | | | | 1.7 | 1.7 | 212 |
| *Pisum sativum*, french peas | C | 2.0 | 1.5 | | | | | | | | 1.5 | 1.5 | 212 |
| *Musa sapientum*, flower | C | 2.0 | 3.0 | | | | | | | | 3.0 | 3.0 | 212 |
| *Brassica oleracea*, cauliflower, broccoli | C | 2.0 | — | | | | | | | | — | — | 212 |
| *Phaeomeria specios*, torch ginger | C | 2.0 | — | | | | | | | | — | — | 212 |
| *Daucus carota*, carrot | C | 2.0 | 1.6 | | | | | | | | 1.6 | 1.6 | 212 |
| *Raphanus sativus*, white radish | C | 2.0 | 1.3 | | | | | | | | 1.3 | 1.3 | 212 |

| | | | | | | | | | | | | | |
|---|---|---|---|---|---|---|---|---|---|---|---|---|---|
| *Curcuma longa*, turmeric | C | 2.0 | 1.1 | | | | | | | | 1.1 | 1.1 | 212 |
| *Allium sativum*, roots | C | 2.0 | 0.8 | | | | | | | | 0.8 | 0.8 | 212 |
| *Pachyrrhizus erosus*, sengkuang | C | 2.0 | — | | | | | | | | — | — | 212 |
| *Pleurotus sajor–caju*, oyster mushroom | C | 2.0 | — | | | | | | | | — | — | 212 |
| **Infant formula** | | | | | | | | | | | | | |
| Milk based infant formula | | | | | | | | | | | | | |
| Powder | A | 2.6 | 14.0 | — | 1.6 | 0.6 | — | — | — | — | 16.2 | 14.2 | 148 |
| | | 2.6 | 13.0 | — | 2.3 | 0.2 | — | — | — | — | 15.4 | 13.2 | 148 |
| | | 1.6 | 10.5 | — | 4.5 | 0.4 | — | — | — | — | 15.4 | 10.9 | 109 |
| | | 1.6 | 10.5 | — | 5.4 | 1.4 | — | — | — | — | 17.3 | 11.1 | 112 |
| | | 2.2 | 15.7 | 0.1 | 2.4 | 0.1 | 1.2 | 0.21 | 1.97 | 0.56 | 22.3 | 16.4 | 119 |
| | | 2.5 | 10.1 | — | — | — | — | — | — | — | 10.1 | 10.1 | 90 |
| | | 1.6 | 11.3 | — | — | — | — | — | — | — | 11.3 | 8.9 | 174[f,i] |
| | | 1.6 | 4.5 | — | — | — | — | — | — | — | 4.5 | 10.1 | 174[f,i] |
| **Powder mean ± SD** | | | 11.2 ± 3.2 | Tr | 3.2 ± 1.6 | 0.5 ± 0.5 | Tr | Tr | Tr | Tr | 14.1 ± 5.4 | 11.0 ± 3.9 | |
| Reconstituted, nonfortified | C | 1.6 | 0.1 | Tr | 1.6 | 0.7 | — | — | — | — | 2.4 | 0.3 | 173 |
| Fortified | A | 1.6 | 1.2 | Tr | 1.5 | 0.7 | — | — | — | — | 3.4 | 1.4 | 173 |
| | | 2.6 | 1.5 | — | — | — | — | — | — | — | 1.5 | 1.0 | 170[f,i] |
| | | 2.2 | 2.3 | — | — | — | — | — | — | — | 2.3 | 1.5 | 171[f,i] |
| **Fortified mean ± SD** | | | 1.7 ± 1.5 | Tr | Tr | Tr | — | — | — | — | 2.4 ± 0.8 | 1.7 ± 0.4 | |
| Whey based infant formula, powder | C | 2.6 | 5.1 | — | 0.4 | 0.1 | — | — | — | — | 5.4 | 5.1 | 148 |

*(continued)*

**TABLE 8.3** *Continued*

| Product | CC[a] | QI[b] | α-T[c] | β-T | γ-T | δ-T | α-T3[d] | β-T3 | γ-T3 | δ-T3 | Total | α-TE[e] mg | Ref. |
|---|---|---|---|---|---|---|---|---|---|---|---|---|---|
| High-protein infant formula, powder | C | 2.6 | 7.8 | — | 3.4 | 0.6 | — | — | — | — | 11.7 | 8.1 | 148 |
| Soy based infant formula, powder | C | 2.6 | 14.0 | Tr | 5.0 | 2.0 | — | — | — | — | 19.3 | 14.4 | 148 |
| **Weaning food** | | | | | | | | | | | | | |
| Rice—mungbean, ungerminated | C | 1.0 | — | 2.4 | 17.9 | 1.2 | — | — | — | — | 21.4 | 3.0 | 149 |
| Rice—mungbean, germinated | C | 1.0 | 0.2 | 0.6 | 16.6 | 1.6 | — | — | — | — | 19.1 | 2.3 | 149 |
| Rice—cowpea, ungerminated | C | 1.0 | — | 0.4 | 12.8 | 18.4 | — | — | — | — | 31.6 | 2.0 | 149 |
| Rice—cowpea, germinated | C | 1.0 | 0.4 | 0.6 | 12.0 | 16.5 | — | — | — | — | 29.4 | 2.4 | 149 |
| Corn—mungbean, ungerminated | C | 1.0 | 1.8 | 0.9 | 32.4 | 1.9 | — | — | — | — | 37.0 | 5.5 | 149 |
| Corn—mungbean, germinated | C | 1.0 | 1.2 | 0.8 | 19.0 | 1.7 | — | — | — | — | 22.7 | 3.5 | 149 |
| Corn—cowpea, ungerminated | C | 1.0 | 1.4 | 1.0 | 14.6 | 15.5 | — | — | — | — | 32.5 | 3.8 | 149 |
| Corn—cowpea, germinated | C | 1.0 | 1.4 | 0.9 | 14.2 | 15.6 | — | — | — | — | 32.1 | 3.7 | 149 |
| **Baby foods** | | | | | | | | | | | | | |
| Applesauce | C | 1.4 | 0.5 | — | Tr | Tr | — | — | — | — | 0.5 | 0.5 | 150 |
| Apricots | C | 1.4 | 0.7 | — | 0.1 | — | — | — | — | — | 0.8 | 0.7 | 150 |
| Bananas | C | 1.4 | 0.2 | — | — | — | — | — | — | — | 0.2 | 0.2 | 150 |
| Beef | C | 1.4 | 0.7 | — | — | — | — | — | — | — | 0.7 | 0.7 | 150 |
| Beef, egg noodles and vegetables | C | 1.4 | 0.3 | — | 0.1 | — | — | — | — | — | 0.4 | 0.3 | 150 |
| Beef liver | C | 1.4 | 0.3 | — | — | — | — | — | — | — | 0.3 | 0.3 | 150 |

| | | | | | | | | | | | | | |
|---|---|---|---|---|---|---|---|---|---|---|---|---|---|
| Beef—vegetable—potato stew | C | 2.6 | 0.3 | Tr | 0.4 | 0.1 | Tr | — | — | — | 0.9 | 0.3 | 139 |
| Beets | C | 1.4 | 0.1 | — | Tr | — | — | — | — | — | 0.1 | 0.1 | 150 |
| Berry purée | C | 1.4 | 0.3 | Tr | 0.1 | Tr | — | — | Tr | — | 0.3 | 0.3 | 139 |
| Carrots | C | 1.4 | 0.6 | — | 0.2 | — | — | — | — | — | 0.8 | 0.6 | 150 |
| Cereal, egg yolk, and bacon | C | 1.4 | 0.2 | — | — | — | — | — | — | — | 0.2 | 0.2 | 150 |
| Chicken | C | 1.4 | 0.3 | — | 0.1 | 0.1 | — | — | — | — | 0.5 | 0.3 | 150 |
| Chicken noodle dinner | C | 1.4 | 0.2 | — | 0.1 | 0.1 | — | — | — | — | 0.4 | 0.2 | 150 |
| Chicken—pork—vegetable stew | C | 2.6 | 0.3 | Tr | 0.4 | 0.1 | Tr | — | Tr | — | 0.9 | 0.3 | 139 |
| Chicken—rice—potato purée | C | 2.6 | 0.1 | Tr | 0.4 | 0.2 | Tr | — | Tr | — | 0.6 | 0.1 | 139 |
| Chicken—vegetable stew | C | 2.6 | 0.1 | Tr | 0.8 | 0.2 | Tr | — | 0.1 | — | 1.2 | 0.2 | 139 |
| Chicken soup, creamy | C | 1.4 | — | — | — | — | — | — | — | — | 0.0 | 0.0 | 150 |
| Chocolate custard pudding | C | 1.4 | 0.2 | — | — | — | — | — | — | — | 0.2 | 0.2 | 150 |
| Corn, creamed | C | 1.4 | 0.2 | — | 0.1 | 0.1 | — | — | — | — | 0.4 | 0.2 | 150 |
| Cottage cheese and pineapple | C | 1.4 | 0.2 | — | — | — | — | — | — | — | 0.2 | 0.2 | 150 |
| Egg yolk | C | 1.4 | 0.6 | — | 0.6 | 0.5 | — | — | — | — | 1.7 | 0.7 | 150 |
| Fish—rice—vegetable stew | C | 2.6 | 0.2 | 0.1 | 1.2 | 0.6 | — | — | — | — | 2.0 | 0.4 | 139 |
| Fish—vegetable stew | C | 2.6 | 0.3 | Tr | 1.6 | 0.7 | — | — | Tr | — | 2.6 | 0.5 | 139 |
| Fish—vegetable purée | C | 2.6 | 0.6 | 0.1 | 1.4 | 0.6 | — | — | — | — | 2.6 | 0.7 | 139 |

*(continued)*

**TABLE 8.3** *Continued*

| Product | CC[a] | QI[b] | α-T[c] | β-T | γ-T | δ-T | α-T3[d] | β-T3 | γ-T3 | δ-T3 | Total | α-TE[e] mg | Ref. |
|---|---|---|---|---|---|---|---|---|---|---|---|---|---|
| Fruit dessert | C | 1.4 | 0.3 | — | — | — | — | — | — | — | 0.3 | 0.3 | 150 |
| Fruit purée | C | 2.6 | 0.4 | — | — | — | — | — | — | — | 0.4 | 0.4 | 139 |
| Garden vegetables | C | 1.4 | 0.6 | — | 0.4 | 0.2 | — | — | — | — | 1.2 | 0.6 | 150 |
| Green beans | C | 1.4 | 0.2 | — | 0.1 | — | — | — | — | — | 0.3 | 0.2 | 150 |
| Gruel | C | 2.6 | 0.8 | Tr | 0.1 | Tr | 0.1 | Tr | 0.1 | Tr | 1.0 | 0.8 | 139 |
| Ham | C | 1.4 | 0.5 | — | Tr | — | — | — | — | — | 0.5 | 0.5 | 150 |
| High-meat, beef with vegetables | C | 1.4 | 0.5 | — | 0.1 | — | — | — | — | — | 0.6 | 0.5 | 150 |
| High-meat, chicken with vegetables | C | 1.4 | 0.2 | — | 0.1 | 0.2 | — | — | — | — | 0.5 | 0.2 | 150 |
| High-meat, ham with vegetables | C | 1.4 | 0.2 | — | 0.1 | — | — | — | — | — | 0.3 | 0.2 | 150 |
| High-meat, turkey with vegetables | C | 1.4 | 0.1 | — | — | — | — | — | — | — | 0.1 | 0.1 | 150 |
| High-meat, veal with vegetables | C | 1.4 | 0.1 | — | Tr | Tr | — | — | — | — | 0.1 | 0.1 | 150 |
| Liver stroganoff | C | 2.6 | 0.4 | Tr | 1.5 | 0.5 | — | — | — | — | 2.4 | 0.6 | 139 |
| Liver–vegetable stew | C | 2.6 | 0.4 | Tr | 1.0 | 0.5 | Tr | — | — | — | 1.9 | 0.6 | 139 |
| Liver–vegetable–rice purée | C | 2.6 | 0.4 | Tr | 0.8 | 0.3 | Tr | — | Tr | — | 1.5 | 0.5 | 139 |
| Macaroni, tomato, and bacon | C | 1.4 | 0.3 | — | 0.1 | 0.1 | — | — | — | — | 0.5 | 0.3 | 150 |
| Mixed cereal with applesauce and bananas | C | 1.4 | 0.2 | — | 0.1 | 0.1 | — | — | — | — | 0.4 | 0.2 | 150 |
| Mixed vegetables | C | 1.4 | 0.2 | — | 0.1 | 0.1 | — | — | — | — | 0.4 | 0.2 | 150 |

| | | | | | | | | | | | | | |
|---|---|---|---|---|---|---|---|---|---|---|---|---|---|
| Oatmeal with applesauce and bananas | C | 1.4 | 0.4 | — | 0.2 | — | — | — | — | — | 0.6 | 0.4 | 150 |
| Orange pudding | C | 1.4 | 0.2 | — | — | — | — | — | — | — | 0.2 | 0.2 | 150 |
| Peaches | C | 1.4 | 1.3 | — | 0.1 | — | — | — | — | — | 1.4 | 1.3 | 150 |
| Pears | C | 1.4 | 0.6 | — | 0.1 | 0.1 | — | — | — | — | 0.8 | 0.6 | 150 |
| Peas | C | 1.4 | 0.2 | — | 0.6 | 0.1 | — | — | — | — | 0.9 | 0.3 | 150 |
| Peas, creamed | C | 1.4 | Tr | — | 0.5 | 0.2 | — | — | — | — | 0.7 | 0.1 | 150 |
| Plums | C | 1.4 | 0.4 | — | 0.1 | 0.2 | — | — | — | — | 0.7 | 0.4 | 150 |
| Pork–beef–vegetable stew | C | 2.6 | 0.3 | Tr | 0.3 | 0.2 | Tr | — | Tr | — | 0.7 | 0.3 | 139 |
| Pork–egg–vegetable–fruit stew | C | 2.6 | 0.2 | Tr | Tr | — | Tr | — | Tr | — | 0.2 | 0.2 | 139 |
| Pork–vegetable purée | C | 2.6 | 0.2 | Tr | 0.1 | 0.2 | Tr | — | Tr | — | 0.4 | 0.2 | 139 |
| Porridge | C | 1.2 | 1.3 | Tr | 0.3 | 0.1 | 0.1 | Tr | 0.1 | Tr | 2.0 | 1.4 | 139 |
| Prunes | C | 1.4 | 0.4 | — | 0.1 | — | — | — | — | — | 0.5 | 0.4 | 150 |
| Rice with applesauce and bananas | C | 1.4 | 0.2 | — | — | 0.1 | — | — | — | — | 0.3 | 0.2 | 150 |
| Rose hip purée | C | 1.2 | 0.5 | Tr | 0.3 | 0.1 | — | — | — | — | 0.9 | 0.5 | 139 |
| Spinach, creamed | C | 1.4 | 1.6 | — | 0.1 | Tr | — | — | — | — | 1.7 | 1.6 | 150 |
| Squash | C | 1.4 | 0.4 | — | 0.3 | — | — | — | — | — | 0.7 | 0.4 | 150 |
| Sweet potato | C | 1.4 | 0.5 | — | 0.1 | — | — | — | — | — | 0.6 | 0.5 | 150 |
| Turkey | C | 1.4 | 0.3 | — | — | — | — | — | — | — | 0.3 | 0.3 | 150 |
| Turkey and rice with vegetables | C | 1.4 | 0.1 | — | Tr | — | — | — | — | — | 0.1 | 0.1 | 150 |
| Veal | C | 1.4 | 0.2 | — | Tr | — | — | — | — | — | 0.2 | 0.2 | 150 |
| Veal–vegetable purée | C | 2.6 | 0.2 | Tr | 0.4 | 0.1 | Tr | — | Tr | — | 0.8 | 0.3 | 139 |

(*continued*)

**TABLE 8.3** *Continued*

| Product | CC[a] | QI[b] | α-T[c] | β-T | γ-T | δ-T | α-T3[d] | β-T3 | γ-T3 | δ-T3 | Total | α-TE[e] mg | Ref. |
|---|---|---|---|---|---|---|---|---|---|---|---|---|---|
| Veal–vegetable stew | C | 2.6 | 0.3 | Tr | 0.8 | 0.2 | Tr | — | Tr | — | 1.4 | 0.4 | 139 |
| Vegetable purée | C | 2.6 | 0.4 | Tr | 1.3 | 0.5 | Tr | — | — | — | 2.2 | 0.6 | 139 |
| Vegetable and chicken | C | 1.4 | 0.1 | — | 0.1 | — | — | — | — | — | 0.2 | 0.1 | 150 |
| Vegetable and lamb | C | 1.4 | 0.3 | — | 0.1 | 0.1 | — | — | — | — | 0.5 | 0.3 | 150 |
| Vegetable and liver | C | 1.4 | 0.3 | — | 0.1 | Tr | — | — | — | — | 0.4 | 0.3 | 150 |
| Vegetable and turkey | C | 1.4 | 0.1 | — | — | — | — | — | — | — | 0.1 | 0.1 | 150 |
| **Legumes** | | | | | | | | | | | | | |
| Bean, unspecified, raw | C | 2.6 | 0.1 | Tr | 0.3 | Tr | — | — | — | — | 0.5 | 0.2 | 145 |
| Bean, baked, tinned | C | 1.0 | 0.3 | — | 0.7 | — | — | — | — | — | 1.0 | 0.4 | 94 |
| Bean, baked, in tomato sauce with pork | C | 2.8 | 0.1 | — | 06 | Tr | — | — | — | — | 0.7 | 0.2 | 88 |
| Cowpeas | | | | | | | | | | | | | |
| Boiled | C | 2.2 | — | — | 1.5 | 1.1 | — | — | — | — | 2.6 | 0.2 | 87 |
| Dried, raw | C | 2.2 | — | — | 5.2 | 6.2 | — | — | — | — | 11.4 | 0.7 | 87 |
| Great northern | | | | | | | | | | | | | |
| Boiled | C | 2.2 | — | — | 1.4 | — | — | — | — | — | 1.4 | 0.1 | 87 |
| Dried, raw | C | 2.2 | — | — | 4.3 | 0.1 | — | — | — | — | 4.4 | 0.4 | 87 |
| Kidney | | | | | | | | | | | | | |
| Boiled | C | 2.2 | Tr | — | 0.9 | Tr | — | — | — | — | 1.0 | 0.1 | 87 |
| Dried, raw | C | 2.2 | 0.1 | — | 3.2 | Tr | — | — | — | — | 3.3 | 0.4 | 87 |
| Lentil | | | | | | | | | | | | | |
| Boiled | C | 2.2 | 0.2 | Tr | 1.0 | — | — | — | — | — | 1.1 | 0.3 | 87 |
| Dried, raw | C | 2.2 | 0.5 | — | 4.2 | — | — | — | — | — | 4.7 | 0.9 | 87 |
| Lima | | | | | | | | | | | | | |
| Boiled | C | 2.2 | Tr | — | 1.9 | 0.1 | — | — | — | — | 2.0 | 0.2 | 87 |
| Canned | C | 2.2 | 0.2 | — | 1.6 | — | — | — | — | — | 1.8 | 0.3 | 87 |

| | | | | | | | | | | | | | |
|---|---|---|---|---|---|---|---|---|---|---|---|---|---|
| Dried, raw | C | 2.2 | 0.1 | — | 5.6 | 0.3 | — | — | — | — | 6.0 | 0.6 | 87 |
| Navy | | | | | | | | | | | | | |
| Boiled | C | 2.2 | — | — | 1.5 | 0.1 | — | — | — | — | 1.6 | 0.2 | 87 |
| Dried, raw | C | 2.2 | 0.1 | — | 2.8 | 0.1 | — | — | — | — | 3.1 | 0.4 | 87 |
| Pea, unspecified, raw | C | 2.6 | Tr | — | 1.6 | Tr | — | — | Tr | — | 1.7 | 0.2 | 87 |
| Pea, chick, canned | C | 2.2 | 1.2 | 0.1 | 6.7 | 0.3 | 0.1 | — | 0.1 | — | 8.5 | 1.9 | 145 |
| Pea, unspecified, dried | C | 2.6 | 0.1 | — | 6.6 | 0.2 | — | — | 0.1 | — | 6.9 | 0.7 | 145 |
| Pea, unspecified, frozen | A | 2.6 | Tr | — | 1.4 | Tr | Tr | — | Tr | — | 1.5 | 0.2 | 145 |
| | | 1.0 | — | — | 0.6 | — | — | — | — | — | 0.6 | 0.1 | 88 |
| | | 2.8 | Tr | — | 0.8 | Tr | — | — | — | — | 0.8 | 0.1 | 87 |
| **Pea mean ± SD** | | | Tr | — | 0.9 ± 0.3 | Tr | Tr | — | Tr | — | 1.0 ± 0.4 | 0.1 ± 0.0 | |
| Pea, split, boiled | C | 2.2 | Tr | — | 1.9 | Tr | — | — | — | — | 2.0 | 0.2 | 87 |
| Pea, split, dried | C | 2.2 | — | — | 4.0 | — | — | — | — | — | 4.0 | 0.4 | 87 |
| Pea, sweet, canned | C | 2.2 | Tr | — | 1.7 | Tr | — | — | 0.1 | — | 1.8 | 0.2 | 87 |
| Pork and beans | C | 2.2 | — | — | 1.2 | — | — | — | — | — | 1.2 | 0.1 | 87 |
| Pulse, Bengal gram | C | 1.0 | 1.7 | 0.1 | 9.2 | 0.4 | — | — | 0.2 | — | 11.6 | 2.7 | 152 |
| Pulse, black gram | C | 1.0 | Tr | — | 6.6 | 0.2 | — | — | — | — | 6.8 | 0.7 | 152 |
| Pulse, green gram | C | 1.0 | 0.1 | Tr | 11.7 | 0.8 | Tr | Tr | Tr | Tr | 12.6 | 1.3 | 152 |
| Pulse, horse gram | C | 1.0 | Tr | — | 6.6 | 0.7 | — | — | — | — | 7.3 | 0.7 | 152 |
| Soybeans, raw | C | 2.2 | 2.1 | — | 16.4 | 4.9 | — | — | — | — | 23.4 | 3.7 | 151 |
| **Nuts and seeds** | | | | | | | | | | | | | |
| Alfalfa seed | C | 1.2 | 33.0 | Tr | 0.9 | — | — | — | — | — | 33.9 | 33.1 | 91 |
| Almond | A | 2.2 | 43.2 | 0.3 | 1.9 | 0.1 | 0.2 | — | — | — | 45.6 | 43.6 | 87 |
| | | 2.6 | 26.4 | 0.2 | 0.8 | Tr | 0.2 | — | Tr | — | 27.7 | 26.7 | 145 |
| | | 1.0 | 34.9 | — | 2.2 | — | — | — | — | — | 37.1 | 35.1 | 153 |
| | | 1.2 | 31.7 | 0.3 | 0.9 | — | 0.5 | — | — | — | 33.4 | 32.1 | 91 |
| | | 2.2 | 29.5 | 0.2 | 1.0 | — | 0.4 | — | — | — | 31.1 | 29.8 | 122 |
| | | 2.8 | 25.1 | 0.2 | 0.8 | — | — | — | — | — | 26.1 | 25.2 | 88 |

*(continued)*

**TABLE 8.3** *Continued*

| Product | CC[a] | QI[b] | α-T[c] | β-T | γ-T | δ-T | α-T3[d] | β-T3 | γ-T3 | δ-T3 | Total | α-TE[e] mg | Ref. |
|---|---|---|---|---|---|---|---|---|---|---|---|---|---|
| **Almond mean ± SD** | | | 31.8 ± 6.0 | 0.2 ± 0.1 | 1.3 ± 0.6 | Tr | 0.2 ± 0.2 | — | Tr | — | 33.5 ± 6.5 | 32.1 ± 6.1 | |
| Brazil nut | C | 2.4 | 8.8 | — | 3.6 | 2.1 | — | — | — | — | 14.5 | 9.2 | 120 |
| Cashew | A | 2.2 | 1.2 | 0.1 | 5.8 | 0.4 | — | 0.2 | — | — | 7.6 | 1.8 | 87 |
| | | 1.0 | — | — | 10.4 | 0.8 | — | — | — | — | 11.2 | 1.1 | 153 |
| | | 2.2 | 1.0 | — | 4.6 | — | — | — | 0.4 | — | 5.9 | 1.4 | 122 |
| | | 1.4 | 2.3 | — | 28.7 | 1.9 | — | — | — | — | 32.9 | 5.2 | 154 |
| **Cashew mean ± SD** | | | 1.1 ± 0.9 | Tr | 12.4 ± 9.7 | 0.8 ± 0.8 | — | 0.1 ± 0.1 | 0.1 ± 0.2 | — | 14.4 ± 10.9 | 2.4 ± 1.6 | |
| Celery seed | C | 1.0 | 6.1 | — | — | — | — | — | — | — | 6.1 | 6.1 | 153 |
| Coconut | C | 2.2 | — | — | 0.1 | — | 0.8 | — | 0.2 | — | 1.0 | 0.2 | 87 |
| Hazelnut, unspecified | A | 2.4 | 19.2 | — | 0.4 | Tr | — | — | — | — | 19.6 | 19.2 | 120 |
| | | 1.0 | 34.1 | Tr | 8.7 | — | — | — | — | — | 42.8 | 35.0 | 153 |
| Whiteheart cultivar | | 1.6 | 23.2 | 1.0 | 9.1 | 0.4 | — | — | — | — | 33.7 | 24.6 | 165 |
| Barcelona cultivar | | 1.6 | 23.8 | 0.6 | 1.6 | 0.1 | — | — | — | — | 26.1 | 24.3 | 165 |
| Butler cultivar | | 1.6 | 19.2 | 0.7 | 1.1 | 0.1 | — | — | — | — | 21.1 | 19.7 | 165 |
| Ennis cultivar | | 1.6 | 10.9 | 0.3 | 1.0 | 0.1 | — | — | — | — | 12.3 | 11.2 | 165 |
| Tonda di Giffoni cultivar | | 1.6 | 25.5 | 0.8 | 1.8 | 0.2 | — | — | — | — | 28.3 | 26.1 | 165 |
| Campanica cultivar | | 1.6 | 17.4 | 0.4 | 1.6 | 0.1 | — | — | — | — | 19.5 | 17.8 | 165 |
| **Hazelnut mean ± SD** | | | 21.7 ± 6.3 | 0.5 ± 0.3 | 3.2 ± 3.3 | 0.1 ± 0.1 | — | — | — | — | 25.4 ± 8.9 | 22.2 ± 6.6 | |
| Macadamia | B | 2.2 | — | — | — | — | 1.36 | — | — | — | 1.4 | 0.4 | 87 |
| | | 2.2 | — | — | — | — | 1.84 | — | — | — | 1.8 | 0.6 | 122 |
| Pecan | A | 2.2 | 1.2 | Tr | 23.7 | 0.1 | — | — | — | — | 25.0 | 3.6 | 87 |
| | | 2.4 | 1.2 | 0.2 | 24.8 | 0.2 | — | — | — | — | 26.4 | 3.8 | 157 |

|  |  |  |  |  |  |  |  |  |  |  |  |  |  |
|---|---|---|---|---|---|---|---|---|---|---|---|---|---|
|  |  | 2.2 | 1.4 | 0.1 | 30.4 | — | — | — | — | — | 31.9 | 4.5 | 122 |
|  |  | 2.8 | 1.4 | 0.5 | 24.6 | 0.3 | — | — | — | — | 26.8 | 4.1 | 88 |
| **Pecan mean ± SD** |  |  | 1.3 ± 0.1 | 0.2 ± 0.2 | 25.9 ± 2.6 | 0.2 ± 0.1 | — | — | — | — | 27.5 ± 2.6 | 4.0 ± 0.3 |  |
| Peanut |  |  |  |  |  |  |  |  |  |  |  |  |  |
| Raw | B | 2.6 | 10.1 | 0.3 | 15.2 | 0.7 | — | — | — | — | 26.2 | 11.8 | 158 |
|  |  | 2.8 | 10.5 | 0.3 | 10.0 | 0.9 | — | — | — | — | 21.7 | 11.7 | 156 |
| Dry roasted | A | 2.6 | 10.9 | 0.3 | 8.4 | 0.2 | — | — | — | — | 19.7 | 11.9 | 145 |
|  |  | 1.0 | 11.2 | 0.8 | 13.3 | — | — | — | — | — | 25.3 | 12.9 | 153 |
|  |  | 2.2 | 5.6 | 0.2 | 10.0 | 0.8 | — | — | — | — | 16.6 | 6.7 | 122 |
|  |  | 2.8 | 5.9 | 0.2 | 9.9 | 0.6 | — | — | — | — | 16.6 | 7.0 | 88 |
|  |  | 2.8 | 7.6 | 0.4 | 8.6 | 0.9 | — | — | — | — | 17.5 | 8.7 | 156 |
| **Peanut, dry roasted Mean ± SD** |  |  | 8.2 ± 2.0 | 0.4 ± 0.2 | 10.0 ± 1.6 | 0.5 ± 0.4 | — | — | — | — | 19.1 ± 3.3 | 9.4 ± 2.2 |  |
| Perilla seed | C | 1.0 | 1.0 | — | 52.6 | 3.1 | — | — | — | — | 56.7 | 6.4 | 159 |
| Pine nut | C | 1.0 | 16.2 | — | 20.8 | — | — | — | — | — | 37.0 | 18.3 | 153 |
| Pistachio, dry roasted | A | 2.2 | 3.1 | 0.2 | 30.2 | 0.8 | 0.5 | — | 4.5 | — | 39.4 | 6.5 | 87 |
|  |  | 1.0 | 3.5 | — | 57.5 | — | — | — | — | — | 61.0 | 9.3 | 153 |
|  |  | 2.2 | 2.3 | Tr | 25.1 | 0.7 | 0.9 | — | 1.9 | — | 30.9 | 5.1 | 122 |
| **Pistachio mean ± SD** |  |  | 3.0 ± 0.5 | 0.1 ± 0.1 | 37.6 ± 14.2 | 0.5 ± 0.4 | 0.5 ± 0.5 | — | 2.1 ± 2.2 | — | 43.8 ± 12.7 | 7.0 ± 1.7 |  |
| Poppy seed | C | 1.0 | 1.2 | — | 31.5 | — | — | — | — | — | 32.7 | 4.4 | 153 |
|  |  | 1.2 | 1.8 | — | 9.2 | — | — | — | — | — | 11.0 | 2.7 | 91 |
| Pumpkin seed | B | 1.0 | Tr | — | 39.0 | — | — | — | — | — | 39.0 | 3.9 | 153 |
|  |  | 2.4 | 3.5 | 0.8 | 23.3 | 1.7 | — | — | — | — | 29.3 | 6.3 | 160 |
| Sunflower seed | B | 2.2 | 21.3 | 1.1 | — | — | — | — | — | — | 22.4 | 21.8 | 87 |
|  |  | 2.2 | 25.9 | 0.9 | 0.3 | — | — | — | — | — | 27.1 | 26.4 | 161 |
| Walnut | A | 2.4 | 1.4 | — | 8.0 | 0.6 | — | — | — | — | 9.9 | 2.2 | 120 |
|  |  | 1.0 | 1.2 | — | 38.4 | 3.1 | — | — | — | — | 42.7 | 5.1 | 153 |

*(continued)*

**Table 8.3** *Continued*

| Product | CC[a] | QI[b] | α-T[c] | β-T | γ-T | δ-T | α-T3[d] | β-T3 | γ-T3 | δ-T3 | Total | α-TE[e] mg | Ref. |
|---|---|---|---|---|---|---|---|---|---|---|---|---|---|
| | | 2.2 | 1.6 | — | 24.8 | 3.5 | — | — | — | — | 29.9 | 4.2 | 162 |
| | | 2.2 | 1.2 | — | 23.5 | 1.8 | — | — | — | — | 26.6 | 3.6 | 122 |
| | | 2.8 | 1.0 | Tr | 18.2 | 1.4 | — | — | — | — | 20.7 | 2.9 | 88 |
| **Walnut mean ± SD** | | | 1.3 ± 0.2 | Tr | 22.6 ± 9.9 | 2.1 ± 1.1 | — | — | — | — | 26.0 ± 10.8 | 3.6 ± 1.0 | |
| Snacks | | | | | | | | | | | | | |
| Candy bar, Snickers | A | 2.8 | 1.1 | Tr | 3.1 | 0.2 | — | — | — | — | 4.4 | 1.4 | 88 |
| | | 2.2 | 1.0 | 0.1 | 5.0 | 0.3 | 0.1 | — | 0.2 | — | 6.7 | 1.5 | 87 |
| Candy bar, Almond Joy | | 2.2 | 1.5 | 0.1 | 3.0 | 0.1 | 0.3 | — | 0.2 | — | 5.2 | 1.9 | 87 |
| Candy bar, Milky Way | | 2.2 | 0.3 | 0.1 | 3.4 | 0.4 | Tr | — | 0.1 | — | 4.3 | 0.6 | 87 |
| **Candy bar mean ± SD** | | | 1.0 ± 0.4 | 0.1 ± 0.0 | 3.6 ± 0.8 | 0.3 ± 0.1 | 0.1 ± 0.1 | — | 0.1 ± 0.1 | — | 5.2 ± 1.0 | 1.4 ± 0.5 | |
| Chocolate, Hershey's, with almond | C | 2.8 | 3.3 | Tr | 4.8 | 0.1 | — | — | — | — | 8.2 | 3.7 | 88 |
| Cookies, chocolate chip | B | 2.2 | 1.4 | 0.3 | 11.6 | 2.1 | 0.1 | — | — | — | 15.4 | 2.8 | 87 |
| Oreo | | 2.2 | 1.1 | 0.2 | 10.6 | 2.1 | 0.1 | — | 0.1 | — | 14.1 | 2.3 | 87 |
| Corn chips | C | 2.2 | 9.3 | 2.2 | 8.9 | 2.1 | — | — | 0.4 | — | 23.0 | 11.3 | 87 |
| Corn puffs | C | 2.2 | 3.7 | 0.2 | 11.9 | 3.1 | — | — | — | — | 18.9 | 5.1 | 87 |
| Crackers, cheese | A | 2.2 | 1.7 | 0.3 | 8.3 | 0.9 | 0.1 | — | — | — | 11.3 | 2.7 | 87 |
| Soft flour | | 2.0 | 0.7 | 0.4 | — | — | 0.2 | 1.9 | — | — | 3.2 | 1.1 | 101 |
| Soft | | 2.0 | 0.4 | 0.3 | 0.1 | Tr | 0.1 | 1.1 | — | — | 1.9 | 0.6 | 101 |
| Saltine | | 2.2 | 1.0 | 0.3 | 8.9 | 1.4 | 0.1 | — | — | — | 11.7 | 2.1 | 87 |
| Wheat Thins | | 2.2 | 1.4 | 0.3 | 7.0 | 1.4 | — | — | — | — | 10.1 | 2.3 | 87 |
| **Crackers mean ± SD** | | | 1.0 ± 0.5 | 0.3 ± 0.0 | 4.9 ± 4.4 | 0.7 ± 0.7 | 0.1 ± 0.1 | 0.6 ± 0.9 | — | — | 7.6 ± 4.2 | 1.8 ± 0.8 | |

| | | | | | | | | | | | | | |
|---|---|---|---|---|---|---|---|---|---|---|---|---|---|
| Popcorn, air-popped | C | 2.8 | 0.4 | Tr | 2.6 | 0.2 | 0.3 | — | 0.2 | — | 3.6 | 0.7 | 125 |
| Potato chips | A | 2.2 | 6.9 | 0.2 | 8.2 | 2.8 | — | — | — | — | 18.0 | 7.9 | 87 |
| | | 2.4 | 4.4 | — | 2.9 | 0.7 | — | — | — | — | 8.0 | 4.7 | 130 |
| | | 2.6 | 5.2 | 0.2 | 14.2 | 1.4 | 0.6 | — | 0.4 | — | 21.9 | 6.9 | 145 |
| | | 2.8 | 10.7 | 0.1 | 5.9 | 0.6 | — | — | — | — | 17.2 | 11.3 | 88 |
| **Potato chips mean ± SD** | | | 6.8 ± 2.4 | 0.1 ± 0.1 | 7.8 ± 4.1 | 1.4 ± 0.9 | 0.2 ± 0.3 | — | 0.1 ± 0.2 | — | 16.3 ± 5.1 | 7.7 ± 2.4 | |
| Tortilla chips | C | 2.4 | 1.3 | — | 1.7 | 0.4 | — | — | — | — | 3.4 | 1.5 | 120 |
| **Spices** | | | | | | | | | | | | | |
| Allspice | C | 1.0 | 1.1 | — | — | 1.1 | — | — | — | — | 2.3 | 1.2 | 153 |
| Aniseed | C | 1.0 | 5.3 | 23.8 | Tr | 8.9 | — | — | — | — | 38.0 | 17.4 | 163 |
| Aniseed, pasteurized | C | 1.0 | 5.0 | 25.4 | Tr | 8.4 | — | — | — | — | 38.9 | 18.0 | 163 |
| Cardamom | C | 1.0 | — | — | — | — | — | — | — | — | 0.0 | 0.0 | 153 |
| Clove | C | 1.0 | 8.5 | — | — | — | — | — | — | — | 8.5 | 8.5 | 153 |
| Coriander | C | 1.0 | Tr | Tr | Tr | — | — | — | — | — | 0.0 | 0.0 | 163 |
| | | 1.0 | — | — | — | — | — | — | — | — | 0.0 | 0.0 | 153 |
| Coriander, pasteurized | C | 1.0 | Tr | Tr | Tr | — | — | — | — | — | 0.0 | 0.0 | 163 |
| Cumin | C | 1.0 | 3.3 | — | — | — | — | — | — | — | 3.3 | 3.3 | 153 |
| Laurel | C | 1.0 | 12.6 | 3.0 | — | — | — | — | — | — | 15.6 | 14.1 | 163 |
| Laurel, pasteurized | C | 1.0 | 12.0 | 2.3 | — | — | — | — | — | — | 14.4 | 13.2 | 163 |
| Nutmeg | C | 1.0 | — | — | 0.5 | — | — | — | — | — | 0.5 | 0.1 | 153 |
| Oregano | | | | | | | | | | | | | |
| Dry | C | 1.0 | 21.4 | 3.4 | 3.7 | 10.4 | — | — | — | — | 38.9 | 23.7 | 163 |
| Pasteurized | C | 1.0 | 18.4 | 3.1 | 3.6 | 10.8 | — | — | — | — | 35.9 | 20.6 | 163 |
| Pepper | | | | | | | | | | | | | |
| Black | C | 1.0 | 0.3 | — | 2.3 | — | — | — | — | — | 2.6 | 0.5 | 153 |
| White | C | 1.0 | 2.7 | 0.3 | 0.1 | — | — | — | — | — | 3.0 | 2.8 | 153 |
| Sweet | C | 2.6 | 2.2 | 0.1 | Tr | Tr | — | — | — | — | 2.3 | 2.2 | 145 |

*(continued)*

**TABLE 8.3** *Continued*

| Product | CC[a] | QI[b] | α-T[c] | β-T | γ-T | δ-T | α-T3[d] | β-T3 | γ-T3 | δ-T3 | Total | α-TE[e] mg | Ref. |
|---|---|---|---|---|---|---|---|---|---|---|---|---|---|
| Rosemary | C | 1.0 | 26.1 | — | — | — | — | — | — | — | 26.1 | 26.1 | 153 |
| Turmeric | C | 1.0 | Tr | Tr | Tr | — | — | — | — | — | 0.0 | 0.0 | 163 |
| Turmeric, pasteurized | C | 1.0 | Tr | Tr | Tr | — | — | — | — | — | 0.0 | 0.0 | 163 |
| Sansho | C | 1.0 | 2.7 | — | 0.3 | — | — | — | — | — | 3.1 | 2.8 | 153 |
| **Miscellaneous foods** | | | | | | | | | | | | | |
| Beer, regular | C | 2.8 | — | — | — | — | — | — | — | — | 0.0 | 0.0 | 88 |
| Chicken nuggets | C | 1.4 | 0.8 | 0.1 | 3.1 | 0.7 | — | — | — | — | 4.7 | 1.2 | 95 |
| Chocolate | C | 2.2 | 0.3 | 3.7 | 0.2 | — | — | — | — | — | 4.1 | 0.7 | 87 |
| Chocolate, baking | C | 2.2 | 0.4 | — | 5.8 | — | — | — | — | — | 6.2 | 1.0 | 87 |
| Cremora creamer | C | 2.2 | 0.6 | — | 0.5 | — | — | — | — | — | 1.1 | 0.6 | 87 |
| Frostings, Chocolate | C | 2.2 | 1.6 | 0.2 | 7.3 | 1.8 | — | — | — | — | 10.7 | 2.4 | 87 |
| Vanilla | C | 2.2 | 2.9 | 0.3 | 12.4 | 1.4 | — | — | — | — | 17.0 | 4.3 | 87 |
| Horseradish sauce | C | 2.2 | 2.4 | 0.3 | 13.9 | 3.8 | — | — | — | — | 20.4 | 4.0 | 87 |
| Mustard spread | C | 2.2 | 0.3 | — | 1.9 | — | — | — | — | — | 2.2 | 0.5 | 87 |
| Orange marmalade | C | 2.6 | 0.2 | Tr | 0.1 | — | — | — | — | — | 0.3 | 0.2 | 145 |
| Protein diet powder | C | 2.4 | 25.6 | — | — | — | — | — | — | — | 25.6 | 25.6 | 120 |
| Strawberry jam | C | 2.6 | 0.1 | Tr | Tr | — | — | — | — | — | 0.1 | 0.1 | 145 |
| Tea leaves from tea bag | C | 2.4 | 7.4 | — | 1.9 | — | — | — | — | — | 9.3 | 7.5 | 120 |

[a]CC, confidence code; [b]QI, quality index; [c]α-T, α-tocophenol; β-T, β-tocophenol; γ-T, γ-tocophenol; δ-T, δ-tocophenol; [d]α-T3, αtocotrienol; β-T3, β-tocotrienol; γ-T3, γ-tocotrienol; δ-T3, δ-tocotrienol; [e]mg α-tocophenol equivalents; [f]only α-tocophenol was assayed; [g]C, corn oil; SB, soybean oil; P, palm oil; SF, safflower oil; SN, sunflower oil; CS, cottonseed oil; CA, canola oil; [h]not assayed by GC or LC; [i]assayed as α-tocophenyl acetate.

**TABLE 8.4** Tocopherol and Tocotrienol Content of Selected Fats and Oils and Their Primary Homologues[a]

| Oil or fat[b] | α-T mg/100 g | Total T + T3 (mg/100 g) | %T | %T3 | Vitamin E homologues |
|---|---|---|---|---|---|
| Wheat germ | 149.2 | 239.8 | 96 | 4 | α-T, β-T, γ-T, γ-T3, δ-T, β-T3, δ-T3 |
| Sunflower | 55.4 | 62.8 | 100 | 0 | α-T, γ-T |
| Safflower | 42.9 | 46.3 | 100 | 0 | α-T, γ-T, β-T |
| Cottonseed | 40.4 | 74.2 | 100 | 0 | α-T, γ-T |
| Canola | 21.9 | 63.6 | 100 | 0 | γ-T, α-T |
| Corn | 18.6 | 93.0 | 100 | Tr | γ-T, α-T, δ-T, α-T3, γ-T3, β-T3 |
| Palm | 14.8 | 53.5 | 28 | 72 | γ-T3, α-T, α-T3, δ-T3, β-T3 |
| Olive | 13.5 | 14.6 | 100 | 0 | α-T, γ-T |
| Peanut | 17.9 | 34.1 | 100 | 0 | α-T, γ-T, δ-T, β-T |
| Soybean | 8.2 | 107.3 | 100 | 0 | δ-T, γ-T, α-T, β-T3 |
| Palm kernel oil | 1.3 | 3.4 | 38 | 62 | α-T3, α-T |
| Lard | 1.0 | 1.1 | 100 | 0 | α-T |
| Coconut oil | 0.3 | 2.5 | 28 | 72 | γ-T3, α-T3, α-T |

[a]In decreasing order of α-T levels.
[b]Data from Table 8.3.
α-T, α-tocopherol; γ-T3, γ-tocotrienol.

α-T level. From this brief table, several generalizations about the vitamin E content of fats and oils are apparent:

1. Oils with the highest α-T content have the highest milligram α-TE values.
2. Of the oils with the greatest world consumption, only palm oil contains tocotrienols in quantity.
3. Total tocopherol plus tocotrienol (T + T3) is not a reliable indicator of milligram α-TE.
4. In some oils, including soybean, peanut, corn, and canola, γ-T is present in large enough quantities to contribute appreciably to milligram α-TE levels.
5. Coconut, cocoa butter, and palm kernel oil contain low amounts of vitamin E.
6. Animal products (butter, lard) contain only low levels of α-T (171).

As discussed in Chapter 1 and Chapter 2, interest in the tocotrienols is dramatically increasing as the knowledge of their specific physiological effects more clearly differentiates them from the effects of the tocopherols. Such effects as hypercholesterolemic activity and anticarcinogenic properties are linked to the inhibition of 3-hydroxy-3-methylglutaryl coenzyme A reductase (HMGR), which is the rate-limiting enzyme in isoprenoid synthesis. Many investigators and nutritionists believe that the tocotrienols are a significant dietary factor apart from $\alpha$-T. Other oils than palm contain tocotrienols. These include oats ($\alpha$-T3, $\beta$-T3), barley ($\alpha$-T3, $\beta$-T3, $\gamma$-T3), coconut oil ($\alpha$-T3, $\beta$-T3, $\gamma$-3), corn oil ($\alpha$-T3, $\gamma$-T3), rice bran oil ($\alpha$-T3, $\gamma$-T3, $\delta$-T3), and wheat germ oil ($\alpha$-T3, $\beta$-T3, $\gamma$-T3). Of these, high-quality rice bran oil matches palm oil in diversity and contains a higher total amount of the tocotrienols. Data are sparse on the vitamin E content of rice bran oil, but work completed in 1999 indicates that heat-stabilized rice bran oil is an excellent source of $\alpha$-T3 with a lesser amount of $\delta$-T3 (108). Palm oil is an excellent source of $\alpha$-T3 and $\gamma$-T3 with measurable amounts of $\beta$-T3 and $\delta$-T3.

**8.3.2.2. Margarines, Salad Oils, Spreads, Shortening, Peanut Butter.** As indicated by previous reviews (33,70,71,72), the vitamin E content of margarine varies greatly, depending upon the types of oils used in formulation. Further, reduced-fat and fat-free margarinelike products contain reduced levels of vitamin E unless fortified (115,117–120). We have organized the compositional data on margarines in Table 8.3 into full-fat, reduced-fat, and fat-free product categories. Product types were further separated into subcategories based on the oil composition of the products. However, except for margarines produced entirely from corn oil or soybean oil, data are too sparse to provide reliable means. In comparing corn oil margarines to soybean oil margarines, the effects of the oil component are readily apparent. The corn oil margarines contained a mean $\alpha$-T level of 18.6 mg/100 g and a mean total tocopherol level of 58.7 mg/100 g. Soybean oil margarines averaged 4.6 mg/100 g of $\alpha$-T with a total vitamin E content of 70.5 mg/100 g. Because of the much higher content of $\alpha$-T, corn oil margarines provide 21.1 mg $\alpha$-TE/100 g compared to 9.7 mg $\alpha$-TE/100 g for soybean oil margarines. This is a simple comparison based on single-component products; however, one can readily see the impact of oil type on the $\alpha$-T level of the margarine. Oils with potential to increase the $\alpha$-T content of margarines because of relatively high $\alpha$-T contents include sunflower, safflower, cottonseed, canola, corn, and palm. Margarines that contain palm oil are sources of tocotrienols ($\alpha$-T3, $\gamma$-T3, and $\delta$-T3).

Studies on the vitamin E composition of margarine published in the late 1990s include Rader et al (118). and Ye et al (115). The Rader et al (118). study clearly showed that reduced-fat and fat-free margarines contained appreciably less vitamin E than 80% fat margarines. $\alpha$-Tocopherol levels varied with total fat content and with the oils used as ingredients. Highest $\alpha$-T contents were present in margarines formulated with corn and sunflower oils. Margarines formulated with soybean oil contained the lowest level of α-T. Ye et al. (115) provided a simple extraction procedure and HPLC determination for application to margarines and reduced-fat products. Their data also showed significantly lower α-T levels in reduced-fat margarines and spreads. The vitamin E content ranged from 4.4 mg α-T/100 g in 64% reduced-fat margarine containing soybean oil as the only oil to 19.3 α-T/100 g in a full-fat margarine containing only corn oil. Earlier work by Slover et al. (91) indicated tocopherol levels were highly variable in margarines. These authors attributed the variability to the natural variability in the oil sources and the effects of processing and storage. α-T levels varied from approximately 1 to 25 mg/100 g.

Limited data are available on the vitamin E content of mayonnaise and salad dressings. University of Georgia studies completed for the USDA Nutrient Composition Laboratory showed that full-fat mayonnaise contained 3.2 mg α-T/100 g whereas a low-fat product contained only trace amounts of α-T.[87,88] The vitamin E content of salad dressings depends predominantly on the oil content and the type of oils used in the formulation. Butter contains only low levels of α-T. α-T levels were reported to range from 1.36 to 1.96 mg/100 g in Bauernfeind's review (72). A more recent study reported 3.2 mg α-T/100 g (94).

Peanut butter, a significant source of α-T in the U.S. consumer's diet, contains 10 mg α-T/100 g according to the data compiled in Table 8.3.

**8.3.2.3. Cereals, Cereal Products, and Baked Products.** A distinguishing characteristic of cereal grains is the presence of tocotrienols. Therefore, because of the quantities of cereals and cereal products consumed in most diets, these foods provide a source of the tocotrienols in Western diets, in which palm oil is not commonly consumed. Although most cereal grains contain less than 2.0 mg α-T/100 g, the amount consumed and the diversity of the vitamin E homologues present make this staple food group a significant source of tocopherols and tocotrienols. Bauernfeind (72) summarized the vitamin E content of baked cereal products with the following points:

1. The vitamin E content of baked grain products originates from the grain fraction (flour, bran) and from the shortening, margarine, or butter added as ingredients.
2. Variability in baked cereal products is due to formulation, processing, handling, and storage.
3. Depending on the recipe and cooking method, baked products are fairly good sources of vitamin E.

Because cereal oils are concentrated in the germ, isolated germ fractions are significantly higher in vitamin E content when compared to the whole grain. Data in Table 8.3 show that the barley germ contains 13 times the α-T content of whole barley grain. Likewise, wheat germ contains approximately 10 times the level found in the whole wheat kernel.

In the review presented by McLaughlin and Weihrauch (33), bleaching of wheat flour was reported to result in a 65% loss of vitamin E. Data in Table 8.3 show that wheat flour contains 0.2 $\alpha$-T/100 g, a level that is considerably lower than that in wheat endosperm (0.4 mg $\alpha$-T/100 g).

**8.3.2.4. Milk, Dairy Products, and Eggs.** Dairy products contain $\alpha$-T at low levels. Dial and Eitenmiller (87) reported 0.07 and 0.1 mg $\alpha$-T/100 g in 2% and whole milk (3.25%), respectively. These values are similar to those reported earlier (33,72). Mature human milk has three to five times the $\alpha$-T level of bovine milk. Vitamin E is not detectable in nonfat dry milk and is only present at trace levels in skim milk since the $\alpha$-T is removed with the butterfat. Because of concentration effects, cheese produced from full-fat milk contains appreciably more $\alpha$-T on a per-gram basis. Full-fat cheese values reported in Table 8.3 range from 0.3 to 0.5 mg $\alpha$-T/100 g.

In eggs, all of the vitamin E is in the yolk (33). Bauernfeind (72) reported that the $\alpha$-T content of egg yolk ranged from 1.6 to 3.9 mg/100 g. These values are much lower than 1998 data provided by Botsoglou et al. (137). These authors reported a range of $<2$ to 113 mg $\alpha$-T/100 g yolk. The mean $\alpha$-T level was 15 for 20 egg yolk samples collected in Greece. The large degree of variability was attributed to differences in diets and the inclusion of vitamin E supplements in some of the diets. Vitamin E transfer from the diet to egg yolk has been demonstrated.[178–180] Widespread use of vitamin E supplementation of layer diets would indicate that older values for the vitamin E content of eggs are invalid. Dial and Eitenmiller (87) assayed six whole egg samples collected from various geographic areas and reported $\alpha$-T levels of 0.6 mg/100 g. Earlier data summarized by Bauernfeind gave a $\alpha$-T level of 0.46 mg/100 g.

**8.3.2.5. Meat, Fish, and Seafood.** Muscle foods almost exclusively contain $\alpha$-T at levels less than 1 mg/100 g. Organ tissues contain slightly higher levels (33). As discussed in detail in Chapter 4, supplementation of the diet of many species can increase vitamin E levels in muscles and organs and, thus, increase oxidative stability of the raw and processed products as well as the nutritive value.

**8.3.2.6. Fruits and Vegetables.** Most fresh fruits and vegetables contain less than 1 mg $\alpha$-T/100 g. $\alpha$-Tocopherol followed by $\gamma$-T are the predominant forms, although $\beta$-T has been reported at trace levels in some fruits and vegetables. Tocotrienols are absent except at low levels in a few products, and $\alpha$-tocotrienol ($\alpha$-T3) is the most commonly occurring tocotrienol. Corn contains

$\gamma$-T3 at higher levels than any other vegetable denoted in Table 8.3. Blueberry, cranberry, and lingonberry have appreciable quantities of $\gamma$-T3.

Various authors have presented the following observations that summarize the vitamin E content of fresh fruits and vegetables:[33,72,145]

1. Vitamin E is more concentrated in leaves than in roots on stems.
2. Vitamin E level is higher in dark green leaves compared to light green tissues.
3. Vitamin E level is higher in mature leaves than in small immature leaves.
4. Vitamin E variation within a plant species depends on cultivar, uneven distribution among different parts of the plant, maturity, growing, harvesting, and marketing conditions.
5. Because of the many factors that influence the vitamin E content of fresh fruits and vegetables and the considerable effect of globalization on supplies throughout the year, it is difficult to obtain a truly representative sample.

Data collected on the vitamin E content of fruits and vegetables since 1970 are of generally high quality with attention being given to sampling protocols. Significant studies include the work of Piironen et al (145). Hogarty et al. (120), and Dial and Eitenmiller (87), and that completed under USDA contract.[87,88]

**8.3.2.7. Infant Formula and Baby Foods.** Information on the vitamin E content of commercial infant formula is hard to interpret because of variation in methods of reporting the concentration. International units are often used instead of milligrams or mg $\alpha$-TE units, values are reported on powder or reconsituted basis, and, often, only *all-rac-$\alpha$-*tocopherol acetate values are provided since this is the form used for formulation. In Table 8.3, we converted all available data to $\alpha$-T on either a 100-g powder basis or a 100-g reconstituted basis. Another confusing convention is to report nutrient concentrations on the basis of 100 kcal since this is the convention used in the Infant Formula Act of 1980 (181), which sets standards for infant formula in the United States. Despite lack of uniformity in reporting of the data, excellent data exist on the vitamin E content of infant formula and reliable methods have been available for its quantification since the 1980s.

Studies by Landen et al. (170,171) Tanner et al. (172) and Thompson and Hatina (173) provide vitamin E levels on commercial formulas produced in the United States and report the levels on a reconstituted basis. The study by Landen et al. (171) is the most comprehensive of all studies completed on vitamin E in infant formulas as a result of the sample size included in the study—46 milk-based and 31 soy-based formulas. This study, however, reported only all-rac-$\alpha$-tocopheryl acetate amounts and did not include natural tocopherol levels originating from the formula ingredients. This condition is not a significant shortcoming since work reported by other investigators shows that natural tocopherols make up only a small percentage of total tocopherols. Thompson and Hatina (173) reported that supplemented *all-rac-$\alpha$*-tocopheryl acetate provided approximately 93% of the $\alpha$-T in the formula they analyzed. Similar indications are present in the data in Table 8.3. The Landen et al (171). study reported mean $\alpha$-tocophenyl acetate levels of 2.3 mg/100 g for reconstituted milk-based formula. Mean vitamin E levels ranged from 97% of label declarations to 118% of label declarations for concentrated formulas.

The study by Tanner et al (172). is significant in that it is the collaborative study for the currently accepted method to determine vitamin E in milk-based formula (see Chapter 7). Values provided for three formulas averaged 10.1 mg $\alpha$-tocopheryl acetate/100 g on a powder basis.

Other vitamin E values reported for milk-based formula on a powder basis were derived from studies by Indyk (109,112), Syväoja et al. (139) Tuan et al. (148) and Woollard et al. (174).

Some data exist on the vitamin E content of weaning foods. Most of the available values originated from work completed at the Food and Nutrition Research Institute, Manila, Philippines, on combinations of rice, cowpea, mungbean, and corn in germinated and nongerminated mixtures of the cereals and legumes (149). In general, germination decreased tocopherol levels, and the largest decreases occurred in the $\gamma$-T fraction of the corn–mungbean mixture.

Quite a large number of baby foods commonly available commercially have been analyzed for vitamin E content. Published data are available in studies by Davis (150) and Syväoja et al (139). The tocopherol and tocotrienol levels are similar to levels noted in like fresh products (fruits, vegetables, meats) and do not seem to show negative processing effects. In the study pertaining to Finnish baby foods (139), mg $\alpha$-T equivalents were 0.46/100 g in fruit-berry products and 0.38/100 g in meat–vegetable combinations. Davis noted as much as twofold differences in $\alpha$-T content between like samples with different processing lot numbers. It was indicated that storage time and conditions were sources of some of the differences found in the study. However, natural variation could also cause such differences. This, again, indicates strict attention to the selection of products to ensure representative sampling. The Finnish study used 30 samples of each product, representing 10 packages of freshly manufactured product, 10 of product stored for about 50% of its shelf life, and 10 of product approaching its best-if-used-date. A composite of the 30 units was used to form a representative sample.

#### 8.3.2.8. Legumes.

Available data on legumes show that most legumes contain less than 0.5 mg $\alpha$-T/100 g. In a study completed for the USDA, Dial and Eitenmiller (87) compared dried legumes to boiled, ready-to-eat products. Boiling had variable effects on vitamin E levels as measured on a dry weight basis, indicating differences in leaching losses of soluble components among the various legumes included in the study. In some cases, total vitamin E level was appreciably higher in boiled products than in dry, uncooked legumes (dry weight basis).

#### 8.3.2.9. Nuts and Seeds

Nuts and seeds represent some of the most concentrated vitamin E sources other than plant oils available to the consumer. Additionally, some, such as pistachios, macadamia, and cashews, contain tocotrienols, adding diversity to the profile of tocopherols and tocotrienols in the diet. Table 8.5 summarizes data from Table 8.3 for some nuts and seeds that are consumed in quantity. Almond shows the highest $\alpha$-T level of any commonly consumed nut and contains mostly $\alpha$-T with small quantities of $\beta$-, $\gamma$-, and $\delta$-T. Peanuts contain an intermediate amount of $\alpha$-T with higher levels of $\gamma$-T. It is significant to note that even though the peanut rates below some nuts and seeds, peanut butter alone accounts for 2.3% of total vitamin E available in the U.S. diet (182). Macadamia is unique in that it contains only $\alpha$-T3, although at less than 2 mg/100 g.

## 8.4. $\alpha$-TOCOPHEROL LEVELS IN FOODS

Because of the specificity of the human for the *2R*-stereoisomeric forms of $\alpha$-T (see Chapter 2), the Institute of Medicine, Panel on Dietary Antioxidants and Related Compounds (36), defined vitamin E only in relation to *RRR*-, *RSR*-, *RRS*-, and *RSS*-$\alpha$-T when setting recommended intakes. Table 8.6 presents mean values

**TABLE 8.5** Tocopherol and Tocotrienol Content of Selected Nuts and Their Primary Homologues

| Nut[b] | $\alpha$-Tmg/100 g | Total T + T3 mg/100 g | %T | %T3 | Vitamin E homologues[a] |
|---|---|---|---|---|---|
| Almond | 31.8 | 33.5 | 99 | 1 | $\alpha$-T, $\gamma$-T, $\alpha$-T3, $\beta$-T |
| Hazelnut | 21.7 | 25.4 | 100 | 0 | $\alpha$-T, $\gamma$-T, $\beta$-T, $\delta$-T3 |
| Peanut, raw | 10.3 | 24.0 | 100 | 0 | $\gamma$-T, $\alpha$-T, $\delta$-T, $\beta$-T |
| Peanut,dry roasted | 8.2 | 19.1 | 100 | 0 | $\gamma$-T, $\alpha$-T, $\delta$-T3, $\beta$-T |
| Pistachio | 3.0 | 43.8 | 95 | 5 | $\gamma$-T, $\alpha$-T, $\gamma$-T3, $\alpha$-T3, $\delta$-T, $\beta$-T |
| Walnut | 1.3 | 26.0 | 100 | 0 | $\gamma$-T, $\delta$-T, $\alpha$-T |
| Pecan | 1.3 | 27.5 | 100 | 0 | $\gamma$-T, $\alpha$-T, $\beta$-T, $\delta$-T |
| Macadamia | — | 1.6 | 0 | 100 | $\alpha$-T3 |

[a]In decreasing order of $\alpha$-T levels.
[b]Data from Table 8.3.
$\alpha$-T, $\alpha$-tocopherol; $\gamma$-T3, $\gamma$-tocotrienol.

**TABLE 8.6** $\alpha$-Tocopherol and Total Tocopherols and Tocotrienols and $\alpha$-Tocopherol Equivalents in Foods[a]

| Food | $\alpha$-T | Total T + T3 |
|---|---|---|
| Wheat germ oil | 149[b] | 240 |
| Sunflower oil | 55.4 | 62.8 |
| Safflower oil | 42.9 | 46.3 |
| Cottonseed oil | 40.4 | 74.2 |
| Almond | 31.8 | 33.5 |
| Canola oil | 21.9 | 63.6 |
| Corn oil | 18.6 | 93.0 |
| Peanut oil | 17.9 | 34.1 |
| Palm oil | 14.8 | 53.5 |
| Olive oil | 13.5 | 14.6 |
| Milk based infant formula, powder | 11.2 | 14.1 |
| Margarine | 10.7 | 50.8 |
| Peanut butter | 10.0 | 20.2 |
| Peanuts, dryroasted | 8.2 | 19.1 |
| Soybean oil | 8.2 | 107.3 |
| Potato chips | 6.8 | 16.3 |
| Shortening | 5.2 | 61.3 |
| Eggs, raw | 2.5 | 3.8 |
| Salmon | 2.0 | 2.0 |
| Spinach | 1.6 | 1.6 |
| Pecans | 1.3 | 27.5 |
| Shrimp | 1.2 | 1.3 |
| Broccoli | 1.2 | 1.5 |
| Peach | 1.0 | 1.0 |
| Wheat, grain | 1.0 | 4.8 |
| Oats, grain | 0.8 | 4.6 |
| Barley, grain | 0.7 | 3.7 |
| Tomato | 0.7 | 0.8 |
| Corn, grain | 0.7 | 4.1 |
| Carrot | 0.6 | 0.6 |
| Grape | 0.6 | 0.9 |
| Lettuce | 0.5 | 1.0 |
| Tuna | 0.5 | 0.7 |
| Coconut oil | 0.4 | 3.3 |
| Cheese, cheddar | 0.3 | 0.3 |
| Bread, wheat | 0.3 | 1.9 |
| Chicken, breast | 0.2 | 0.3 |
| Apples | 0.2 | 0.2 |
| Milk, bovine, whole | 0.1 | 0.1 |
| Potato | 0.1 | 0.1 |
| Peas | Trace | 1.0 |

[a]Data represents mean values from Table 8.3.
[b]In milligrams per 100 g.
$\alpha$-T, $\alpha$-tocopherol; $\gamma$-T3, $\gamma$-tocotrienol.

of $\alpha$-T and total tocopherol values for the broad range of foods presented in Table 8.3. This table provides a summary of the $\alpha$-T quantities in foods on a high to low ranking based on the mean values derived from current literature.

## 8.5. QUALITY EVALUATION OF ANALYTICAL DATA

Table 8.7 presents the mean quality index (QI) for the 14 food categories represented in Table 8.3. Although the oils and fats category contains the largest number of observations represented in Table 8.3, this category has a relatively low QI of 1.7. This low quality score for the most significant vitamin E source for the human is troubling, yet, if one studies the data sources in detail, understandable. The low score is attributable to the following factors: (a) major studies were completed before quality evaluation of data was given high priority in compositional studies; (b) attention was not given to sample numbers, complete sample descriptions, or the general area of planning to ensure representative sampling; (c) many of the data originated from method development studies in which sampling was not a high-priority part of the research; (d) in some cases, quality control of the analytical approach was not apparent.

If one keeps in perspective the problems involved with the collection of meaningful food compositional data, the deficiencies still apparent in the available vitamin E data are not surprising. The QI comparisons in Table 8.7 also show several food categories such as fruits, vegetables, and margarines that have

**TABLE 8.7** Quality Indexes for Vitamin E Composition Data by Food Category

| Food category | Quality index |
|---|---|
| Animal feed | 1.7 |
| Cereal and cereal products | 2.1 |
| Fruits | 2.4 |
| Infant formula and weaning foods | 1.7 |
| Legumes | 2.1 |
| Margarine | 2.5 |
| Meat, fish, and seafood | 2.2 |
| Milk, egg, and dairy products | 1.9 |
| Nuts and seeds | 1.9 |
| Oils and fats | 1.7 |
| Snacks | 2.3 |
| Spices | 1.1 |
| Vegetables | 2.4 |
| Miscellaneous foods | 2.3 |

relatively high QI evaluations. For the most part, these studies were recently completed with few sampling or analytical problems. It is encouraging to realize that worldwide efforts of many individuals and organizations that stress improvement of food compositional studies are having a positive effect. Food composition researchers in all areas of food composition research are now generating meaningful values and not just numbers. This fact is readily apparent in recently published work on vitamin E composition.

## REFERENCES


1. Kovac, M.; Holikova, K. Editorial. J. Food Comp. Anal. **2002**, *15*, 335–337.
2. INFOODS Food Composition. http://www.fao.org.infoods/index-em.stm, 2003.
3. Charrondiere, U.R.; Vignat, J.; Moller, A.; Ireland, J.; Becker, W.; Church, S.; Farram, A.; Holden, J.; Klemm, C.; Linardou, A.; Mueller, D.; Salvini, S.; Serra-Mjerm, L.; Skeie, G.; van Stavern, W.; Unwin, I.; Westenbrink, S.; Slimani, N.; Bole, E.R. The European nutrient database (ENDB) for nutritional epidemiology. J. Food Comp. Anal. **2002**, *15*, 435–451.
4. Klensin, J.C. *INFOODS Food Composition Data Interchange Handbook*; The United Nations University: Tokyo, Japan, 1992.
5. INFOODS Food Component Tags. www.fao.org/infoods/tags/newtags.text, 2001.
6. Murphy, S.P. Dietary reference intakes of the U.S. and Canada: update on implications for nutrient databases. J. Food Comp. Anal. **2002**, *15*, 411–417.
7. U.S. Department of Agriculture, Agricultural Research Service. *Composition of Foods: Dairy and Egg Products; Raw, Processed, Prepared. Agric. Handb.*; No. 8–1; 1976.
8. U.S. Department of Agriculture, Agricultural Research Service. *Composition of Foods: Spices and Herbs: Raw, Processed, Prepared. Agric. Handb.*; No. 8–2, 1977.
9. U.S. Department of Agriculture, Agricultural Research Service. *Composition of Foods: Baby Foods: Raw, Processed, Prepared. Agric. Handb.*; No. 8–3, 1978.
10. U.S. Department of Agriculture, Agricultural Research Service. *Composition of Foods: Fats and Oils: Raw, Processed, Prepared. Agric. Handb.*; No. 8–4, 1979.
11. U.S. Department of Agriculture, Agricultural Research Service. *Composition of Foods: Poultry Products: Raw, Processed, Prepared. Agric. Handb.*; No. 8–5, 1980.
12. U.S. Department of Agriculture, Agricultural Research Service. *Composition of Foods: Soups, Sauces, and Gravies: Raw, Processed, Prepared. Agric. Handb.*; No. 8–6, 1980.
13. U.S. Department of Agriculture, Agricultural Research Service. *Composition of Foods: Sausages and Luncheon Meats: Raw, Processed, Prepared. Agric. Handb.*; No. 8–7, 1982.
14. U.S. Department of Agriculture, Agricultural Research Service. *Composition of Foods: Breakfast Cereals: Raw, Processed, Prepared. Agric. Handb.*; No. 8–8, 1982.

15. U.S. Department of Agriculture, Agricultural Research Service. *Composition of Foods: Fruits and Fruit Juices: Raw, Processed, Prepared. Agric. Handb.*; No. 8–9, 1982.
16. U.S. Department of Agriculture, Agricultural Research Service. *Composition of Foods: Pork Products: Raw, Processed, Prepared. Agric. Handb.*; No. 8–10, 1982.
17. U.S. Department of Agriculture, Agricultural Research Service. *Composition of Foods: Vegetables and Vegetable Products: Raw, Processed, Prepared. Agric. Handb.*; No. 8–11, 1984.
18. U.S. Department of Agriculture, Agricultural Research Service. *Composition of Foods: Nut and Seed Products: Raw, Processed, Prepared. Agric. Handb.*; No. 8–12, 1984.
19. U.S. Department of Agriculture, Agricultural Research Service. *Composition of Foods: Beef Products: Raw, Processed, Prepared. Agric. Handb.*; No. 8–13, 1990.
20. U.S. Department of Agriculture, Agricultural Research Service. *Composition of Foods: Beverages: Raw, Processed, Prepared. Agric. Handb.*; No. 8–14, 1986.
21. U.S. Department of Agriculture, Agricultural Research Service. *Composition of Foods: Finfish and Shellfish Products: Raw, Processed, Prepared. Agric. Handb.*; No. 8–15, 1987.
22. U.S. Department of Agriculture, Agricultural Research Service. *Composition of Foods: Legumes and Legume Products: Raw, Processed, Prepared. Agric. Handb.*; No. 8–16, 1986.
23. U.S. Department of Agriculture, Agricultural Research Service. *Composition of Foods: Lamb, Veal, and Game Products: Raw, Processed, Prepared. Agric. Handb.*; No. 8–17, 1989.
24. U.S. Department of Agriculture, Agricultural Research Service. *Composition of Foods: Baked Products: Raw, Processed, Prepared. Agric. Handb.*; No. 8–18, 1992.
25. U.S. Department of Agriculture, Agricultural Research Service. *Composition of Foods: Snacks and Sweet: Raw, Processed, Prepared. Agric. Handb.*; No. 8–19, 1991.
26. U.S. Department of Agriculture, Agricultural Research Service. *Composition of Foods: Cereal Grains and Pasta: Raw, Processed, Prepared. Agric. Handb.*; No. 8–20, 1989.
27. U.S. Department of Agriculture, Agricultural Research Service. *Composition of Foods: Fast Foods: Raw, Processed, Prepared. Agric. Handb.*; No. 8–21, 1988.
28. U.S. Department of Agriculture, Agricultural Research Service. *Composition of Foods: Raw, Processed, Prepared Agric. Handb.*; No. 8. Supplement, 1990.
29. U.S. Department of Agriculture, Agricultural Research Service. *Composition of Foods: Raw, Processed, Prepared Agric. Handb.*; No. 8. Supplement, 1991.
30. U.S. Department of Agriculture, Agricultural Research Service. *Composition of Foods: Raw, Processed, Prepared Agric. Handb.*; No. 8. Supplement, 1992.
31. U.S. Department of Agriculture, Agricultural Research Service. *Composition of Foods: Raw, Processed, Prepared Agric. Handb.*; No. 8. Supplement, 1993.
32. United States Department of Agriculture Agricultural Resarch Service USDA Nutrient Database for Standard Reference, Release 16, Nutrient Data Laboratory Home Page. http://wwww.nal.usda.gov/fnic/foodcomp. Riverdale, MD: Nutrient Data Laboratory, USDA, 2003.

33. McLaughlin, J.; Weihrauch, J. Vitamin E content of foods. J. Am. Diet. Assoc. **1979**, *75*, 647–665.
34. National Research Council. *Recommended Dietary Allowances*, 9th Ed.; National Academy of Sciences: Washington DC, 1980.
35. Eitenmiller, R.R.; Landen, W.O., Jr. *Vitamin Analysis for the Health and Food Sciences*; Boca Raton: CRC Press, FL, 1999.
36. Food and Nutrition Board Institute of Medicine. *Dietary Reference Intakes for Vitamin C, Vitamin E, Selenium, and Carotenoids*; National Academy Press: Washington, DC, 2000; 186–283.
37. Roe, M.A.; Finglas, P.M.; Church, S.M. Eds. *McCance and Widdowson's The Composition of Foods*, 6th Ed.; The Royal Society of Chemistry and Food Standards Agency: Summary London, 2002.
38. UK Nutrient Database. http://wwwrsc.org/is/database/nutsabou.htm. Royal Society of Chemistry: Cambridge, 2003.
39. Cashel, K.; English, R.; Lewis, J. *Composition of Foods Australia*; Australian Government Publishing Service: Canberra, 1989.
40. Cashel, K.; English, R.; Lewis, J. *Composition of Foods Australia: 2. Cereals and Cereal Products*; Australian Government Publishing Service: Canberra, 1990.
41. Lewis, J.; English, R. *Composition of Foods Australia: 3. Dairy Products, Eggs and Fish*; Australian Governement Publishing Service: Canberra, 1990.
42. English, R.; Lewis, J. *Composition of Foods Australia: 4. Fats and Oils, Processed Meats, Fruit and Vegetables*; Australian Government Publishing Service: Canberra, 1990.
43. Lewis, J.; English, R. *Composition of Foods Australia: 5. Nuts and Legumes, Beverages, Miscellaneous Foods*; Australian Government Publishing Service: Canberra, 1990.
44. Lewis, J.; Holt, R.; English, R. *Composition of Foods Australia: 6. Infant Foods and Dairy Foods Update*; Australian Government Publishing Service: Canberra, 1992.
45. Miller, J.B.; James, K.W.; Maggiore, P.M.A. *Tables of Composition of Australian Aboriginal Foods*; Aboriginal Studies Press: Canberra, 1993.
46. Lewis, J.; Brooke-Taylor, S.; Stenhouse, F. The databases of the Australian national food authority. In *Quality and Accessibility of Food-Related Data*; Greenfield, H., Ed.; AOAC International: Arlington, VA, 1995.
47. Cashel, K.; Greenfield, H. Population nutrition goals and targets for Australia: influences of new Australian food composition data. J. Food Comp. Anal. **1997**, *10*, 176–189.
48. Burlingame, B.A.; Milligan, G.C.; Spriggs, T.W.; Athar, N. *The Concise New Zealand Food Composition Tables*, 3rd Ed.; Crop and Food Research, Ltd: Palmerston North, New Zealand, 1997.
49. Visser, F.R.; Burrows, J.K. *Composition of New Zealand Foods: 1. Characteristic Fruits and Vegetables, DSIR Bulletin 235*; Science Information Publishing Centre: Wellington, New Zealand, 1983.
50. Visser, F.R.; Hannah, D.J.; Bailey, R.W. *Composition of New Zealand Foods: 2. Export Fruits and Vegetables*; The Royal Society of New Zealand: Wellington, New Zealand, 1990.

51. Visser, F.R.; Gray, I.; Williams, M. *Composition of New Zealand Foods: 3. Dairy Products*; Design Print: Wellington, New Zealand, 1991.
52. Gibson, J.; West, J.; Diprose, B. *Composition of New Zealand Foods: 4. Poultry*; Electronic Publishing: Wellington, New Zealand, 1993.
53. Monro, J.; Humphrey-Taylor, V. *Composition of New Zealand Foods: 5. Bread and Flour*; Wellington, New Zealand, 1993.
54. Dignan, C.A.; Burlingame, B.A.; Arthur, J.M.; Quigley, R.J.; Milligan, G.C. *The Pacific Islands Food Composition Tables*; South Pacific Commission, New Zealand Institute for Crop and Food Research Ltd and International Network of Food Data Systems, 1994.
55. Pennington, J.A.T. Book review–the Pacific islands food composition tables. J. Food Comp. Anal. **1996**, *9*, 91–92.
56. Pennington, J.A.T. *Bowes and Church's Food Values of Portions Commonly Used*, 17th Ed.; Lippincott: New York, 1998.
57. Souci, S.W.; Fachmann, W.; Kraut, H. *Food Composition and Nutrition Tables*, 6th Ed.; CRC Press: Boca Raton, FL, 2000.
58. Kirchhoff, K. On-line publication of the German food composition table "Souci–Fachmann–Kraut" on the Internet. J. Food Comp. Anal. *15*, 465–472.
59. Slover, H.T. Tocopherols in foods and fats. Lipids **1970**, *6*, 291–296.
60. Harris, R.S.; Wool, I.G.; Marrian, G.F.; Thimann, K.V. Influences of storage and processing on the retention of vitamin E in foods. *Vitamins and Hormones*; Academic Press: New York, 1962; *20*, 603–619.
61. Draper, H.H. The tocopherols. In *Fat-Soluble Vitamins*; Morton, R.A., Ed.; Pergamon Press: New York, 1970.
62. Dicks, M.W. Vitamin E content of foods and feeds for human and animal consumption. Bulletin 435, University Wyoming Agric. Exp. Sta, 1965.
63. Harris, P.L.; Quaife, M.L.; Swanson, W.J. Vitamin E content of foods. J. Nutr. **1950**, *40*, 367–381.
64. Brown, F. The tocopherol content of farm feeding-stuffs. J. Sci. Food Agric. **1953**, *4*, 161–165.
65. Mahon, J.H.; Chapman, R.A. Detection of adulteration of butter with vegetable oils by means of the tocopherol content. Anal. Chem. **1954**, *26*, 1195–1198.
66. Green, J. The distribution of tocopherols during the life-cycle of some plants. J. Sci. Food Agric. **1958**, *9*, 801–812.
67. Mason, E.L.; Jones, W.L. The tocopherol contents of some Australian cereals in flours milling products. J. Sci. Food Agric. **1958**, *9*, 524–527.
68. Booth, V.H.; Bradford, M.P. Tocopherol contents in vegetables and fruits. Brit. J. Nutr. **1963**, *17*, 575–581.
69. Herting, D.C.; Drury, E.E. Vitamin E content of vegetable oils and fats. J. Nutr. **1963**, *81*, 335–342.
70. Ames, S.R.; Tocopherols. V. Occurrence in foods. In *The Vitamins*; Sebrell, W.H., Jr., Harris, R.S., Eds.; Academic Press: New York, 1972; Vol. *V*, 233–248.
71. Bauernfeind, J.C. The tocopherol content of food and influencing factors. Crit. Rev. Food Sci. Nutr. **1977**, *8*, 337–382.

72. Bauernfeind, J.C.; Tocopherols in foods. In *Vitamin E. A Comprehensive Treatise*; Machlin, L.J., Ed.; Marcel Dekker, New York, 1980.
73. Sheppard, A.J.; Weihrauch, J.L.; Pennington, J.A.T. The analysis and distribution of vitamin E in vegetable oils and foods. In *Vitamin E in Health and Disease*; Packer, L., Fuchs, J., Eds.; Marcel Dekker, New York, 1992.
74. Mangels, A.R.; Holden, J.M.; Beecher, G.R.; Forman, M.R.; Lanza, E. Carotenoid content of fruits and vegetables; an evaluation of analytical data. J. Am. Diet Assoc. **1993**, *93*, 284–296.
75. Holden, J.M.; Schubert, A.; Wolf, W.R.; Beecher, G.R. A system for evaluating the quality of published nutrient data: selenium, a test case. http://www.unu.edu/unupress/unupbooks/80633e,80633E00.htm#contents.
76. Schubert, A.; Holden, J.M.; Wolf, W.R. Selenium content of a core group of foods based on a critical evaluation of published analytical data. J. Am. Diet Assoc. **1987**, *87*, 285–276, 299.
77. Lurie, D.G.; Holden, J.M.; Schubert, A.; Wolf, W.R.; Miller-Ihli, N.J. The copper content of foods based on a critical evaluation of published analytical data. J. Food Comp. Anal. **1989**, *2*, 298–316.
78. Bigwood, D.W.; Heller, S.R.; Wolf, W.R.; Schubert, A.; Holden, J.M. SELEX: an expert system for evaluating published data on selenium in foods. Anal. Chim. Acta **1987**, *200*, 411–419.
79. Holden, J.M.; Eldridge, A.L.; Beecher, G.R.; Buzzard, I.M.; Bhazwat, S.A.; Davis, C.S.; Douglass, L.W.; Gebhardt, S.; Haytowitz, D.; Schakel, S. Carotenoid Content of U.S. foods: an update of the database. J. Food Comp. Anal. **1999**, *12*, 169–196.
80. Holden, J.M.; Bhagwat, S.A.; Patterson, K.Y. Development of a multi-nutrient data quality system. J. Food Comp. Anal. **2002**, *15*, 339–348.
81. Carpenter, D.L.; Lehmann, J.; Mason, B.S.; Slover, H.T. Lipid composition of selected vegetable oils. JAOCS **1976**, *53*, 713–718.
82. Muller-Mulot, W. Rapid method for the quantitative determination of individual tocopherols in oils and fats. JAOCS **1976**, *53*, 732–736.
83. Govind, M.K.; Rao Perkins, E.G. Indentification and estimation of tocopherols and tocotrienols in vegetable oils using gas chromatography-mass spectrometry. J. Agric. Food Chem. **1972**, *20*, 240–245.
84. Thompson, J.N.; Erdody, P.; Maxwell, W.B. Chromatographic separation and spectrophotofluorometric determination of tocopherols using hydroxyalkoxypropyl sephadex. Anal. Biochem. **1972**, *50*, 267–280.
85. Syväoja, E.L.; Piironen, V.; Varo, P.; Koivistoinen, P.; Salminen, K. Tocopherols and tocotrienols in Finnish foods: oils and fats. JAOCS **1986**, *63*, 328–329.
86. Rammell, C.G.; Hoogenboom, J.L. Separation of tocols by HPLC on an amino–cyano polar phase column. J. Liq. Chromatogr. **1985**, *8*, 707–717.
87. Dial, S.; Eitenmiller, R.R. Tocopherols and tocotrienols in key foods in the U.S. diet. In *Nutrition, Lipids, Health, and Disease*; Ong, A.S.H., Nike, E., Packer, L., Eds.; AOCS Press: Champaign, IL, 1995.
88. Eitenmiller, R.R.; Lee, J. University of Georgia Data, USDA Contract Report, Studies on vitamin E content of foods, USDA Nutrient Data Laboratory, Riverdale, MD, 1988–2001.

89. Chase, G.W., Jr.; Akoh, C.C.; Eitenmiller, R.R. Analysis of tocopherols in vegetable oils by high-performance liquid chromatography: comparison of fluorescence and evaporative light-scattering detection. JAOCS **1994**, *71*, 877–880.
90. Taylor, P.; Barnes, P. Analysis for vitamin E in edible oils by high performance liquid chromatography. Chemistry and Industry (London) 722–726, 1981.
91. Slover, H.T.; Lehmann, J.; Valis, R.J. Vitamin E in foods: determination of tocols and tocotrienols. JAOCS **1969**, *46*, 417–420.
92. Whittle, K.J.; Pennock, J.F. The examination of tocopherols by two-dimensional thin-layer chromatography and subsequent colorimetric determination. Analyst **1967**, *92*, 423–430.
93. McBride, H.D.; Evans, D.H. Rapid voltammetric method for the estimation of tocopherols and antioxidants in oils and fats. Anal. Chem. **1973**, *45*, 446–449.
94. Christie, A.A.; Dean, A.C.; Millburn, B.A. The determination of vitamin E in food by colorimetry and gas-liquid chromatography. Analyst **1973**, *98*, 161–167.
95. Simonne, A.H.; Eitenmiller, R.R. Retention of vitamin E and added retinyl palmitate in selected vegetable oils during deep-fat frying and in fried breaded products. J. Agric. Food Chem. **1998**, *46*, 5273–5277.
96. Desai, I.D.; Bhagavan, H.; Salkeld, R.; J.E. Dutra De Oliveira. Vitamin E content of crude and refined vegetable oils in southern Brazil. J. Food Comp. Anal. **1988**, *1*, 231–238.
97. Van, P.J.; Niekerk Burger, A.E.C. The estimation of the composition of edible oil mixtures. JAOCS **1985**, *62*, 531–538.
98. Speek, A.J.; Schrijver Schreurs, H.P. Vitamin E composition of some seed oils as determined by high-performance liquid chromatography with fluorometric detection. J. Food Sci. **1985**, *50*, 121–124.
99. Carpenter, A.P. Determination of tocopherols in vegetable oils. JAOCS **1979**, *56*, 668–671.
100. Abe, K.; Yuguchi, Y.; Katsui, G. Quantitative determination of tocopherols by high-speed liquid chromatography. J. Nutr. Sci. Vitaminol. **1975**, *21*, 183–188.
101. Slover, H.T.; Lehmann, J.; Valis, R.J. Nutrient composition of selected wheats and wheat products. III. Tocopherols. Cereal. Chem. **1969**, *46*, 635–641.
102. Padlaha, O.; Eriksson, A.; Toregard, B. An investigation of the basic conditions for tocopherol determination in vegetable oils and fats by differential pulse polarography. JAOCS **1978**, *55*, 530–532.
103. Waters, R.D.; Kesterson, J.W.; Braddock, R.J. Method for determining the $\alpha$-tocopherol content of citrus essential oils. J. Food Sci. **1976**, *41*, 370–371.
104. Lehmann, J.; Martin, H.L.; Lashley, E.L.; Marshall, M.W.; Judd, J.T. Vitamin E in foods from high and low linoleic acid diets. J. Am. Diet. Assoc. **1986**, *86*, 1208–1216.
105. El-Agaimy, M.A.; Neff, W.E.; El-Sayed, M.; Awatif, I.I. Effect of saline irrigation water on olive oil composition. JAOCS **1994**, *71*, 1287–1289.
106. Sturm, P.A.; Parkhurst, R.M.; Skinner, W.A. Quantitative determination of individual tocopherols by thin layer chromatographic separation and spectrophotometry. Anal. Chem. **1966**, *38*, 1244–1247.

107. Rogers, E.J.; Rice, S.M.; Nicolosi, R.J.; Carpenter, D.R.; McClelland, C.A.; Romanczyk, L.J., Jr. Identification and quantitation of $\gamma$-oryzanol components and simultaneous assessment of tocols in rice bran oil. JAOCS **1993**, *70*, 301–307.
108. Ye, L.; Eitenmiller, R.R. University of Georgia, Unpublished data, 1999.
109. Indyk, H.E. Simplified saponfication procedure for the routine determination of total vitamin E in dairy products, foods and tissues by high-performance liquid chromatography. Analyst **1988**, *113*, 1217–1221.
110. Barnes, P.J.; Taylor, P.W. The composition of acyl lipids and tocopherols in wheat germ oils from various sources. J. Sci. Food Agric. **1980**, *31*, 997–1006.
111. Clough, A.E. The determination of tocopherols in vegetable oils by square-wave voltammetry. JAOCS **1992**, *69*, 456–460.
112. Indyk, H.E. Simultaneous liquid chromatographic determination of cholesterol, phytosterols and tocopherols in foods. Analyst **1990**, *115*, 1525–1530.
113. Jawad, I.M.; Kochhar, S.P.; Hudson, B.J.F. The physical refining of edible oils. 2. Effect on unsaponfiable components. Lebensm. Wiss. Technol. **1984**, *17*, 155–159.
114. Gutfinger, T.; Letan, A. Quantitative changes in some unsaponifiable components of soya bean oil due to refining. J. Sci. Food Agric. **1974**, *25*, 1143–1147.
115. Ye, L.; Landen, W.O.; Lee, J.; Eitenmiller, R.R. Vitamin E content of margarine and reduced fat products using a simplified extraction procedure and HPLC determination. J. Liq. Chromatogr. Rel. Technol. **1998**, *21* 1227–1238.
116. Carpenter, D.L.; Slover, H.T. Lipid composition of selected margarines. JAOCS **1973**, *50*, 372–376.
117. Slover, H.T.; Thompson, R.H., Jr.; Davis, C.S.; Merola, G.V. Lipids in margarines and margarine-like foods. JAOCS **1985**, *62*, 775–786.
118. Rader, J.I.; Weaver, C.M.; Patrascu, L.; Ali, L.H.; Angyal, G. $\alpha$-Tocopherol, total vitamin A and total fat in margarines and margarine-like products. Food. Chem. **1997**, *58*, 373–379.
119. Konings, E.J.M.; Roomans, H.H.S.; Beljaars, R. Liquid chromatographic determination of tocopherols and tocotrienols in margarine, infant foods, and vegetables. JAOAC Int. **1996**, *79*, 902–906.
120. Hogarty, C.J.; Ang, C.; Eitenmiller, R.R. Tocopherol content of selected foods by HPLC/fluorescence quantitation. J. Food Comp. Anal. **1989**, *2*, 200–209.
121. Waltking, A.E.; Kiernan, M.; Bleffert, G.W. Evaluation of rapid polarographic method for determining tocopherols in vegetable oils and oil-based products JAOAC Int. **1977**, *60*, 890–894.
122. Lee, J.; Landen, W.O., Jr.; Phillips, R.D.; Eitenmiller, R.R. Application of direct solvent extraction to the LC quantification of vitamin E in peanuts, peanut butter and selected nuts. Peanut. Sci. **1998**, *25*, 123–128.
123. Budin, J.T.; Brene, W.M.; Putnam, D.H. Some compositional properties of seeds and oils of eight *amaranthus* species. JAOCS **1996**, *73*, 475–481.
124. Peterson, D.M. Barley tocols: effects of milling, malting, and mashing. Cereal. Chem. **1994**, *71*, 42–44.
125. Piironen, V.; Syväoja, E.L.; Varo, P.; Salminen, K.; Koivistoinen, P. Tocopherols and tocotrienols in cereal products from Finland. Cereal. Chem. **1986**, *63*, 78–81.

126. Cort, W.M.; Vicente, T.S.; Waysek, E.H.; Williams, B.D. Vitamin E content of feedstuffs determined by high-performance liquid chromatographic fluorescence. J. Agric. Food Chem. **1983**, *31*, 1330–1333.
127. Hakkarainen, J.; Pehrson, B. Vitamin E and polyunsaturated fatty acids in Swedish feedstuffs for cattle. Acta. Agric. Scand. **1987**, *37*, 341–346.
128. Davis, K.R.; Litteneker, N.; Le, D.; Tourneau Cain, R.F.; Peters, L.J.; McGinnis, J. Evaluation of the nutrient composition of wheat. I. Lipid constituents. Cereal. Chem. **1980**, *57*, 178–184.
129. Peterson, D.M. Oat tocols: concentration and stability in oat products and distribution within the kernel. Cereal. Chem. **1995**, *72*, 21–24.
130. Slover, H.T.; Lehmann, J. Effects fumigation on wheat in storage. IV. Tocopherols. Cereal. Chem. **1972**, *49*, 412–415.
131. Hakansson, B.; Jagerstad, M. The effect of thermal inactivation of lipoxygenase on the stability of vitamin E in wheat. J. Cereal. Sci. **1990**, *12*, 177–185.
132. Hakansson, B.; Jagerstad, M.; Oste, R. Determination of vitamin E in wheat products by HPLC. J. Micronutr. Anal. **1987**, *3*, 307–318.
133. Balz, M.K.; Schulte, E.; Thier, H.P. Simultaneous determination of α-tocopherol acetate, tocopherols and tocotrienols by HPLC with fluorescence detection in foods. Fat. Sci. Technol. **1993**, *6*, 215–220.
134. Herting, D.C.; Drury, E.E. Vitamin E content of milk, milk products, and simulated milks: relevance to infant nutrition. Am. J. Clin. Nutr. **1969**, *22*, 147–155.
135. Kanno, C.; Yamauchi, K.; Tsugo, T. Occurrence of γ-tocopherol and variation of α- and γ- tocopherol in bovine milk fat. J. Dairy Sci. **1968**, *51*, 1713–1719.
136. Pennock, J.F.; Neiss, G.; Mahler, H.R. Biochemical studies on the developing avian embryo. Biochem. J. **1962**, *85*, 530–537.
137. Botsoglou, N.; Fletouris, D.; Psomas, I.; Mantis, A. Rapid gas chromatographic method for simultaneous determination of cholesterol and α-tocopherol in eggs. JAOAC Int. **1998**, *81*, 1177–1183.
138. Moffatt, P.A.; Lammi-Keefe, C.J.; Ferris, A.M.; Jensen, R.G. Alpha and gamma tocopherols in pooled mature human milk after storage. J. Pediatr. Gastr. Nutr. **1987**, *6*, 225–227.
139. Syväoja, E.L.; Piironen, V.; Varo, P.; Koivistoinen, P.; Salminen, K. Tocopherols and tocotrienols in Finnish Foods: human milk and infant formulas. Int. J. Vitam. Nutr. Res. **1985**, *55*, 159–166.
140. Syväoja, E.L.; Salminen, K. Tocopherols and toctrienols in Finnish foods: fish and fish products. JAOCS **1985**, *62*, 1245–1115.
141. Erickson, M.C. Extraction and quantitation of tocopherol in raw and cooked channel catfish. J. Food Sci. **1991**, *56*, 1113–1114.
142. Erickson, M.C. Variation of lipid and tocopherol composition in three strains of channel catfish (*Ictalurus punctatus*). J. Sci. Food Agric. **1992**, *59*, 529–536.
143. Ackman, R.G.; Cormier, M.G. α-Tocopherol in some Atlanta fish and shellfish with particular reference to live-holding without food. J. Fish Res. Bd. Canada **1967**, *24*, 357–373.

144. Ang, C.Y.W.; Searcy, G.C.; Eitenmiller, R.R. Tocopherols in chicken breast and leg muscles determined by reverse phase liquid chromatography. J. Food Sci. **1990**, *55*, 1536–1539.
145. Piironen, V.; Syväoja, E.L.; Varo, P.; Salminen, K.; Koivistoinen, P. Tocopherols and tocotrienols in Finnish foods: vegetables, fruits, and berries. J. Agric. Food Chem. **1986**, *34*, 742–746.
146. Sawamura, M.; Kuriyama, T.; Li, Z. Rind spot, antioxidative activity and tocopherols in the flavedo of citrus fruits. J. Hortic. Sci. **1988**, *63*, 717–721.
147. Hassapidou, M.N.; Manoukas, A.G. Tocopherol and tocotrienol composition of raw table olive fruit. J. Sci. Food Agric. **1993**, *61*, 277–280.
148. Tuan, S.; Lee, T.F.; Chou, C.C.; Wei, Q.K. Determination of vitamin E homologues in infant formulas by HPLC using fluorometric detection. J. Micronutr. Anal. **1989**, *6*, 35–45.
149. Marero, L.M.; Payumo, E.M.; Aguinaldo, A.R.; homma, S.; Igarashi, O. Vitamin E constituents of weaning foods from germinated cereals and legumes. J. Food Sci. **1991**, *56*, 270–271.
150. Davis, K.C. Vitamin E content of selected baby foods. J. Food Sci. **1973**, *38*, 442–446.
151. Guzman, G.J.; Murphy, P.A. Tocopherols of soybean seeds and soybean curd (Tofu). J. Agric. Food Chem. **1986**, *34*, 791–795.
152. Gopala, A.G.; Krishna Prabhakar, J.V.; Aitzetmuller, K. Tocopherol and fatty acid composition of some Indian pulses. JAOCS **1997**, *74*, 1603–1606.
153. Fukuba, K.; Murota, T. Determination of tocopherols in foodstuffs, especially nuts and spices, by high-performance liquid chromatography. J. Micronutr. Anal. **1985**, *1*, 93–105.
154. Toschi, T.G.; Caboni, M.F.; Penazzi, G.; Lercker, G.; Capella, P. A study on cashew nut oil composition. JAOCS **1993**, *70*, 1017–1020.
155. Shukla, V.K.S.; Jensen, O.H. Fatty acid composition and tocopherol content of Amazonian palm oils. J. Food Lipids **1996**, *3*, 149–154.
156. Chun, J.; Lee, J.; Eitenmiller, R.R. University of Georgia, Unpublished Data, 1999.
157. Yao, F.; Dull, G.; Eitenmiller, R.R. Tocopherol quantification by HPLC in pecans and relationship to kernel quality during storage. J. Food Sci. **1992**, *57*, 1194–1197.
158. Hashim, I.B.; Koehler, P.E.; Eitenmiller, R.R. Tocopherols in runner and Virginia peanut cultivars at various maturity stages. JAOCS **1993**, *70*, 633–635.
159. Shin, H.S.; Kim, S.W. Lipid composition of perilla seed. JAOCS **1994**, *71*, 619–622.
160. Murkovic, M.; Hillebrand, A.; Winkler, J.; Pfannhauser, W. Variability of vitamin E content in pumpkin seeds (*Cucurbita pepo* L.). Z. Lebensm. Unters. Forsch. **1996**, *202*, 275–278.
161. Nagao, A.; Yamazaki, M. Lipid of sunflower seeds produced in Japan. JAOCS **1983**, *60*, 1654–1658.
162. Lavedrine, F.; Ravel, A.; Poupard, A.; Alary, J. Effect of geographic origin, variety and storage on tocopherol concentrations in walnuts by HPLC. Food Chem. **1997**, *58*, 135–140.
163. Marero, L.M.; Homma, S.; Aida, K.; Fujimaki, M. Changes in the tocopherol and unsaturated fatty acid constituents of spices after pasteurization with superheated steam. J. Nutr. Sci. Vitaminol. **1986**, *32*, 131–136.

164. Osuna-Garcia, J.A.; Wall, W.M.; Waddell, C.A. Endogenous levels of tocopherols and ascorbic acid during fruit ripening of new Mexican-type Chile (*Capsicum annuum* L.) cultivars. J. Agric. Food Chem. **1998**, *46*, 5093–5096.
165. Savage, G.P.; McNeil, D.L.; Dutta, P.C. Lipid composition and oxidative stability of oils in hazelnuts (*Corylus avellana* L.) grown in New Zealand. JAOCS **1997**, *74*, 755–759.
166. Wang, L.; Newman, R.K.; Newman, C.W.; Jackson, L.L.; Hofer, P.J. Tocotrienol and fatty acid composition of barley oil and their effects on lipid metabolism. Plant Foods Hum. Nutr. **1993**, *43*, 9–17.
167. Ap, R.; Ferrari Schulte, E.; Esteves, W.; Bruhl, L.; Mukherjee, K.D. Minor constituents of vegetable oils during industrial processing. JAOCS **1996**, *73*, 587–592.
168. Dionisi, F.; Prodolliet, J.; Tagliaferri, E. Assessment of olive oil adulteration by reversed-phase high-performance liquid chromatography/amperometric detection of tocopherols and tocotrienols. JAOCS **1995**, *72*, 1505–1511.
169. Kanner, J.; Harel, S.; Mendel, H. Content and stability of $\alpha$-tocopherol in fresh and dehydrated pepper fruits (*Capsicum* annuum L.) J. Agric. Food Chem. **1979**, *27*, 1316–1318.
170. Landen, W.O., Jr. Application of gel permeation chromatography to high performance liquid chromatographic determination of retinyl palmitate and $\alpha$-tocopheryl acetate in infant formulas. J. Assoc. Off. Anal. Chem. **1982**, *65*, 810–816.
171. Landen, W.O., Jr.; Hines, D.M.; Hamill, T.W.; Martin, J.I.; Young, E.R.; Eitenmiller, R.R.; Soliman, A.G.M. Vitamin A and Vitamin E content of infant formulas produced in the United States. J. Assoc. Off. Anal. Chem. **1985**, *68*, 509–511.
172. Tanner, J.T.; Barnett, S.A.; Mountford, M.K. Analysis of milk-based formula: phase V. Vitamins A and E, folic acid, and pantothemic acid: food and Drug Administration-Infant Formula Council: collaborative Study. JAOAC Int. **1993**, *76*, 399–412.
173. Thompson, J.N.; Hatina, G. Determination of tocopherols and tocotrienols in foods and tissues by high performance liquid chromatography. J. Liq. Chromatogr. **1979**, *2*, 237–344.
174. Woollard, D.C.; Blott, A.D.; Indyk, H. Fluorometric detection of tocopheryl acetate and its use in the analysis of infant formula. J. Micronutr. Anal. **1987**, *3*, 1–14.
175. Harris, P.L.; Embree, N.O. Quantitative consideration of the effect of polyunsaturated fatty acid content of the diet upon the requirements for vitamin E. Am. J. Clin. Nutr. **1963**, *13*, 385–392.
176. Bunnell, R.H.; Keating, J.; Quaresimo, A.; Parman, G.K. Alpha-Tocopherol Content of Foods. Am. J. Clin. Nutr. **1965**, *17*, 1–10.
177. Eitenmiller, R.R. Vitamin E content of fats and oils—nutritional implications. Food Technol. **1997**, *51*, 78–81.
178. Surai, P.; Ionov, I.; Buzhin, A.; Buzhima, N. Vitamin E and egg quality. Proceedings of the VI European Symposium on the Quality of Eggs and Egg Products, In Briz, R.C., Ed.; Zarazoza, Spain, 1995, 387–391.

179. Frigg, M.; Whitehead, C.; Weber, S. Absence of effects of dietary $\alpha$-tocopherol on egg yolk pigmentation. Br. Poul. Sci. **1992**, *33*, 347–353.
180. Jiang, Y.H.; McGeachin, R.B.; Bailey, C.A. $\alpha$-Tocopherol, $\beta$-carotene, and retinol enrichment of chicken eggs. Poul. Sci. **1994**, *73*, 1137–1143.
181. Infant Formula Act of 1980 Public Law 96–359.
182. Haytowitz, D. United States Department of Agriculture, Personal Communication, 2000.
183. Palm Oil Research Institute of Malaysia. Palm Oil and Human Nutrition. Bandar Baru Bangi, Malaysia 1991.
184. Bonvehi, J.S.; Coll, F.V.; Rius, I.A. Liquid Chromatographic determination of tocopherols and tocotrienols in vegetable oils, formulated preparations, and biscuits. AOAC Int. **2000**, *83*, 627–634.
185. Velasco, L.; Goffman, F.D. Chemotaxonomic significance of fatty acids and tocopherols in boraginaceae. Phytochemistry **1999**, *52*, 423–426.
186. Psomiadou, E.; Tsimidou, M.; Boskou, D. $\alpha$-Tocopherol content of Greek virgin olive oils. J. Agric. Food Chem. **2000**, *48*, 1770–1775.
187. Velasco, L.; Goffman, F.D. Tocopherol, plastochromanol and fatty acid patterns in the genus Linum. Plant Syst. Evol. **2000**, *221*, 77–88.
188. Aparicio, R.; Roda, L.; Albi, M.A.; Gutierrez, F. Effect of various compounds on virgin olive oil stability measured by rancimat. J. Agric. Food Chem. **1999**, *47*, 4150–4155.
189. Savage, G.P.; Dutta, P.C.; McNeil, D.L. Fatty acid and tocopherol contents and oxidative stability of walnut oils. J. Am. Oil Chem. Soc. **1999**, *76*, 1059–1063.
190. Median-Juárez, L.A.; Gámez-Meza, N.; Ortega-García, J.; Noriega-Rodriguez, J.A.; Angulo-Guerrero, O. Trans fatty acid composition and tocopherol content in vegetable oils produced in Mexico. J. Am. Oil Chem. Soc. **2000**, *77*, 721–724.
191. Abushita, A.A.; Daood, H.G.; Biacs, P.A. Change in carotenoids and antioxidant vitamins in tomato as a function of varietal and technological factors. J. Agric. Food Chem. **2000**, *48*, 2075–2081.
192. Abidi, S.L.; List, G.R.; Rennick, K.A. Effect of genetic modification on the distribution of minor constituents in canola oil. J. Am. Oil Chem. Soc. **1999**, *76*, 463–467.
193. Dolde, D.; Vlahakis, C.; Hazèbroek, J. Tocopherols in breeding lines and effects of planting location, fatty acid composition, and temperature during development. J. Am. Oil Chem. Soc. **1999**, *76*, 349–355.
194. Oomah, B.D.; Ladet, S.; Godfrey, D.V.; Liang, J.; Girard, B. Characteristics of raspberry (*Rubus idaeus* L.) seed oil. Food Chem. **2000**, *69*, 187–193.
195. Goffman, F.D.; Möllers, C. Changes in tocopherol and plastochromanol-8 contents in seeds and oil of oilseed rape (*Brassica napus* L.) during storage as influenced by temperature and air oxygen. J. Agric. Food Chem. **2000**, *48*, 1605–1609.
196. Grela, E.R.; Jensen, S.K.; Jakobsen, K. Fatty acid composition and content of tocopherols and carotenoids in raw and extruded grass pea (*Lathyrus sativus* L). J. Sci. Food Agric. **1999**, *79*, 2075–2078.
197. Murcia, M.A.; Martínez-Tomé, M.; del, I.; Cerro Sotillo, F.; Ramírez, A. Proximate composition and vitamin E levels in egg yolk: losses by cooking in a microwave oven. J. Sci. Food Agric. **1999**, *79*, 1550–1556.

198. Bennink, M.R.; Ono, K. Vitamin B12, E and D content of raw and cooked beef. J. Food Sci. **1982**, *47*, 1786–1792.
199. Bonvehi, J.S.; Coll, F.V.; Ruis, I.A. Liquid chromatographic determination of tocopherols and tocotrienols in vegetable oils, formulated preparations, and biscuits. J. AOAC Int. **2000**, *83*, 627–634.
200. Jo, C.; Ahn, D.U. Volatile and oxidative changes in irradiated pork sausage with different fatty acid composition and tocopherol content. J. Food Sci. **2000**, *65*, 270–275.
201. Lazos, E.S.; Tsaknis, J.; Lalas, S. Charateristics and composition of tomato seed oil. Grasas Aceites **1998**, *49*, 440–445.
202. Gogolewski, M.; Nogala-Kalucka, M.; Szeliga, M. Changes of the tocopherol and fatty acid contents in rapeseed oil during refining. Eur. J. Lipid Sci. Technol. **2000**, *102*, 618–623.
203. Bagorogoza, K.; Bowers, J.; Okot-Kotber, M. The effect of irradiation and midified atmosphere packaging on the stability of intact chill-stored turkey breast. J. Food Sci. **2001**, *66*, 367–372.
204. Demir, C.; Cetin, M. Determination of tocopherols, fatty acids and oxidative stability of pecan, walnut and sunflower oils. Dtsch Lebensmittel Rundschau **1999**, *95*, 278–282.
205. Okogeri, O.; Tasioula-Margari, M. Changes occurring in phenolic compounds and $\alpha$-tocopherol of virgin olive oil during storage. J. Agric. Food Chem. **2002**, *50*, 1077–1080.
206. Koski, A.; Psomiadou, E.; Tsimidou, M.; Hopia, A.; Kefalas, P.; Wähälä, K.; Heinonen, M. Oxidative stability and minor consituents of virgin olive oil and cold-pressed rapeseed oil. Eur. Food Res. Technol. **2002**, *214*, 294–298.
207. Goffman, F.D.; Galletti, S. Gamma-linoleinic acid and tocopherol contents in the seed oil of 47 accessions from several *Ribes* species. J. Agric. Food Chem. **2001**, *49*, 349–354.
208. Goffman, F.D.; Becker, H.C. Genetic analysis of tocopherol content and composition in winter rapeseed. Plant Breeding **2001**, *120*, 182–184.
209. Normand, I.; Eskin, N.A.M.; Przybylski, R. Effect of tocopherols on the frying stability of regular and modified canola oils. JAOCS **2001**, *78*, 369–373.
210. Bereau, D.; Benjelloum-Mlayah, B.; Delmas, M. Letters to the editor *Maximiliana maripa* drude mesocarp and kernel oils: fatty acid and total tocopherol compositions. JAOCS **2001**, *78*, 213–214.
211. Alpaslan, M.; Tepe, S.; Simsek, O. Effect of refining processes on the total and individual tocopherol content in sunflower oil. Int. J. Food Sci. Technol. **2001**, *36*, 737–739.
212. Ching, L.S.; Mohamed, S. Alpha-tocopherol content in 62 edible tropical plants. J. Agric. Food Chem. **2001**, *49*, 3101–3105.
213. Kallio, H.; Yang, B.; Peippo, P.; Tahvonen, R.; Pan, R. Triacylglycerols glycerophospholipids tocopherols and tocotrienols in berries and seeds of two subspecies (*ssp sinensis*and *mangolica*) of sea buckthorn (*Hippophae rhamnoides*). J. Agric. Food Chem. **2002**, *50*, 3004–3009.
214. Goffman, F.D.; Bohme, T. Relationship between fatty acid profile and vitamin E content in maize hybrids (*Zea mays L*). J. Agric. Food Chem. **2001**, *49*, 4990–4994.

# Index